T0251865

Barasi's HUMAN NUTRITION

A Health Perspective

THIRD EDITION

Mike Lean
Emilie Combet
The University of Glasgow, UK

CRC Press
Taylor & Francis Group
Boca Raton London New York

CRC Press is an imprint of the
Taylor & Francis Group, an **informa** business

CRC Press
Taylor & Francis Group
6000 Broken Sound Parkway NW, Suite 300
Boca Raton, FL 33487-2742

Printed and bound by CPI Group (UK) Ltd, Croydon, CR0 4YY on acid-free paper
Version Date: 20160122

International Standard Book Number-13: 978-1-4441-3720-0 (Paperback)

Library of Congress Cataloging-in-Publication Data

Names: Lean, M. E. J. (Michael Ernest John), author. | Combet, Emilie, author. | Barasi, Mary E. Human nutrition. Preceded by (work):
Title: Barasi's human nutrition : a health perspective / Michael E.J. Lean and Emilie Combet.
Other titles: Human nutrition
Description: Third edition. | Boca Raton : Taylor & Francis, 2017. | Preceded by Human nutrition / Mary E. Barasi. 2nd ed. c2003. | Includes bibliographical references and index.
Identifiers: LCCN 2016002285 | ISBN 9781444137200 (alk. paper)
Subjects: | MESH: Nutritional Requirements | Nutrition Processes | Diet | Food | Food Habits | Nutrition Disorders
Classification: LCC QP141 | NLM QU 145.3 | DDC 613.2--dc23
LC record available at http://lccn.loc.gov/2016002285

Visit the Taylor & Francis Web site at
http://www.taylorandfrancis.com

and the CRC Press Web site at
http://www.crcpress.com

Barasi's

HUMAN NUTRITION

A Health Perspective

THIRD EDITION

Contents

SECTION I Foods, Nutrient Requirements and Nutrition

SECTION II Nutrition through the Life Cycle

SECTION IV Eating Behaviour and Nutritional Epidemiology

SECTION V Dietary and Nutritional Assessment

SECTION VI Applied Nutrition

Preface

This third edition of Barasi's classic textbook has been a long time coming, after a period of great change. The reasons, translated into the needs behind this revised textbook, are multiple:

- There is a major new emphasis on a joined-up translational approach across all bio-medical sciences, with a view to generate shifts in human behaviours to improve health. A great deal of perfectly good previous research failed in real life to have the impact suggested by clinical trials. Massive government and industry investments to develop new drugs looked diminished when consistent evidence emerged that many people do not want to take drugs. For example, around 30% of prescriptions for diabetes are not used, even when the drugs are provided for free by a national health service.
- For human nutrition, we have a huge amount of solid information on the effects of nutrients, and nutrient balance, on physiology and disease risks. However, despite extensive health education and reports, population eating habits and nutrition-related diseases have changed very little. The three most frustrating research questions have always been (1) 'What do people (really) eat?' (2) 'Why do people eat What they eat?' and (3) 'What is needed to change the way they eat, sustainably?'
- A translational approach has pointed to the complexity of the food environment, a concatenation of environments and the policies behind them – physical, agricultural, educational, social, but dominated by the commercial and marketing environment.
- Population demographics have changed, to present greater emphasis on the needs of the elderly and young children in smaller families. Food provision for populations is clearly vital, but policies affecting national food provision have rarely included assessment of nutritional adequacy. They are mainly driven by the quest for commercial profit, thus, if possible, to buy cheap and sell expensive. This ethos has exaggerated the impact on the health of people at the extremes of age.
- The wider recognition of the blindingly obvious – that food and nutrition define human growth, development, mental and physical health, and thus susceptibility to most diseases – has begun to register as a responsibility and accountability for carers and caterers, as well as for the medical and health professions.
- In an era when healthcare is becoming hard to sustain, disease prevention enjoyed a renewed interest, with policy makers and health professionals beginning to accept that education does not solve the problem, since commercial food and drink marketing beats education every time. While 'Health by Stealth' has been hailed as one of the only sustainable solutions, a better term is needed. We can anticipate, in the next decade, great investment into preventive measures based on covert reformulation of foods and meals, to ensure that all people are presented with foods and meals that provide nutrients in recommended proportions for optimal health. This applies particularly to the more vulnerable, at the extremes of age and through social and educational limitations. These are people whose health and well-being can only depend on decisions made by others – on nutritional knowledge and guidance provided to their carers and caterers.

These changes come at a time when the media and the Internet are essentially unregulated, and the profusion of information or apparent information available or even thrust on people can be bewildering. Sifting truth, that is, secure, statistically sound evidence-based information, from plausible claims has become exceedingly difficult even for trained individuals.

Another change to the world of nutrition was the early loss of Mary Barasi in 2008. Mary was a renowned leader and teacher of nutrition and dietetics, holding posts in Scotland, Wales, England

and Japan. She generated a buzz wherever she was, and her 'road to Damascus' was probably stepping out to take an Open University degree in business administration. She saw the potential of the still very new Open University to spread education in what was still a very neglected field and designed a nutrition course for it, and that was the impetus behind her writing the first edition of this book.

We are honoured to have been invited to prepare the third edition by the publishers (and by Mary's husband Steven). We hope this new edition retains the common-sense attitude toward science that Mary instilled. There are now many more courses in nutrition, with many more students being trained in human nutrition, and the University of Glasgow master's in human nutrition has become one of the most popular. For the third edition, we have updated every chapter of the book and altered the structure to better match the evolving needs of students, with six cross-referenced sections taking the reader from chapters on basic nutritional science (nutrients and requirements, nutrition through the life cycle, digestion and absorption of nutrients, eating behaviour and nutritional epidemiology) to chapters introducing key fields of applied nutrition (dietary and nutritional assessment, clinical nutrition, obesity and weight management, sports nutrition and public health nutrition).

The two co-authors have different but complementary training and expertise, and they have had great support in preparing this third edition from several colleagues in Glasgow.

Acknowledgements

For this revised third edition, we have welcomed the help of colleagues Christina Buckton, Maira Bouga and Po San Lam. We thank them for their input, which has helped shape the book in the context of nutrition as a body of integrative sciences.

Authors

Dr. Emilie Combet trained in analytical biology and biochemistry at Université Claude Bernard in Lyon, France, and later at the Horticulture Research International research station in Wellesbourne, United Kingdom (now Warwick University). She has lectured in human nutrition at the University of Glasgow since 2009, and her research focuses on foods, nutrition and the life cycle, with special interest in nutrition and stress (ageing, oxidation, nitrosation, obesity and inflammation) and key periods of development (conception, pregnancy and infancy).

Professor Mike Lean trained in medicine at Cambridge University and St Bartholomew's Hospital in London. He has held the chair of human nutrition at the University of Glasgow since 1993, leading a newly established department, covering the full span from basic science, through clinical and community interventions to epidemiology, in a city that has led the way in nutrition research, particularly its social dimension, for almost 100 years. His main areas of personal research include obesity, diabetes and cardiovascular risk.

Dr. Combet and Professor Lean have enjoyed collaboration on a variety of research topics, notably to develop the world's first nutritionally balanced meal – a pizza developed with local business EatBalanced, now being served in Scottish school dinners.

Section I

Foods, Nutrient Requirements and Nutrition

1 Introduction
What Is Nutrition?

AIMS

The aims of this chapter are to

- Define nutrition as a discipline and reflect on its importance and contribution to evidence-based biomedical sciences.
- Encourage the reader to think about food intake, and their own and others' perceptions of nutrition.
- Consider the nutrition of populations and how it is (i) included in, or (ii) impacted by government in nutrition policies.

DEFINITIONS OF NUTRITION

Everybody has their own experience of food and eating, so it is likely that people will have different ideas about what is meant by nutrition. Some may see eating primarily as a means of meeting our basic physiological needs and warding off hunger, others as a pleasurable experience in its own right and something to share, anticipate and plan. These represent the two extremes implied by the sayings '*eat to live*' and '*live to eat*'.

In reality, eating is far more complicated than this, involving aspects of our psychological make-up and current state of mind, our genetic blueprint, the social environment of which we are a part, our economic situation and external factors relating to the availability, presentation and marketing of the food. Eating is certainly necessary to keep us alive and provide for the demands our lives generate. When insufficient food or specific nutrients are supplied, some physiological adaptation may occur to minimize the consequences. Eventually, however, a deficiency state will arise.

Factors influencing eating behaviours are covered in Chapter 13, pp. 255–268.

At the beginning of the twentieth century, the science of nutrition, indeed most medical research, was directed at discovering the essential nutrients, studying the effects of insufficient intakes and determining the quantities needed to prevent deficiency states. Since then, it has gradually been recognized that good nutrition is not simply a matter of providing enough of all the nutrients. We now realize that diets in the affluent Western countries, although apparently containing all the necessary nutrients, are probably contributing to many of the diseases afflicting these populations. Much research has focused on finding which nutrients are linked to which diseases, to promote change in the dietary intake and hence an improvement in health. Since the 1970s, a great deal of advice has been aimed at encouraging people to eat a healthier balance of foods, thereby reducing disease. The emphasis in the twenty-first century has started to move towards promoting positive health through diet, known as optimum nutrition. However, nutritionists recognize that altering people's food intakes is complicated because food choices and eating are influenced by many factors other than the need to eat and the desire for well-being.

Defining nutrition is far from straightforward, and different definitions have been suggested:

- *'the study of nutrients vital to health and how the body uses these to promote and support growth, maintenance and reproduction of cells'*
- *'the study of the relationship between people and their food'*

The first definition deals only with nutrients, what happens to them within the body and what the results are at a cellular level if insufficient amounts are provided. These are essential topics, but a lot goes on before nutrients reach cells. People do not eat nutrients; they eat foods and meals. Multiple external factors play a crucial role in our approach to food and eating. These factors are different for each individual, depending on cultural background and the circumstances of a person's life.

The second definition may look unfocussed but actually takes a more mature 'broad-focus' perspective, from the supply of food and all the influences thereon through the individual's food selection and, finally, to the physiological and biochemical effects of the nutrients in the normal human body and the consequences for health and survival. A 'broad-focus' view of nutrition recognizes that nutritionists do not only study the effects of nutrients on biochemical and physiological functioning; they have an additional responsibility to translate their knowledge for those who produce, process and market the foods. Furthermore, nutritionists must be involved in the formulation of policies that determines the access to food for consumers. Finally, consumers need the help of nutritionists to make the best of the food available. Only by broadening our definition of the subject across the full range of human relationships with food can nutrition have its justified place in human well-being.

Evidence-Based Nutrition

The dietary recommendations made in the United Kingdom are based on evidence that relates both food and nutrients to health. In 2012, the Scientific Advisory Committee on Nutrition set out a framework for the evaluation of scientific evidence. Scientific evidence that is applicable to the UK population is (i) gathered systematically, (ii) evaluated and (iii) used to draw conclusions serving to make any of the dietary recommendations for the UK population. The possible risks associated with the recommendations are also assessed. This is known as evidence-based nutrition.

WHY IS NUTRITION IMPORTANT?

To answer this question, it is perhaps useful to consider the various levels at which nutrition can be studied. The core principles of nutrition form a cognate field of science which is not taught and seldom understood by those in other disciplines. However, the 'broad-focus' integrative definition of nutrition means that (i) actions in many other spheres impact on food availability and food choice and (ii) that altered nutritional supply potentially affects every organ function and human activity overall.

Human nutrition is a body of integrated science underpinning much of biomedical and health research with broad implications for public health and related policies and commercial activities.

Table 1.1 illustrates some applications of nutritional science in other fields of study. In each case, nutrition plays a specific role, and the emphasis required may differ from its application in all other roles. Thus, nutrition is a science with many different applications and meanings to different specialists. Nevertheless, each of these specialists, working in their own particular field of expertise, needs to have knowledge of nutrition in order to apply the findings of their work to the nutritional context.

TABLE 1.1
Understanding of Nutrition Is Required by All Involved in Studying and Applying Nutrition

Level of Study	Examples of Research Activities	Speculations and Outcomes
Macro/population	Government statistics (for formulation of policy, e.g. about agriculture, social or health) Policy and strategy analysis (to identify cross-cutting effects on nutrition from other government departments) Epidemiology (to study influence on and relationships between diet and disease) Sociology (to study patterns of behaviour related to food)	Ministry and government and civil services, food industry – Better monitoring + Matching of food supply to health
Individual/whole person	Psychology (to explore knowledge, attitudes and beliefs about food and models of behavioural change) Food science/technology (to identify changes in individual preferences for food; sensory qualities) Sports science (to identify links between diet and performance) Medicine (to study influences of diet on the health of the individual and recovery from illness)	Delivering reliable information and guidance, e.g. psychologists, training, doctors, nurses (all sub-specialties), journalists
Micro/laboratory	Physiology (to understand the role of nutrients in functioning of body systems) Biochemistry (to investigate the biochemical role of nutrients in normal and abnormal functioning) Molecular biology (to study gene–nutrient interactions) Imaging (detailed study of body composition)	Define best methods for surveys, monitoring and individual assessment Laboratory

There has been an upsurge of general interest in nutrition in the last 20–30 years in the scientific community, and also among the general population. Why has this happened?

See Chapter 23 for more on food innovation in the context of nutrition and health, pp. 431–444.

First, dietary intakes have been changing rapidly. In the Western world, an ever-increasing selection of foods is available. People can now eat every day the foods our ancestors had only on special occasions. New foods are appearing, some conceived and developed by food technologists; sometimes these contain unusual ingredients, which provide nutrients in unexpected amounts (this can be a problem for the nutritionist in giving advice). New processing techniques, such as irradiation, may affect the nutrients in food.

In modern society, meal patterns have become less rigid and many people no longer eat meals at regular mealtimes. The members of a family may each have an independent meal at different times of the day, and the traditional family meal is a rare event.

Concerns about food safety and environmental issues have resulted in changes in dietary habits, notably the rise in vegetarianism in the United Kingdom and increasing demand for organically-grown food. Nevertheless, the great majority of food now comes from large retail supermarkets that exert a major limiting influence over customer choice. There may be 50 brands of butter, but most if not all are salted. Fruit is selected by supermarkets on size, colour and shelf life, not on flavour or any nutritional criteria.

Health issues have a great deal of prominence in the media. Western populations have excess mortality (i.e. death rates) and morbidity (i.e. rates of illness) from many diseases related to diet, such as diabetes, cardiovascular disorders, bowel diseases and cancers, as well as high prevalence of obesity and related disability. At the same time, we are often shocked by images of starvation in other parts of the world where conflict, drought and other disasters still result in millions of people suffering acute malnutrition and starvation.

The media are very sensitive to public concern, so that news about nutritional findings receives a great deal of publicity. Unfortunately, the style of reporting may distort the scientific detail, so that what is eventually presented by the media may not accurately represent the findings. Moreover, excessive prominence may be given to very minor and insignificant findings, especially if they appear to contradict earlier results. These stories are commonly led by commercial interests, which may not be apparent to consumers. Consequently, rather than being better informed, the public may become confused. It is essential, therefore, that those trained in nutrition have a clear understanding of nutritional issues and are able to disentangle some of the inaccuracies presented by the media. Public health nutrition is now a discipline in its own right, with a specific remit of promoting health through good (evidence-based) nutrition. Consensus is being reached on how diet is involved in Western diseases, and advice can now be based on much firmer evidence. However, new research may require current advice to be modified.

Public Health Nutrition is introduced fully in Chapter 19, pp. 363–381.

WHAT DO WE EAT?

Different dietary patterns around the world are determined by many factors: food availability, traditional practices and beliefs and any religious prescriptions (which often relate to health outcomes from food consumption).

The basis of the diet is the meal or 'eating occasion'. Traditionally, this is usually three times a day. The basis of each meal is a core food, referred to as the 'staple', around which meals are constructed. Without the staple, a meal would not be perceived as a meal. There are usually only a very few core foods in any one culture, sometimes only one. They are generally starchy foods, cereals, or roots and tubers, and the main source of energy.

The concepts of the meal as the smaller unit of nutrition and the nutritionally-balanced diet are covered in Chapter 2, pp. 11–29.

Secondary foods are less important as energy sources and enhance the meal, endowed with specific properties of their own (protein-rich foods, such as meat or antioxidants, fruit and vegetables). They may be believed to maintain bodily forces in balance ('hot' and 'cold' foods as in some Eastern cultures). In addition, some secondary foods may be important at particular life stages.

The third category of foods in Western diets is peripheral foods, often considered non-essential, but pleasant to eat. Examples include biscuits, cakes, confectionery, preserves, sauces and puddings. Meals may also include flavourings and seasonings. It is interesting that these foods tend to rely on sugar and spices, which are 'new' foodstuffs, only imported to Western countries from the seventeenth century.

It is interesting to reflect that many traditional diets evolved, using locally available foods, to achieve excellent overall nutritional balance. For example, although the best individual protein sources, to provide essential amino acids, are meats, eggs and dairy foods, these were not accessible for whole populations. The same balance could be achieved by combing cereals with legumes, as is the traditional meals of many countries. Similarly, milk, yoghurt or cheese form a vital source of calcium, and were adopted somehow by populations across the world. Similarly, populations adopted the incorporation of vegetables and fruit into all meals, long before any scientist observed the consequences of their omission or identified their essential vitamin contents.

Thus, despite the huge diversity of foods eaten around the world, it is possible to identify common patterns in the foods that people eat. In general, a greater part of the diet comes from the staple in the poorer parts of the world, when the peripheral foods are not consumed, but they make an excessively large contribution in richer countries. Clearly, the core and secondary foods in any national or cultural diet must supply the essential nutrients in appropriate amounts to sustain life and promote health. Some diets appear to achieve this better than others, as is shown by the fact that mortality rates from diseases that can be attributed to diet are lower in some countries of the world than in others.

HOW IS INFORMATION ABOUT PEOPLE'S DIETS COLLECTED?

To permit any exploration of the role of food in the health and welfare of the whole individual, rather than its biochemical effect at the system or cellular level, it is necessary to investigate what people eat. It is relatively straightforward for individuals to think about their own food intake and to keep some sort of diary of what they have eaten. Most people can identify foods that they like or dislike, that they eat often, rarely or never. However, for most people, keeping a detailed food record over a period sufficient to be representative of usual habitual eating is difficult.

Many of us would also be able to make statements about the food intake of members of our family or close friends. However, this information would inevitably be less detailed than our own, as we can rarely know about absolutely everything someone else has eaten. For a nutritionist, trying to find out what people eat poses a number of problems and requires varied approaches.

Dietary assessment methods, for groups and individuals, are covered in Chapter 18, pp. 343–347.

Population and Household Information

Information about the diet of a population can be obtained either in a very general way or with progressively more detailed techniques. In many countries, data are collected together in 'food balance sheets', which estimate the amount of food moving into and leaving a country, in much the same way as monetary transactions on a financial balance sheet. This can provide an overview of the theoretical availability of food in a country. Such statistics are collated and published by the United Nations' Food and Agriculture Organization for most countries of the world and are used to provide an overview of food availability, or 'food disappearance'. Assumptions and adjustments have to be made about wastage, re-exporting after processing argumentation from non-purchased sources (e.g. gardening), but these data can give indications of changes in per capita food consumption.

In Europe, several Household Budget Surveys exist, each providing valuable data about dietary intakes in the specific country. The Data Food Networking initiative (DAFNE) is a collaborative effort across Europe to develop a bank of regularly updated and comparable data in order to assess and monitor trends in dietary patterns.

In the United Kingdom, data have been collected by the Household Food Consumption and Expenditure Survey, and in particular, the National Food Survey (produced annually by the Ministry of Agriculture, Fisheries and Food) since 1940. This has provided a continuous surveillance of the food coming into households for consumption, together with money spent on food according to household composition, economic status and geographical location. In 1994, the Survey started to collect data about food eaten outside the home, a reflection of the growing importance of eating out. The National Food Survey in this form ended in March 2001 and was replaced by the Expenditure and Food Survey (EFS), published by the Department for Environment, Food and Rural Affairs, known as the Living Costs and Food Survey since 2008. Information about food consumption, nutrient intakes and food expenditure from a study of this nature, however, cannot tell us the intake of an individual. All of the data are collected with the household as the unit, and the total divided by the number of household members. More information is required on food distribution patterns within households. The EFS will continue to publish information at the level of the household, although individual members keep their own diaries, to try to reduce underreporting and increase accuracy. The Diet and Nutrition Survey in England and Scottish Health Surveys are designed as regular nationally representative surveys which collect food frequency data, together with detailed demographic and health data.

Surveys which require the engagement of individuals to collect or provide information are always limited by the need for consent. This can result in a lack of information about the most vulnerable population sectors – the very young, the very old, the educationally and intellectually limited, the suspicious and the busy. Response rates are often low, so results can be seriously biased. Even when individuals do agree to participate, misreporting, even intentionally, is very common.

The use of supermarket till receipts collected over 4 weeks, together with 4-day individual diaries, has been used to assess patterns of fat and energy intake and has been shown useful as it can include individuals and/or households who are not able or willing to provide dietary intake information and can be related to location and social deprivation measures. The involvement of supermarket checkout data to obtain information about population dietary patterns has potential in dietary surveys, but concerns about ethics and commercial sensitivity limit their use.

STUDYING NUTRITION

In order to understand nutrition, it is important to consider

1. Foods and their nutrients and bioactive dietary components.
2. The nutrient requirements, how these are established and applied, and how they underpin the concept of a nutritionally-balanced diet.
3. The functions of nutrients in the body.
4. The role of nutrition through the life cycle, from pregnancy and birth through to old age.
5. The aspects of physiology and biochemistry essential for the human body to utilize nutrients and dietary components present in foods.
6. The factors influencing eating behaviours.
7. Nutritional epidemiology and the role of diet in disease prevention.
8. The concepts of energy needs, intake, and expenditure and how they relate to energy balance and body composition.
9. The concepts of dietary and nutritional assessments.
10. Specialists areas of applied nutrition, including public health nutrition and health promotion, obesity and weight management, sport nutrition, clinical nutrition and food innovation.

These are presented in turn in this textbook. However, nutrition is a fast-paced research field, and the study of each chapter is only complete when the published primary literature is taken in consideration and critically appraised.

SUMMARY

1. Nutrition is a very broad discipline, relevant to people from a variety of backgrounds, who can also make useful contributions to its knowledge base.
2. There has been a huge increase in interest in nutrition in the last decade and people want to be better informed.
3. Nutrition underpins most fields of biomedical and health research.
4. Nutrition has broad implications for public health and related policies and commercial activities.

ACTIVITY

1.1 Why are you studying nutrition?
At what level will you be applying your nutritional knowledge?
At what level might the following specialists be using nutrition:

Nurse	Pharmacist
Dietitian	Journalist
Obstetrician	Parent
Home economist	

Try to think of some other examples of people working with nutrition, at each of the different levels in Table 1.1.

2 Nutrient Requirements and the Nutritionally Balanced Diet

AIMS

The aims of this chapter are to

- Explain the concepts of diet quality and nutritional balance.
- Describe the basis and application of dietary reference values for individual nutrients.
- Discuss some of the food labelling and dietary planning tools that aim to promote food choices for an optimally balanced diet.

While it may be easier for us to choose what to eat according to our particular desires at a specific time, the increased variety makes it more difficult to achieve consistency in terms of nutrient balance. Many people, despite being offered 6000–9000 different items in a major supermarket, are consistently selecting only a very narrow range of foods.

DIET QUALITY AND THE NUTRITIONALLY BALANCED DIET

Several components of diet quality exist and are often confused. Terms such as 'healthy' have no definition and are used mostly for marketing, with the implication of an effect on body weight. The term 'nutritionally balanced' refers to diets, or meals, which have nutrient compositions which approximate to the dietary needs for optimal health. The meal is the smaller unit of nutrition which ought to be considered. Therefore, it is not useful to consider nutritional balance of individual foods or ingredients, which must be combined in different proportions to make up meals.

For foods, the concept of 'nutrient density' can be valuable in nutritional science, referring to the density of nutrients per unit energy (per 1000 kcal). This is different from the concept of density of nutrient per unit weight, as used in food science. A high-quality diet has several cultural and economic features and so might be based on meals built on a wide, seasonal, locally sourced, unprocessed selections of nutrient-rich foods, to match the reference intakes (RI) for all nutrients but without exceeding the reference energy intake. These concepts will be discussed further in the following text, as well as in subsequent chapters.

Consumers and Health Claims

Consumers are faced with overt health claims, or more covert promotion of specific foods on health grounds with the presentation of selected nutrient contents on labels, and with a bewildering range of guidance, or promotion, of different dietary principles, with little to help them distinguish between the scientific, the mythical or the religious. People are often keen to attribute magical properties to foods, and most health claims fall into this category. Newspapers, TV and magazines are full of assertive promotions of dietary principles which have little or no evidence for any benefit. For example, there is consistent observational evidence and very limited experimental proof that a vegetarian, plant-based diet will reduce heart disease. However, the effect size is small, and there are many other influences of the physical, mental and social health of individuals and populations, such that the imposition, or blind pursuit of vegan diets, for example, would impair the health of many. The extrapolation to a vegan (purely plant food diet) presents major social obstacles, although a minority of people enjoy an essentially religious basis for their food choices. There is no evidence for any health benefit from following biblical, hallal, macrobiotic or other 'religious diets', although many claims are made.

The promotion of vitamin supplement has the same distorted origin. It is the duty of nutritionists and dieticians to guide people out of the world of myths and marketing towards health.

A variety of 'diets' are promoted to people with specific health problems – commonly chronic or fluctuating condition such as arthritis, anxiety/depression, cancers and diabetes. There is little or no evidence that dietary advice for such people should be different from the general population. The difficulty is that conventional healthful eating advice is not as exciting or marketable as whacky (or fad) diets aimed at vulnerable consumers.

A number of fad diets are regularly promoted because so many members of the public have come to believe in them. Examples include diets which avoid wheat and gluten and 'anti-candida' diets. There is no evidence at all that wheat/gluten or candida is the cause of disease (outside rare medical conditions such as coeliac disease or drug chemotherapy) or that these diets do any good. Organically produced food has no demonstrated effect on the health of consumers. Some may feel temporarily 'better' on these diets if their restrictive nature leads to weight loss. The same applies to some diets for arthritis. Where there is evidence for a particular dietary pattern, for example a low GI diet, to improve diabetes and blood lipids, marketing claims often go way beyond the evidence. Examples include, far-reaching claims for effects on weight loss and dietary principles with modest benefits promoted as critical, or a cure-all.

NUTRITIONALLY BALANCED DIET: WHICH FOODS TO CHOOSE?

If we are interested in and committed to taking care of ourselves and others, the 'healthfulness' of our selection of food needs to be considered. However, 'health' is not the only feature we look for in our food. Most of us would be very reluctant to eat an unfamiliar food just because we were told it was healthful; the property of healthiness would be included in the general consideration of the food in deciding whether or not to include it in the diet.

However, the foods commonly compiled into a 'nutritionally balanced diet' are not very different from those which make up a less nutritionally balanced diet – it is the balance of the parts making up the total meal or diet that is important. As such, there are no 'bad' foods; it is their place in the general picture of the diet that is important. Some foods provide only a very narrow range of nutrients. If such foods comprise a substantial part of the daily intake, the consumer will run the risk of not meeting nutritional requirements for a range of nutrients. The greater the range of foods, the less likely are there to be 'gaps' in the nutrient intake, and the more likely it is that consumers will meet their nutritional needs.

What Is the Difference between Meals and Snacks?

A meal generally contains a selection of different separate items, usually eaten with utensils (although in some cultures this is not usual), and takes some time to prepare and to eat. Traditionally, this would be eaten in a designated eating place, for example, at a table. Sociologists have attempted to identify what it is that makes food into a meal. There are usually several food groups included, often with more than one dish or course. The presence of a 'staple' food such as potato, rice or pasta, confers meal status for some. The inclusion of meat, and specifically grazing, has been used as an indicator of meal status, but burgers are now promoted as between-meal snacks. The two- or three-course meal is clearly a limited middle-class Western model, and the 'sweet after savoury' model was a French seventeenth-century development. A more pragmatic, functional definition of a meal used by the Food Standards Agency (FSA), for example, as a basis for school meals, is an eating occasion which provides about a third of daily energy requirement. For adults, this would be 600–800 kcal. However, many meals are much larger than this.

A snack is an eating occasion where just one type of food is eaten, perhaps accompanied by a drink, and might include biscuits, chocolate or sandwich. Often, this is eaten in an informal setting or perhaps in the street or while travelling. Historically, a snack was food eaten when for some reason a meal was missed, for example, by mountaineers, to tide them over. It was small and portable, usually a source of energy with a piece of fruit and a drink. More recently, the power of marketing has elevated the position of the high-energy item and high-energy drink, and fruit is no longer considered part of a snack. In the last 20 years, more informal eating has been adopted, as lifestyles become more flexible and a vast industry has emerged to take advantage of this. In some instances, all of the food taken during the course of a day may be classified as 'snacks', with perhaps as many as 10 or more convenient products being consumed. This 'grazing' is particularly prevalent among young people and causes concern to nutritionists, as some of the snack foods are low in micronutrients but contain substantial amounts of fat and/or sugar. Not all snack foods are nutritionally poor: sandwiches, fruit, nuts and drinks, such as milk or fruit juice, can provide useful nutrients.

NUTRITIONALLY BALANCED DIET: HOW MUCH TO EAT?

In addition to deciding what foods to eat, each person makes a decision about the quantity to consume. From experience, individuals have learned what an adequate serving size is at a particular time, and this obviously varies according to recently eaten meals, activities and anticipated food availability.

Our ability to assess how much of a food we would like to eat relies on learned responses added to whenever a new food or a new situation has been introduced. Reflex hormonal and neural pathways, linked to the metabolic consequences of the meal, may be part of the regulatory process. It is believed that this type of learning is an important component of the control of food intake.

See Chapter 9 for more on the physiological regulation of food intake, pp. 186–190.

The variability of 'normal' serving sizes between individuals is a dilemma for those studying food intakes in populations. There is no single serving size, which would apply to everyone. However, for the sake of expediency, such a measure is quoted and used in many contexts, most notably in 'snack bars' and ready meals. For other foods, different people will have 'large' or 'small' servings. Interpretations of these are also subjective and, therefore, variable.

Dieticians try to resolve this issue using replica foods or photographs, which generally represent an 'average' serving. Patients may then indicate whether the amount they would consume is similar to this or different. There is always, of course, the tendency to claim that one's intake follows the average.

The amount of food habitually eaten at a snack or meal has its first impact on energy intake, and thus energy balances. Given the relatively modest variation in metabolic rates and energy meals of normal-weight people, there are arguments for standardizing the energy contents of pre-prepared snacks and meals to be appropriate for most, assuming that they would prefer not to gain or lose weight. The UK FSA has suggested that main meals should contain about 30% of daily energy need, and breakfast 5%, leaving 15% for two or three snacks. If this is based on the energy need of an average woman (2000 kcal/day), a reasonable starting point would be as follows:

Breakfast	300–500 kcal
Lunch	500–700 kcal
Dinner	500–700 kcal
Plus two snacks at	150 kcal

This would be appropriate for children from age 10, but men would generally need about 20% more and athletes in training a further 20%–30%.

WHAT ARE THE FEATURES OF A NUTRITIONALLY BALANCED DIET?

This question is likely to produce a number of different responses from people, depending on their level of interest in nutrition and their understanding of the principles of health. In fact, people have a very different understanding of common words used to describe nutritional concepts. This is an issue for health promotion, as the message put forward must be consistent and understood by as wide a section of the population as possible. Answers will fall into one or several of the following categories:

- Eating more or less of particular foods
- Eating more or less of particular nutrients
- Eating specific foods that are believed to have 'health' properties (this may include taking nutritional supplements or eating organically produced food)
- Adopting particular diet-related practices as well as lifestyle changes
- Having a 'balanced diet'

Eating More or Less of Particular Foods

This response derives from the belief that there are 'good' foods and 'bad' foods. Unfortunately, it is not a straightforward matter to classify foods in this manner; individual foods are less important than the way in which they are combined in diets. However, foods that contain a lot of fat or sugar, or those which have been extensively refined or processed, are likely to be of less value in a complete diet, since they reduce the nutrient density. The remaining foods in the diet must contain more of the micronutrients to compensate, and there is a limit to achieving this compensation.

Incorporating low-nutrient-density foods can be a particular problem in people who have relatively small appetites, such as the elderly, or who are sedentary and, therefore, have low energy needs, since their potential intake of the more nutritious foods in the diet will be limited. Alcoholics can consume 2000–3000 kcal/day purely from alcohol. This satisfies their appetites without normal foods, and a range of nutrient deficiencies develop.

Energy intake and balance are covered in Chapters 16 and 17, pp. 313–330; 331–342.

Eating More or Less of Particular Nutrients

The aim of dietary guidelines is to promote a particular balance of nutrients, but people eat foods and not nutrients. Foods (with a very few exceptions) are not simply a source of one nutrient, and, therefore, changing the intake of a certain group of nutrients by excluding particular foods from the diet may have consequences for other nutrients also found in those foods. For example, if milk and dairy products are excluded because of their fat content, this can have serious implications for intakes of calcium, iodine and riboflavin. Furthermore, if specific foods are excluded, people's appetites will always be satisfied with other sources of energy, so nutrient balances will be further upset.

Some foods contain a nutrient in quite large amounts, which is used for promotion. For example, ordinary hard cheese (such as Cheddar cheese) is recognized by most people as a source of protein and calcium, important for growing children and for bones. However, it is also very rich in fat. In listing sources of fat, many people would omit to mention cheese and will continue to eat it often in quite large amounts. If changes are made only to the most obvious sources of visible fat, such as the spreading fats, cooking oils and full-fat milk, but other sources including cheese, pastries, biscuits and cakes are not reduced, then the overall impact on total fat intakes will be small.

As a consequence, more recent dietary guidelines directed at consumers have moved away from this focus on nutrients and have reverted to giving advice on foods or 'food groups' containing interchangeable foods, which should be included in the diet. These current guidelines urge greater consumption of fruits and vegetables, reduced fat dairy products, and breads and cereals, and decreased the use of high-fat dairy products, processed meat products and fats. However, there are still some nutrients whose consumption is largely controlled by food manufacturing processes. To optimize the diets of populations, there are, therefore, actions required by manufacturers, caterers and retailers to modify the nutrient content of the food supply. Nutrient profiling aims to provide such answers, by scrutinising the nutrient levels in foods, and less often meals, to draw conclusions on the food supply and potential food reformulation required. For example, sodium (salt) consumption is currently two- to threefold about recommended levels, and 70–80% of all salt is already added to foods (e.g. bread, cereals, spreads) before purchase. It is impossible for the population to achieve recommended levels (to cut hypertension and strokes) without major changes in the food supply. Similarly, the very high intakes of sugar by some children (up to 50% of energy requirement by some toddlers) is maintained by the manufactures of very sweet drinks, containing 10% by weight of sugar (or equivalent artificial sweeteners), together with addictive caffeine. Manufacturers need to reduce sweetness and to remove the caffeine of soft drinks to help improve the nutrient intakes of children.

Eating Specific Foods That Are Believed to Have 'Health-Promoting' Properties

There is a perception that only certain foods are healthy, and they should be included in the diet. Linked to this is the notion that, provided these foods are present, it does not matter what else the diet contains. Thus, in practice, an individual might be eating all the wrong proportions of macronutrients, but believes the diet is healthy because it includes a high-fibre breakfast cereal and semi-skimmed milk, or extra so-called superfoods. Clearly there is some confusion here. A single food or two cannot make a diet healthy, although they can possibly contribute to redress an unbalanced diet.

Another example in this category is the inclusion of nutritional supplements to correct (perceived) deficiencies in the diet consumed. Although some aspects of the nutritional content of a diet may be improved by the micronutrients commonly found in supplements, the balance of macronutrients may still be unhealthy. Again, the consumer has a mistaken perception that they are eating healthily. Micronutrients, for example, vitamins and minerals are only required in minute amounts; 'they only confer benefit if there is a frank deficiency'. They cannot rescue a poor diet or confer health otherwise.

Including 'organically' grown products in the diet may reduce the level of agricultural chemicals consumed, but again does not make the diet nutritionally better balanced or healthful.

The remedy for an unbalanced diet that contains unhealthy proportions of the macronutrients and perhaps inadequate amounts of the micronutrients lies in a change in the foods consumed and an alteration in the proportions of the different food groups.

WHAT NUTRIENTS ARE NEEDED AND IN WHAT AMOUNTS?

In practice, most people have no idea about the actual quantities of nutrients they require each day, and yet most manage to obtain approximately sufficient amounts to maintain adequate health. Whether their health is as good as it could be (i.e. 'optimal') and remains optimal into the future or whether health could be enhanced by changes to their diets is a matter for debate. Long-term health includes physical, mental, social and even genomic elements, and there are many other factors which interact with diet and nutrition.

Moreover, measured health (e.g. in terms of blood pressure, blood glucose) or future outcomes such as strokes or cancers can be related to dietary factors, but what people experience is perceived health, which they couple with dietary beliefs and attributions. Most people perceive their diets as balanced. Nutritionists require more specific information on which to base scientific and reasonable evaluation and advice. The starting point for these figures is the nutritional requirement.

Nutritional Requirement

Each individual uses or loses a certain amount of each nutrient daily; this amount must, therefore, be made available to the tissues either from the daily diet or from the body stores of that nutrient. If the nutrient is taken from body stores, it must be replaced at a later stage; otherwise, the stores will gradually become depleted and the person will be totally reliant on their daily intake. Eventually, a deficiency state might develop, if the intake is insufficient. Excess intakes may be accommodated by increased storage, but this can increase costs, and some essential nutrients can even be toxic in excess (for example, iron). There may then be a range of intakes compatible with good health.

The amount of each nutrient used by the body daily is the physiological requirement. It is defined as the amount of a nutrient required by an individual to prevent signs of clinical deficiency. This amount varies between individuals; it could differ from day to day due to different levels of energy expenditure. It may also alter with the composition of the diet owing to changes in efficiency of absorption or utilization of nutrients.

There are, however, a number of inherent problems with this definition. First, it is argued that this approach, based as it is on the very least amount needed to survive without developing a deficiency, leaves no margin of safety. Consideration could be given to the provision of a nutrient store to act as a reserve in time of physiological stress or reduced intake. Second, it gives no guidance on how to determine the requirement for nutrients for which there is currently no easily recognized clinical deficiency. This applies to fats (except essential fatty acids) and sugars. Third, there are no universally agreed criteria of when clinical deficiency exists. This is because a clinical deficiency reflects one end of a continuum, making it difficult to define precisely, as indicated in Figure 2.1.

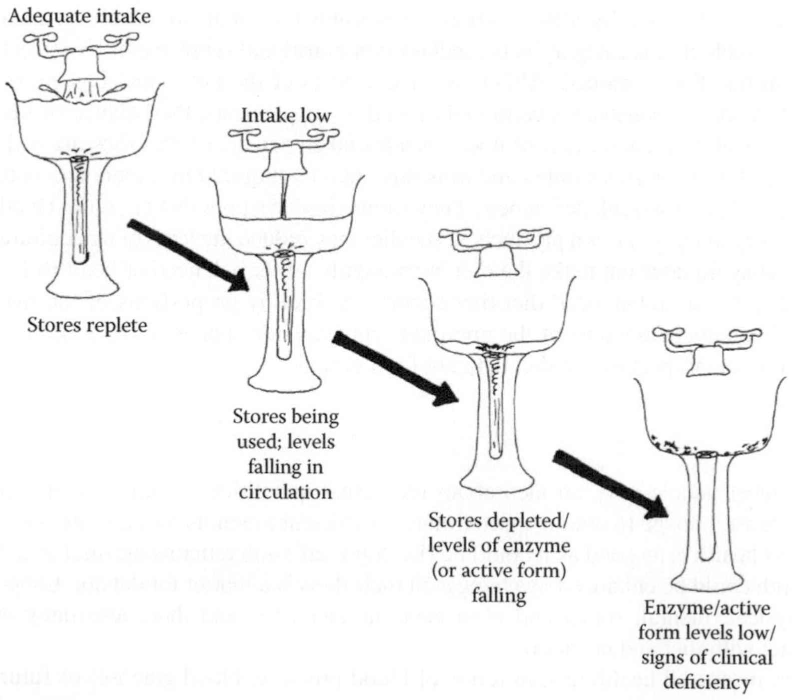

FIGURE 2.1 The stages of development of a clinical deficiency. This is a general guide to the progression from adequacy to deficiency. In some cases, the biochemical end point may be very difficult to identify or there may be no specific signs associated with deficiency.

When intake of a nutrient falls, there may be secondary metabolic adaptation to allow continued function for a time. However, this reduction adaptation may incur collateral costs to health.

It is cumbersome to obtain individual values for each nutrient requirement. One solution is to look at the average requirements of groups of similar people and to define a reasonable minimum level. The age of the child is taken as a basis for defining 'similar' children; for pregnant women, the stage of pregnancy is taken as the common basis; for other groups of the population, age and gender are common criteria. This is the approach used by the Panel on Dietary Reference Values of the Committee on Medical Aspects of Food Policy, which produced the most recent set of data for the United Kingdom in 1991 (DoH, 1991). This panel derived information about nutritional requirements in a number of ways. These included the following:

- Measures of the actual intakes of particular nutrients in populations that are apparently healthy
- The intakes of nutrients that are required to maintain balance in the body
- Amounts of a nutrient needed to reverse a deficiency state
- Amounts needed for tissue saturation, normal biochemical function or an appropriate level of a specific biological marker

The appropriate method has to be selected for each nutrient, taking into account its metabolic activity, mode of excretion, storage in the body and the availability of suitable biochemical indicators. None of the criteria used in determining the level of requirement is deemed perfect, but is the best available with the current state of knowledge. The classical nutritional approach to determine sufficiency requires a series of metabolic balance studies at different levels of intake of the nutrient. This type of experiment is potentially hazardous, risking deficiency. It also produces a rather hypothetical value, since in practice it is rare for a diet to be deficient in just one isolated nutrient. In real life, diets usually become more marginal and then deficient for a range of nutrients, often including energy, and a variety of adaptive mechanisms come into play.

Defining nutritional requirements is then usually based on collating data from a range of observations, none precise, and many depend on dietary intake assessment, with all its limitations.

DISTRIBUTION OF NUTRITIONAL REQUIREMENTS IN A POPULATION

When measurements of requirements are obtained from a sufficiently large population, the results are usually assumed to follow a typical 'normal' distribution curve. If the group is sufficiently large, then half will fall above the sample mean and half below it; this is simply a property of the distribution and not something peculiar to nutrition or requirements. Within a group or population, some individuals, or subgroups, may have different relative requirements for certain nutrients. There may, for example, be relatively high requirement for folate, defined by metabolic and genetic factors. Nutrient requirements are also affected by disease status and even by insufficiency of other nutrients, so nutrient requirements are not fixed characteristics. If the normal distribution of requirements can be determined for each nutrient, it is possible to define the level of intake, two standard deviations above the mean of requirements, above which almost all individuals will be adequately supplied. This is one of the scientific principles behind the UK dietary reference values (DRV) (Reference values, DoH, 1991). Individuals whose requirements are above this level (about 2.5% of people) will need a greater intake. A 'safety margin' is therefore added.

It is important to note that just as there is a normal distribution of nutrient requirements, within the population, there is an approximately normal distribution of actual intakes of each nutrient. It is possible that individuals who happen to have unusually high requirements, for metabolic or genetic reasons, may for social or other reasons have unusually low intakes. This is a potential source of disease which would not be identified if only mean values are considered.

FROM REQUIREMENTS TO RECOMMENDATIONS: DIETARY REFERENCE VALUES

Having established the range of nutritional requirements for a particular nutrient, several options might be available to define the level of intake which should be recommended (Figure 2.2). Setting the level at a point A, which is above the range of individual requirements, would ensure that everyone's needs were met but might pose a risk in terms of excessive intakes, if the nutrients were harmful in large amounts. There would also be cost implications – should people be encouraged to buy so much food to meet this high level? An alternative might be to set the level at point B, which is the mean. By definition, this would imply that this level of intake would be sufficient for half of the population, but would be inadequate for the other half. This would not be satisfactory as a recommended intake for most nutrients. However, energy point B, which is defined as the estimated average requirement (EAR), is used as the reference value since for energy each individual has a rather precise average daily requirement, to remain in energy balance. The reference values are intended for use by groups. Within a group, there will be some whose energy needs are above and some below the EAR. If the food provided, or consumed, contains an amount of energy that reaches the EAR, and the individuals eat to appetite without weight change, then one can assume that their energy needs are being met. If the mean energy provided or consumed lies below the EAR, this suggests that some of the group may not be reaching their EAR. Conversely, a mean intake above the EAR implies an excessive intake of energy among some members of the group, manifested in weight gain. Judgements about individuals cannot be made by comparison with the EAR figure, as this is a group mean.

For most nutrients, the DRV uses a point towards the upper end of the distribution curve of nutritional requirements, at the mean + 2 standard deviations (SD). Because of the particular characteristics of this type of distribution curve, this point (C) covers the requirement figures for 97.5% of the population. It could be argued that this leaves 2.5% of the population outside the limits and, therefore, at risk of an inadequate intake. However, in practice, it was felt that an individual would not have extremely high requirements for all nutrients, and it was thus unlikely that anyone would consistently fail to meet the requirements across the range. Eating to satisfy appetite would be likely to ensure adequate intake.

Therefore, to summarize, point C was identified as the reference nutrient intake (RNI). In addition, the panel identified point D, the lower reference nutrient intake (LRNI) at the lower end of the requirement range. This represents the mean – 2 standard deviations, and covers the requirements of only 2.5% of the population, who fall below this level. Again, it is possible that there are

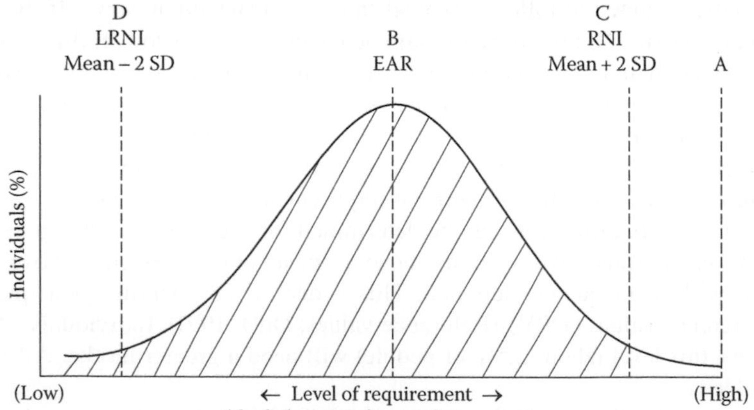

FIGURE 2.2 The normal distribution curve of nutrient requirements in a population and levels used for setting dietary recommendations. LRNI, lower reference nutrient intake; EAR, estimated average requirement; RNI, reference nutrient intake; SD, standard deviations.

some people who have nutritional requirements consistently below this point and who may, therefore, meet their needs at this level of intake. However, it is more probable that, if a population has a mean intake as low as this, most individuals are not meeting their nutritional requirement. It effectively represents the lowest level that might be compatible with an adequate intake.

The DRV tables (UK Department of Health as Report 41; DoH, 1991), therefore, provide three distinct figures for the majority of nutrients: the LRNI, EAR and RNI, which can be used to give a guide on the adequacy of diets. The term recommended daily amount (RDA), which was used previously, was considered too prescriptive, suggesting that the amounts given referred to what individuals must consume and implying that intakes below the RDA-indicated deficiency.

The DRVs were designed to provide greater nutritional understanding for assessing dietary adequacy on groups or population and changing the diets of individuals. In addition, the DRV tables contain guidance on dietary requirements for fats and carbohydrates, in order to improve health of population, and on some micronutrients for which little information was available. The DRVs apply largely to the 'essential' nutrients and do not address the potential value of non-essential nutrients in pursuit of optimal health.

Fats and Carbohydrates

The approach to dietary requirements based on deficiency is not appropriate for nutrients having no specific associated clinical deficiency. Consequently, in the past, no RDA figures were set for fats and carbohydrates. There is now considerable public health interest in fat and carbohydrate intakes, and a desire for guidance on intake levels. The DRV panel used their judgement, therefore, based on research evidence of health risks at particular levels of intake, to arrive at population average figures for the components of dietary fats and carbohydrates as well as non-starch polysaccharides. Since these nutrients contribute to dietary energy, their exact level must vary to maintain different individuals in energy balance. Rather than giving absolute figures, the DRV values are expressed in terms of the percentage of total energy, which should come from the various components (Table 2.1).

TABLE 2.1

Dietary Reference Values for Fat and Carbohydrate for Adults, as a Percentage of Daily Total Food Energy Intake (Excluding Alcohol)

	Individual Minimum	Population Average	Individual Maximum
Saturated fatty acids		11	
cis-polyunsaturated fatty acids		6.5	10
n-3	0.2		
n-6	1.0		
cis-monounsaturated fatty acids		13	
trans-fatty acids		2	
Total fatty acids		32.5	
Total fat		35	
Non-milk extrinsic sugars	0	11	
Intrinsic and milk sugars		39	
Total carbohydrate		50	
Non-starch polysaccharides (g/day)	12	18	24

Source: Reproduced from DoH (UK Department of Health), Dietary reference values for food energy and nutrients in the United Kingdom, Report on Health and Social Subjects No. 41, Report of the Panel on Dietary Reference Values of the Committee on Medical Aspects of Food Policy, HMSO, London, UK, 1991. With permission.

Recognizing that a range of intakes is comparable with good health, individual minimum and maximum values are cited for some of the components.

Less-Studied Micronutrients

In the case of some of the micronutrients, insufficient data were available to establish a normal distribution of requirements and thence derive values for LRNI and RNI. In these cases, on the basis of all available evidence, a single 'safe intake' figure is provided, sufficient to fulfil most people's needs, but not so high that there is a risk of undesirable effects.

In the United States, a similar approach has been adopted in the revision of the Recommended Daily Allowances (RDA) that had been set in 1989. Since 1998, the National Academy of Sciences has constituted a number of expert panels to prepare a comprehensive set of reference values for nutrient intakes for healthy U.S. and Canadian populations. A number of reports have presented Dietary Reference Intakes (DRI) for vitamins and some minerals. These parallel the DRV figures published by DoH (1991) in the United Kingdom. The DRI includes a number of values as follows:

- RDA, which covers the needs of most individuals in a particular life stage and gender group.
- EAR, which represents the mean requirement of the individuals in a population.
- Adequate intake, which represents an amount for a nutrient that is believed to satisfy needs, but for which there is insufficient evidence to describe the full range of RIs.
- Tolerable upper intake level (UL), which represents the highest level of a nutrient intake that is likely to pose no risk of adverse health effects for almost all individuals in the general population. As intake increases above UL, the risk of adverse effects increases.

Although the figures presented in the U.S. tables are not always the same as those in the United Kingdom, they provide similar guidance on the range of nutrient intakes compatible with health.

If the UK tables are compared with those produced by the Food and Agriculture Organization/World Health Organization (FAO/WHO) or by other countries, differences are found both in the range of nutrients listed and the amounts advised. This implies two things: first, there are differences in needs between peoples of certain countries, as a result of different lifestyles and perhaps different genetic make-up of the population. Therefore, when tables of reference values are used, they should be those relating to the country in question. Second, opinions differ between the committees drawing up the tables in different countries, as to the safety margins that should be added to the figures. As a result, final figures also differ. This does not mean that some are more 'correct' than others; it reflects differences in emphasis and serves to underline the uncertainty surrounding such figures. It is important to remember that these figures are never an 'absolute' when their uses are considered. They are basically the 'best judgement' based on the physiological and nutritional data available at the time.

Practical Applications

For Individuals

It is important to remember that the DRV tables were not primarily designed for use to judge individual nutritional intakes for their adequacy. They were designed to be applied to groups of healthy individuals. However, since in practice they are used to assess individual diets, some words of caution are necessary.

Most people are unlikely to consume an amount of each nutrient to match their personal requirement exactly. However, it is probable that those with higher needs consume more than those whose needs are lower. The higher the correlation of intake and needs, the lower the risk of deficiency there is in any one individual. Unfortunately, the information about individual needs is not available and judgement must be used. The higher the intake level (i.e. the closer it is to the RNI), the lower the risk that it is inadequate. On the other hand, intakes approaching the LRNI level are likely to carry a high risk of being inadequate.

Thus, a firm statement about an individual diet is only possible when the intake falls outside the range of RNI to LRNI. Nevertheless, the DRV panel estimated that the risk of deficiency is about 15% with an intake at the EAR and falls to negligible levels when the intake approaches the RNI. However, it rises sharply at low levels of intake, approaching 100% at the LRNI.

A major practical problem is that there is no method available to measure the intakes of nutrients of individuals. For some nutrients, for example, sodium, excretion rates in the urine, skin and faeces are normally assumed to be the same as intakes but the amount is difficult and demands high cooperation from subjects. For others, estimates of nutrient intakes are commonly made from reported food consumption or from food frequency questionnaires, linked to databases of average nutrient compositions of common foods. There are many sources of error and bias – notably from over- or under-reporting of 'habitual' food consumptions.

For Groups of Individuals

The principle use of DRVs is to asses or plan the diets of groups of people. When a group's mean intake exceeds the RNI, the likelihood of many members of the group having intakes substantially below the RNI is small. The lower the mean intake, with respect to the RNI, the greater the chance that some members have an inadequate intake. For dietary energy group, the mean EAR cannot be exceeded without weight gain.

For Dietary Planning

DRVs can be used in institutions in planning diets for groups of individuals. Achieving a mean intake above the RNI for each essential nutrient should be taken as the target. Similarly, if a dietary prescription for an individual is being planned, then the RNI should be the target, unless there is no other information about the actual needs of the individual, for example, if there is any degree of malabsorption or a need to replenish stores of a nutrient.

The exception as always is dietary energy; unless there is a need to gain or lose weight, the energy intake must match the specific energy requirement (i.e. the energy expenditure) of each individual. For groups, energy intakes must thus match the EAR. It is best to plan diets on the basis of measured or calculated energy requirements using DRVs rather than basing diets on reported dietary intakes because of misreporting errors.

Food Labelling

Nutritional labelling of foods serves several purposes. Information about nutrient contents per serving or per 100 g can be used for dietary analysis, or planning, if the same information is available for all foods. Comparisons between similar, exchangeable, products can guide food choices by discerning consumers. Various attempts, using different systems, have been made to provide consumers with simple guidance about the health implications of particular foods, or products. It is possible to assess the nutrient comparison of a food, or meal, in relation to its energy content and to express how well, or how badly, it matches DRVs and dietary recommendations. However, this makes little sense for individual foods, or ingredients, because they are not consumed exclusively or in isolation. The nutrients in the totality of the diet, or the meal, define healthfulness, and individual foods or ingredients do not matter.

However, to provide some guidance on how specific foods should be used, their nutrient contents have been classified using traffic-light systems (United Kingdom), Green Keyhole system (Sweden) or others.

In Europe, the Reference Intakes now replace the Guideline Daily Amounts. They are based on the predicted daily consumption of an average consumer (female) eating a diet conforming to UK DRV (DoH, 1991) recommendations. The agreed RI are as follows:

Energy	8400 kJ/2000 kcal
Total fat	70 g
Saturated fat	20 g
Carbohydrates	260 g
Sugar	90 g
Proteins	50 g
Salt	6 g

Other labelling directives, related to EU rulings, use RDA as the basis for guidance. The RDA figures on some foods are not necessarily the same as the RNI or EAR figures. Thus, several yardsticks are in operation, each providing somewhat different information to the consumer.

DIETARY PLANNING

It is important that those who use figures from the DRV tables should understand how they have been derived and, therefore, what are their uses and limitations. In practice, however, this is not always possible, and, therefore, a means to translate the scientific information contained in the DRV tables into more accessible format is needed.

Most people recognize three main meals, through the day, often with snacks about 2 hours after the main meal. One way to achieve a healthful, nutritionally balanced day's intake and diet is to apply nutritional guidelines to each of three meals. The meals (or 'eating episode') can be taken to include also an item held back a snack before the next meal: defined in this way, the meal is the smallest 'unit' of diet to which nutritional guidelines for health can or should be applied. If all three meals are well planned to be nutritionally balanced, then the whole day's diet is of course also healthful. If one meal is in some way unbalanced, it is possible to compensate with the other meals, but only to a limited degree. Designing nutritionally balanced meals requires knowledge of portion sizes and reference to tables of nutritional composition. Consumers can use RIs to help planning, but most people find this too complicated for regular use. This is a problem compounded by the currently chaotic nutritional composition of ready meal (see Celnik et al., 2012).

MEAL PLANNING TOOLS

Many countries in the West have used meal selection guides for a number of years to help their consumers with healthful eating. Food guides provide a framework to show how foods can be combined together in a day's eating to provide an overall intake, which contains the appropriate range of nutrients. They achieve this by

- Grouping together foods that provide (generally) similar nutrients and that may be interchangeable in the diet
- Making a quantitative statement about the number of 'servings' of foods from each food group to be taken daily

Health-directed food guides were first devised in the United States in 1916, based on five food groups – milk and meat, cereals, vegetables and fruits, fats and fat foods and sugars and sugary foods. At that time, there was no specific evidence, and vitamins were still unrecognized. Further developments occurred between the 1940s, stimulated by scientific evidence linking food and health, gathered during the Second World War, and 1970s, when evidence linking dietary fats and heart disease emerged. Changes to the number and components of the groups reflected an increase in the understanding of the role of diet in health and disease prevention.

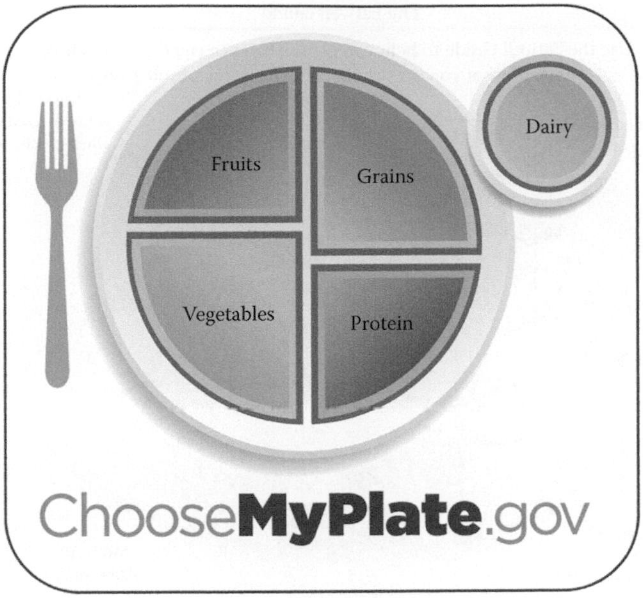

FIGURE 2.3 The USDA MyPlate model, illustrating the five food groups. (www.ChooseMyPlate.gov)

Most countries that have developed a food guide use either the concept of a pyramid or a circle to illustrate that there are various components making up a whole diet. The most recent version of the U.S. food guide is a plate, which replaced the pre-existing pyramid in 2011 (Figure 2.3). The food guide does not imply that any single food is essential in the diet and no food group alone provides all the necessary nutrients. What is important, however, is to include variety in the diet. In this way, shortcomings in one food are likely to be compensated by an adequate intake in another food. Australian research has shown that a healthful nutrient balance is most easily consumed by people with the greatest variety of foods in their diet. Diets with very limited variety are more often unhealthful and have nutrient deficiencies, for example, through poor food availability or poor choice, as often seen in autism.

Most children in the United States have been found not to meet the guidelines that were depicted in the pyramid, especially with respect to the grains, fruit and dairy groups. This is resulting in concern about nutritional intakes, especially of sugars and saturated fats and very low calcium intakes. In addition, the rising prevalence (i.e. the numbers of people affected in the population) of weight gain and obesity that now affects over 20% of children in the United States has led to this initiative, in an attempt to influence eating habits at a young age.

In the United Kingdom, a national food guide (the Balance of Good Health) subsequently renamed the Eatwell plate (and now Eatwell Guide since 2016) was launched for the first time in 1994 (Figure 2.4). The evolution of the guide is discussed by Buttriss (2016). The design is a 'tilted plate' incorporating five food groups in the following proportions:

Segment size as percent of whole plate (2016 adjustments)

Bread, other cereals and potatoes	37
Fruit and vegetables	39
Meat, fish, beans, pulses and alternatives	12
Milk and dairy foods and dairy alternatives	8
Oil and spreads	1
Biscuits, sweets, foods to eat less often	3

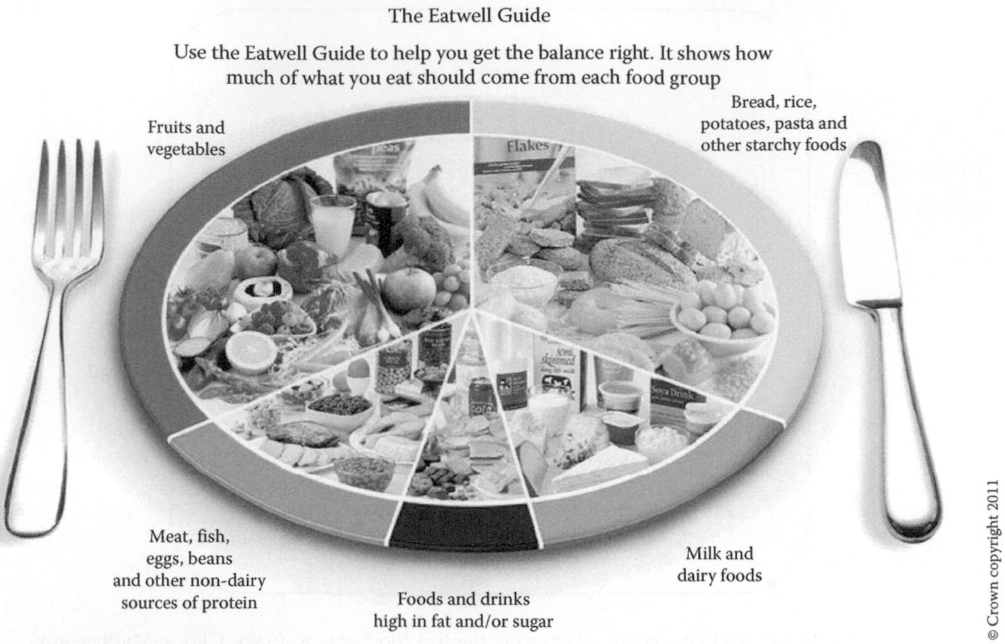

FIGURE 2.4 The Eatwell Guide. (From Department of Health in association with the Welsh Assembly Government, the Scottish Government and the Food Standards Agency in Northern Ireland.)

Eatwell Guide – the main dietary messages

- Eat at >=5 portions of a variety of fruit and vegetables every day.
- Base meals on potatoes, bread, rice, pasta or other starchy carbohydrates; choose wholegrain versions where possible.
- Have some dairy or dairy alternatives (such as soya drinks); choosing lower fat and lower sugar options.
- Eat some beans, pulses, fish, eggs, meat and other proteins (including 2 portions of fish every week, one of which should be oily).
- Choose unsaturated oils and spreads and eat in small amounts.
- Drink 6–8 cups/glasses of fluid a day.
- If consuming foods and drinks high in fat, salt or sugar have these less often and in small amounts.

The nutritional details of the groups used in the Eatwell Guide are presented in Table 2.2.

The foods which are portrayed in the Eatwell Guide are meant to be the representative of the main food groups – not prescriptive or restrictive. The actual proportions shown were originally intended to show the appropriate amounts needed to make up a nutritionally balanced diet for one person for a week; however, the picture cannot be followed exactly.

Although well recognized by the public, individuals have not been able to translate it into practical actions to modify their diets. To do this in a new project, the FSA and the University of Glasgow have developed the 'Eatwell Week' which provides interchangeable meals for several days, which satisfy the requirements for a nutritionally balanced diet.

TABLE 2.2

Nutritional Details of the Five Groups in the Eatwell Guide

Name of Food Group	Composition of Food Group	Key Nutrients Found in Group
Potatoes, bread, rice, pasta and other starchy carbohydrates	All breads made with yeast and other breads	Carbohydrate NSP
	Cereals, including wheat, oats, barley, rice, maize, millet and rye together with products made from them, including breakfast cereals and pasta	Vitamin B complex Calcium Iron
	Potatoes in the form usually eaten as part of a meal (but not as a snack, e.g. crisps)	(Recommend: Low-fat methods of cooking and sauces/dressings and spreads High-fibre varieties to maximize micronutrients)
Fruits and vegetables	Fresh, frozen, chilled and canned fruit and vegetables	Vitamins C and E and carotenes (antioxidant vitamins), folate
	Fruit juices	Minerals: potassium, magnesium, trace minerals
	Dried fruit	Carbohydrate
	Not included: potatoes, pulses, nuts	
Beans, pulses, fish, meat and other proteins	Carcass meats, meat products (but not pastries and pies)	Protein B vitamins (especially B_{12}) Minerals: phosphorus, iron, zinc, magnesium
	Fish and fish products	NSP (from pulses only)
	Poultry	Long-chain polyunsaturated fatty acids (in oily fish).
	Eggs	Meat and its products that may be significant contributors to fat intake (low-fat alternatives available)
	Pulses, beans and nuts	NSP, protein, iron
Dairy and alternatives	All types of milk	Protein, iodine
	Yoghurt	Calcium
	Cheese	Fat-soluble vitamins (except in low-fat varieties) B vitamins (riboflavin, B_{12})
	Not included: butter and eggs	
Oil and spreads	Butter, margarine, fat spreads, oils and other fats	Energy, essential fatty acids, fat-soluble vitamins Fat
	Cream	Sugar

Notes: Does not include composite dishes. These should be allocated to groups according to their main ingredients. Cakes, ice cream, sugar, savoury and sugary snacks (including crisps, biscuits, pastries, sweets) sit aside from the tilted plate and should be consumed less often and in small amounts.

As with any other food planning guide, the Eatwell Guide and eatwell week do not take into account the needs of those on special diets, infants and children under 5 years or frail elderly people. Individuals in these groups may need to pay greater attention to the nutrient density of the foods consumed if their intakes are small.

NUTRITION INFORMATION

There are numerous booklets and leaflets now available to the consumer produced by food companies, retailers, hospital trusts and many other organizations. How should these be viewed and what is the quality of the information they contain? Many of them are sound and very informative. Some, however, can be misleading, often not by what they actually include but by judicious omission of key points.

When reading nutrition information leaflets, ask yourself the following questions:

- Is the dietary advice being offered compatible with a balanced diet, defined under current nutritional guidelines?
- Is the advice stressing the importance of selected essential nutrients to the neglect of others?
- Is a particular product or brand being promoted?
- Is there bias in the advice being given because of other interests that the sponsor of the leaflet may have?
- Does the leaflet promise realistic outcomes?
- Are health claims legal, with explicit support from agencies such as EFSA?
- Is scientific evidence being quoted, including references, representative of the totality of reputable sources of information?
- Is the advice being given sustainable and appropriate to you and your lifestyle?
- Is the leaflet written by a registered nutritionist or dietician?
- Is there an address from which further information can be obtained?

It is commonly said, but simply not true, that nutrition professionals are continuously changing their views and advice, as the media claim. Scientific debate is an important way of moving knowledge forward, and without it, a subject stagnates and becomes dated. The majority of nutrition experts do agree on the basic principles about healthy eating, and they have changed very little over the past 50 years. Where there is disagreement, it usually reflects small points of emphasis in dietary advice and how best to achieve the nutritional goals which are agreed. The media tend to report the views of self-publicists as equal to those of trained experts and to report the results of isolated conflicting results as 'food scares', without references to the totality of the evidence.

THE QUESTION OF ALCOHOL

The consumption of alcohol is not discussed in the basic guidance on a balanced diet, as it is not an essential component of the diet and does not feature in all diets. Yet, the consumption of alcohol is prevalent. Almost 90% of people in Europe consume alcohol at some time each year. Alcoholic beverages are consumed as part of many social activities, but consumption can also become excessive and result in physical, psychological and social harm to the individual as well as those around them. Alcohol is a potent cell toxin, and excessive consumption soon depletes the diet of essential nutrients. Economic estimates suggest that health and other problems related to alcohol consumption, including time away from work, represent a heavy financial burden. However, there is also very substantial revenue to the government from the taxes levied on alcoholic beverages and a powerful industry which tends to modify health advice.

In order to quantify amounts of alcohol drunk from a variety of different sources, a standard 'unit' of alcohol has been developed. In the United Kingdom, this is equivalent to 8 g or 10 mL of ethanol. Approximately, this amount of ethanol is found in the following measures of common drinks:

- ½ pint of standard-strength beer (284 ml)
- 1 measure of spirit (25 ml)
- 1 glass of wine (125 ml)

Many other drinks are available on the market that do not fit exactly into these categories; labelling information must be used to identify exactly how many units are present in a drink.

To complicate matters, the definition of a unit differs between countries and, in the United States, equals 14 g of alcohol (AIM sensible drinking guidelines, 2012).

Benchmarks for safe levels of intake of alcohol have been published, using the concept of a unit. These are that men should not exceed 3–4 units per day with a limit of 21 units per week and women should not exceed 2 3 units per day or 14 units per week. In addition, there should be some drink-free days during the week.

With progressively higher alcohol intakes, there is a greater risk of harm occurring. Consequences of excessive alcohol consumption include damage to every system of the body, including the liver, digestive system, heart, brain and nervous system. In addition, nutritional intake is likely to be affected and chronic overconsumption is associated with a number of specific nutritional deficiencies. Even at moderate intakes, alcohol at 7 kcal/g contributes to total energy supply and may cause weight gain. Social consumption of alcohol accompanying meals has been shown to be associated with a larger food intake as well as the consumption of higher levels of fat. This means that alcohol is an obstacle to weight management or slimming.

However, moderate alcohol consumption has also been linked to beneficial effects, particularly in the protection against coronary heart disease. There is a J-shaped relationship between overall mortality and alcohol consumption, with abstainers and heavier drinkers having higher mortality rates than those seen in moderate drinkers. Maximum health advantage for coronary heart disease lies at levels of intake between 1 and 2 units per day. The reasons for the shape of this curve are still not agreed. In addition, the J-shaped relationship is now known to apply predominantly to men over the age of 35 years and women after the menopause, with benefits increasing in older age groups. The level at which no harm is caused by alcohol also increases with age, so that the younger drinker is most at risk. Mortality risk is increased in young drinkers at levels of alcohol consumption normally considered to be 'safe', through accidents and violence, rather than the long-term physical damage caused by alcohol itself.

On a population basis, there is no recommendation to increase alcohol consumption, for although abstainers might benefit from a small amount of alcohol, the extra harm that could ensue from increased drinking among heavier consumers would not translate into an overall improvement in health.

SUMMARY

1. Diet quality is not synonymous to including specific 'health-giving' foods to the diet, using specific food preparation techniques, avoiding additives or taking nutritional supplements. None of these will make the diet healthy, and health claims may confuse the consumers.
2. Choosing a nutritionally balanced diet requires knowledge on foods, how to select them and in what quantities.
3. Adequate amounts of food must be consumed to meet nutrient requirements. These are expressed as DRVs and cover the needs of most of the population.
4. Dietary planning tools show how a balanced diet can be created, by choosing from a wide range of foods, in appropriate quantities.

STUDY QUESTIONS

1. What is the smallest number of different foods which are needed to construct a healthful balanced day's diet for a man?
2. For what reasons might a vegetarian diet be considered more healthful than an omnivorous diet?
3. Explain why a nutritional deficiency state can be difficult to define precisely. What different end points are used to delineate deficiency?
4. How is an individual's nutritional requirement different from the reference nutrient intake for a particular nutrient (e.g. vitamin C)?

ACTIVITIES

2.1 Make a list of foods that you usually eat during the course of a week. Divide them up into four columns: foods eaten at breakfast, lunch, evening meal and snack foods.

- Is this easy to do? If so, you have got strong ideas about what foods are appropriate at what times, and in what meals. If you found it quite hard to do, this may be because you have a much 'freer' food structure, and the items in your diet may serve several roles.
- Check with a partner how easy their list was to write into columns.
- Finally, check how much agreement there is between your list and your partner's – do you consider the same foods as appropriate at particular times?

2.2 1. *Observation*: During the next few days, use any opportunities you may have to observe people at mealtimes. Notice whether the amounts of food items they consume are similar to or greater/smaller than you would choose.

2. *Quantitative assessment*: If you have access to dietary or household weighing scales, make measurements of the typical serving size that you select of everyday foods. Ask members of your family or your colleagues/friends to do the same. Collate the information from as many different people as possible.
   - How much variation do you find?
   - Are portion sizes for some foods more variable than others?
   - Can you offer explanations for this?
   - What are the health implications of people's different concepts of 'appropriate' serving size?

2.3 Now carry out a similar exercise on your own food intake. You may have already kept a record of a typical day or several days' food intake. Make an assessment of the proportions of your diet coming from the various groups.

- What groups are overrepresented?
- Are some underrepresented?

Use the Eatwell Guide to suggest alternatives in the diet that could make the balance better.

Figure 2.5 shows the results of a riboflavin intake study in a large group of boys. Three boys in this group (boys A, B and C) were found to have intakes of A, B and C mg, respectively. The following conclusions can be drawn from the results:

- With an intake of A mg, we can be fairly sure that boy A is not reaching his nutritional requirement for riboflavin, since it falls at the level of the LRNI. He may already be showing signs of clinical deficiency, such as dermatitis. If not, he should be investigated, and given advice on increasing his riboflavin intake.
- Boy B's riboflavin intake, of B mg, is below the EAR for the group. However, this does not necessarily imply that he is receiving an inadequate intake. He may simply be a child

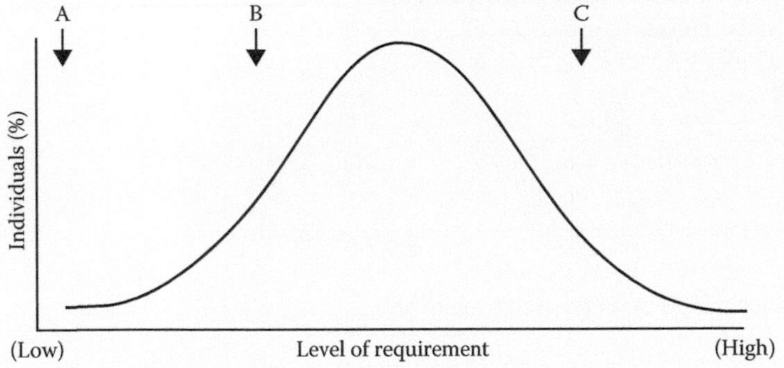

FIGURE 2.5 Distribution of riboflavin intakes in a population of 12-year-old boys.

with a low individual requirement. On the other hand, if he is not growing normally or showing signs of ill health, his needs are probably not being met and his intake should be increased.

- At first sight, boy C's intake of C mg seems to be quite adequate, as it almost reaches the RNI; it is quite likely that this is the case. However, the possibility could exist that he has a very high requirement, which is not being met by the current intake, even though it appears quite high. It can only be assumed that his intake is sufficient, if there is no evidence of inadequacy.

BIBLIOGRAPHY AND FURTHER READING

Buttriss, J. L. 2016. The Eatwell Guide refreshed. *Nutrition Bulletin* 41(2), 135–141.

Celnik, D., Gillespie, L. and Lean, M.E.J. 2012. Time-scarcity, ready-meals, ill-health and the obesity epidemic. *Trends in Food Science and Technology* 27(1), 4–11.

DoH (UK Department of Health). 1991. Dietary reference values for food energy and nutrients in the United Kingdom. Report on Health and Social Subjects No. 41. Report of the Panel on Dietary Reference Values of the Committee on Medical Aspects of Food Policy. London, UK: HMSO.

DoH (UK Department of Health). 1995. Sensible drinking. The Report of an Inter-Departmental Working Group. London, UK: HMSO.

Fairweather-Tait, S.J. 1993. Optimal nutrient requirements: Important concepts. *Journal of Human Nutrition and Dietetics* 6, 411–417.

Hunt, P., Gatenby, S. and Rayner, M. 1995. The format for the National Food Guide: Performance and preference studies. *Journal of Human Nutrition and Dietetics* 8, 335–351.

Institute of Grocery Distribution. 1995. *Voluntary Nutrition Labelling Guidelines to Benefit the Consumer.* Watford, U.K.: Institute of Grocery Distribution.

Johnson, R.K. 2000. The 2000 dietary guidelines for Americans: Foundation of US nutrition policy. *British Nutrition Foundation Nutrition Bulletin* 25, 241–248.

Lachat, C. and Tseng, M. 2013. A wake-up call for nutrition labelling. *Public Health Nutrition* 16(03), 381–382.

MAFF (Ministry of Agriculture, Fisheries and Food). 1990. *Eight Guidelines for a Healthy Diet.* London, UK: Food Sense.

Mela, D.J. 1993. Consumer estimates of the percentage energy from fat in common foods. *European Journal of Clinical Nutrition* 47(10), 735–740.

Nestle, M. 1999. Animal v plant foods in human diets and health: Is the historical record unequivocal? *Proceedings of the Nutrition Society* 58, 211–218.

Perez, R. and Edge, M.S. 2014. Global nutrition labeling: Moving toward standardization? *Nutrition Today* 49(2), 77–82.

Public Health England. 2016. The Eatwell Guide - Helping you Eat a Healthy, Balanced Diet. London:HMSO.

3 Macronutrients in Foods and Diets

Proteins, Carbohydrates and Fats

AIMS

The aims of this chapter are to

- Describe the composition and nature of proteins and identify protein-providing foods in the diet.
- Discuss the concept of indispensable amino acids and how this is reflected in measurement of protein quality.
- Describe the carbohydrates that are important in human nutrition, including simple and complex carbohydrates.
- Consider the desirable levels of carbohydrate in the diet.
- Describe the nature and characteristics of fats important in human nutrition.
- Discuss the role of fat in the diet and trends in fat consumption.

PROTEINS

The word 'protein' is derived from the Greek language and means 'holding first place'. Proteins are essential in the structure and function of all living things. Their importance, however, lies principally in the amino acids of which they are composed.

Some people associate protein with strength and muscle power and perceive meat as being the most valuable source of protein. This view is only partly true; proteins are an essential component of muscles, but this is only one of their many functions in the body. Meat is a source of protein, but so are also many other foods, both of plant and animal origin.

There are millions of different proteins – plant, animal and human – but all are built up from the same 20 amino acids. The particular sequence and number of amino acids contained in a protein determine its nature. With 20 different amino acids to choose from, and chains which include perhaps several hundred different amino acids, the variety is almost endless. The variety of proteins that exist is far greater than that of carbohydrates and fats. However, each protein has its own particular sequence of amino acids, which is crucial for its properties and functions. If even one amino acid is missing or misplaced in the chain, the properties of the protein will alter. The sequence of amino acids is controlled by the genetic machinery of our cells, encoded in the DNA and RNA chains. This critical relationship between the number of units (the amino acid) contained and the protein function does not apply in the case of carbohydrates: they may contain more or fewer of the particular component unit (usually a monosaccharide) without significant changes in properties.

The majority of amino acids originate from plants, which are able to combine nitrogen from the soil and air with carbon and other substances to produce amino acids. These are then built into proteins by plants. Humans obtain their proteins directly either by eating plant foods or by eating the animals (and their products), which have themselves consumed the plants. The proteins that we eat are broken down into their constituent amino acids and are rebuilt, or some new amino acids are first made, before new proteins are made in our bodies. Our bodies are able to make some amino acids from others, but certain amino acids (called essential or indispensable) cannot be synthesized *de novo* by the body and must, therefore, be supplied by the diet. Essential amino acids are phenylalanine, valine, threonine, tryptophan, isoleucine, methionine, leucine, lysine and histidine. Conditional amino acids are indispensable in certain circumstances (such as in neonates, during growth and in case of trauma/metabolic stress). These are cysteine, tyrosine, arginine, taurine and glutamine.

Protein digestion and absorption are covered in Chapter 10, p. 193, and amino acid metabolism in Chapter 10, p. 193.

It is our need for these amino acids that makes it vital to have adequate amounts of protein in our diet. If an individual fails to eat sufficient amounts of protein, the body's own structural proteins are broken down to meet metabolic needs for repair. In addition, other protein-requiring functions can also fail, with resulting illness and possible death. To judge the needs of an individual for protein, it is important to understand how proteins are used in the body and the magnitude of the daily turnover.

Amino Acids: The Building Blocks

Amino acids have all the same basic structure – a carbon (known as the α carbon), with four groups of atoms attached to it:

- An amino group ($-NH_2$)
- An acid group ($-COOH$) always present
- A hydrogen atom ($-H$)
- A fourth group, which varies between different amino acids and characterizes each one. This is the side chain, identified as $-R$ in the 'generic' formula of an amino acid:

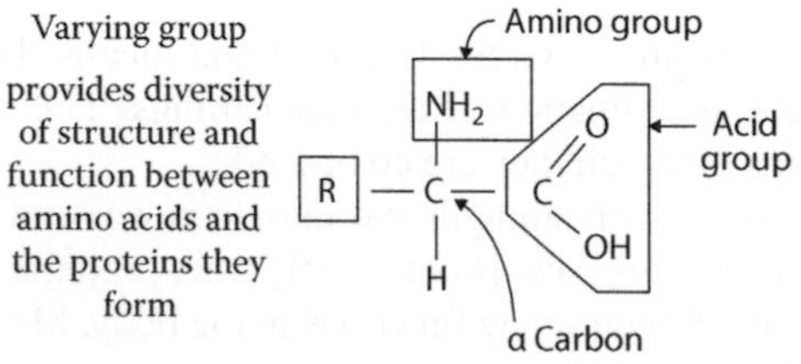

The simplest amino acid is glycine, in which the side chain R is a H atom. Thus, the formula for glycine is

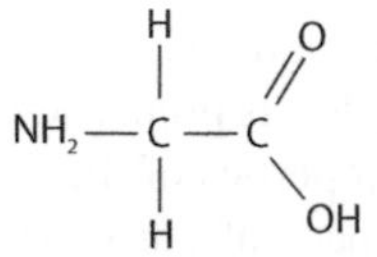

or CH_2NH_2COOH

The nature of the side chain will determine some of the properties of the amino acid, and of proteins that contain a high proportion of these acids. Side chains may be aliphatic (open-chain structure) or aromatic (i.e. unsaturated ring structure) or acidic or basic (Table 3.1).

Except for the case of glycine, in which the α carbon has two H atoms attached, all other amino acids have four different groups attached to the α carbon. This implies that the molecule so formed can exist as two optically active isomers that are the mirror image of one another: D and L forms. This also occurs in monosaccharides, as discussed later on in this chapter. The majority of amino acids in nature exist in the L form; however, some D amino acids do exist in foods, and a few can

TABLE 3.1
Amino Acids Classified According to the Nature of Their Side Chains

Aromatic Amino Acids	Aliphatic Amino Acids		Acidic Amino Acids and Their Amides	Basic Amino Acids
Phenylalanine	Glycine		Aspartic acid	Lysine
Tyrosine	Alanine		Asparagine	Arginine
Tryptophan	Valine Leucine Isoleucine	Branched-chain amino acids	Glutamic acid Glutamine	Histidine
	Serine Threonine	OH in side chain		
	Cysteine Cystine Methionine	S groups in side chain		
	Proline			

be metabolized by the body. Generally, metabolic reactions in the body distinguish between L and D forms of amino acids and D forms are used less well. Some transamination of D-methionine and D-phenylalanine can take place to their respective L forms.

When amino acids combine to form proteins, they do so through the $-NH_2$ group of one amino acid reacting with the $-COOH$ group of the adjacent amino acid, splitting off $H \cdot OH$ (water) in the process. The link is known as a peptide link, and the proteins formed are known as polypeptides or peptide chains. The polypeptide backbone does not differ between different protein chains; it is the side chains (R–) that provide the diversity.

A chain of amino acids may be written as

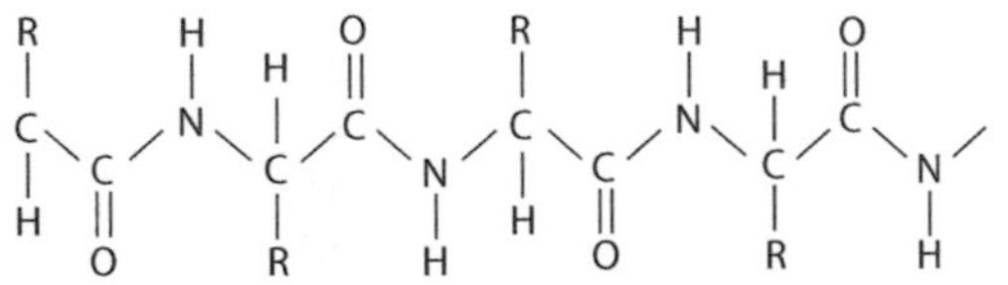

When the whole chain is put together in three-dimensional space, the R– side chains are packaged in a structure depending on affinity between all amino acids: some are attracted to each other and some are repelled. Side chains consisting of only carbon and hydrogen tend to come together, for they exclude water. Side chains with oxygen or $-NH_2$ groups will be more hydrophilic and will tend to occupy adjacent places. Thus, the nature and location of the side chains within a polypeptide chain will determine its arrangement. It will fold or coil in an attempt to bring together compatible side chains. In addition, other weaker bonds (e.g. hydrogen bonds) also form to provide further levels of organization of the protein structure. These will determine the strength and rigidity of the protein as well as dictating its final shape. Proteins with different roles in the body will have different shapes, most appropriate to their function. Their shape may, for example, be thread-like, helical or globular.

In addition, the shape of the protein may be altered by changes in its environment, such as heat or pH change, which affect its stability. Once the change in shape has passed a certain point, the protein is said to be denatured. This means that specific properties of the protein, such as antibody or enzyme activity, are lost. However, the nutritional value remains unchanged, as the amino acids themselves are still present and unchanged.

Cooking processes cause denaturation of protein – the change from raw to cooked forms is something with which we are familiar. For example, there is a noticeable difference between a raw and cooked egg or the curdling of milk in the presence of acid or bacteria in the production of many dairy products. These changes occur because of the loosening of the weaker bonds holding the protein in shape so that its natural shape is lost, and some of the molecules rearrange themselves in new positions. Usually, cooking or food preparation processes do not affect the basic peptide bonds.

Proteins in Food

The overall proportions of amino acids in plant foods are different from those needed by humans; those in foods of animal origin are more similar. The main sources of protein in the Western diet are meat, milk, bread and cereals. However, protein can also be provided by other animal products, such as eggs, dairy products (cheese and milk-based desserts) and fish. Plant foods that are useful sources of protein include all cereals and their products (including pasta and breakfast cereals), legumes, nuts and seeds. In vegetarian diets, the plant foods are the only sources of protein; clearly, they can provide an adequate supply of protein. Roots and tubers do not have high protein content but, if they constitute a substantial proportion of the diet, this protein can make an important contribution.

Table 3.2 highlights the amounts of protein contained in a range of foods. As most protein sources do not contain all of the amino acids required by humans, it is important that a range of protein sources is consumed to allow compensation between sources. This is discussed in the next section on 'Protein Quality'.

TABLE 3.2
Sources of Protein

Food	Protein (g/100 g)	Protein (g/Average Serving)	Energy from Protein (%)
Wholemeal bread	9.4	3.4	17.3
White bread	7.9	2.8	14.4
Cornflakes	7.9	2.4	8.4
Boiled rice	2.6	4.7	7.5
Semi-skimmed milk	3.4	6.8	29.5
Yogurt, low fat	4.2	5.3	21.5
Cheddar cheese	25.4	10.2	24.4
Egg	12.5	6.3	34.0
Beefburger	28.5	25.7	34.7
Beef, stewed	15.1	39.3	44.4
Roast chicken	27.3	27.3	61.7
Pork chop	31.6	44.2	49.2
Cod in batter	16.1	29.0	26.1
Peanuts, salted, roast	24.5	6.1	16.2
Peanut butter	22.6	4.5	14.9
Baked beans	5.2	7.0	24.8
Peas	6.0	4.2	35
Potatoes, boiled	1.8	3.2	10
Cheese and tomato pizza	14.4	33.1	20.8

Sources: Data calculated from Food Standards Agency, *Food Portion Sizes*, 3rd edn., The Stationery Office, London, UK, 2002a; Food Standards Agency, *McCance and Widdowson's The Composition of Foods*, 6th summary edn., Royal Society of Chemistry, Cambridge, UK, 2002b.

TABLE 3.3
Use of Complementary Foods to Make Up for Limiting Amino Acids in Some Plant Foods

Plant Food	Limiting Amino Acid	Useful Complementary Food	Example of Meal
Grains (or cereals)	Lysine, threonine	Legumes/pulses	Beans on toast
Nuts and seeds	Lysine	Legumes/pulses	Hummus (chickpeas with sesame seeds)
Soya beans and other legumes/pulses	Methionine	Grains; nuts and seeds	Lentil curry and rice
Maize	Tryptophan, lysine	Legumes	Tortillas and beans
Vegetables	Methionine	Grains; nuts and seeds	Vegetable and nut roast

Protein Quality

A protein is most useful to the body if it supplies all of the indispensable amino acids in appropriate amounts. If this is not the case, any protein synthesis that is required can only take place by breaking down existing proteins. Alternatively, limited synthesis may take place until all of the amino acid present in least amounts has been used up. The body cannot synthesize incomplete proteins; therefore, synthesis is limited by this amino acid. Such an amino acid is termed 'limiting', and the protein from which it comes would be described as having low quality. How can this be quantified?

Milk or egg proteins have traditionally been used as the 'reference proteins', as their amino acid pattern most nearly conforms to that of total body protein. Most recently, the amino acid pattern of human milk has been set as the standard against which all other proteins can be judged for their efficiency of meeting human needs.

Different sources of protein have been shown to match the required amino acid pattern to varying extents, and combining different plant foods, for example, makes it possible to obtain the necessary amino acids from several sources and achieve an overall balance (Table 3.3). Populations have naturally been doing this for generations; there is nothing new about it and many traditional dishes reflect this.

In addition, it is possible to complement protein foods of plant origin with foods derived from animals to compensate for the limiting amino acid. In particular, milk and its products provide good complementary protein to partner the plant foods. Examples of such traditional mixtures include bread and cheese, macaroni cheese, rice pudding, cereal and milk.

Measuring Protein Quality

Chemical Score

This compares the amount of each indispensable amino acid in the test protein with the amount of this amino acid in the reference protein; the chemical score is the value of this ratio for the limiting amino acid.

$$\text{Chemical score} = \frac{\text{Amount of amino acid in test protein (mg/g)}}{\text{Amount of amino acid in reference protein (mg/g)}} \times 100$$

The reference scoring pattern for the most frequently limiting amino acids was developed by the FAO/WHO/UNU (1985):

Amino Acid	Reference Score (mg/g Protein)
Leucine	19
Lycine	16
Threonine	9
Valine	13
Methionine + cystine	17

The calculation does not take into account the digestibility of the protein and is, therefore, a very theoretical value. Digestibility is particularly an issue for many plant-based diets and some cereals, for example, millet and sorghum, and needs to be considered especially for children in developing countries. A variation to this calculation, the protein digestibility-corrected amino acid score (PDCAAS) takes in consideration a correction factor for the faecal digestibility (tested in rats) of the test protein.

$$\text{PDCAAS}(\%) = \frac{\text{mg of limiting amino acid in 1 g of test protein}}{\text{mg of same amino acid in 1 g of reference protein}} \times \text{faecal true digestibility}(\%) \times 100$$

Biological Value

The biological value (*BV*) of a protein is a measure of how effectively a protein can meet the body's biological need. To make this measurement, the test protein is fed to an experimental animal as the sole source of protein, and the nitrogen retention and loss are measured. The greater the nitrogen retention, the more of the protein has been used (remember that, if a protein cannot be used because it contains limiting amino acids, it cannot be stored and, therefore, is broken down and the nitrogen excreted as urea).

$$BV = \frac{\text{Nitrogen retained} \times 100}{\text{Nitrogen absorbed}}$$

or more precisely

$$BV = \frac{\text{Dietary nitrogen} - (\text{urinary nitrogen} + \text{faecal nitrogen}) \times 100}{\text{Dietary nitrogen} - \text{faecal nitrogen}}$$

For egg protein, *BV* is 100, and for fish and beef, the value is 75. It is generally agreed that a *BV* of 70 or more can support growth, as long as energy intake is adequate.

For both *BV* and chemical score, the result for a single food is of relatively little relevance because most people consume a mixture of foods in their daily diet.

Millward (1999) showed that, even with revised amino acid scoring methods, the problem of inadequate protein or severely limiting amino acids is not as widespread as commonly assumed.

Protein Requirements

Requirements for protein are calculated on the basis of nitrogen balance studies, which estimate the amount of high-quality milk or egg protein needed to achieve equilibrium. The safe level of protein intake was established by FAO/WHO/UNU (1985) as 0.75 g/kg body weight per day. In addition to nitrogen balance results, increments were included for growth in infants and children, calculated from estimates of nitrogen accretion. In pregnancy, protein retention in the products of conception

TABLE 3.4
Dietary Reference Values for Protein for Adults

Gender/Age	Estimated Average Requirement (g/Day)	Reference Nutrient Intake (g/Day)
Males		
19–50 years	44.4	55.5
50+ years	42.6	53.3
Females		
19–50 years	36.0	45.0
50+ years	37.2	46.5

Source: Reproduced from DoH (UK Department of Health), Dietary reference values for food energy and nutrients in the United Kingdom, Report on Health and Social Subjects No. 41, Report of the Panel on Dietary Reference Values of the Committee on Medical Aspects of Food Policy, HMSO, London, UK, 1991. With permission.

and maternal tissues was calculated, and, for lactation, the protein content of breast milk in healthy mothers was used to obtain the reference value.

Uncertainty is expressed about the accuracy of these balance studies because they give results that are considerably higher than minimum nitrogen losses in adults on protein-free diets. Also the duration of the studies may not be sufficient for adaptation to occur. Finally, it is unclear how the amount of energy given to the subjects affects the results.

Figures recommended in the United Kingdom (DoH, 1991) for adults are calculated on the basis of 0.75 g protein/kg body weight per day [reference nutrient intake (RNI)]. Values obtained using reference body weights for adults are shown in Table 3.4. Current intakes in the United Kingdom are considerably higher than the values recommended here. The Family Food module of the Living Costs and Food Survey (DEFRA, 2011) shows that the mean daily total protein intake was 78.6 g, of which 69.1 g was consumed in the household and 9.5 g consumed outside the home (eating out). Approximately 42 g of the protein consumed in household was of animal origin. The mean household protein intake represents 150% of the mean RNI for protein (170% when the figure for protein intake from foods consumed outside the home, compared to 175% in 2007). Similar figures are reported in the National Diet and Nutrition Survey (DoH/FSA 2008/2012) with a daily protein intake of 88.1 g for men and 65.4 g for women (adults aged 19–64).

Major food groups providing protein were shown (in percent of total protein intake):

Meat and meat products	40% (♂)	35% (♀)
Cereals and cereal products	22% (♂)	23% (♀)
Milk products and cheese	13% (♂)	15% (♀)

It is assumed that, in the United Kingdom, there is a sufficient variety of different protein sources to eliminate concerns about protein quality. However, for those individuals whose diet contains a considerable amount of unrefined cereal and vegetable, a correction for digestibility of 85% is to be applied.

Report 41 (DoH, 1991) suggests that it is prudent to avoid protein intakes that are in excess of an 'upper safe limit' of 1.5 g/kg per day, suggesting that such high intakes may contribute to bone demineralization and a decline in kidney function with age. It has been found that there is a linear relationship between increases in animal protein intake and calcium loss in the urine, although the relationship with bone demineralization is still unclear. More recent evidence has largely failed to support concerns about effects of high protein intakes on kidney function, unless there is preexisting renal disease. A number of cross-sectional studies in the United States and Britain have shown an inverse relationship between protein intakes and blood pressure and stroke. However, the possible mechanisms involved are yet to be discovered, and interventional studies have been unable to replicate these effects.

Finally, it should be noted that those individuals with high energy needs, such as athletes, consuming a typical Western diet are likely to ingest protein in excess of this 'upper safe limit', unless they make adjustments to the balance of macronutrients in their diet. This should preferably be achieved through consuming more carbohydrate, rather than more fat, but may be impractical in terms of the volume of food required.

Many questions remain to be resolved and new issues are continually being raised in this field. Some of these are briefly discussed in the following:

- New research on individual amino acids suggests that requirement figures for indispensable amino acids may need to be increased, and therefore, the safe level of protein intake may need to be revised upwards. Given the prevalence of undernutrition in the world, such a revision would have enormous implications in terms of global food policies.
- The distinction between essential and non-essential amino acids may become less clear-cut, as studies have shown that there is some potential for amino acid synthesis from urea residues, by the colonic bacteria. Factors that might influence this synthesis and availability to the host may need to be considered in the future.
- It is already clear that needs for specific amino acids vary between individuals and at different times of life and conditions. The ability to cope with these life situations may also depend on optimal amino acid availability and the presence of other nutrients.

CARBOHYDRATES

WHAT ARE CARBOHYDRATES?

Carbohydrates are a group of substances found in both plants and animals, composed of carbon, hydrogen and oxygen in the ratio of 1:2:1 (C—H_2O carbohydrate). The name 'carbohydrate' was first used in 1844 by Schmidt, but the sweet nature of sugar had already been recognized for many centuries. It is said that sugar was extracted as early as 3000 BC in India; Columbus is credited with introducing sugar cane into the New World in the fifteenth century, and in the sixteenth century, Elizabeth I is reported to have developed rotten teeth owing to excessive consumption of sugar.

Carbohydrates are the main structural and energy storage components of most plants, and carbohydrate-rich foods are the cheapest sources of energy in the world (1 g provides 16 kJ/3.75 kcal). Carbohydrates provide most of the energy in human diets – commonly a half of all calories and a major total economic factor for both small farmers and food companies.

The simple forms of carbohydrates are the sugars, which are generally present as 6-carbon single units called monosaccharides ($C_6H_{12}O_6$) or as double units called disaccharides. Chains of simple sugars with 3–10 monosaccharide units are termed oligosaccharides. Longer and more complex chains are polysaccharides. Foods may also contain sugar alcohols, which are hydrogenated sugars, for example, sorbitol.

Most of the carbohydrates in the diet come from plants, synthesized from carbon dioxide and water, with energy provided by sunlight, by the process of photosynthesis. The disaccharide sucrose accumulates as the major product of photosynthesis in the chloroplast. Germinating seeds can also convert fat and amino acids into sugar. All plant cells are also able to convert glucose and fructose into sucrose. Animals cannot synthesize sugars from any non-carbohydrate source except from the 3-carbon glycerol (e.g. in triglyceride).

Monosaccharides

Monosaccharides are the simple sugars. Each molecule usually consists of four, five or, most often, six carbon atoms, generally in a ring form. In the hexoses (six-carbon monosaccharides, most common in the diet), the "ring" contains one oxygen atom and all but one of the carbon atoms- the remaining carbon, hydrogen and oxygen atoms are located 'above' or 'below' the ring (Figure 3.1). Monosaccharides are classified as aldose (such as glucose) or ketose (such as fructose), bearing either, respectively, an aldehyde group or a ketone. It is important to note that glucose can exist in two isomeric forms: D-glucose and L-glucose (known as stereoisomers). However, only D-glucose ('dextrose') is used in the body. Fructose and galactose are the other nutritionally important 6-carbon monosaccharides or hexoses ('hex' meaning six, '-ose' being the standard ending used for carbohydrates). They can also exist as stereoisomers. Fructose and galactose have the same empirical formula as glucose but differ in the way the atoms are arranged in the ring. Other arrangements are possible and are found in various plant and bacterial carbohydrates.

Monosaccharides, disaccharides and sugars in general can be either reducing or non-reducing depending on the presence of an aldehyde group in the open-chain form. Reducing sugars are not limited to aldose, as ketose can produce aldehyde in solution via tautomeric reactions. Reducing monosaccharides include glucose, galactose, lactose and maltose. In this case, the anomeric carbon bears an aldehyde group in the open-chain configuration. However, sucrose is a non-reducing sugar: the anomeric carbon, bearing the functional group (aldehyde), is located in between the two monosaccharide units and cannot be exposed in the open-chain configuration-it is not "free". Practically, reducing sugars can reduce chemical entities (taking part in redox reactions), and this can be tested with the Benedict's reagent.

Glucose is the main carbohydrate in the body, although it only constitutes a small part of dietary carbohydrate intake. It is a fundamental component of human metabolism, being an 'obligate fuel' (i.e. essential under normal circumstances) for a number of organs, most notably the brain. Consequently, the levels of glucose in the blood are controlled within narrow limits by a number of hormones. It is naturally present in small amounts in honey, fruits, fruit juices and vegetables (as an intrinsic sugar). It is also present in larger amounts in soft drinks, confectionary, cakes, biscuits and ice cream as an industrial product extracted from starch as corn syrup and by the hydrolysis of sucrose (from beets or cane) into its constituent glucose and fructose (a process known as 'invertion') – glucose/fructose added in confectionary products contributes to the non-milk extrinsic sugars (NMES) in the diet. The latest Scientific Advisory Committee on Nutrition (SACN) report (2015) proposed that the term 'free sugars' replaces the term 'non-milk extrinsic sugars', since NMES is a term predominantly used in the United Kingdom, encompassing added sugars as well as sugars in unsweetened juices and honey, and half of the sugar found in dried/stewed/canned fruits. *Free sugars* include added sugars, sugars present in unsweetened juices and honey (but not half the sugar in dried/stewed/canned fruits).

Fructose (also called laevulose) is not present in large amounts in the human diet. Naturally occurring sources include honey, fruit and some vegetables. However, in recent years, high fructose corn syrup has increasingly been used as a sweetening agent in beverages and processed foods,

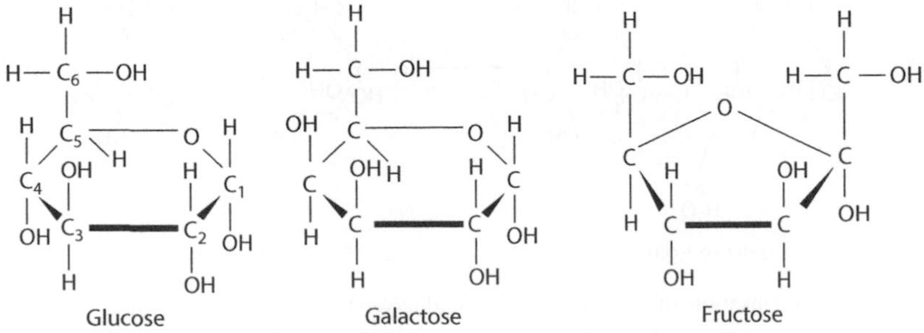

FIGURE 3.1 Structural formulae for three simple sugars.

especially in the United States. This is derived from the hydrolysis of starch obtained from corn, initially to glucose and then by subsequent conversion to fructose. The syrup thus produced is inexpensive and often replaces sucrose in products such as soft drinks, canned fruit, jams, jellies, preserves and some dairy products. The major advantages of this syrup are that it does not form crystals at acid pH, and it has better freezing properties than sucrose. These changes are making fructose one of the major simple sugars in the Western diet.

After absorption, fructose (derived directly from the diet or from sucrose hydrolysis) is transported to the liver, where it is metabolized rapidly. The products can include glucose, glycogen, lactic acid or fat, depending on the metabolic state of the individual. Following exercise, fructose increases glycogen stores rapidly. In the fed (or overfed) state, it increases fat (triglyceride) store.

Galactose is not usually found free in nature, being part of the lactose disaccharide in milk. However, fermented milk products may contain some galactose that has been released. Once absorbed into the body, galactose may be incorporated into nerve tissue in growing infants, or, if not required, is transformed either into glucose or glycogen for storage. In lactating (breastfeeding) women, galactose is synthesized from glucose and included as lactose in the milk secreted by the mammary glands.

Carbohydrate digestion and absorption are covered in Chapter 10, pp. 197–199, and their metabolism in Chapter 11, pp. 228–231.

Other monosaccharides occasionally found in foods include xylose and arabinose in white wine and beer, mannose in fruit and fucose (a methyl pentose sugar) in human milk and bran.

Sugar alcohols may also be present in food. The three most commonly found are sorbitol, mannitol and xylitol. They are absorbed and metabolized to glucose more slowly than the simple sugars. This confers the advantage of a slower rise in blood glucose levels, which is why 'diabetic' foods are sometimes sweetened with sorbitol. Although the rate of absorption is slower, the amount of energy that they ultimately provide is the same as from the simple sugar, so they are of no benefit where energy reduction is required. However, the sugar alcohols are useful in reducing dental caries, since they are not fermented by the bacteria in the mouth and, therefore, do not contribute to acid production. For example, xylitol has been shown in a number of studies to have a cariostatic (caries-preventing) effect when included in chewing gum. The slow rate of absorption of the sugar alcohol can, however, result in diarrhoea if large amounts are consumed in a short time.

Disaccharides

Disaccharides are formed when monosaccharides combine in pairs. Those of importance in nutrition are sucrose, lactose and maltose. In each case, a molecule of water is lost when the two constituent monosaccharides combine, in a condensation reaction. This is illustrated in Figure 3.2, showing the formation of maltose.

Sucrose (*sometimes called invert sugar*) is the most widespread and best-known disaccharide in the human diet. It is the main transport sugar of plants and the main sugar in honey, formed by the condensation of

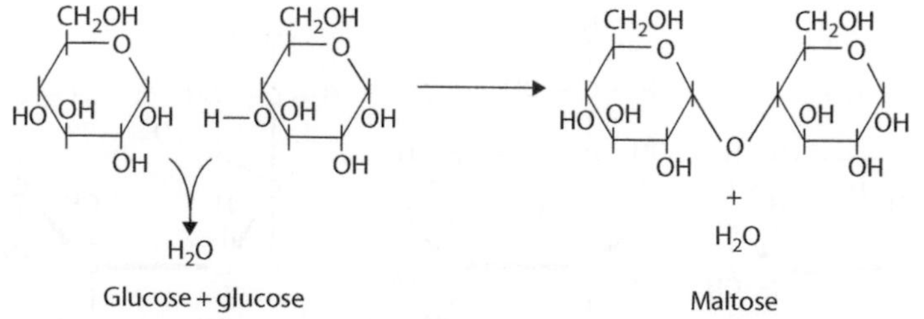

FIGURE 3.2 The condensation of two molecules of glucose to form maltose. First, an OH group from one glucose and a H atom from another glucose combine to create a molecule of H_2O. Then, the two glucose molecules bond together with a single O atom to form the disaccharide maltose.

glucose with fructose. It is obtained commercially from sugar beet or sugar cane, both of which contain sucrose as 10%–15% by weight of the plant. The juice extracted from these plants is purified and concentrated, and the sucrose is crystallized out and removed. The by-products of this process include molasses, golden syrup and brown sugar. Sucrose is also contained in honey and maple syrup. Naturally occurring sucrose is also found in small amounts in fruit, vegetables and some cereal grains.

Lactose (*milk sugar*) is present in the milk of mammals. In the West, most of the lactose is provided by cows' milk and its products. In addition, any foods that contain milk powder or whey, such as milk chocolate, muesli, instant potato, biscuits and creamed soups, will contain some lactose. It is the main energy source in mammalian and human milk. Lactose consists of glucose and galactose, which must be hydrolyzed as part of intestinal digestion with the enzyme lactose. Lactose which is not hydrolyzed is not absorbed and instead provides energy to the colonic bacteria (i.e. it functions as dietary fibre).

Maltose (*malt sugar*) is mainly found in germinating grains, as their starch store is broken down. Its major source is sprouted grain, such as barley or wheat used in the manufacture of beer. The 'malt' produced by the sprouting is then acted on by yeasts to produce the familiar fermented product. Small amounts of maltose may also be found in some biscuits and breakfast cereals and in malted drinks. Maltose consists of two glucose units.

Oligosaccharides

Compounds made up from 10 or less sugar units, linked into a single molecule, are known as oligosaccharides. They are present in a number of plant foods including leeks, garlic, onions, Jerusalem artichokes, lentils and beans. Both the galactosyl-sucroses (raffinose, stachyose and verbascose) contained in legume seeds and the fructosyl-sucroses in onions, leeks and artichokes are resistant to digestion in the upper gastrointestinal tract. Consequently, they pass largely unchanged into the colon, where they are fermented by colonic bacteria, resulting in the production of volatile short chain fatty acids and gases, which can cause flatulence. This can be uncomfortable and may discourage the consumption of these foods. Nevertheless, there are health benefits from this fermentation, and oligosaccharides have been studied and developed as possible components of prebiotics or functional foods, which provide a substrate for the gut microbiota.

Polysaccharides

Polysaccharides are complex sugars containing over 10 monosaccharide units, arranged in straight or branched and coiled chains. They may be made up of hexoses and pentoses or a mixture of these, sometimes with other constituents, such as uronic acid.

Traditionally, a distinction has been made between polysaccharides that are digestible and nutritionally 'available' (i.e. those digested in the small bowel and absorbed as sugars), such as starch, and the 'unavailable' indigestible forms, which were also termed 'dietary fibre'. However, research has shown that digestibility of starch can vary substantially, with cooking and storage, into 'retrograded starch', which is not digested but remains fermentable by bacteria in the colon. Starch forms the main energy store for plants, while other polysaccharides, grouped together as 'non-starch polysaccharide' (NSP), form the structure of plants. The NSP includes cellulose, hemicellulose, lignin and also 'soluble fibre' such as pectin, which is fermentable by bacteria, and these have been more clearly differentiated into

- Starches
- NSPs

Both of these groups of polysaccharides are of plant origin, comprising the store of energy in the plant and its structural framework, respectively. A comparable carbohydrate store in animals is in the form of glycogen, but its content in the diet is negligible.

Starch

Starch consists of linked glucose units arranged in either straight or branched chains. Amylose is the straight-chain form of starch. It contains several hundred glucose molecules linked by alpha-glycosidic bonds between carbons 1 and 4 of adjacent glucose molecules. The linkage is formed by a condensation reaction, with the loss of a molecule of water. The branched-chain component of starch, amylopectin, contains some alpha bonds between carbons 1 and 4, with additional bonds linking carbons 1 and 6, at intervals, to produce side branches. In this way, amylopectin may contain thousands of glucose units in one polysaccharide unit (see Figure 3.3). Most of the common starchy foods such as potatoes, cereals and beans contain approximately 75% amylopectin and 25% amylose. The presence of a large amount of amylopectin allows the starch to form a stable gel with good water retention. Along with naturally occurring starches in foods, such as cereals, roots, tubers and pulses, food processing may add two further sources of starch into the diet. These are extruded starch products, such as savoury snacks and breakfast cereals, and modified starches, which are added to foods as emulsifiers and stabilizers. Their structures and metabolism are different from native starch in foods.

Processed Starches In general, the processing of starchy foods is carried out to make a more attractive product for human consumption. For example, the grinding of wheat grains to make flour makes it possible to produce bread, cakes, biscuits, etc. Such rigorous processing disrupts the starch granules, releasing amylose and making it readily available to digestive enzymes, and thus increases digestibility without the need for prolonged cooking prior to consumption.

Retrograded starch: If moist starchy foods are heated and then cooled, the sols formed by amylose and amylopectin during the heating stage will become gels on cooling, which retrograde on further cooling into insoluble precipitates. Amylose gels retrograde more readily than amylopectin gels, so their relative proportions are an important determinant of the physical properties of the cooked food. Some retrograded starch can still be digested, albeit more slowly. Retrograded amylose particles are especially resistant to digestion and form an important part of the starch that escapes digestion in the small intestine, so they pass into the colon where it is fermented by bacteria.

Resistant starch: The components of dietary starch that are resistant to the normal enzymatic digestion process in the small intestine originate in three possible ways:

- The physical structure of the food may prevent access to digestive enzymes if the starch is surrounded by fat or is in large lumps owing to inadequate chewing. Once these barriers are removed during digestion, the starch can be broken down.
- The nature of the cell walls around the starch granules may impede digestion. Walls in cereals may be partly broken down by milling and grinding, in potatoes by mashing, but the cell walls in legumes are thicker and constitute a more resistant barrier. When starchy foods are eaten with little disruption of cell walls, digestion will be slowed.
- Where the starch has become retrograded by heating and cooling, the enzymes are no longer able to break the bonds. This starch will travel undigested into the colon, where, together with the NSPs in dietary fibre, it plays a positive, beneficial role in health.

'Dietary Fibre' and Non-Starch Polysaccharides

Dating back particularly from the 1970s, a group of well-meaning and influential doctors proposed that refined foods and a lack of 'dietary fibre' were responsible for a wide range of diseases prevalent in Western societies, including bowel diseases, such as appendicitis and diverticular disease, diabetes, heart disease and even varicose veins. When properly investigated, it turned out that these were mostly associations, without any causal relationship, and they were based on erroneous suppositions about the dietary fibre content of traditional diets. When proper measurements were made, it was clear that dietary fibre or NSP contents of traditional diets were not very different from those in Western societies. Weak relationships exist between soluble fibre and lower rates of diabetes, and cereal fibre does generally help prevent constipation, but myths about supposed hazards from highly refined foods, and supposed benefits of dietary fibre, persist.

Unfortunately, the term 'dietary fibre' is misleadingly simple. The original definition included all material undigested by the endogenous secretions of the human digestive tract. This collective

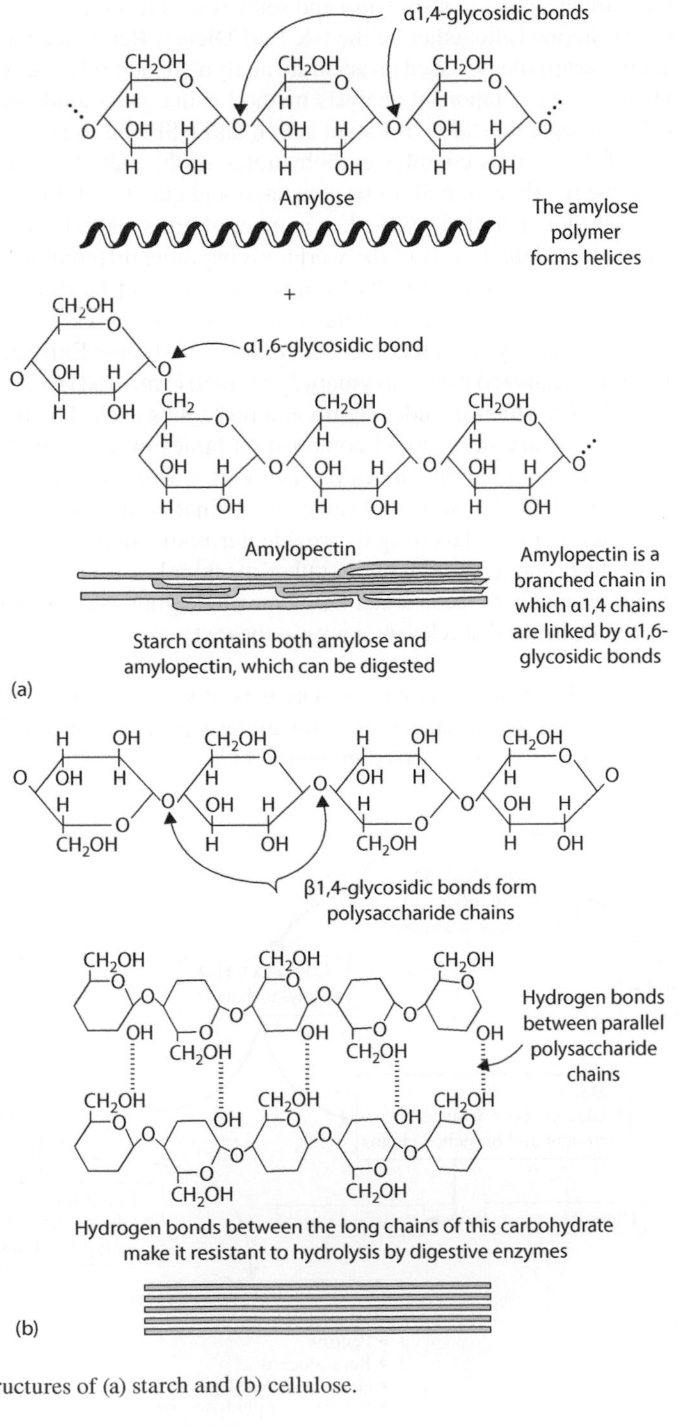

FIGURE 3.3 Structures of (a) starch and (b) cellulose.

term covered a number of very diverse compounds, in plants, but with different physiological and physical properties. A further problem arises with the analysis and quantification of 'dietary fibre' in foods, to allow proper scientific study. One of the initial methods of analysis (Southgate method) included unavailable carbohydrate but also lignin and some resistant starch.

The term 'fibre' was dropped altogether for the UK 1991 Dietary Reference Values (DoH, 1991), and much more precise terminology, based on accurate analytical methods, was used. The Englyst method determines NSP by a component analysis method using gas–liquid chromatography. In this way, it is possible to separate starch, resistant starch and NSP and to define the physical and chemical properties of the various complex carbohydrates in the diet. The method also allows the soluble and insoluble fractions of NSP to be separated and quantified. From this, the specific biological effects will be more readily identified. A number of other methods for the measurement of fibre have been used in different parts of the world, giving quite different results in any single commodity and increasing confusion. Results from studies may not be directly comparable, if different analytical methods have been used to quantify the dietary fibre.

This terminology is not widely accepted; the United States and some European countries continue to use 'dietary fibre', analyzed by an enzymatic/gravimetric method (Association of Official Analytical Chemists, 2000), which includes lignin and resistant starch. The results obtained by AOAC are termed 'total dietary fibre'. Food composition tables in the United Kingdom (Food Standards Agency, 2002b) provide NSP values for all foods where these are available. There is additional information available about AOAC values for a smaller number of foods. It is recommended that these are used in food labelling to provide harmonization across Europe.

Although the term 'high-fibre diet' is actually rather meaningless scientifically, it represents a concept recognized by the public to mean a diet based on whole grain cereals, legumes and pulses and as such will, therefore, be used at relevant points in the text.

Constituents of NSP NSPs include a number of polymers of simple sugars, together with uronic acid. They are broadly divided into cellulose and non-cellulosic polysaccharides. Their relationship to total carbohydrate in the diet is summarized in Figure 3.4.

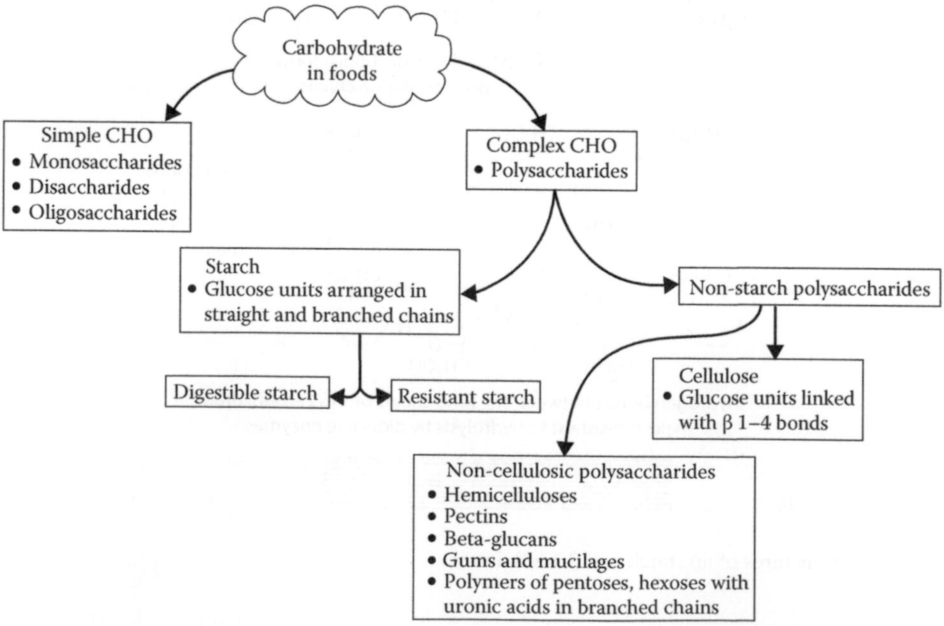

FIGURE 3.4 The relationship of non-starch polysaccharides to other sources of carbohydrate.

TABLE 3.5
Non-Starch Polysaccharide Content of Some Common Foods, Showing Soluble and Insoluble Fractions

Food	Total NSP (g/100 g)	Soluble NSP (g/100 g)	Insoluble NSP (g/100 g)
White bread	1.5	0.9	0.6
Wholemeal bread	5.8	1.6	4.2
Weetabix	9.7	3.1	6.6
Oatcakes	5.9	3.5	2.4
Rice, white	0.2	Trace	0.2
Apples	1.6	0.6	1.0
Bananas	1.1	0.7	0.4
Peanuts	6.2	1.9	4.3
Baked beans	3.5	2.1	1.4
Lentils	1.9	0.6	1.3
Potatoes	1.2	0.7	0.5
Carrots	2.5	1.4	1.1

Source: Adapted from Englyst, H.N. et al., *J. Hum. Nutr. Diet.*, 1, 247, 1988. Reproduced with kind permission of Blackwell Science Ltd.

Cellulose is the principal component of cell walls in plants. It is made up of glucose units, linked by beta 1–4 linkages, which are resistant to digestion and to fermentation by colonic bacteria. It has a very stable crystalline structure, which gives it low reactivity (see Figure 3.3). Cellulose is, however, fermented in the rumen of farm animals.

The non-cellulosic NSPs comprise hemicelluloses, pectins, beta-glucans, gums and mucilages. The sugars they contain include arabinose, xylose, mannose, fucose, glucose, galactose and rhamnose. Those NSPs that contain predominantly cellulose tend to be insoluble; an increasing content of uronic acids increases solubility. Wheat bran and, therefore, whole grain wheat products contain a high proportion of insoluble NSP and only traces of uronic acids. Cereals such as oats and barley, however, are particularly good sources of beta-glucans, which are water-soluble polymers of glucose. Fruit and vegetables, in general, have more uronic acids and pectin in their NSPs and thus a higher proportion of soluble fibre than cereals.

Gums and mucilages are generally found in the human diet as a result of manufacturing processes. Gums are extracted, for example, from the acacia tree or the Indian cluster bean, and are used as thickeners, stabilizers and emulsifiers by the food industry. Mucilages from algae and seaweeds are also used by the food industry as stabilizers and thickeners.

The soluble and insoluble NSP contents of some common foods are shown in Table 3.5. It should be noted, however, that the separation into soluble and insoluble fractions is not chemically very distinct and depends on the method of extraction used.

How Much Carbohydrate Should We Have?

The intake of dietary carbohydrate must not only be sufficient to provide the necessary energy for the survival of the body but must also contain sufficient specific sugars to allow the synthesis of essential complex molecules. However, this is difficult to quantify; it is much easier to calculate the amount of protein needed by the body to maintain nitrogen balance, and the amounts of fat to supply the essential fatty acids.

The only true requirement for carbohydrates that current knowledge has identified is for the prevention of ketosis. Estimates of the minimum amount of carbohydrate needed by an adult are in the range of 150–180 g carbohydrate per day which is around 30% of our daily energy needs. However, this does not necessarily need to be supplied entirely from the diet: up to 130 g could be synthesized by gluconeogenesis, with the remaining 50 g provided exogenously from food. Below this, ketosis will develop with a range of possible hazards.

Studies on pregnant rats indicate that a minimum amount of carbohydrate, up to 12% of glucose, is needed to sustain pregnancy and lactation and avoid high mortality rates in the offspring. This points to other specific requirements for synthesis of carbohydrate-containing complexes.

In the United Kingdom, the recommendations made about carbohydrates use an 'optimal' intake approach, which includes an amount sufficient to prevent ketosis, avoid starvation but not induce obesity, avoid adverse effects on the large intestine and on lipid and insulin metabolism and avoid dental caries. In addition, the intake should contribute to an enjoyable diet. The dietary reference values report suggests that

- Dietary carbohydrate should supply about 50% of energy
- Sugars not contained within cellular structures (the NMES) should constitute no more than 11% of daily energy intake. The most recent (2015) SACN report however advocates for an upper level of 5% contribution to energy intake for added sugars.
- The balance should be made up from complex carbohydrates and other sugars, such as those in fruits and milk

Dietary guidelines published in other countries, on the whole, adopt a similar approach to sugar intake with a level of approximately 10% being recommended. Some scientists believe that the low level recommended by SACN (5%) is not achievable alongside the goal to lower-fat intakes. A reciprocal relationship exists between intakes of fat and refined sugars and that lowering the sugar intake is likely to cause an increase, rather than the desired reduction, in the intake of fats. This highlights one of the dilemmas associated with looking at individual nutrient components of the diet to compile 'whole diet' guidelines.

The National Food Surveys and Family Food/Living Costs and Food Surveys (DEFRA, 2001, 2011) showed the reciprocal trend in carbohydrate and fat reported in the foods being purchased in the United Kingdom over the past 60 years, with a decreasing percentage of the energy from carbohydrate being accompanied by an increased percentage from fat. The estimated total intake of carbohydrates was 253 g from household food (a further 26 g of carbohydrate was consumed from foods eaten outside the household) – overall 279 g. Specifically, household foods contained 153 g of starch and 125 g of total sugars (including 82 g of NMES).

In the National Diet and Nutrition Survey (DoH/FSA Rolling programme 2008/2010), major food groups providing carbohydrates were shown (in percent of total protein intake):

Cereals and cereal products	44% (♂)	43% (♀)
Vegetables and fruit	19% (♂)	21% (♀)
Beverages (including alcoholic)	12% (♂)	9% (♀)

The most recent survey (Family Food/Living Costs and Food Survey, 2010; DEFRA, 2011) showed that carbohydrates provided, overall, 47.2% of total energy, including 13.9% of total energy actually provided by NMES. There are, however, substantial differences between the age groups. For instance, breastfed and bottle-fed infants may obtain 40% of their total energy from milk sugars. Contribution of milk and milk products towards daily carbohydrate intake was 16% for children aged 1.5–3 years, decreasing progressively for all other age groups (5%–9%) (NDNS, 2008/2010).

Meanwhile, the average British diet contained 15.3 g of NSP (reported as 'fibre') per day. In keeping with all such surveys, this represents an underestimate of about 20% below true intakes, so 17 g/day might be about 'correct'. Vegetarians and vegans tend to have greater intakes of NSP. Mean values of NSP intake for the United States are 15 g/day, with a higher intake recorded in men. Other urban populations in affluent countries are reported to have similar intakes, but slightly higher intakes have been recorded in rural populations. This probably reflects a greater energy intake, related to higher energy expenditure levels.

According to the National Diet and Nutrition Survey (DoH/FSA Rolling programme, 2008/2012), the major food groups providing NSP in the United Kingdom are as follows:

Cereals and cereal products	44% (♂)	43% (♀)
Vegetables and potatoes	32% (♂)	32% (♀)
Fruit	8% (♂)	10% (♀)

According to the latest SACN report (2015), the dietary reference value for dietary fibre intake (carbohydrates not digested or absorbed in the small intestine and which have a degree of polymerization of three or more, including lignins) should be 30 g/day for adults.

Overall, these figures show that the proportions of carbohydrates consumed in the United Kingdom do not match the dietary guidelines. From a nutritional perspective, 'extrinsic' and 'non-extrinsic' sugars are exactly the same and glucose released from starch becomes the same, so the current guidelines may to some extent be continuing a 'demonization' of sugar. A more relaxed approach to dietary sugars may be preferred if it helps to reduce saturated fat consumption. However, the adverse effects of fructose (from sucrose) in elevating serum triglycerides need to be considered.

FATS

All living cells, including plant cells, contain some fat in their structure, since fatty acids are essential components of cell walls and intracellular membranes. In addition, mammals and birds store fat throughout the body, especially between the muscles, around internal organs and under the skin. Many fish have fat stored exclusively in the liver, but in the oily fish (like herring and mackerel), it is present throughout the flesh. In the plant kingdom, fats are found in the fruits of various plants such as olives, maize, nuts and avocados. Plants manufacture fats by photosynthesis, the same process that they use to make carbohydrates. Animals use or store the fat they ingest or can synthesize fat from surplus energy taken in as carbohydrates or proteins. This does not generally apply in humans under normal circumstances. Advice on healthy eating encourages us to reduce our intake of certain types of fats and increase others. Names such as cholesterol, polyunsaturates and omega-3s are used by food manufacturers and can be very confusing for many people. To be able to understand the rationale and the details of this advice, it is necessary first to understand the nature of fats and how this is related to their behaviour in the body. Only then can we interpret the advice both for ourselves and others.

WHAT ARE FATS?

Fats are substances that are insoluble in water but soluble in organic solvents like acetone. In addition, fats are greasy/waxy in texture. When we think about fats in the diet, most people make a distinction between fats, which are solid at room temperature, and oils, which are liquid. Chemically, however, these two groups are similar; the major attributes that produce the differences in solubility are size of the molecule and types of bonds present. To the chemist and biochemist, all of these compounds are 'lipids'. In nutrition, the most important lipids are triglycerides (or triacylglycerols), which constitute more than 95% of the fat we consume. In addition, there are phospholipids, sterols and fat-soluble vitamins in the diet and body tissues. If we consider an average fat intake of 100 g/day, this would be made up as follows:

90–95 g	Triglycerides
4–8 g	Phospholipids
1 g	Glycolipids
350–450 mg	Cholesterol

Like carbohydrates, lipid molecules contain carbon, oxygen and hydrogen atoms linked in a specific and unique way. The simplest lipids are the neutral fats (triacylglycerols or triglycerides).

Triglycerides

Triglycerides are made up of a backbone of glycerol to which three fatty acids are attached. Glycerol is a very simple molecule. When a fatty acid combines with glycerol, the linkage occurs between the —OH group on the glycerol and the —COOH group of the acid by esterification, with the loss of a molecule of water.

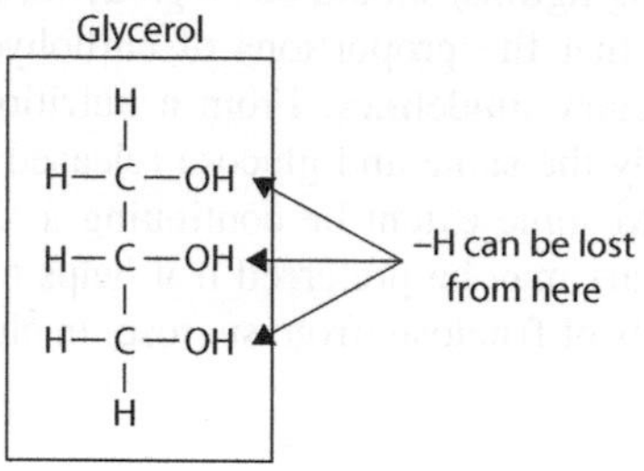

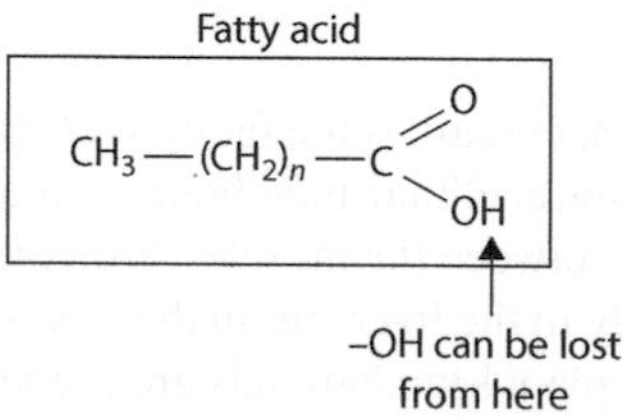

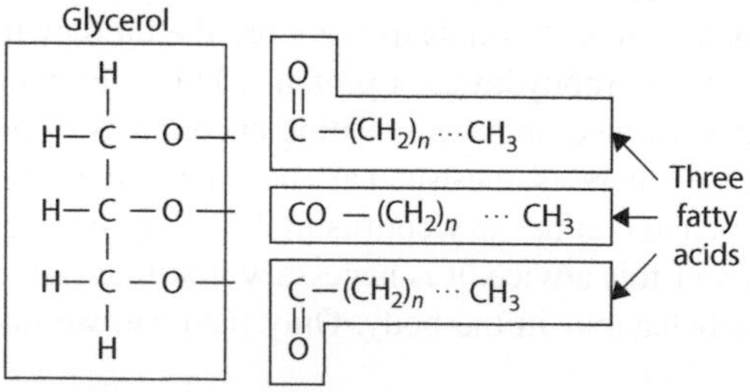

Usually, three different fatty acids are attached to the glycerol molecule, creating a wide diversity of triglycerides.

Triglycerides are readily broken down and resynthesized. A fatty acid can also be removed from the glycerol molecule by de-esterification, which occurs during the digestion of fats. Resulting products are diglycerides and monoglycerides, containing two or one fatty acid, respectively (see Chapter 11). Fatty acids can be replaced on glycerol molecules by re-esterification. These two processes create particular triglycerides to meet the specific needs of the body.

Fat digestion and absorption are covered in Chapter 11, pp. 195, and fat metabolism in Chapter 12, pp. 220–227.

Fatty acids are chains of carbon atoms with hydrogen attached in the form of methylene ($-CH_2$) groups. At one end of the chain is a methyl group ($-CH_3$), and at the other end is an acid group ($-COOH$). The simplest is the two-carbon fatty acid (acetic acid) with the formula $CH_3 \cdot COOH$. Most naturally occurring fatty acids contain even numbers of carbons in their chain, normally ranging from 4 to 24 carbons. Thus, the basic formula for a fatty acid is $CH_3 \cdot (CH_2)_n \cdot COOH$, where n is any number between 2 and 22.

Fatty acids with 6 or fewer carbons may be described as 'short-chain', those containing 8–12 carbons are 'medium-chain', and those in which the chain is 14 carbons or more are 'long-chain' fatty acids. The human diet contains mostly long-chain fatty acids, with less than 5% coming from those having fewer carbons. The most commonly occurring chain lengths are 14 and 16.

No fat consists of a single type of triglyceride. In butter, for example, the main fatty acids attached to glycerol are butyric (4:0), oleic (18:1) and stearic (18:0) acids, although there are 69 different fatty acids actually present.

It is the identity of the fatty acids present within a triglyceride that determines its physical characteristics. Thus, a triglyceride made up predominantly of short-chain fatty acids is likely to be a hard fat (like butter), whereas one consisting of long-chain fatty acids will have a lower melting point and may even boil at room temperature. In addition, the proportions of saturated and unsaturated fatty acids present will also affect its hardness.

Types of Fatty Acids

Fatty acids occurring in nature can be divided into three categories:

- Saturated fatty acids
- Monounsaturated fatty acids (MUFAs) with one double bond
- Polyunsaturated fatty acids (PUFAs) with at least two double bonds

In a saturated fatty acid, the carbon atom holds as many hydrogens as is chemically possible; it is said to be 'saturated' in terms of hydrogen. In an unsaturated fatty acid, there are one or more double bonds along the main carbon chain, known as ethylenic bonds. Each double bond replaces two hydrogen atoms. If there is just one double bond, the acid is monounsaturated; if two or more double bonds are present, the fatty acid is polyunsaturated.

Implications of Unsaturation

The location of double bonds in a PUFA is not random. Multiple double bonds are separated by a methylene group, as follows:

$$-CH{=}CH-CH_2-CH{=}CH-$$

If the location of the first double bond is identified, the remainder can be predicted from this. Unsaturated fatty acids are classified according to the position of their first double bond (counting from the carboxylic end for the Δ nomenclature or from the methyl end for the omega/*n-x* nomenclature). The omega (also known as *n-*) nomenclature, with families 3, 6 and 9, is used a lot in nutrition. The families of the common fatty acids are given in Table 3.6, together with the number of carbon atoms, and, in the case of the unsaturated fatty acids, the number of double bonds present. Fatty acids from one family cannot be converted into another family; any interconversion can only occur within the same family.

Where double bonds exist, there is a possibility of *cis* or *trans* geometric isomerism, which affects the properties of the fatty acid. Most naturally occurring forms are the *cis* isomers [or *zusammen* (Z),

TABLE 3.6

Classification of Fatty Acids by Saturation, Chain Length and Family

Type of Fatty Acid	Name	Number of Carbon Atoms [Double Bonds (Fatty Acid Family)]
Saturated	Butyric acid	4
	Caproic acid	6
	Caprylic acid	8
	Capric acid	10
	Lauric acid	12
	Myristic acid	14
	Palmitic acid	16
	Stearic acid	18
	Arachidic acid	20
Monounsaturated	Palmitoleic acid	16:1
	Oleic acid	18:1 (*n*-9)
	Eicosenoic acid	20:1 (*n*-9)
	Erucic acid	22:1 (*n*-9)
Polyunsaturated	Linoleic acid	18:2 (*n*-6)
	Alpha-linolenic acid	18:3 (*n*-3)
	Arachidonic acid	20:4 (*n*-6)
	Eicosapentaenoic acid (EPA)	20:5 (*n*-3)
	Docosahexaenoic acid (DHA)	22:6 (*n*-3)

Notes: In the shorthand system used in the table, the number of carbon atoms precedes the colon; the number of double bonds follows. The allocation to specific fatty acid families occurs on the basis of the position of the first double bond in the molecule, counting from the methyl end. Thus in the *n*-3 family, the first double bond occurs on the third carbon from the methyl end, and in the *n*-6 and *n*-9 families, these occur on the sixth and ninth carbons, respectively.

together], in which the hydrogen atoms are on the same side of the double bond. Figure 3.5 shows the structural arrangement of different fatty acids types. In *cis* configurations, the molecule is folded back, kinked or bent into a U-shape. In this arrangement, fatty acids pack together less tightly, increasing, for example, the fluidity of membranes. When the hydrogen atoms are arranged on opposite sides of the double bond in *trans* configuration [or *entgegen* (E), opposite], the molecule remains elongated and similar to a saturated fatty acid. This allows the *trans* fatty acid molecules to pack more tightly together and raises the melting point of the fat. To the consumer, this means that the fat is harder.

Trans fatty acids are produced as a result of processing and are thus found in products containing hardened fats, such as hard margarine, pastries, biscuits and meat products. In addition, *trans* fatty acids are produced during transformations by anaerobic bacteria in the rumen of sheep and cows, so that some *trans* fatty acids may be found in meat and products from these animals, such as milk and dairy products. Evidence is accumulating that *trans* fatty acids have adverse effects in the body. In the UK, major food businesses agreed, in 2012, to remove artificial trans fat from their products.

A further consequence of unsaturation, particularly in PUFAs, is that the spare electrons are highly reactive and vulnerable to oxidation. In the presence of free radicals, such as 'singlet' oxygen or reactive hydroxyl groups, the double bonds can be attacked, leading to the formation of lipid oxides or peroxides. These change the properties of the fat and may lead to malfunction and disease. Free radicals arise in the body as part of normal metabolic processes and can thus readily attack PUFAs. The resulting products

The concept of antioxidant is covered in Chapter 4, pp. 65–79., and Chapter 23, pp. 431–434.

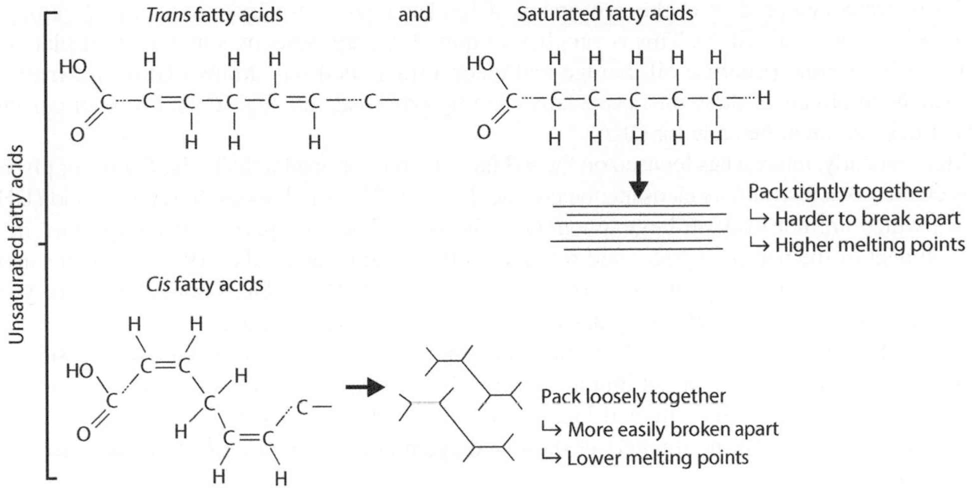

FIGURE 3.5 Spatial configuration of saturated, *cis* and *trans* unsaturated fatty acids.

are themselves highly reactive, triggering a chain reaction and producing more highly reactive products. The body has a complex defence mechanism against such reactions in the form of antioxidants, which exist both intracellularly and extracellularly and whose function is to react with the free radicals and thus inactivate them.

Essential Fatty Acids

Fatty acid manipulation in foods is covered in Chapter 23, pp. 431–441.

Although the body can synthesize most of the fat it requires, it has been known since the early part of the twentieth century that certain of the PUFAs cannot be synthesized and must be supplied in the diet. If they are excluded, a deficiency syndrome will develop, which in animals has been shown to include retarded growth and skin lesions, such as dermatitis. This deficiency can also occur in humans. Consequently, these fatty acids are known as 'essential fatty acids'. Occasionally, you will find them referred to as 'vitamin F'.

The essential fatty acids are linoleic (18:2, *n*-6) and alpha-linolenic (18:3, *n*-3) acids. Vertebrates lack enzymes to introduce double bonds at the *n*-3 and *n*-6 position and cannot, therefore, synthesize members of these fatty acid families. However, if acids containing these double bonds (i.e. the essential fatty acids) are provided in the diet, other members of the family can then be produced by a series of desaturation (adding a double bond by removing hydrogen) and elongation (adding two carbon atoms) reactions.

Diet → 18:2 (*n*-6) Linoleic acid → 18:3 (*n*-6) Gamma-linolenic acid → 20:3 (*n*-6) Dihomo-gamma-linolenic acid → 20:4 (*n*-6) Arachidonic acid

Diet → 18:3 (*n*-3) Alpha-linoleic acid → 18:4 (*n*-3) … 20:5 (*n*-3) Eicosapentaenoic acid (EPA) → 22:6 (*n*-3) Docosahexaenoic acid (DHA)

(Note: Some of the intermediate acids have been omitted from the n-3 series, for clarity.)

Moreover, there is competition between the fatty acid families for the enzymes involved, with the result that a predominance of one family (e.g. *n*-6 acids) in the diet can limit the synthesis of some of the larger members of the *n*-3 family. For this reason, both *n*-6 and *n*-3 fatty acids should be supplied in sufficient amounts in the diet.

An intermediate product in the conversion of linoleic acid to arachidonic acid (*n*-6 family) is gamma-linolenic acid (GLA). This is supplied in quite large amounts by some unusual plant oils, particularly evening primrose oil, borage and blackcurrant seed oils. Many claims are made for the beneficial effects of these oils, especially evening primrose, although there does not currently appear to be an identified role for GLA.

More recently, interest has focused on the *n*-3 fatty acids contained in fish oils. These supply very long-chain *n*-3 acids, such as eicosapentaenoic acid (EPA) (20:5) and docosahexaenoic acid (DHA) (22:6), which are not made in large amounts in the body. They are particularly important in the development of the nervous system and retina in young infants, and a dietary source is needed in very early life. The ability to convert the smaller *n*-3 acids to EPA and DHA does exist in the young infant, but probably is not sufficiently active to produce adequate amounts.

Normally, breast milk produced by mothers consuming mixed diets would supply sufficient amounts of DHA, but formula-fed infants may receive inadequate quantities, and some milks are now being formulated with additional long-chain PUFAs. Preterm babies are particularly vulnerable to receiving insufficient amounts of these and again need to obtain a fortified feed to ensure their intake.

The relative proportions of *n*-6 and *n*-3 acids in the Western diet have changed in the last 30 years for a number of reasons:

- There has been an increase in the consumption of vegetable oils, such as corn and sunflower oil as a result of healthy eating initiatives, to replace the traditional consumption of butter and other animal fats.
- The total intakes of meat from ruminant animals (beef and lamb) that are a source of *n*-3 fatty acids have fallen. Furthermore, the *n*-3 acid content of the meat has also declined as the animals are fed less on grass and more on alternative concentrates to maximize production.
- Consumption of oily fish (and total fish) has been declining over this period, resulting in lower intakes of *n*-3 acids.

Consequently, there is concern that insufficient quantities of *n*-3 acids can be synthesized in the body, as there is too much competition from the *n*-6 acids. This has potential implications for the metabolic products derived from these acids and their effects in the body. There may be consequences within membranes throughout the body, as well as effects on neurotransmitter functions in the brain and on mood.

Evidence from a number of studies across Europe indicates that the ratio of *n*-6 to *n*-3 acids is approximately 6:1. Proposals have been made in the United States and Europe that the intake of *n*-3 acids should increase, without any further increases in *n*-6 acids, to reduce this ratio. Strategies to achieve this and safety considerations need to be considered.

Further discussion on the metabolic role of *n*-3 fatty acid is found in Chapter 11, pp. 226–228, and information on enriched products is found in Chapter 23, pp. 435–437.

Conjugated Linoleic Acid

A group of isomers of linoleic acid, containing different geometrical double-bond configurations, have become of interest. The double bonds are conjugated or contiguous, rather than methylene-separated, as they are in linoleic acid. The two double bonds can be in carbon positions 8 and 10, 9 and 11, 10 and 12, or 11 and 13. Each of the double bonds can also be in the *cis* or *trans* configuration, and this results in a number of possible isomers. The most studied of these is C18:2 c9t11 isomer. This isomer has also been called rumenic acid, as it is predominantly produced in the rumen of cows and sheep. The main dietary sources of this acid are, therefore, dairy products and meat from ruminants. Conjugated linoleic acid (CLA) has been reported to have anticarcinogenic, antiatherogenic and immune-modulating potential, although the mechanisms are unclear. Body weight gain, with reduced fat mass and increased protein, has been shown in mice. CLA appears to be safe at doses up to 10 times those normally found in the diet. Research into its bioavailability and potential benefits of naturally occurring or supplemented CLA is ongoing.

Other Lipids

Phospholipids are closely related to triglycerides, as they contain a glycerol backbone and two fatty acids. However, the third fatty acid is replaced by a phosphate group and a base. The most common phospholipid lecithin (also called phosphatidylcholine) contains choline as the base. It is widely distributed in cell membranes throughout the body and is also a component of the surfactant in the lungs, which facilitates breathing by reducing surface tension in the alveoli. Other bases found in phospholipids include serine, inositol and ethanolamine.

All phospholipids serve an essential function in the body, as their structure contains both a hydrophobic (water-hating) and a hydrophilic (water-loving) area. This allows them to associate with both lipid and aqueous compounds in the body and to serve as an emulsifying agent, allowing these two dissimilar parts to coexist. Their role is particularly important in cell membranes, and high concentrations are found in the brain and nervous system. Sphingomyelin is a phospholipid occurring in the myelin sheath of nerve fibres. All the phospholipids can be synthesized in the body and are, thus, not essential in the diet.

Sterols are ringed structures containing carbon, hydrogen and oxygen. The most prevalent example of this group in animals is cholesterol (Figure 3.6), which is a waxy substance that can be synthesized by the body from acetyl coenzyme A. The main site of synthesis is the liver, although all cells of the body can make it. The human body typically contains about 100 g of cholesterol, of which 7% is found in the blood and the remainder distributed in all cells of the body. Here, cholesterol plays a number of roles:

- Maintenance of the structure and integrity of cell membranes
- Regulation of the fluidity of cell membranes
- Facilitation of the communication between the cell and its environment, including transport across the membrane
- Limiting the leakage of Na and K ions across the membrane
- Synthesis of bile acids, which are needed for fat absorption
- Synthesis of hormones, including the sex hormones, steroids and vitamin D

In the diet, cholesterol is only found in foods derived from animals. Plant foods contain phytosterols, the most important being beta-sitosterol, which is found in nuts, cereals, fats and oils. Vegetarian diets are low in cholesterol, unless they include some animal products, like milk and eggs. Body cholesterol levels in an individual are kept fairly constant, with synthesis decreasing as dietary intake increases and

Diet and the prevention of cardiovascular diseases are covered in Chapter 14, pp. 269–292.

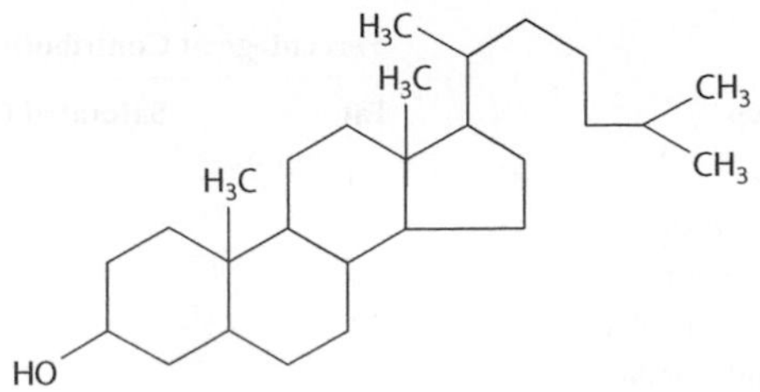

FIGURE 3.6 Chemical structure of cholesterol.

vice versa. Absorption of cholesterol is variable, ranging from 15% to 60% of dietary intake. Large intakes of phytosterols may inhibit cholesterol absorption, and this has been utilized in a number of functional products developed to lower cholesterol levels. Cholesterol is excreted from the body in the faeces, having been secreted into the digestive tract in the bile produced by the liver.

Levels of cholesterol in the blood are partly genetically determined, so that effects of dietary intake may be quite variable. Plasma cholesterol levels in some individuals respond minimally to changes in dietary intake of cholesterol, while in others, the response is much greater. Raised blood cholesterol levels are a major risk factor in the development of cardiovascular disease, and for this reason, a great deal of research has been undertaken to discover the factors which affect them.

Fats in the Diet

Sources of Fat in the Diet

Visible fats are those that can be clearly seen in our food; these include the spreading fats, cooking oils and the fat around pieces of meat. As this fat is obvious, the consumer can quite readily make an effort to reduce it – using less spread on bread, not using oil in frying and by trimming the fat off meat.

Invisible fat is often integral in a food product, for example, the fat in egg yolk, the fat contained within tissues in meat and fish, in nuts and, particularly, in processed and manufactured foods, such as sausages, burgers, pies, biscuits, cakes, pastries and chocolate. It is clearly more difficult to reduce this fat – either via process alteration or total elimination from the diet. Some success has been achieved by food producers in promoting lower-fat milk and dairy products and lower-fat versions of some processed foods. A major difficulty is that the consumer often does not appreciate how much fat is contained in a food, because it cannot be seen. Moreover, the labelling of foods may be often confusing, with essentially meaningless slogans, such as '90% fat free' or '30% less fat', providing little information on the actual fat content.

Table 3.7 shows the main sources of fat and saturated fatty acids in the British diet, based on data from the National Diet and Nutrition Survey (2008/2009–2011/2012). There have been some advances in the breeding and particularly butchering of animals in the last decade, so that new analyses of meat available in the United Kingdom show reductions in the fat content of lamb, beef and pork, with the greatest reductions achieved in pork. To an extent, it has also been possible to alter the fatty acid composition of the fat in meat by manipulating the types of fats fed to animals. This is more successful in non-ruminants, such as pigs and poultry, than in ruminants, as these tend to saturate fat by bacterial action in their rumen.

TABLE 3.7

Sources of Fat and Saturated Fatty Acids in the British Diet [Calculated from National Diet and Nutrition Survey (2008/2009–2011/2012)]

	Percentage of Contribution to Total	
Food Group	**Fat**	**Saturated Fatty Acids**
Fat spreads	10	10
Fish and fish dishes	5	3
Eggs and egg dishes	4	3
Meat and meat products	24	24
Milk and milk products	13	22
Cereals and cereal products	19	20

Sources of Essential Fatty Acids

The parent acid of the n-6 PUFA family, linoleic acid, occurs in meat, eggs and nuts (walnuts, Brazil nuts, almonds and peanuts). It also occurs in seeds used for oils and spread, such as sunflower, soya, corn, sesame and safflower. The parent of the n-3 PUFA family, alpha-linolenic acid, is found in dark green, leafy vegetables and meat from grass-fed ruminants. Oils derived from nuts and seeds are also a source of this acid (as well as the nuts themselves). Examples include walnuts, peanuts, almonds, soya, rapeseed and linseed. The longer members of the n-3 family are found in oil-rich fish, such as sardines, pilchards, salmon, trout, herrings, mackerel and fresh (not canned) tuna. Cod liver oil is also a rich source, although not a common component of the diet.

Trends in Intakes of Fats

Historical records suggest that fat intakes in many parts of Europe increased quite markedly at the start of the twentieth century, rising from a level of around 20% of the total energy in the late nineteenth century to values around 30% by the 1920s. Studies from this era are not necessary comparable with today's methods, but they do indicate a rapid increase over a relatively short time. Expressed as a percentage of the total energy intake, fat intake has risen steadily since data have been collected by the National Food Surveys and Family Food/Living Costs and Food Surveys. Levels in the 1940s were around 34% of total energy. Throughout the 1950s and 1960s, they rose to reach 41% and continued at a slower rate to reach 43% by the mid-1980s. Levels have gradually been falling since this time, and in 2010, the Family Food/Living Costs and Food Survey (DEFRA, 2011) reported that fat contributed 38.6% of total energy intake. It is worth noting that carbohydrate intakes have mirrored this trend, with an initial fall, followed by a rise in the percentage of energy from carbohydrate.

The figures discussed earlier reflect the percentage of energy from fat in the total energy intake. The actual amount of fat consumed has been decreasing, as noted by successive National Food Survey/Family Food/Living Costs and Food Survey reports. There has been a greater reduction in fat intakes in the higher than in the lowest income group, so that fat intakes are now marginally greater in this latter group. The data are shown in Table 3.8. On average, the difference in fat intake between social groups, regions and families within the United Kingdom is relatively small.

TABLE 3.8

Trends in Total Fat (g) and Energy (Calories) Intakes, per Person per Day, Showing Mean Population Figures and Intakes in the Highest and Lowest Income Groups Studied by the National Food Survey (DEFRA, 1950–2000) and Food Family Module of the Living Costs and Food Survey (DEFRA, 2000–2011)

	Population Mean		Highest Income Group[c]		Lowest Income Group[c]	
Year	Fat (g)	Energy (Cal)	Fat (g)	Energy (Cal)	Fat (g)	Energy (Cal)
1950[a]	101	2474	109	2542	97	2379
1960[a]	115	2630	120	2600	106	2540
1970[a]	121	2600	124	2520	108	2470
1980[a]	106	2230	106	2150	105	2240
1990[a]	86	1870	86	1710	86	1890
2000[a]	74	1750	68	1600	75	1720
2010[b]	84	1981	82	1965	78	1933

[a] 1950–2000, the figures do not include confectionery and soft or alcoholic drinks.

[b] The figures do not include alcoholic drinks and are relative to household foods.

[c] Lowest income group, group D in HFS 1950–2000 and equivalized income deciles 1&2 in LCFS; highest income group, group A in HFS 1950–2000 and equivalized income deciles 9&10 in LCFS.

TABLE 3.9
Percentage of Energy from the Main Groups of Fatty Acids

Year	Saturated Fatty Acids	Monounsaturated Fatty Acids	Polyunsaturated Fatty Acids
1972	19.3	15.9	4.3
1980	18.9	16.0	4.6
1990	16.7	15.3	6.7
2000	15.0	13.5	6.9
2010	14.5	14.2	7.1

Much greater differences are seen if culturally different societies are compared (with white British households obtaining 14% of their energy intake from saturated fatty acids in 2010, compared to 12% for Asian and Asian British households).

One should remember, however, that there has been a progressive trend towards eating outside the home, which is more frequent in higher income households. Therefore, the recorded intakes do not include all of the food consumed by individuals. Eating out was measured for the first time in 1994, and the National Food Survey reports show that foods eaten out have a higher percentage fat content than those eaten at home.

In addition to changes in the total fat intake, there has also been an alteration in the balance of the saturated, monounsaturated and PUFAs in the diet. The changes reported by DEFRA (2001, 2011) in the percentage of energy from the main groups of fatty acids are shown in Table 3.9. These values reflect trends in food consumption patterns, with a decline in the consumption of whole milk, butter, margarine and lard and an increase in the intake of oils and spreads made from vegetable oils. Many of these changes have been prompted by advice on healthy eating in the last two decades and the response of food manufacturers.

The implication of change in the dietary fat for cardiovascular diseases is covered in Chapter 14, pp. 281–285.

How Much Fat Should We Have in the Diet?

For many nutrients, the answer to such a question would entail a consideration of the prevention of deficiency of the particular nutrient. However, in the case of fat, there is no recognized deficiency state that develops from the absence of fat in general. The only problem arises from an absence of the essential fatty acids. It should, therefore, be possible to set levels for guidance on intake of these fatty acids, in order to prevent deficiency. An evidence of the need for essential fatty acids comes from reports of linoleic acid deficiency in children and in clinical situations in adults. The dietary reference values report (DoH, 1991) recommends that linoleic acid should provide at least 1% of total energy and alpha-linolenic acid at least 0.2%. This amounts to between 2 and 5 g of essential fatty acids daily, which can be readily achieved from a serving of fish, seed oil used in cooking or green leafy vegetable. Since the publication of this report, there has been more interest in the possible health benefits of *n*-3 fatty acids and the implications of the ratio of *n*-6 to *n*-3 fatty acids. There are no firm recommendations on a desirable ratio, but it has been proposed that linoleic acid (*n*-6) should comprise a maximum of 3% of energy intake and total *n*-3 acids should be 1.3% of energy. Thus, the ratio of *n*-6 to *n*-3 fatty acids should be between 2:1 and 3:1. Specific interest has focused on the diets of pregnant women, where the status of long-chain PUFAs is correlated with those in the baby. The importance of *n*-3 acids for neurological development in the fetus and infant has been discussed earlier in this chapter, and women whose diets contain high levels of *n*-6 acids or minimal amounts of *n*-3 acids may be unable to supply their baby with adequate levels of *n*-3 acids, either via the placenta or in breast milk. Premature infants may be especially at risk, although term babies also need an adequate supply. The addition of long-chain fatty acids to formula milk is now permitted by European and UK legislation, to improve intakes in infants. There is a need for more research in this area.

The recommended levels of total fat and the distribution of this fat into saturated, monounsaturated and polyunsaturated fats are based on our knowledge of intakes in populations and evidence on the incidence of disease in these populations, that is, an optimum health approach. The main diseases that are considered in advice on fat are atherosclerosis and cancer, and much of the guidance on fat intakes aims to reduce the incidence of these diseases. Consequently, the recommended levels in the United Kingdom are that total fatty acid intake should average 30% of dietary energy including alcohol. Of this, 10% of total energy should be provided by saturated fatty acids, 12% by monounsaturated fatty acids, an average of 6% from PUFAs and 2% from *trans* fatty acids. When calculated as total fat (including glycerol), these figures amount to 33% of total dietary energy including alcohol or 35% of energy from food.

SUMMARY

Proteins

1. Proteins are composed of combinations of amino acids, creating a wide diversity of proteins.
2. Twenty different amino acids occur in proteins. The body uses these very efficiently and is able to convert some of the amino acids into others. However, eight of them cannot be made in the body and must be provided in the diet; they are the essential amino acids.
3. Dietary sources of protein may be of animal or plant origin. The ability of the body to make full use of the amino acids supplied depends on the energy intake and the pattern of the amino acids in the protein. An inadequate amount of one amino acid may limit the usefulness of the whole protein, unless it is combined with a complementary source, which provides the limiting amino acid.
4. Protein requirements are based currently on nitrogen balance studies. Intake of protein in the United Kingdom is above the RNI in healthy adults.

Carbohydrates

1. Carbohydrates may be classified by size and by digestibility; the basic building blocks for carbohydrate are monosaccharides.
2. Starches may be digestible or resistant. The digestible starches release glucose more slowly than simple sugars. In addition, food sources of starch generally contain other nutrients.
3. NSP can be classified as soluble or insoluble.
4. Carbohydrates should supply approximately 50% of the daily energy needs, of which no more than 11% should be supplied by sugars.

Fats

1. The diet contains saturated and unsaturated fatty acids, arranged in triglycerides of varying composition. The nature of the fatty acids (chain length, saturation) influences the physical characteristics of the dietary fat. In addition, the diet contains small amounts of cholesterol and phospholipids.
2. Fat intakes in the United Kingdom have fallen in absolute terms in the last 40 years, but in relation to the total energy intake, levels remain at about 40% of food energy. The majority of fat intake comes from fats, oils, meats and meat products.
3. Fats increase the palatability of the diet and can contribute to overconsumption of energy, because of the high energy content per unit weight.
4. Advice for the population in general is to reduce total fat intakes.

STUDY QUESTIONS

1. Consider the sources of proteins for an individual following
   a. An omnivorous diet
   b. A vegetarian diet
   c. A vegan diet
   Discuss the practical challenges met to secure an adequate protein intake.
2. Healthy eating advice recommends a reduction in the intake sugars to 11% of total energy.
   a. What changes in the diet would be needed to achieve this?
   b. What effect might these changes have on other components of the diet?
   c. Suggest practical and realistic ways in which an increase in starchy carbohydrates intake might be promoted.
   d. What other benefits might follow from the changes you suggest?
3. Both gamma-linolenic acid and alpha-linolenic acid contain 18 carbon atoms and three double bonds. In what ways are they different and why is this important?
4. What are the functions of the phospholipids and how does this relate to their structure?
5. Suggest some explanations for the finding of the National Food Survey that food eaten outside the home has a higher fat content than that eaten at home. What do your explanations imply about promotion of healthy eating?

ACTIVITY

3.1 The three-dimensional conformation of proteins is essential for their activity and function. Draw a diagram illustrating the changes occurring to the three-dimensional protein shape during cooking. What happens when the mixture is cooled?

BIBLIOGRAPHY AND FURTHER READING

Association of Official Analytical Chemists. 2000. *Official Methods of Analysis*, 17th edn. Gaithersburg, MD: AOAC.

Conning, D. (ed.). 1993. *Biological Functions of Carbohydrates*. London, UK: British Nutrition Foundation.

DEFRA (UK Department for Environment, Food and Rural Affairs). 2001. National food survey 2000. Annual report on food, expenditure, consumption and nutrient intakes. London, UK: The Stationery Office.

DEFRA (UK Department for Environment, Food and Rural Affairs). 2011. *Family Food 2010*. London, UK: National Statistics Publication.

DoH (Public Health England). 2014. National diet and nutrition survey: Results from years 1–4 (combined) of the rolling programme (2008/2009–2011/2012). London, UK: PHE.

DoH (UK Department of Health). 1991. Dietary reference values for food energy and nutrients in the United Kingdom. Report on Health and Social Subjects No. 41. Report of the Panel on Dietary Reference Values of the Committee on Medical Aspects of Food Policy. London, UK: HMSO.

Englyst, H.N., Bingham, S.A., Runswick, S.A. et al. 1988. Dietary fibre (non starch polysaccharides) in fruits, vegetables and nuts. *Journal of Human Nutrition and Dietetics* 1, 247–286.

FAO (Food and Agriculture Organization). 1998. Carbohydrates in human nutrition. Report of a joint FAO/WHO Expert Consultation. Rome, Italy: FAO.

FAO/WHO/UNU. 1985. Energy and protein requirements. Report of a joint FAO/WHO/UNU Expert Consultation. WHO technical report no. 724. Geneva, Switzerland: WHO.

Food Standards Agency. 2002a. *Food Portion Sizes*, 3rd edn. London, UK: The Stationery Office.

Food Standards Agency. 2002b. *McCance and Widdowson's The Composition of Foods*, 6th summary edn. Cambridge, UK: Royal Society of Chemistry.

Food Standards Agency. 2006. *FSA Nutrient and Food Based Guidelines for UK Institutions*. London, UK: The Stationery Office.

Jackson, A.A. 1992. Sugars not for burning. In Eastwood, E., Edwards, C. and Parry, D. (eds.). *Human Nutrition: A Continuing Debate*. London, UK: Chapman & Hall, pp. 82–99.

Jackson, A.A. 2003. Human protein requirement: Policy issues. *Proceedings of the Nutrition Society* 60, 7–11.

Macdiarmid, J.I., Cade, J.E. and Blundell, J.E. 1994. Dietary fat: Grams or percentage energy? Analysis of the dietary and nutrition survey of British adults and the Leeds high fat study. *Proceedings of the Nutrition Society* 53, 232A.
Millward, D.J. 1999. The nutritional value of plant-based diets in relation to human amino acid and protein requirements. *Proceedings of the Nutrition Society* 58, 249–260.
Morton, G.M., Lee, S.M., Buss, D.H. et al. 1995. Intakes and major dietary sources of cholesterol and phytosterols in the British diet. *Journal of Human Nutrition and Dietetics* 8(6), 429–440.
Sanderson, P., Gill, J.M.R., Packard, C.J. et al. 2002. UK Food Standards Agency cis-monounsaturated fatty acid workshop report. *British Journal of Nutrition* 88, 99–104.
Schaafsma, G. 2005. The protein digestibility-corrected amino acid score (PDCAAS) – A concept for describing protein quality in foods and food ingredients: A critical review. *Journal of AOAC International* 88, 988–994.
Scientific Advisory Committee on Nutrition. 2008. *The Nutritional Wellbeing of the British Population*. London, U.K.: The Stationery Office.
Scientific Advisory Committee on Nutrition. 2015. *Carbohydrate and Health*. London, U.K.: The Stationery Office.
Scrimshaw, N.S., Waterlow, J.C. and Schurch, B. (eds.). 1996. Energy and protein requirements, *Proceedings of an IDECG Workshop*, November 1994, London, UK, Supplement of the *European Journal of Clinical Nutrition* (IDECG, 1994, 198 p.). *European Journal of Clinical Nutrition* 50: 1.
Simopoulos, A.P. 2003. Importance of the ratio of omega-6/omega-3 essential fatty acids: Evolutionary aspects. *World Review of Nutrition and Dietetic* 92, 1–22.
Wise, A. and McPherson, K. 1995. The relationship between individual beliefs and portion weights of fat spreads. *Journal of Human Nutrition and Dietetics* 8(3), 193–200.

4 Vitamins and Phytochemicals

AIMS

The aims of this chapter are to

- Identify food sources of particular vitamins and describe the role of water-soluble and fat-soluble vitamins in the body and discuss interactions between vitamins.
- Describe the main phytochemicals in foods.
- Identify the population groups who may be at risk of inadequate intake and discuss the reasons for this.

VITAMINS

Throughout the body, there are catalysts acting on a host of chemical reactions within living cells. Most of these are proteins acting as enzymes; some of these require additional 'cofactors' to complete their function. Some of these cofactors are minerals, such as magnesium, calcium and copper. There are also organic cofactors that must be consumed in the diet because the body (in general) is unable to synthesize them for itself. These are the vitamins.

See Chapter 12 for more details on minerals as cofactors, pp. 244–252.

Vitamins possess a number of specific characteristic features.

- They are organic and, unlike the minerals, can be readily destroyed.
- They are essential and, in their absence, particular functions of the body fail and may cease. Ultimately, deficiency of a vitamin can be fatal.
- They generally work individually in a particular aspect of metabolism. However, some vitamins work in cooperation with one another. They may have similar effects and can thus replace one another (up to a point). They may be involved at different stages of the same pathway and a lack of one member may prevent the others being used.
- They are present in food in small amounts, usually in both plant and animal foods. They vary in their chemical composition. Vitamins can be synthesized in the laboratory and can be taken as supplements, which function in a similar way to those found in foods, since they are chemically identical.
- They are needed by the body in small amounts and measured in milligram or microgram quantities. In some cases, excessive amounts of a vitamin are harmful. The body has varying capacity to store the vitamins; thus, for some, a regular intake is needed.

As vitamins occur in such small quantities in foods, their discovery was a slow process. Traditional cultures had many practices incorporated into their food habits, which ensured that vitamins were adequately supplied, although they would not have been able to offer an explanation. These include the making of drinks from pine-needle infusions to supply vitamin C and soaking maize in lime water to liberate niacin. Limes were included in the cargo on long sea voyages in the eighteenth century in response to a perceived lack of 'a nutritional factor' in the remaining provisions, which had traditionally resulted in death among sailors.

Identification of the vitamins in the early twentieth century came from studies observing people and animals eating poor or restricted diets. Some of the substances that cured the signs and symptoms were found to be fat soluble; others were water soluble. In the beginning, these vitamins, as they were initially known, were allotted names according to the letters of the alphabet: A, B, C, etc. As the knowledge of the vitamins expanded and they were chemically isolated and identified, it became more sensible to call them by their proper names. Nevertheless, the alphabetic naming is still used, particularly when there are several members of the group having similar properties, where using individual names would be cumbersome.

There have continued to be new findings about the functions of the vitamins ever since their original discovery. Clearly, our understanding of the vitamins is still incomplete and new findings will continue to be made. In addition, some of the vitamins have been found to have pharmacological properties when present in amounts much greater than those required for their metabolic function and have, therefore, been used as medication, both therapeutically and prophylactically. Further understanding of this role is also needed.

Fat-Soluble Vitamins

As a group, these vitamins share several properties:

See Chapter 11 for more details on digestion and absorption of fat, pp. 220–228, and Chapter 12 on metabolism of key nutrients, pp. 236–252.

- They are found in the fat or oily parts of foods and are, therefore, absent from foods that are devoid of fat.
- Their absorption and transport from the digestive tract requires the secretion of bile and normal fat absorption mechanisms. On the whole, they are absorbed with the digested fats into chylomicrons and transported in the lymph ultimately to reach the blood.
- Their transport in the blood requires carriers that are lipid soluble.
- They are stored in lipid fractions of the body, for example, in the adipose tissue or in association with lipid components of cells.
- Because of their insolubility in water, they are not excreted in the urine and accumulate in the body, especially in the liver and adipose tissue. Large stored amounts, particularly of vitamin A and D, may be harmful, and, therefore, care must be taken to avoid high intake levels.

Vitamin A

Vitamin A was the first fat-soluble vitamin to be identified; it is now known that there are several related compounds that have vitamin A activity; hence, the name vitamin A will be used. The deficiency associated with inadequate levels of vitamin A in the body, night blindness, has been recognized for many centuries.

Three forms of vitamin A possess activity in the body: retinol, retinal and retinoic acid; collectively, they are called the retinoids. There is interconversion between the first two forms, but once the acid has been formed, it cannot be reconverted. In addition, there are provitamin A compounds, the carotenoids, which can be converted, with varying degrees of efficiency into retinol (Figure 4.1). The most important of these is beta-carotene.

Vitamin A in Foods

Foods derived from animals mostly contain preformed vitamin A, usually in the form of retinyl palmitate, which is easily hydrolyzed in the intestine. Good sources are eggs, butter, milk and milk products, liver and fish or fish oils. Margarines contain vitamin A added as a legal requirement to domestic size packs in the United Kingdom.

Plant foods contain carotenoids, which are red or yellow pigments found in many fruit and vegetables. In the United Kingdom, most of the provitamin is in the form of beta-carotene, although,

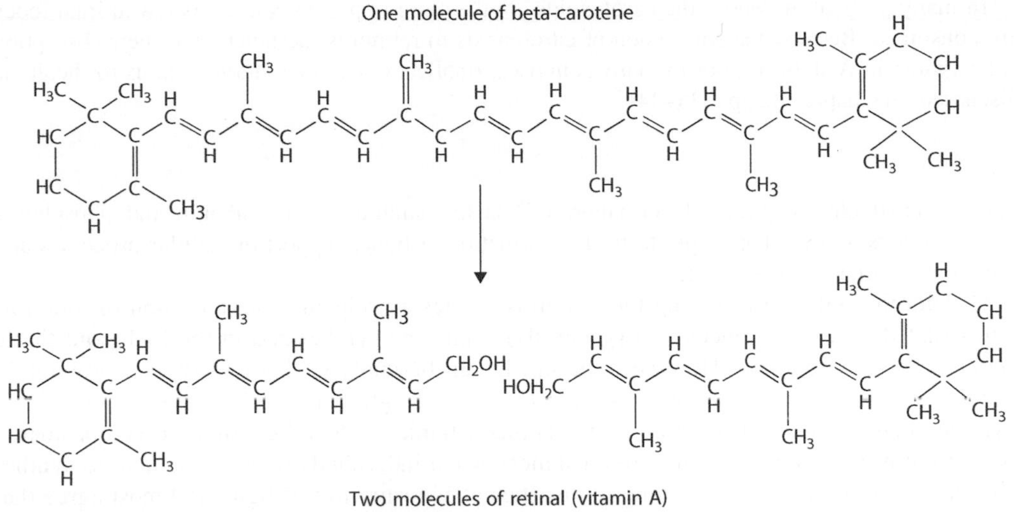

FIGURE 4.1 Conversion of beta-carotene to retinol.

in other parts of the world, alpha- and gamma-carotenes may be important. Red palm oil used in parts of Africa is rich in alpha-carotenes. Rich sources of carotenoids in the West include carrots, dark green leafy vegetables, broccoli, red peppers and tomatoes; in addition, apricots, peaches and mango are good sources.

Ordinary cooking processes do not damage either retinol or the carotenoids. Cooking of carrots, for example, enhances their digestibility and so makes more of the carotene available for absorption.

In order to obtain an estimate of the total amount of vitamin A activity consumed from both preformed retinol and carotenoids, it is necessary to devise a combined unit. This is the retinol equivalent, which represents the amount of retinol consumed + (the amount of beta-carotene ÷ 6). This accounts for losses in both absorption and conversion to the active vitamin.

Requirement for Vitamin A

Report 41 (DoH, 1991) based its reference values on the amounts needed to maintain an adequate pool of the vitamin in the liver at a concentration of 20 μg/g wet weight. On this basis, the reference nutrient intake (RNI) for men and women was set at 700 and 600 μg/day, respectively. Upper limits for regular intakes are also given, at 9000 μg/day in men and 7500 μg/day in women.

In the United Kingdom, mean total retinol intakes have been found (Bates et al., 2014) to be 946 μg retinol equivalents/day, which represents 152% of the mean RNI. Intakes have fallen quite sharply in the last 10 years as a result of lower fat intakes (e.g. from whole milk and spreads), and, in several groups within the population, particularly households with three or more children, the mean intake is less than the RNI.

The major food contributors overall are as follows:

Vegetables (mostly carrots)	32%
Meat (mostly liver)	16%
Fats	13%
Milk and cheese	14%

The contribution of preformed vitamin A is approximately 64% of the total intake, and the remainder being provided by carotenoids.

In many parts of the world, the carotenoids are the more important source as few animal foods are consumed. Because the conversion of carotenoids to retinol is inefficient and their absorption is low, vitamin A status is poor in many countries. Implications of low vitamin status for health is discussed in Chapter 12, pp. 235–244.

Vitamin D

The principal physiological role of vitamin D is to maintain serum calcium and phosphorus concentrations at a level appropriate for the formation of bone, support of cellular processes and functioning of nerves and muscles.

Considering vitamin D among the vitamins creates a problem. The definition of vitamins states that they are substances that (generally) cannot be synthesized in the body and that a dietary intake is required. However, vitamin D can be made in the skin from a provitamin under the influence of ultraviolet (UV-B) light of wavelength between 290 and 320 nm. There has been considerable debate, therefore, whether vitamin D should continue to be considered as a vitamin. However, there are circumstances when individuals may not be able to synthesize the vitamin, for example, owing to insufficient exposure to UV light, and most agree that a dietary source is required. In the United Kingdom, no synthesis occurs in the skin between October and March because light in correct wavelength does not reach the earth's surface. Consequently, synthesis that has taken place during the summer months has to provide the body's vitamin D needs during the winter. In addition, those who are housebound or those living in an environment with high levels of air pollution may have to depend on a dietary source all year round.

There are two potential provitamins for vitamin D: 7-dehydrocholesterol (vitamin D_3) and ergosterol (vitamin D_2). The former is present in animal fats, including the skin of humans, having been made in the body from cholesterol. Ergosterol is found in yeast and fungi and is used as a source of commercial vitamin production.

Vitamin D in the Diet

There are few sources of vitamin D that are consumed on a regular basis. Butter, spreading fats (including margarine, low-fat spreads), eggs and milk are the most regularly consumed sources. Levels in the dairy products vary with the seasons and are higher in the summer months. Where vitamin D is added by law as fortification, for example, to margarine, levels are constant throughout the year. In the United Kingdom, 7.05–8.82 μg/100 g margarine is the prescribed level added to margarine. Low-fat spreads may be fortified at the manufacturers' discretion. Meat has, relatively recently, been found to be a useful source of the vitamin. Other sources include oily fish and liver, although these may occur rarely in the diet. A number of manufactured foods may also be fortified with vitamin D, for example, breakfast cereals, evaporated milk, bedtime drinks, yoghurts and infant foods. Fish oil supplements are a rich source of vitamin D.

Recorded intake level of vitamin D is 2.85 μg/day; there is no RNI figure for the majority of the population. The main food groups contributing to dietary vitamin D are reported by Bates (2014), shown as follows:

Meat and meat products	31%
Fats and oils	20%
Fish	17%
Fortified breakfast cereals	13%
Milk and cheese	5%

Dietary Reference Value

A dietary reference value (DRV) is difficult to establish for vitamin D because, for the majority of the population with a normal lifestyle who are able to synthesize the vitamin in the skin, a dietary source is unnecessary. However, children under the age of 3 years have high needs to sustain rapid growth, which may not be met readily from the diet or by exposure to sunlight and, therefore, an RNI value of 8.5 μg/day up to 6 months and 7 μg/day from 6 months to 3 years is given. Pregnant or lactating women may also benefit from a regular intake of vitamin D to sustain calcium metabolism. Older adults, who may have a reduced ability to synthesize the vitamin, or who are less likely to spend time outside may also benefit from a dietary source of the vitamin. For both of these groups, the RNI is given as 10 μg/day (DoH, 1991). People of Asian origin, for whom vitamin D status may be marginal for cultural or dietary reasons, may also benefit from additional vitamin D, but no RNI has been specifically given. A draft report has been prepared by the Scientific Advisory Committee for Nutrition in July 2015, with consultation closing in September 2015. It should be noted that an intake of 10 μg/day is difficult to achieve through dietary means, and a supplement may be needed. Results from the National Dietary and Nutrition Survey (NDNS) rolling programme in 2008/2009 and 2009/2010 highlighted that only 27% of children aged 1–3 and 33% older adults aged 65 and over achieved the RNI.

Increased requirements in pregnancy are covered in Chapter 6, pp. 104–109, while increased requirements in older age are covered in Chapter 8, pp. 153–177.

Most people in the United Kingdom obtain vitamin D by skin synthesis during the summer months on exposure to UV light from the sun. The day does not have to be sunny nor the skin completely uncovered for synthesis to occur, as the light can penetrate thin cloud and light clothing. There is now greater awareness of the dangers of exposure to solar radiation with respect to skin cancer, with recommendations to cover the skin with sunscreening creams or clothing. It is likely that this reduces the potential synthesis of vitamin D. A balance between the harmful (cancer risk) and beneficial outcomes (vitamin D synthesis) is required; it has been suggested that about half an hour per day of exposure to sunlight (avoiding the hottest part of the day) can achieve the beneficial synthesis, without risking harmful consequences.

Vitamin E

Vitamin E was first identified as an anti-sterility substance, necessary for normal reproductive performance in rats. The rats could be successfully treated with whole wheat. This role has, however, been difficult to identify in humans. In recent years, it has become clear that vitamin E is possibly the most important antioxidant vitamin in the body, playing an essential protective role against free radical damage.

It is now known that vitamin E consists of a group of substances belonging to two closely related families: tocopherols and tocotrienols (Figure 4.2), with each existing in a number of isomeric forms, alpha, beta, gamma and delta, making a total of eight different members of the group. The most important member, with the greatest biological potency and accounting for 90% of the vitamin activity in the tissues, is alpha-tocopherol. It is this form that is often taken as the representative of the whole group.

Vitamin E in Food

Animal foods provide only alpha-tocopherol, whereas plant foods may contain the other isomeric forms of tocopherol and the tocotrienols as well. Among plant foods, vegetable oils are the most important sources. The germ of whole cereal grains contains vitamin E (a rich source of tocotrienols). In addition, some is found in green leafy vegetables, fruits and nuts. Margarines manufactured from vegetable and seed oils contain some vitamin E, although amounts vary. Breakfast cereals may be fortified with the vitamin, but specific information should be sought

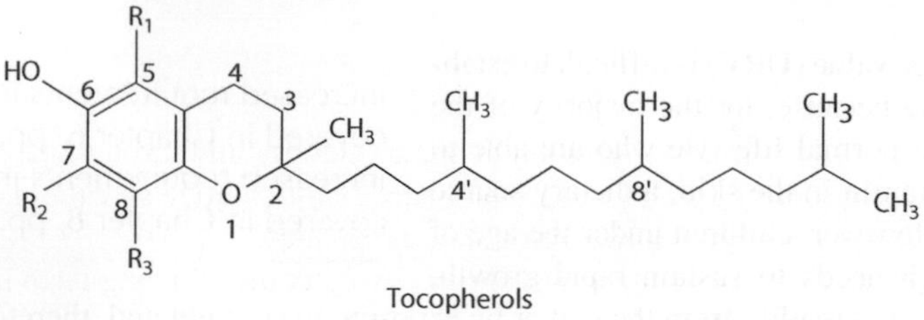

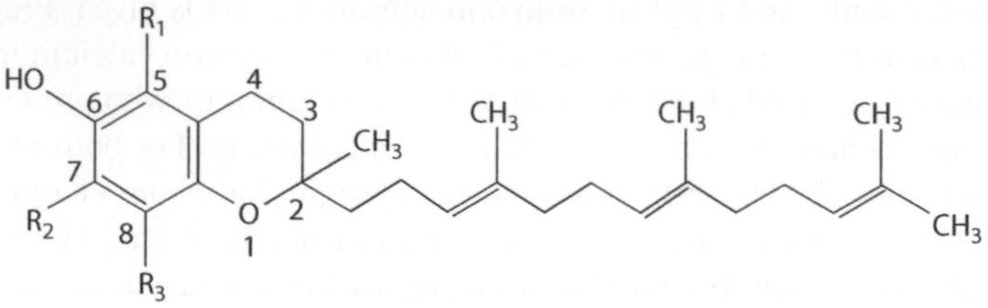

FIGURE 4.2 Structures of tocopherols and tocotrienols.

on the label. Animal foods generally are not rich sources of vitamin E, although small amounts occur in poultry, fish and eggs.

Dietary Reference Value

The vitamin E requirement depends on the polyunsaturated fatty acid (PUFA) content of the diet. Based on current levels of PUFA intake, it is proposed that intakes of 4 and 3 mg/day for men and women, respectively, are adequate. An alternative used in other countries relates the vitamin E intake to the PUFA content of the diet in the ratio of 0.4 mg tocopherol/g of dietary PUFA. In the United Kingdom, the average diet provides a ratio of 0.6 mg tocopherol/g PUFA. Some authors have suggested that intakes should be considerably higher than this, up to 87–100 mg/day, to protect against cardiovascular disease. More work in this area is needed.

In the NDNS Survey (Bates, 2014), the mean vitamin E intake is shown to be 9.2 mg/day. Most important contributors are the following:

Cereals and cereal products	20%
Meat and meat products	14%
Fats	11%
Vegetables	8%
Potatoes and potato products	7%

Vitamin K

This vitamin was initially isolated as a factor involved in blood clotting, with a haemorrhagic disease observed in its absence. A number of compounds are now recognized as having vitamin K activity, all related by their structure as members of the naphthoquinone family. The most important naturally occurring members are phylloquinone (K_1) (Figure 4.3) and menaquinone (K_2); there is also a synthetic compound, menadione (K_3), which is water soluble and, therefore, has advantages in absorption.

Sources of Vitamin K

The menaquinones are synthesized by bacteria, including those which reside in the human terminal ileum and colon. It is, therefore, possible to obtain some of the vitamin requirement from synthesis in the gastrointestinal tract. Very little is known about the site or mechanisms of absorption of this

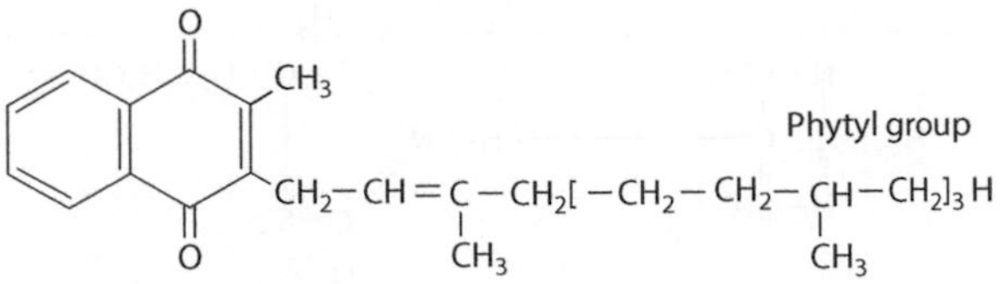

FIGURE 4.3 Phylloquinone (vitamin K_1) is derived from plants and is lipid soluble.

potentially large pool of vitamin K. It is unlikely that this can meet all the needs; therefore, a dietary source is also required. If the colonic bacteria are eliminated, for example, by antibiotic use, the individual is totally dependent on dietary supplies. Phylloquinones are obtained from plant foods, with rich sources being the green leafy vegetables (such as broccoli, cabbage, spinach, Brussels sprouts) and peas. Green vegetables supply about 50% of the total dietary intake of vitamin K_1. Vegetable oils and margarines together with foods that contain these, such as biscuits and cakes, provide a further 20%–25% of the intake. Menaquinones occur in animal foods, especially liver; meat and dairy products contain smaller amounts. Generally, vitamin K is widely distributed in foods and a dietary deficiency is rare. Tea also contains a useful amount of vitamin K.

Dietary Reference Value

This is difficult to set because of an indeterminate amount of bacterial synthesis in the colon. The Department of Health (DoH, 1991) uses normal blood clotting factor concentrations as an indicator of adequate status. This can be achieved with an intake of 1 μg/kg per day in adults. It has been suggested that a higher level of vitamin K than this may be needed for optimal bone function, but evidence to propose a new level is lacking. Prophylactic vitamin K is recommended in all infants. Meanwhile, the Institute of Medicine has set adequate intake values for the United States at 120 and 90 μg/day for men and women, respectively.

Menaquinones intake in the British diet is unknown and likely to represent only a small portion of the overall vitamin K intake (10% in the Netherland). Phylloquinones account for most of the vitamin K intake in the United Kingdom, which were found to be 86 and 94 μg/day in men and women aged 18–64, respectively. The study highlighted significant overall decrease in phylloquinones intake for all age and gender groups between 1986/1987 and 2000/2001, mainly due to a lower consumption of cooked leafy green vegetables, which contributed 60% of the total intake in 2000/2001 versus 68% in 1986/1987 (Thane et al., 2006).

Water-Soluble Vitamins

With the exception of vitamin C, the water-soluble vitamins belong to the B-complex group. Many of the B vitamins share similar functions and often work together; they can be broadly described as cofactors in metabolism. They facilitate the use of energy and are involved in the interconversion between different groups of metabolites. Folate and vitamin B_{12} are involved in cell division.

Owing to their chemical nature, the water-soluble vitamins have different characteristics from the fat-soluble vitamins:

- They are absorbed into the portal blood after digestion.
- When present in excess, they are excreted in the urine.
- The body has limited storage capacity for these vitamins (with the exception of vitamin B_{12}); most reserves in the body are found in association with enzymes where the vitamin plays a cofactor role.
- They are more readily lost during food preparation processes, since they are soluble in water (in particular, this occurs on heating, especially in water and also on exposure to light and air).

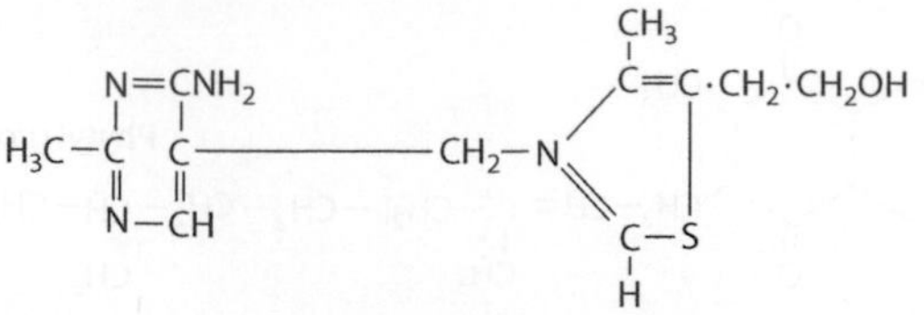

FIGURE 4.4 Structure of thiamin.

Thiamin (Vitamin B_1)

The deficiency disease associated with thiamin, beriberi, has been known for 4000 years, although the name was first used in the seventeenth century. The nutritional links were first recognized at the beginning of the twentieth century in Japan. The water-soluble agent was eventually isolated in 1911 and named vitamin B to differentiate it from the first fat-soluble vitamin – A.

The structure of thiamin is unusual in that it contains a sulphur group in the thiazole ring (Figure 4.4).

Sources of Thiamin

The most important sources of thiamin in the British diet are cereals, which provide 45% of the intake. The whole cereal grain is rich in the vitamin but losses on milling are high, as most is concentrated in the outer layers; thus white flour and polished rice are low in thiamin. However, thiamin is added to white flour at the rate of 2.4 mg/kg, which restores the level. Many breakfast cereals are also enriched with thiamin and, therefore, provide a useful source. Beans, seeds and nuts are also rich in thiamin and may provide an important amount in the diet, especially in vegetarian populations. In rice-eating countries, they are one of the main sources of thiamin.

Meat is generally not rich in the vitamin, with the exception of pork and liver, and meat and meat products provide only 15% of dietary thiamin. Milk and related products provide 8% of total intake and potatoes provide 9%. Both of these have low concentrations but, as they are consumed frequently, their contribution can be useful.

Dietary Reference Value

Thiamin requirements are related to energy metabolism and, therefore, to energy intake. Deficiency occurs when intakes fall below 0.2 mg/1000 cal. The dietary reference value report (DoH, 1991), therefore, based its RNI at 0.4 mg/1000 cal to allow for variance and provide a margin of safety. Excessive intakes above 3 g/day are reported to be toxic and should be avoided.

Mean daily intake in the United Kingdom is 1.43 mg, which represents 169% of the RNI (Bates, 2014). Thiamin is one of the more unstable vitamins, especially in alkaline conditions, and at temperatures above 100°C. Estimates suggest an average of 20% is lost in domestic food preparation. The presence of sulphur dioxide as a preservative accelerates destruction of thiamin.

Riboflavin (Vitamin B_2)

Riboflavin (Figure 4.5) was originally identified as a growth-promoting substance, rather than a factor to cure a specific deficiency disease. It was isolated from a number of food substances, including

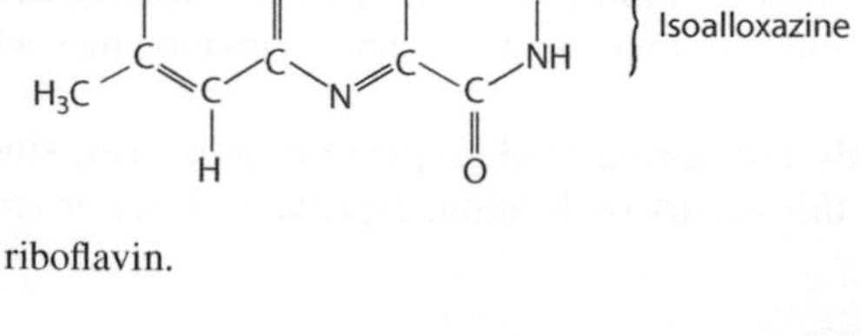

FIGURE 4.5 Structure of riboflavin.

milk, eggs and yeast, and for a time was known as 'vitamin G'. One of its most characteristic features is that the crystalline substance has a yellow-orange colour.

Riboflavin in Foods

The diet contains both free riboflavin and its two phosphorylated forms, flavin adenine dinucleotide and flavin mononucleotide. Foods rich in riboflavin include milk and milk products, meat (especially liver) and eggs. The major sources in the British diet derive from milk and dairy products (43% of total intake), cereal products that contain milk and eggs (27% of total) and meat (14% of total). Cereals alone are not a good source of the vitamin, unless enriched. A small amount of riboflavin is supplied by tea. Fruits and most vegetables are not important sources of the vitamin, although the dark green leafy vegetables may be important contributors, if eaten regularly.

Dietary Reference Value

Intakes of 0.55 mg/day over a period of 4 months have been reported to result in riboflavin deficiency. Earlier recommendations had been based on levels producing tissue saturation. The upper range of glutathione reductase activity is now considered a more sensitive indicator of saturation. Surveys have shown that intakes in the United Kingdom achieve this level. The RNI was set at 1.3 mg/day for men and 1.1 mg/day for women. Excessive intakes of riboflavin are poorly absorbed and, therefore, no evidence exists of potential harmful effects.

Mean intakes of riboflavin in Britain are 1.56 mg/day; this represents 136% of RNI. Riboflavin is more stable to heat and less soluble than many of the B vitamins, but may be lost in cooking water. It is also destroyed by exposure to sunlight. Leaving milk exposed to sunlight in glass bottles will result in the loss of 10% of the vitamin per hour. Paper and plastic cartons are better for protecting the vitamin content of milk.

Nicotinic Acid (Niacin, Vitamin B_3)

The deficiency disease associated with niacin is pellagra, Italian name for 'rough skin'. The disease was recognized as endemic among maize-eating populations, and its occurrence spread with the introduction of maize throughout Europe and into Africa. In the early twentieth century, it reached epidemic proportions in the southern states of America. A dietary cause was suspected in the 1920s, and a protein-free extract of meat or yeast was found to prevent the deficiency. The association with maize was not explained for a further 20 years. The pellagra-preventing factor in yeast and meat extract, nicotinic acid, can be made in the human body from the amino acid tryptophan. The conversion is very inefficient, with only 1 mg of vitamin produced from 60 mg of tryptophan. However, tryptophan is the limiting amino acid in maize protein, so none is available for vitamin synthesis. In addition, the nicotinic acid in maize is present in a bound and unabsorbable form. These two factors make a deficiency of the vitamin likely when the diet is poor and mainly composed of maize.

Nicotinic acid and its amide nicotinamide (Figure 4.6) are nutritionally important and are collectively termed niacin.

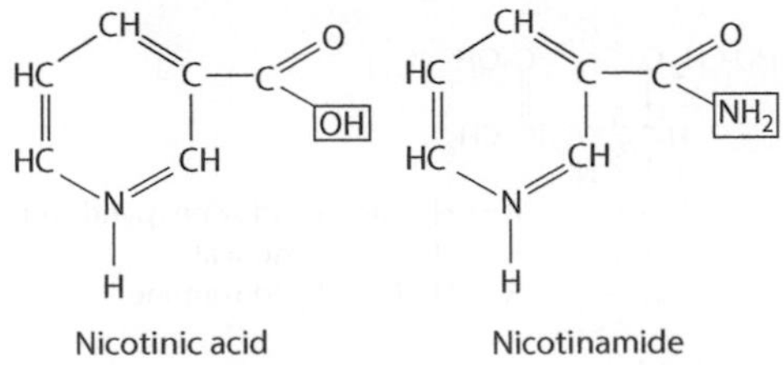

FIGURE 4.6 Structures of nicotinic acid and nicotinamide, collectively known as niacin.

Sources of Niacin

In addition to niacin provided as preformed vitamin, the body makes a certain amount of niacin by conversion from tryptophan. In the West, the large amount of protein in the diet probably supplies enough tryptophan to meet the whole of the need for niacin and a dietary intake of preformed niacin may not be needed. However, if protein intakes are low, insufficient tryptophan may be available to meet the need for niacin.

Food composition tables provide an estimate of the amount of niacin supplied from tryptophan, given as 'nicotinic acid equivalents'. (This is calculated as 1/60 of the tryptophan content.) Adequate amounts of vitamin B_6 and riboflavin are required for this conversion. An overall figure for total niacin equivalents can then be obtained by adding preformed niacin + nicotinic acid (or niacin) equivalents from tryptophan.

Rich sources of niacin equivalents are meat (especially liver), fish, peanuts and cereals (especially if fortified). In the British diet, meat is the main source (38% of total intake), followed by cereals (25% of total), milk and dairy products (13% of total) and vegetables (including potatoes) (11% of total). It is also worth noting that coffee and cocoa provide some niacin.

In some foods, niacin is bound to complex carbohydrates or peptides, which makes it largely unavailable. This is particularly a problem with maize, but to a lesser extent applies to other cereal grains. However, soaking of maize in lime water releases the bound niacin, making it available. This is a traditional practice in Mexico, and, consequently, although maize is the staple food in this country, pellagra does not occur.

Since most of the niacin in the diet is in the form of its coenzymes, it is relatively stable to light, heat and air and losses on cooking occur only by leaching into water.

Dietary Reference Value

The level of niacin needed to prevent or cure deficiency is 5.5 mg/1000 cal. On this basis, the RNI has been set at 6.6 mg/1000 cal for adult men and women. High doses of nicotinic acid (in excess of 200 mg/day) may cause vasodilatation, flushing and a fall in blood pressure.

Large doses (1 g/day) have been used in the treatment of hypercholesterolaemia; however, side effects, which include flushing, gastrointestinal discomfort and possible damage to the liver, mean that this is not a treatment of choice. At other times, niacin has been used as a treatment for chilblains and schizophrenia, although the benefits are uncertain. The total amount of niacin equivalents in the UK diet is reported as 36.95 mg (Bates, 2014), which represents 263% of the RNI.

Vitamin B_6

This vitamin was isolated as a cure for a scaly dermatitis seen in rats fed on purified diets. It is now clear that there are three closely related compounds that have biological activity. These are pyridoxine (found predominantly in plant foods), pyridoxal and pyridoxamine (both of which are present in animal foods, generally in the phosphorylated form) (Figure 4.7).

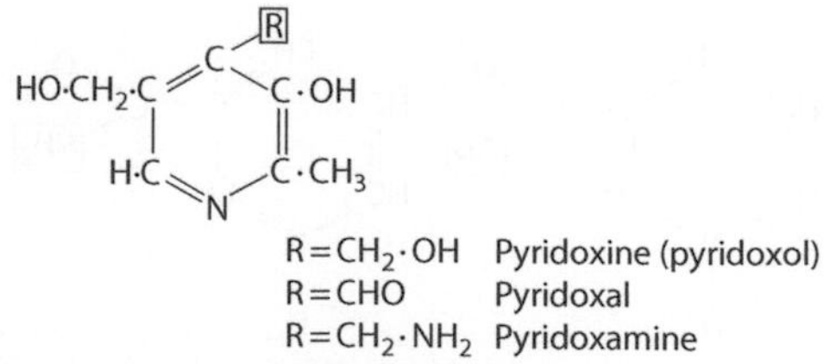

FIGURE 4.7 Structures of the three closely related compounds known as vitamin B6: pyridoxine, pyridoxal and pyridoxamine.

Sources of Vitamin B_6

Vitamin B_6 is widely distributed in small quantities in all animal and plant tissues. Rich sources are liver, whole cereals, meat (including poultry), peanuts, walnuts, bananas and salmon. Moderate amounts are found in vegetables, such as broccoli, spinach and potatoes. The availability from animal sources of the vitamin may be greater than that from plant sources, because of binding to glucoside. Vitamin B_6 is also susceptible to processing losses in heating, canning and freezing. It is estimated that between 10% and 50% may be lost in this way. Main contributors in the total diet are vegetables (32% of total), meat (30% of total) and cereals (25% of total). Beer may also make a useful contribution to the total intake of the vitamin.

Dietary Reference Value

Depletion studies have shown that deficiency develops faster on high protein intakes. The RNI has been set in relation to protein intake at 15 μg/g protein for both men and women. The elderly may have poorer rates of absorption and metabolism, but currently there is insufficient evidence to set a higher RNI.

Care should be taken with supplement use, as some cases of sensory neuropathy have been reported with chronic intakes of 100–200 mg/day. Mean daily intakes in the United Kingdom are 2.2 mg (Bates, 2014) accounting for 172% of the RNI.

Folate

This vitamin was originally identified as a factor present in yeast extract, which could cure a type of anaemia that had been described in pregnant women. This anaemia was similar to pernicious anaemia, with large macrocytic cells, but the lesions of the central nervous system were absent. The active agent was found in crude liver extract and in spinach and was thus named folate (from *foliage*).

Folate is now used as the generic name for the group of substances with related vitamin activity; this includes the synthetic form of the vitamin folic acid (or pteroyl glutamic acid) (Figure 4.8) and various polyglutamate forms (containing several glutamic acid residues) that are commonly present in foods, including the 5-methyl- and 10-methyltetrahydrofolates, which are the coenzyme forms of the vitamin.

Folate in Foods

Food is analyzed for folate content using a microbiological growth assay with *Lactobacillus rhamnosus* (formerly *Lactobacillus casei*). This may not always give an accurate measurement of the amount of folate obtainable by humans on ingestion of the food. New methods continue to be developed, for example, high-performance liquid chromatography and antibody-based techniques. Reference standards have also been developed, which should contribute to more reliable assays. However, at present, there is still uncertainty about the validity of figures for folate contents. The majority of food sources contain polyglutamates, with probably less than 25% being present as monoglutamate. Folic acid itself does not occur in nature and is used only in supplements and fortification.

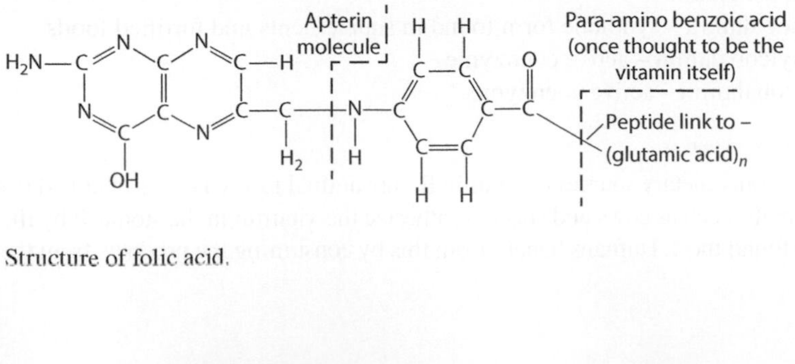

FIGURE 4.8 Structure of folic acid.

The richest dietary sources are green leafy vegetables (spinach, Brussels sprouts) and liver, with lower but useful amounts in broccoli, cabbage, cauliflower, parsnips, fortified cereals and bread, oranges and whole wheat. Folate intakes are, in general, correlated with income; families on a high income may have substantially more folate in their diet than those on a low income. Folate intake also correlates with vitamin C intakes, as many of the sources provide both of these vitamins. The main foods contributing to total intakes include cereals and cereal products, mainly as a result of fortification (31% of total intake) and vegetables, including potatoes (28% of total). Milk and fruit both provide small amounts (7% each). Beer intake can contribute important amounts of folate, as a result of its yeast content.

Folate in foods is susceptible to cooking losses; it is less soluble in water than many of the B vitamins, but is sensitive to heat, and, therefore, most cooking procedures will cause a loss of some of the vitamin. Keeping food hot for periods of time or reheating is particularly damaging and can destroy all of the folate originally present. The extent of loss will depend on the particular form of the folate in food. Folic acid itself is more stable chemically than natural folates in foods.

Dietary Reference Values

On the basis of surveys of habitual intakes of folate, liver and blood levels of folate and amounts that prevent deficiency, the RNI (DoH, 1991) is 200 μg/day for both men and women. A folate supplement of 400 μg is now recommended prior to and for the first 12 weeks of pregnancy. Mean intakes in studies in the United Kingdom were found to be 258 μg/day (Bates, 2014). Levels have increased since the mid-1980s with the gradual introduction of fortified products, especially breakfast cereals, and the increased consumption of fruit juices. The mean intake achieves 135% of the mean RNI, but there are groups identified by the National Food Survey, in whom the mean intake is just 100% of RNI. These are particularly found in large households and those with three or more children.

Increased requirements in pregnancy are covered in Chapter 6, pp. 104–109, while the folic acid supplementation campaign is covered in Chapter 19, pp. 377–379.

Vitamin B_{12}

The existence of vitamin B_{12} had been accepted since the 1920s, when it was found that a protein- and iron-free extract of liver given by injection could cure pernicious anaemia. However, the biologically active agent was not isolated and identified until 1948. An additional finding was the requirement for a factor in gastric juice, which would enable the vitamin B_{12} to be absorbed when it was given by mouth. For this reason, dietary treatment with liver previously had to use very large amounts (of raw liver) on a daily basis to provide any improvement. Even at this stage, there was some confusion with folate, as some of the signs of deficiency are similar for both the vitamins. It is now recognized that vitamin B_{12} is needed to release folate from its methyl form so that it can function as a carrier of single-carbon units. However, not all of the functions of vitamin B_{12} are associated with folate.

Vitamin B_{12} is the name given to a group of compounds called the corrinoids; their characteristic feature is the presence of an atom of cobalt in the centre of four reduced pyrrole rings. Four important forms are recognized:

- Hydroxocobalamin
- Cyanocobalamin – synthetic form found in supplements and fortified foods
- Adenosylcobalamin – active coenzyme
- Methylcobalamin – active coenzyme

Vitamin B_{12} in Foods

For humans, the only dietary sources of vitamin B_{12} are animal foods; none is obtained from plant foods. Ruminant animals, such as cows and sheep, synthesize the vitamin in the stomach by the actions of the bacterial flora found there. Humans benefit from this by consuming the products from these animals.

Trace amounts of the vitamin may occur in a plant-only diet, resulting from contaminating yeasts, bacteria or faecal contamination of water sources. The richest sources are animal livers, where the vitamin is stored in life. Meat, eggs, milk and dairy products contain smaller concentrations.

It is essential that vegans, who exclude all animal foods from their diet, should have an alternative source of vitamin B_{12}. Most vegans are aware of this and supplement their diet either with a specific vitamin supplement or vitamin-enriched products. Excess amounts of vitamin C can interfere with vitamin B_{12} availability, converting it to an inactive form; care needs to be taken with high levels of intake.

Dietary Reference Value

Turnover of the vitamin is very slow and conservation is very efficient; thus, it is difficult to induce deficiency. Evidence for the level of requirement is based on habitual intakes and responses to the treatment in pernicious anaemia. The RNI has, therefore, been set at 1.5 mg/day for adult men and women; this is believed to be sufficient to produce stores that would allow the subject to withstand a period of low intake. Mean intake in the United Kingdom is 5.15 μg/day (or 369% of the RNI). This is predominantly derived from meat and fish (38% of total intake) and milk and cheese (45% of intake).

Pantothenic Acid (Vitamin B_5)

The name for this member of the B group of vitamins derives from the Greek word for *everywhere*, suggesting that it is widespread. Biochemically, it is part of the coenzyme A molecule, which plays a role in the metabolic pathways for all the macronutrients. It is, therefore, central to energy transformations in the cell.

Deficiency has only been studied when induced experimentally. It includes a diverse and unspecific number of symptoms. An abnormal sensation in the feet and lower legs, termed 'burning foot syndrome', has been attributed to pantothenic acid deficiency in malnourished patients, as it responded to the treatment with the vitamin. In rats, pantothenic acid deficiency was associated with loss of colour from the fur, and the vitamin is still included in some shampoos as an anti-grey hair factor, although there is no evidence that it has this role in humans.

No dietary reference value has been set, although it has been noted that mean intake in the United Kingdom is 5.4 mg/day. Main sources are meat, cereals and vegetables.

Biotin (Vitamin B_7)

Deficiency of biotin (a member of the B group of vitamins) can be induced experimentally by the feeding of raw egg white. This contains avidin, which has a high binding affinity for biotin and makes it unavailable for absorption. The clinical signs include loss of hair and a fine scaly dermatitis. Biotin is needed as a cofactor for several carboxylase enzymes, which carry carbon dioxide units in metabolic pathways. Carboxylases occur in the metabolism of all the major macronutrients, and hence biotin has a widespread role.

Biotin occurs in many foods: the richest sources are egg yolks, liver, grains and legumes. There is also significant synthesis of biotin by the bacterial flora in the colon, although whether this is available or not is unclear.

Occasional cases of biotin deficiency have been reported in subjects with unusual dietary practices and unbalanced total parenteral nutrition or in severe malabsorption consequent on bowel disease or alcoholism. Deficiency has also been reported in epileptics treated with some of the common anticonvulsant drugs.

Intakes of biotin in Britain average 26–39 mg/day; in the absence of deficiency, these appear to be adequate. Main contributors to the diet are cereals, eggs, meat and milk (together with beer, usually greater in men).

Vitamin C

The function of vitamins as antioxidants are covered in Chapter 14, pp. 271–289, in relation to cardiovascular disease; in Chapter 15, pp. 293–310, in relation to cancer; and in Chapter 22, pp. 421–431, in relation to sport and exercise.

As early as 1601, it was known that oranges and lemons or fresh green vegetables could protect a person against scurvy, a disease that broke out after several months of a diet devoid of fresh vegetables or fruit. The disease was a particular problem for sailors in the sixteenth to eighteenth centuries, when long sea voyages of discovery were being made. Classical experiments by James Lind in 1747 compared the curative properties of cider, hydrochloric acid, vinegar, seawater and oranges and lemons in sailors suffering from scurvy. Only those eating the citrus fruits recovered, within 1 week. However, the inclusion of citrus fruits and attention to adequate fresh vegetables was by no means routine thereafter in expeditions, and even Scott's expedition to the South Pole at the beginning of the twentieth century came to a tragic end because of scurvy. Populations in Europe throughout the Middle Ages suffered scurvy during the winter months, and it was probably the introduction and rapid rise in popularity of the potato in the sixteenth century that contributed most to the decline of this disease.

It is important to remember, however, that scurvy is still present nowadays among refugees around the world, in relief camps where the diet does not provide adequate vitamin C, but also in developed countries, especially among most deprived groups. It has been reported among teenagers eating highly refined diets and among the homeless of Britain.

Two forms of the vitamin have biological activity: these are ascorbic acid (Figure 4.9) and its oxidized derivative, dehydroascorbic acid. The two forms are interconvertible and are collectively termed vitamin C. If further oxidation takes place, the vitamin loses its potency.

Vitamin C is unique among the vitamins in that it is essential as a vitamin for only a few animal species; most members of the animal kingdom can synthesize vitamin C from glucose and have no dietary requirement for it. The exceptions are the primates, including humans, and the guinea pig, together with a fruit-eating bat and a rare bird. It has been calculated that primates originally had the gene to perform this synthesis, but the ability was lost some 70 million years ago.

Sources of Vitamin C

Most dietary vitamin C is supplied by fruit and vegetables. Only very small amounts come from animal sources, mostly from milk, although levels here may be reduced by pasteurization and other processing.

Among the fruits, the richest sources are blackcurrants and rosehips, but for the general population, oranges (and orange juice) probably provide most of the vitamin. Other sources are mangoes, papayas and strawberries. Vegetable sources include green peppers, broccoli, cauliflower and Brussels sprouts. Potatoes have a varying content of vitamin C: new potatoes are rich in the vitamin, but content declines as the storage time increases. Traditionally, potatoes have been a very important source of the vitamin in UK diets. However, potato consumption has fallen markedly in Britain, and other sources of vitamin C, notably fruit juice, have become more common, resulting in a changing profile of vitamin C intake.

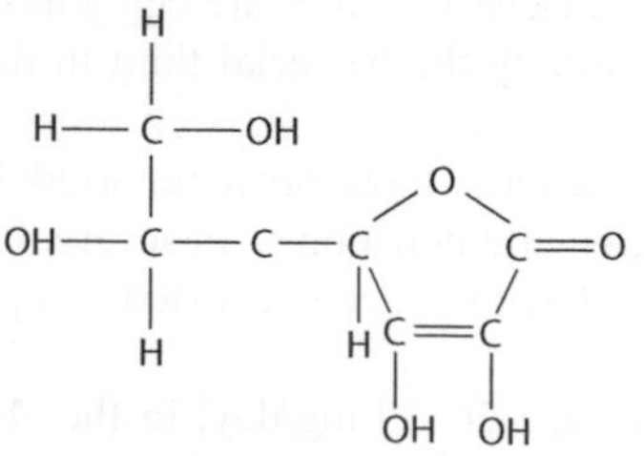

FIGURE 4.9 Structure of ascorbic acid.

Vitamin C is readily lost on cooking and processing. It is probably the least stable of all the vitamins, and its destruction is accelerated by exposure to light, alkali, air and heat. Therefore, most parts of the food preparation process may cause some loss of the vitamin. Anyone who is involved in preparing fruit and vegetables should consider the following ways of conserving vitamin C:

- Handle food with care, with minimum bruising when cutting, to prevent release of oxidizing enzymes.
- Immerse vegetables directly into boiling water to destroy the enzymes and thus protect the vitamin; this is also true of immersion into hot fat (e.g. in the cooking of potato chips).
- Cover the saucepan with a lid to reduce exposure to air.
- Use a small volume of water, or preferably steam, to minimize the leaching of vitamin into water; if the cooking water can subsequently be used, then the vitamin C may still be included in the meal.
- Avoid adding sodium bicarbonate, which enhances the green colour of some vegetables but destroys much of the vitamin C.
- Avoid keeping vegetables hot after cooking, as this continues the destruction of the vitamin, so that almost none may remain after 1 hour. This is a particular problem when food is cooked in bulk and kept hot on serving counters during a service period which may span 1–2 hours.

Vitamin C in fruit is subject to much less destruction, as the lower pH in acidic fruits protects the vitamin. However, fruit juice loses its vitamin content if left to stand in the refrigerator after squeezing or after opening of a carton. The best way to maximize intake of vitamin C from fruit and vegetables is to consume as many as possible in their raw form.

Dietary Reference Value

The requirement for vitamin C may be defined in terms of the amount needed to prevent scurvy: the majority of studies agree that an intake of 10 mg/day will be preventive. Further increases in intake do not increase plasma levels until the intake reaches 40 mg/day, when measurable amounts start to appear in the plasma. This level of intake has, therefore, been set as the RNI by the DoH (DoH, 1991), as indicative of sufficient supply of the vitamin to distribute to the tissues.

In the United Kingdom, the mean vitamin C intake is 83 mg/day, which represents 213% of the mean RNI (Bates, 2014). Intakes were lowest in Scotland, Northern Ireland and North West England and also in lower income households. There is a recommendation that smokers should consume up to 80 mg/day more than the RNI, to allow for the increased needs. In terms of optimal intakes, 200 mg/day has been suggested, which will achieve a saturation level of the vitamin in the plasma. More work is needed to support this proposal.

Contributors to vitamin C intake were as follows:

Vegetables	28.5%
Soft drinks	22%
Fruit	20%
Potatoes	8.5%
Milk	6%

PHYTOCHEMICALS

Vegetables and fruit have been promoted as part of a healthy diet for many years, and, since the 1990s, there has been specific advice to include five portions, or 400 g, of these in the daily diet. Both fruit and vegetables contain a number of valuable nutrients, but, in addition, it has been recognized that they are rich in non-nutritive substances, known as phytochemicals (sometimes referred to as vitamin P). These occur in plants and plant-based foods and products made from plants at varying concentrations. Amounts are relatively low in the storage parts of plants, higher in the fruiting parts, and highest in the seeds and parts that are dried and concentrated for use as herbs and spices. The latter, however, are generally used in small amounts and, therefore, may not represent an important dietary source. Several different mechanisms of action have been identified; these are briefly reviewed in the following sections.

Phenolic Compounds, Including Flavonoids

Higher concentrations of phenolic compounds are generally found in young sprouting plants or seedlings than in the mature plant, in line with their role as protection against predators. Immature fruit, such as apple or grapefruit, are very bitter because of the presence of these compounds.

There are over 5000 different flavonoids, many of which are responsible for the colour of flowers, leaves and fruit. They are generally bitter or astringent. The various flavonoids differ according to their molecular structure and occur in different sources. Flavonols, including rutin and quercetin, are found in apple skins, broccoli, grapes, olives, onions and parsley. Quercetin, which mainly occurs in foods as a glycoside, is the most important contributor to the estimated intake of flavonoids, mainly from the consumption of apples and onions. Flavanones, including hesperetin, are predominantly found in citrus fruit and their peel and contribute to the bitterness of these fruit. The catechins occur in green and black tea, cocoa and red wine (from both the seeds and skins of grapes). Finally, included in this group are anthocyanins, which occur in blue and purple coloured fruit such as berries, cherries, grapes. Isoflavones are mainly found in soy-based products and include daidzein and genistein (more detail in the next section). Other minor flavonoid subclasses include the flavones, coumarins, chalcones and aurones. Non-flavonoid polyphenols include the phenolic acids, the hydroxycinnamic acids (such as chlorogenic, caffeic and ferulic acid) and the stilbenes (including resveratrol).

In addition, high-molecular-weight polyphenols, also known as tannins, are found in sorghum, millet, barley, peas, dry beans and legumes, fruit, tea and wine. Tannins form insoluble complexes with proteins and starches and can reduce the nutritional value of foods.

While often researched in the past for their antioxidant activity, limiting the production of reactive oxygen species and scavenging free radicals, recent research has shifted focus towards the potential of polyphenolics and their metabolites as regulator of transcription, particularly in relation to inflammation. Further evidence also points toward a potential prebiotic (bifidogenic) effect. More research on phenolic compounds and flavonoids is required, together with more information about the bioavailability of the compounds and the development of sensitive techniques for the measurement of intake and excretion levels.

Digestion and absorption of polyphenolics is covered in Chapter 10, pp. 212–213.

In the meantime, it is important that the known dietary sources of these compounds are encouraged in the diet, to maximize the diversity of intake and potential derived benefits.

Dietary Phytoestrogens

Phytoestrogens are present in plant foods; the two major subclasses are isoflavones and lignans. The majority of interest has been focused on the isoflavones, of which the major examples are genistein and daidzein, which are found in soya beans and products derived from them including textured vegetable protein, tofu and soya milk. The richest source of lignans is flaxseed (linseed); however, many fibre-rich foods contain small amounts, including lentils, sweet potato and oat bran. More accurate analytical data are still needed. A more potent phytoestrogen has recently been discovered in hops, and more sources may yet be discovered.

Phytoestrogens have been shown to exert a wide range of hormonal and non-hormonal effects in animal and *in vitro* studies. In addition, epidemiological evidence indicates that, in Asian countries, where the habitual daily intake of isoflavones is between 20 and 50 mg/day, there is a lower incidence in women of many hormone-dependent diseases, such as coronary heart disease, menopausal symptoms, osteoporosis and breast cancer. Women in communities where soya beans are eaten tend to have longer menstrual cycles, by 1–2 days. This can relate to 2 fewer years of menstruating life, less ovarian activity and possibly reduced breast cancer risk. In Japanese men, the incidence of clinical prostate cancer is significantly lower than in American men, and prostatic tumours develop more slowly. Benefits in terms of coronary heart disease and osteoporosis also apply in men.

Interest in the phytoestrogens arose because of their structural similarity to mammalian oestrogen. The compounds were shown to act both as oestrogen agonists (mimicking the effects of the hormone), as well as antagonists (blocking the action of the hormone). The varying effects are attributable to the existence of two different oestrogen receptors in specific tissues, which result in varied responses. Target tissues include the breast, ovaries and uterus, brain, bone, lungs, blood vessels, kidneys, adrenals, testes and prostate. In addition to oestrogen-related responses, phytoestrogens have also been shown to alter steroid metabolism, increase sex hormone binding in the blood, act as antioxidants and reduce thrombogenesis. At present, these effects have not been fully tested in clinical studies, although small short-term studies have reported benefits in menopausal symptoms and bone loss. There is much to discover about the bioavailability of the phytoestrogens from dietary sources, the levels achieved in the blood and at active sites and the amounts required to produce a clinical effect. Studies also indicate that there is considerable individual variation in the metabolic fate of the compounds, and this may make recommendations about dosage very difficult to predict. These compounds represent a challenge to the functional food market, in trying to balance a beneficial health effect with acceptability and safety. One of the problems with soya products is their bitterness; the food industry makes attempts to reduce this, but may at the same time remove the beneficial isoflavones.

Phytosterols

Phytosterols are compounds that are structurally similar to cholesterol and are currently being used in a range of products as cholesterol-lowering agents. Phytosterols are thought to have been present in the diet of our ancestors in much greater amounts than occurs currently. Intakes of naturally occurring plant sterols are higher in vegetarians than in omnivores. The plant sterols currently used are extracted from soya bean oil or pine tree oil and are esterified to increase solubility. The most common are sitosterol, campesterol and stigmasterol. Products may contain plant sterol (unsaturated) or plant stanol (saturated) esters, and evidence shows that both have a similar capacity to lower circulating total and low-density lipoprotein (LDL) cholesterol levels.

These effects are achieved with relatively small doses of the phytosterols. As little as 1 g/day may have an effective lipid-lowering effect, although a dose of 1.6 g/day of plant sterol is recommended. There appears to be a plateau effect with no further reduction of cholesterol seen at intakes above 3 g/day. The average reduction in cholesterol levels is in the region of 5%–8% from spread alone, and, when combined with other lipid-lowering measures in the diet, or drug treatments, levels of cholesterol may be reduced by 10%–15%. The dispersal of the phytosterol within the food product appears to be the key determinant of its effectiveness.

Although developed as an aid to the management of blood lipids levels in cardiovascular disease reduction, new evidence suggests that the plant sterols may also have a role in inhibition of tumour growth.

Plant sterols and stanols are currently marketed as a range of spreads, dairy goods, such as yogurt and cream cheese, and salad dressing.

Glucosinolates

These compounds occur mostly in the cruciferous vegetables (cabbage family), including broccoli, cauliflower, turnips, Brussels sprouts, cabbage and kale. *In vitro* studies suggest that glucosinolate compounds, such as sinigrin and progoitrin, induce enzymes that inactivate carcinogens by neutralizing their toxic properties and speeding their elimination from the body. In addition, products derived from glucosinolates during digestion, including isothiocyanates, are also reported to block the effects of carcinogens. Clinical studies have so far not been able to support these findings. However, diets high in cruciferous (and other) vegetables are linked in epidemiological studies with lower cancer rates, including lung and alimentary tract. One of the major practical problems for food scientists is the bitter taste of many of the vegetables in this family. Selective breeding, genetic modification and alteration of growing conditions are all being used to decrease bitterness and increase consumer acceptability, while protecting the content of active agents.

Carotenoids

Carotenoids are fat-soluble pigments found in many fresh fruit and vegetables. Initially, they were of nutritional interest because of the role of beta-carotene as a major precursor of vitamin A in the body; other carotenoids have lower levels of provitamin A activity. The total amount of carotenoids taken up from the diet is relatively small and a regular intake appears to optimize absorption. It is now known that some 600 carotenoids exist and at least 40 have been isolated in foods. The association between plasma levels of beta-carotene and cardiovascular disease has been reported in a number of epidemiological studies. However, supplementation trials using beta-carotene have not replicated the beneficial results. For example, the Carotene and Retinol Efficacy Trial study in smokers resulted unexpectedly in a higher incidence of lung cancer and heart disease (Omenn et al., 1996). Mechanisms behind the deleterious effect of beta-carotene in supplementation trials in smokers have not been fully elucidated and may involve beta-carotene acting as a pro-oxidant.

It should be remembered that antioxidants donate an electron to stabilize a free radical. In so doing, the antioxidant itself becomes unstable, with the potential to become a free radical and propagate a chain reaction. It is essential, therefore, that there are other antioxidants to repair and maintain the system. One such agent is believed to be vitamin C. This illustrates the importance of having adequate and comparable levels of various antioxidants in the body and may explain why large amounts of one of these may be more harmful than protective. Thus, any supplement that provides additional carotenoids should also contain adequate vitamin C.

Lycopene, an acyclic form of beta-carotene, has been found to be a more potent antioxidant than beta-carotene itself. *In vitro* studies suggest that it protects LDL against oxidation. Lycopene is one of the major carotenoids in the Western diet, being found in tomato and tomato products. Intake levels are lower in developing countries. Other sources include pink grapefruit, watermelon, guava and apricot. An epidemiological association has been reported between low plasma levels of lycopene and prostate cancer in the United States. A study in Finland recently reported an excess incidence of acute coronary events and stroke in association with low levels of lycopene.

Lutein is a major pigment in chloroplasts and, as such, is one of the five most common carotenoids in the diet. Together with zeaxanthin (which is similar in structure), it is found in the macular region of the eye, which is the region of the highest visual discrimination, but also the most light-sensitive area. This area is, therefore, very vulnerable to damage by free radicals produced by light interacting with oxygen in the blood. Over time, this can result in macular generation (age-related macular degeneration) and blindness. This is the most common cause of blindness in Western society. It is particularly common in smokers, in whom levels of lutein have been shown to be lower than the population average. Lutein absorbs blue light and, as an antioxidant, quenches free radicals. Lutein cannot be synthesized in the body and, therefore, a dietary intake is needed to maintain serum levels;

active transport mechanisms concentrate lutein in the macula. There are high levels of lutein in breast milk. In addition, lutein is found in green leafy vegetables and in orange/yellow fruit and vegetables.

All of the phytochemicals discussed earlier have potential roles in risk reduction and health promotion. The evidence for most of them is, at present, based largely on *in vitro* or animal studies, with a limited number of clinical studies. However, epidemiological data support the link between intakes of fruit and vegetables in the prevention of a number of diseases. Food scientists can develop varieties in which the active agents are enhanced, but, in the mean time, five servings a day of fruit and vegetables remains sound nutritional advice.

USE OF VITAMIN AND OTHER NUTRITIONAL SUPPLEMENTS

Use of vitamin and other nutritional supplements may be indicated in very some specific instances, for example, where there is clinical deficiency as seen in iron deficiency anaemia; due to a disease state where requirements are enhanced or absorption compromised, as in Crohn's disease; or at a particular stage of life when physiological factors can affect needs, as seen with folate requirements in pregnancy. However, for most healthy individuals, there is very little evidence to suggest that use of supplements can promote health and performance or protect against future chronic diseases such as cardiovascular disease and cancer. There is some epidemiological evidence to suggest associations between the use of supplements and disease prevention; however, the quality of evidence is low, and the limited number of randomized control trials in this area has failed to support such findings. Indeed there is evidence to suggest that use of supplements could actually be harmful, particularly for high doses of antioxidants and multivitamins which have been linked positively to all-cause mortality.

The evidence for and against the use of nutritional supplements is by no means conclusive and is often dependent on the baseline nutritional status, health and lifestyle of study participants. The nutritional advice remains that a nutritionally balanced diet can (and should) provide all the essential vitamins and minerals the human body requires, and this in combination with our capacity to tightly regulate micronutrient levels through homeostatic processes can ensure optimal micronutrient levels in the body.

SUMMARY

1. The fat-soluble vitamins perform diverse functions, acting as regulators of metabolic reactions (vitamin D and K), protective agents (vitamin E) or constituents of essential chemicals in the body (vitamin A).
2. New roles are emerging for these vitamins as metabolic regulators at the nuclear level, perhaps involved in gene expression.
3. Adequate levels of these vitamins are required, although excessive amounts are stored in the body and may be toxic.
4. The water-soluble vitamins perform many key functions in the body; without them, there is a considerable risk of failure of specific metabolic functions. Several of the vitamins act cooperatively, for example, folate and vitamin B_{12}, riboflavin and niacin, and vitamin B_6 and niacin.
5. Many of the water-soluble vitamins are sensitive to cooking procedures and may be lost in substantial amounts. Care should be exercised when preparing foods that are important sources of these vitamins.
6. Several of the vitamins occur in similar foods:
   - Meats provide thiamin, niacin, riboflavin and vitamin B_{12}.
   - Milk and dairy products are important sources of riboflavin and vitamin B_{12}.
   - Cereals provide thiamin, niacin and folate and vitamin E.

- Fruits and vegetables are important sources of vitamin C and folate, as well as carotenes and vitamin K.
- Thus, omitting one of these groups of foods can have implications for more than one nutrient. A balanced diet, prepared with care, will ensure that all of these vitamins are supplied.

7. Supplementation with some vitamins, for example, folate, may have positive health benefits and more research is ongoing in this area.
8. Plant products are rich in polyphenolic compounds and other phytochemicals, which may exert a range of beneficial effect on heath and disease. However, more research is required to understand their mode(s) of action.

STUDY QUESTIONS

1. A 25-year-old mother with three young children, aged 2, 4 and 6 years, is concerned that she is not giving them a balanced diet, as most of what they eat is made up of simple convenience foods. She herself tends to eat with the children and often finishes their leftovers. She feels tired and depressed. She asks if the whole family should take supplements of vitamins and/or minerals. What do you think?
2. Consider the various reasons why the following may not meet their vitamin requirements:
   a. A college student, living in self-catering accommodation
   b. A middle-aged man, working long hours and living alone
   c. A recently bereaved, elderly woman
3. Construct tables to compare common features (e.g. functions, sources, signs of deficiency) of the following pairs of vitamins:
   a. Riboflavin and niacin
   b. Vitamin B_{12} and folate
   c. Vitamins C and E
4. Can you identify any other vitamins that might share features in common with any of the pairs in Q.3?

ACTIVITY

4.1 Build a mind map articulating the arguments for and against whole population supplementation with Vitamin D in Scotland (United Kingdom), France and the Seychelles.

BIBLIOGRAPHY AND FURTHER READING

Bates, B., Lennox, A., Prentice, A., Bates, C., Page, P., Nicholson, S. and Swan, G. 2014. National diet and nutrition survey results from years 1, 2, 3 and 4 (combined) of the rolling programme (2008/2009–2011/2012). London, UK: Public Health England.

Bjelakovic, G., Nikolova, D. and Gluud, C. 2013. Meta-regression analyses, meta-analyses, and trial sequential analyses of the effects of supplementation with beta-carotene, vitamin A, and vitamin E singly or in different combinations on all-cause mortality: Do we have evidence for lack of harm? *PLoS One* 8(9), e74558.

Bogan, K.L. and Brenner, C. 2008. Nicotinic acid nicotinamide and nicotinamide riboside: A molecular evaluation of NAD(+) precursor vitamins in human nutrition. *Annual Review of Nutrition* 28, 115–130.

Carpenter, T.O., Herreros, F., Zhang, J.H. et al. 2012. Demographic, dietary, and biochemical determinants of vitamin D status in inner-city children. *American Journal of Clinical Nutrition* 95, 137–146.

Cashman, K.D., Fitzgerald, A.P., Kiely, M. et al. 2011. A systematic review and meta-regression analysis of the vitamin D intake-serum 25-hydroxyvitamin D relationship to inform European recommendations. *British Journal of Nutrition* 106, 1638–1648.

Combet, E. and Buckton, C. 2015. Micronutrient deficiencies, vitamin pills and nutritional supplements. *Medicine* 43(2), 66–72.

D'Ambrosio, D.N., Clugston, R.D. and Blaner, W.S. 2011. Vitamin A metabolism: An update. *Nutrients* 3, 63–103.

European Food Safety Authority, Scientific Committee on Food. 2006. Tolerable upper intake levels for vitamins and minerals. Available at: http://www.efsa.europa.eu/en/ndatopics/docs/ndatolerableuil.pdf (accessed June 2015).

Expert Group on Vitamins and Minerals. 2003. *Safe Upper Levels for Vitamins and Minerals.* Food Standards Agency Publications, London, UK.

Okarter, N. and Liu, R.H. 2010. Health benefits of whole grain phytochemicals. *Critical Reviews in Food Science and Nutrition* 50, 193–208.

Scientific Advisory Committee on Nutrition. 2005. *Review of Dietary Advice on Vitamin A.* London, UK: The Stationnary Office.

Scientific Advisory Committee on Nutrition. 2006. *Folate and Disease Prevention.* London, UK: The Stationnary Office.

Shea, M.K. and Booth, S.L. 2008. Update on the role of vitamin K in skeletal health. *Nutrition Reviews* 66, 549–557.

Thane, C.W., Bolton-Smith, C. and Coward, A. 2006. Comparative dietary intake and sources of phylloquinone (vitamin K1) among British adults in 1986–7 and 2000–1. *British Journal of Nutrition* 96, 1105–1115.

Thane, C.W., Paul, A.A., Bates, C.J. et al. 2002. Intake and sources of phylloquinone (vitamin K1): Variation with socio-demographic and lifestyle factors in a national sample of British elderly people. *British Journal of Nutrition* 87, 605–613.

Webb, A.R., Kift, R., Durkin, M.T. et al. 2010. The role of sunlight exposure in determining the vitamin D status of the U.K. white adult population. *British Journal of Dermatology* 163, 1050–1055.

Zamora-Ros, R., Knaze, V., Lujan-Barroso, L. et al. 2011. Estimated dietary intakes of flavonols, flavanones and flavones in the European Prospective Investigation into Cancer and Nutrition (EPIC) 24 hour dietary recall cohort. *British Journal of Nutrition* 106, 1915–1925.

5 Minerals, Electrolytes and Fluid

AIMS

The aims of this chapter are to

- Identify the major elements found in the human body and main food sources.
- Describe the functions of each element and consider the interactions between certain elements.
- Examine the importance of fluids and discuss the body's need for fluid and how this can be met.
- Discuss the causes of an inadequate intake of specific minerals in certain groups of the population.
- Describe the rationale for the levels of inorganic minerals given as reference values.

MINERALS

This chapter considers the substances that appear in food analyses as ash. These are the substances that are left behind when the carbon, hydrogen and nitrogen have all been burnt away in the presence of oxygen as, for example, in a bomb calorimeter. Commonly called minerals, these substances occur in nature in water, in the soil and in rocks and are taken up by the roots of plants and thereby find their way into animals. Humans, therefore, consume minerals both from plant and animal sources, although foods of animal origin generally have a higher content as the minerals have been concentrated in the tissues.

The body contains about 22 known minerals, of which the majority are believed to be essential to life. Those that are considered to be nutritionally important are shown in Table 5.1. Their amounts in the human body and in food have an extraordinarily wide range, from over 1 kg of calcium in an adult to 5–10 mg of chromium. Altogether, they account for 4% of the weight of the body.

Some of the minerals are present in the body as contaminants from the environment and, as far as is known at present, have no essential function in the body. These include vanadium, arsenic, mercury, silicon, tin, nickel, boron, lithium, cadmium and lead.

The major minerals are those present in amounts greater than 5 g; this applies to calcium and phosphorus. Also of great importance, although present in rather smaller quantities, are the electrolytes, namely sodium, potassium and chlorine (as chloride ion). Although sulphur is listed, it does not occur freely in the body but is an essential component of the sulphur-containing amino acids.

In addition, there are the trace minerals that together amount to approximately 15 g. Although present in small amounts, those trace substances are vital for particular functions in the body.

The minerals have several features in common:

- They exist in the body in one of two forms:
  - As biological components – in the skeleton, in haemoglobin, in thyroid hormones and in many enzymes.
  - In their ionized state in the body fluids, where they serve to maintain homeostasis. Whichever of these forms occurs, the minerals retain their chemical identity.

TABLE 5.1
Average Amounts of Minerals Found in the Adult Human Body

Minerals	Total Body Content
Major minerals	
Calcium	1200 g
Phosphorus	780 g
Potassium	110–137 g
Sulphur	175 g
Sodium	92 g
Chloride	84 g
Magnesium	25 g
Trace minerals	
Iron	4.0 g
Zinc	2.0 g
Manganese	12–20 mg
Copper	80 mg
Iodide	15–20 mg
Chromium	<2.0 mg
Cobalt	1.5 mg
Selenium	3–30 mg

- Once in the body, it is sometimes difficult for the mineral to be excreted. Those that dissolve in water can be excreted in the urine; others are excreted in the faeces, either by being secreted into the digestive tract (usually in bile) or by being lost when cells are shed from the intestinal lining. Toxic minerals are harmful in the body because they may be difficult to excrete without the use of dedicated drugs to chelate and remove them. In addition, those that are similar in size and properties to the essential minerals may displace them. This is what happens when strontium and caesium find their way into bones and milk in place of calcium.
- Minerals are generally resistant to heat, air and acid, which is why they remain when a food has been burned in a bomb calorimeter. This also means that they are rarely lost during food preparation procedures, although the ones that are water soluble can be lost into cooking water.
- A problem with some minerals is that they are found in food as large complexes attached to a number of different compounds. Probably the most prevalent is inositol hexaphosphate (phytate), which is found in cereals, legumes and nuts and which binds calcium, iron and zinc. This interferes with their absorption in the digestive tract, reducing their bioavailability. A similar problem can occur where minerals are present in foods containing large amounts of dietary fibre (non-starch polysaccharides [NSPs]).
- Some minerals interfere with the absorption of other minerals, competing for the same carrier mechanism in the digestive tract. For example, large amounts of calcium may interfere with the absorption of iron and magnesium, and zinc can reduce absorption of iron and copper. For these reasons, taking supplements of one mineral may cause an imbalance of other minerals in the body.

Details on absorption of minerals are covered in Chapter 10, pp. 204–210, while the role of the minerals in the body, and in health and diseases, is covered in Chapter 12, pp. 244–251.

Major Minerals

Calcium

Calcium is the most abundant mineral present in the body, amounting to almost 40% of the total mineral mass. The majority is present in bone where, together with phosphorus (as hydroxyapatite $Ca_{10}(PO_4)_6(OH)_2$), it plays an essential part in hardening the skeleton and teeth. In addition, this calcium is a reserve of the mineral for its role in body fluids as ionic calcium, which is essential for nerve impulse transmission, muscle contraction and blood clotting.

See Chapter 8 for a detailed account on the role of calcium in bone health through the life cycle, pp. 165–168.

Sources of Calcium

The main dietary sources of calcium are milk and dairy products. For vegetarians who do not use dairy products, tofu set with calcium salts or calcium-enriched soya milk may be important sources of calcium. In addition, cereals and cereal products may supply a reasonable amount of calcium, although this may be less well absorbed from wholegrain cereals owing to the presence of NSP and phytate. All wheat flour in the United Kingdom, with the exception of wholemeal has, since 1943, been fortified with calcium carbonate by law and provides the equivalent of 94–156 mg calcium/100 g of flour. Although a number of expert reports have in recent years considered this addition to be no longer necessary, it currently remains in force. Green leafy vegetables, such as spinach, broccoli and kale, contain good amounts of calcium, but its absorption may be inhibited by the presence of oxalates.

Other sources of calcium may include small fish, such as sardines, whose bones (when eaten) supply calcium, dried figs, nuts (e.g. almonds, Brazil nuts), parsley, watercress and black treacle. Unless these foods form a major part of the diet, their contribution to the total dietary intake will be small.

In parts of the world where the water is hard (i.e. contains many dissolved salts), it can supply a significant amount of calcium to the day's intake.

Dietary Reference Values

These are difficult to determine, as there is no single satisfactory approach. The figures recommended in Report 41 (DoH, 1991) are, therefore, based on the factorial approach, taking into account needs for growth and maintenance. The average absorption is assumed to be 30%; the reference nutrient intake (RNI) for adults is 700 mg/day. There are no specific recommendations made to take into account possible health implications.

Calcium in the British Diet

Daily intakes in the United Kingdom, reported by the National Diet and Nutrition Survey Results of the Rolling Programme (2008/2009–2011/2012), are 825 mg. This represents 118% of the mean RNI; however, 14% of children 11–18 years do not meet the lower reference nutrient intake (LRNI). The main contribution comes from cereals and cereal products (37%) and milk and milk products (35%).

Calcium Excretion

Calcium is lost from the body via the faeces and urine, with very small amounts lost in sweat. Loss in the faeces represents the calcium unabsorbed from the diet, together with endogenous calcium from digestive secretions, especially bile and cells shed into the digestive tract, amounting to approximately 100 mg/day. Total losses in the faeces, therefore, depend on the amount consumed.

Urinary calcium represents the final adjustment of plasma calcium levels, with the majority (up to 97%) of the calcium filtered being reabsorbed by the renal tubules.

Levels of Urinary Calcium Are Increased	Levels of Urinary Calcium Are Decreased
By a high protein diet	In old age
On a high calcium intake	By a high potassium intake
By high sodium intake	By a high magnesium intake
In women at the menopause	By a high phosphorus intake

Phosphorus

Phosphorus is often considered together with calcium, as both are present in the bone. In blood, they have a reciprocal relationship and are controlled by similar mechanisms. Phosphorus is widely available in both animal and plant foods including meat, poultry, fish, eggs and dairy products and in cereals, nuts and legumes. Small amounts occur in tea and coffee. It is widely present as a food additive in bakery goods, processed meats and soft drinks.

Phosphorus in the Body

Second only to calcium, phosphorus is abundant in the human body with about 85% found in the bones and teeth. It is found as hydroxyapatite in calcified tissues, as phospholipids in biological membranes, and in nucleotides and nucleic acid. Phosphorus is also needed for the maintenance of normal pH, storage and transfer of energy and the activation of catalytic enzymes by phosphorylation.

As such, it is required for the growth, maintenance and repair of all tissues and cells and for the production of the genetic material DNA and RNA.

Intakes of phosphorus in the United Kingdom average 1.2–1.3 g/day; a minimum intake of 400 mg/day had been proposed to maintain adequate plasma phosphate levels. The RNI (DoH, 1991) is given as 550 mg/day for adults, based on an equimolar ratio with calcium intakes. Intakes may be low in premature infants, vegans, alcoholics and people who use aluminium-containing antacids regularly.

Magnesium

The human body contains approximately 25 g of magnesium, of which 60% is found in the bones, the remainder in the soft tissues, with 1% in the extracellular fluid. It is the most abundant divalent intracellular ion.

The food sources of magnesium include whole grain cereal, nuts, legumes, seafoods, coffee, tea, cocoa and chocolate. Chlorophyll found in green leafy vegetables contains magnesium. Intakes in the United Kingdom are reported to be around 289 mg/day.

Magnesium in the Body

The magnesium found in bones is thought to act as a reservoir to sustain plasma levels. The remaining magnesium is largely found in the muscle and other soft tissues. It occurs as part of cell membranes but is also an essential activator of more than 300 enzyme systems. Most notably, it is involved in all enzyme systems utilizing ATP. In addition, magnesium is involved in protein synthesis, energy production, muscle contraction and nerve impulse transmission.

Sulphur

Sulphur enters the body as the sulphur-containing amino acids methionine and cysteine. The sulphur-containing side chains in these amino acids can link to each other forming disulphide bridges, which give great strength to the peptide produced. These bonds are found in proteins that form the hard parts of the body, such as the skin, nails and hair. Sulphur is also present in the vitamins thiamin and biotin.

These amino acids are required for the synthesis of proteins and connective tissue constituents, such as chondroitin sulphate. Sulphur also has an important role in the detoxifying pathways used by the liver for the removal of waste products and participates in the acid-base balance.

A mixed diet is unlikely to be short of sulphur as most proteins contain more than 1% sulphur. Egg and milk proteins are particularly rich in methionine, which is especially important in tissue growth and regeneration after illness and injury.

Microminerals or Trace Elements

Iron

Iron is part of the haemoglobin molecule in blood and, as such, accounts for two-thirds of the body's iron content. In this role, combined with the protein globin, it is the carrier of oxygen from the lungs to the tissues and, therefore, plays a vital role in survival. In addition, some is found in myoglobin, which is the pigment found in muscles that has a high affinity for oxygen.

The remainder is used in enzymes (especially cytochromes, which are essential in oxidation–reduction reactions), is stored in the body or is found in the blood, being carried between sites in the body.

The total amount of iron present in the body varies with the body weight, gender and long-term nutrition. It is also affected by the state of health, growth and pregnancy. On average, the body iron content averages 50 mg/kg of body mass in men and 38 mg/kg in women.

Dietary Sources of Iron

Iron occurs in the diet in two forms: as haem iron, mainly in foods of animal origin, and non-haem or inorganic iron, predominantly in plant foods. The richest sources of haem iron are meat and fish (the liver is one of the richest sources of iron, although many people never eat it). Cereals contain inorganic iron, which may also be bound to insoluble compounds such as phytate. However, fortification of white bread flour with iron does ensure that some additional iron is available without competition from phytate, which is removed in the milling process. Legumes and green vegetables also provide iron, although the availability of this is much less than from the animal sources. Other sources of iron include nuts and dried fruits. Milk and dairy products are very low in iron, and intakes of large amounts of milk may be linked to poor iron status. The main contributors in the United Kingdom to iron intakes are cereal products (48%), meat (15%) and vegetables (15%).

Iron supplements are widely available. They contain a variety of iron salts – sulphate, succinate, gluconate and fumarate – and have varying levels of bioavailability. It is stated that in people taking supplements, these contribute 7.5 mg/day of iron.

Dietary Reference Values

Report 41 (Reference values, DoH, 1991) takes into account the obligatory losses of iron and estimates of the average absorption rates for iron. Assuming this to be 15% from mixed diets, the RNI for adult men is 8.7 mg and for women is 14.8 mg. However, it is accepted that there will be some 10% of the female population whose needs will be greater than this and who may need supplements. After the menopause, the RNI for women falls to the same level as that of men.

See Chapter 8 for a detailed account on the importance of iron during the life cycle, pp. 153–174.

No additional increment is proposed for pregnancy, although it is recognized that there are increased iron requirements amounting to 680 mg over the whole pregnancy. It is assumed that women will have adequate stores of iron on which to draw, and there is also a saving on daily iron balance from the cessation of the menses. Some women with inadequate stores may, however, require additional iron. Levels of haemoglobin that fall below 10 g/L in pregnancy have been shown to be associated with progressively increasing risk to the baby, preterm delivery and associated complications. Iron absorption may increase between five- and ninefold during pregnancy as needs increase. It is, therefore, difficult to make predictions of the exact dietary needs at this time, and serum ferritin or haemoglobin levels should be monitored.

Iron in the Diet

Average intakes of iron in the United Kingdom are 11.8 mg/day, which represents 117% of the average RNI (Bates, 2014). However, several of the groups studied in the Family Food module of the Living Costs and Food Survey had mean intakes that fell below 100% of the RNI, and households with no children achieved intakes of 100% or more of the RNI. In the *Health Survey for England 1994* (Colhoun and Prescott-Clarke, 1996), low iron stores (measured as plasma ferritin) were reported for 4% of men and 26% of women. Meanwhile, the recent National Diet and Nutrition Survey reported a median plasma ferritin concentration of 32 μg/L (mean 53 μg/L) for adult women (median 127 μg/L/ mean 155 μg/L for adult men) indicative of low iron stores in a proportion of women.

Zinc

Sources of Zinc

Dietary intake of zinc is correlated with the protein content of the diet because zinc occurs complexed with proteins and their derivatives. Particularly, good sources are lean meat (especially offal), seafoods and dairy products. Pulses and whole grains are a moderate source but are of importance in vegetarian diets. Low levels of zinc occur in leafy vegetables, fruits, fats, alcohol and refined cereals. As with other divalent minerals, bioavailability is a determinant of the usefulness of particular dietary sources. Animal sources of zinc are generally more readily available than plant sources.

Dietary Reference Value

Figures for the daily turnover of zinc are used as the basis for setting dietary reference values. In adults, systemic needs appear to be 2–3 mg/day, and these can be converted into RNI, using an estimate of 30% for absorption of dietary zinc. Thus, RNIs for adult men and women are 9.5 and 7.0 mg/day, respectively. No additional increment is recommended in pregnancy, since it is assumed that metabolic adjustment takes place to provide the extra zinc.

Excessive intakes of zinc may cause nausea and vomiting and at 50 mg/day may interfere with immune responses and the metabolism of iron and copper. Caution should, therefore, be exercised in taking zinc-containing supplements.

Zinc in the Diet

The average daily intake in the United Kingdom is 9.5 mg (Bates, 2014), equating to 116% of the RNI. The main contributors of zinc in the British diet are meat and meat products (35%), cereal products (25%) and dairy products (15%). In many groups, especially in households with three or more children, the average intake fell below 100% of the RNI, indicating some groups at risk of low intakes.

Copper

There are approximately 100 mg of copper in the adult human body and the amount decreases with age. Deficiency of copper is well known in animals and results in anaemia and failure to mature. In humans, deficiency has been recognized for many years, but the diagnosis and significance of any suboptimal status in populations are still uncertain.

Sources of Copper

The content of copper in plant foods varies with soil conditions and food processing techniques. However, liver, shellfish, nuts, seeds (including cocoa) and legumes together with the outer parts of cereals are reported to be the richest sources (0.3–2.0 mg/100 g). Bananas, potatoes, tomatoes and mushrooms have intermediate levels (0.05–0.3 mg/100 g). Low levels are found in milk, bread and breakfast cereals. Drinking water can be an important source, where copper piping is used, and can provide up to 6 mg/day.

Estimated mean daily intakes of copper in the United Kingdom were 1.16 mg/day in British adults (Bates, 2014), the range for developed countries being 0.6–1.6 mg/day. Intakes among vegetarian populations have been reported to range from 2.1 to 3.9 mg/day. Analyzed values are reported to be higher than those calculated from food composition tables, reflecting the variability in foods. Meat and meat products (27%), together with cereal products (27%), are the main contributors of copper in the UK diet.

Selenium

The amount of selenium present in the body varies with the local environment, as its content in soil is variable. Levels are low where soils are acid and rainfall is heavy. In some countries, for example, Finland, fertilizers contain added selenium to enhance the content in the soil. In recent years, there has been a reduction in the dietary intake of selenium in some parts of the world, including Britain, and epidemiological evidence suggests a possible link between selenium and certain diseases. As a result, more attention has been paid to this trace element.

The selenium content of foods is related to the protein level, since it is found as selenocysteine (in animal products) or selenomethionine (in cereals). However, it should be remembered that the actual content within a particular sample of food will depend on the level in the soil or in the diet of the animal, and variation may be up to 100-fold. In addition, many Western diets contain foods from different parts of the world. This makes it very difficult to calculate selenium intakes accurately using food tables. Only where there is dependence on local products, a more accurate prediction of selenium intake can be made.

In the United Kingdom, Brazil nuts are the richest dietary source, with fish (especially shellfish), and offal (kidney and liver) providing a moderate source. Meat and eggs also provide moderate amounts of the element. Cereals and cereal products can provide a useful source, depending on their origin. In the United Kingdom, bread was an important source in the past, when flour was imported from North America. Presently, European flour is used, and the selenium levels in bread have fallen considerably. It is believed that this has had a major effect on average selenium intakes in the British diet, which have fallen from an average of 62 μg/day in the late 1980s to 48 μg/day in 2008/2010 (DoH/FSA, 2011). Fruits and vegetables are generally low in selenium. In the United Kingdom, selenium intakes derive mostly from meat and eggs (39%), cereals (22%), dairy products (15%) and fish (13%). Intakes in vegetarians have been found to be lower than the average in the United Kingdom. Selenium is also consumed in the form of supplements.

Iodine

Iodine exists in the body as iodide, which is a less toxic form. Any iodine ingested in food is rapidly converted to iodide in the gut. Iodide is necessary for the production of the thyroid hormones, which maintain the metabolic pattern of most cells in the living organism. In addition, the hormones play a key role in the early growth and development of organs, especially that of the brain. In humans, this occurs in fetal and early postnatal life. Therefore, iodine deficiency at this time of life, if it is severe enough to affect thyroid function, can cause hypothyroidism, brain damage and mental retardation. In the adult, an absence of iodide results in during pregnancy an enlargement of the thyroid gland (goitre) with major consequences during pregnancy.

Sources of Iodine

Most of the iodine in the world is in the oceans, since the land masses have had the iodine leached from them by glaciation, rain and floods. Thus, soils which are mountainous, landlocked or subject to frequent flooding, together with the crops grown on them, are most likely to be devoid of iodine. This is true of many of the central regions of large continental land masses.

Milk is the major source of iodide, as a result of an increased use of cattle-feed supplements containing iodine as well as iodine in medications and disinfectants used in animal husbandry. In addition, seafoods are a rich source, particularly haddock, whiting and herring. Plaice and tuna have a lower iodine content. Seaweed and products made from them may be rich in iodine, although not all have a high content. Vegans who rely on these sources should ensure that the intake is adequate. In the United States, bread contains iodine from improvers used in the baking industry. Iodized salt is an important source of iodine in areas where food sources are low in mineral. Salt in the United Kingdom is not fortified with iodine, and together with several other European countries (Belgium, Italy, Czech Republic, Hungary and Romania), low urinary excretion of iodine is observed.

Report 41 (DoH, 1991) states that an intake of 70 μg/day appears to protect populations against the occurrence of goitre; with a margin for safety, the RNI is stated to be 140 μg/day for adults. The World Health Organization recommends a daily iodine intake of 150 μg/day for adults, with an increase to 250 μg/day in pregnancy (WHO, 2007). The European Food Safety Authority also recommends iodine intake for adults 150 and 200 μg/day for pregnant and lactating women. However, the UK DoH does not recommend any increment for pregnancy and lactation.

Mean intake of iodine in adults in the United Kingdom is 167 μg/day (median 150 μg/day) (Bates, 2014). Iodine status of a population is best established using quantification of iodine in urine, with 100 μg/L the cut-off for iodine sufficiency in the adult population. In the United Kingdom, iodine status was considered adequate, until new evidence indicated that the United Kingdom may be iodine insufficient, with a median iodine excretion of 75 μg/L (Vanderpump et al., 2011).

Chromium

Chromium can exist in either trivalent or hexavalent form, with the former being more biologically active. Both forms appear to exist in tissues and may interconvert.

The richest sources of chromium are spices, brewer's yeast, meats (especially beef), whole grains, legumes and nuts. However, doubts have been expressed about the accuracy of some of the analytical methods used to assay chromium in foods, and values may need to be revised when better techniques are developed. Refining of foods causes a significant reduction in levels of chromium, and consuming a refined diet results in a very low intake of chromium. It has also been suggested that sugars may stimulate loss of chromium in the urine.

Chromium is excreted mainly in the urine, at levels of 1 μg/day. Chromium deficiency is not clearly defined, with many people apparently consuming less than the requirement for chromium. Glucose tolerance is improved by chromium supplementation at levels of 150 μg/day of chromium. In general, levels of chromium in Western populations decline with age. There are a very small number of reported cases of chromium deficiency in patients maintained on intravenous nutrition for long periods. Symptoms included impaired glucose tolerance or hyperglycaemia. Chromium is available as a supplement, and suggested roles include amelioration of diabetes and gestational diabetes, lipid abnormalities and insulin resistance. Doses of trivalent chromium up to 1000 μg/day appear to be safe.

Report 41 (DoH, 1991) suggests a 'safe intake' for chromium of more than 25 μg/day, for adults.

Fluoride

Fluoride intake is largely determined by the level in the water supply, as few foods contain significant amounts. Tea and seafoods are the major dietary sources.

Fluoride is essential for the production of hard, caries-resistant enamel in the teeth, but, when present in water supplies in amounts greater than 2–3 mg/L, it causes mottling of the dental enamel.

Even though these teeth are discoloured, they are still resistant to caries. Where naturally occurring levels are low, fluoride has been added to the water supply of parts of the world for more than 50 years as part of the effort to reduce the incidence of dental caries. In addition, fluoride toothpastes are widely available in many countries. These can provide an additional source of fluoride, especially for children, who may swallow significant amounts from the toothpaste.

In communities where fluoride is present in the water supply at recommended levels of 1 mg/L, there is at least a 50% reduction in tooth decay when compared with areas that have no fluoride. There has been considerable controversy about the desirability of adding fluoride to water supplies, and human rights cases have been heard by the courts. The safety of the procedure has been thoroughly investigated, and, at present, there are no scientific data to support the claim that fluoridation is harmful to health. The widespread availability and use of fluoride toothpaste has made a significant difference to caries incidence in most European countries. For individuals who regularly use this, there are few additional advantages from fluoridated water. However, in every society, there are sectors for whom tooth cleaning and the use of toothpaste are not a habit; in these cases, fluoridated water can make an important contribution to dental health.

There appear to be no other requirements for fluoride apart from this role in dental health promotion.

ELECTROLYTES

Sodium and Chloride

These two minerals are considered together, because they occur together in foods and in the body, as well as in seawater and the earth's crust.

Together with potassium, sodium and chloride contribute in large measure to the osmolality of the body fluids, which, in turn, determines their distribution and balance. Changes in osmolality may involve changes in the content of minerals or of water. Restoration of a normal balance activates mechanisms that regulate mineral excretion or water loss via the kidney, by means of hormonal control, and through aldosterone, rennin–angiotensin or antidiuretic hormone, as appropriate.

Sodium is the major cation of extracellular fluid (with an extracellular concentration of approximately 140 mM), comprising over 90% of the cations in the blood. Some 40% of the body's sodium is present in bone as an integral part of the mineral lattice, but it is not clear how readily this can be mobilized to maintain sodium levels in extracellular fluids.

Sodium plays a crucial role in

- Maintaining osmolality of body fluids
- Maintaining the extracellular fluid, and hence the blood volume
- Acid-base balance
- Maintaining the electrochemical gradients across cell membranes

The electrochemical gradients are especially important in nerve and muscle cells, where they are vital for the propagation of nerve impulses and for muscle contraction. They are also important in the absorption of substances across cell membranes against concentration gradients, for example, in the digestive tract and kidneys. The maintenance of electrochemical gradients at all times in the body consumes the greatest part of the daily energy requirement for life, as the ATP pumps move the ions across cellular membranes maintaining a low intracellular concentration (5–15 mM).

Since sodium is essential to homeostasis, it is clear that the levels of sodium in the body must be carefully regulated, regardless of levels of intake. Further, there is no functional store of sodium, so the daily needs must be met by control of excretion when intake is variable.

Chloride occurs generally in association with sodium as the major anion in extracellular fluid, but it is not found in bone. It can also associate with potassium in intracellular fluids and can readily cross the cell membrane. In addition to its role in electrolyte balance associated with sodium, it is also essential for the transport of carbon dioxide in red blood cells and in the formation of hydrochloric acid secreted by the stomach. Chloride is the major secretory electrolyte of the whole digestive tract. Losses of digestive juices, especially in vomiting, can deplete the levels of chloride in the body.

Sodium and Chloride in Foods

Most foods naturally contain a low level of sodium: plant foods contain very little sodium, while animal foods contain low to moderate levels. The majority of sodium in the diet comes from foods that have undergone some processing and to which salt has been added. In addition, sodium comprises 39% by weight of sodium chloride, the major source of sodium in the diet. In general, the greater the consumption of processed foods, the higher will be the sodium intake. Not surprisingly, sodium intakes are very variable, both within a population and between people in different countries.

Sodium (usually as chloride) is used in food processing and manufacture because of its properties as a

- Preservative (e.g. in meats, dairy products, preserved vegetables)
- Flavouring agent (e.g. in breakfast cereals, crisps, packet soups, bread)
- Texture enhancer (e.g. in cheese, preserved meats)

Other sodium salts are used as raising agents.

Dietary Reference Value

The RNI for sodium is 1.6 g/day for adults, with an LRNI of 575 mg/day. The majority of people in the United Kingdom consume levels in excess of the RNI. There appears to be no physiological advantage to this, and in the light of evidence of the relationship with blood pressure, it is suggested that current intakes are needlessly high and should decrease. A reduction in the salt content of manufactured foods would make a significant contribution to reducing salt intakes in the population.

Special care should be taken with sodium intakes in young infants, as their ability to regulate sodium levels in the body is not well developed in the first weeks of life. In addition, if there is vomiting and diarrhoea, serious depletion can result.

In the United Kingdom, estimated average daily sodium intakes are 2.83 g, although this does not include table salt (DEFRA, 2011). The main food sources to the total intake in the United Kingdom are cereals and cereal products (36%) and meat and meat products (28%). If no salt is added to foods, the sodium intake from natural sources would be between 0.5 and 1 g/day. Thus, it is evident that the greater part of our intake originates from added salt.

It is not easy to measure sodium intakes, as there is so much variability between individuals, and a proportion of that used in cooking may be discarded before consumption, for example, in cooking water. A more reliable approach is to measure 24 hour urinary sodium excretion, which closely mirrors the intake (lithium can also be used as a marker of cooking or table salt and measured in the urine).

The 2008 urinary sodium survey of the UK population assessed total daily intakes of sodium chloride (salt), with an average intake of 7.7 g in women and 9.7 g in men. The Scientific Advisory Committee on Nutrition recommended in 2003 that average salt intake for adults should not exceed 6 g/day (equivalent to 2.4 g of sodium). Based on this figure, 82% of men and 65% of women are over the recommended intake.

Potassium

Potassium is the major intracellular cation of the body, with almost all of the body's content found within the cells, the majority of it bound to phosphate and protein. Like sodium, potassium is essential for cellular integrity and the maintenance of fluid, electrolyte and acid-base balance. It is also involved in the propagation of the nerve impulse and muscle contraction. Potassium that leaks out into the extracellular fluids is quickly pumped back to maintain the differential between the composition of the fluids outside and inside cells, on which much of the cellular function depends. Intracellular concentration of potassium is approximately 140 mM, while extracellular concentration is approximately 5 mM.

Dietary Reference Value

The RNI for adults has been set at 3.5 g/day, although it is recognized that intakes may be much higher than this. Toxicity is unlikely, however, at normal dietary levels. Intakes in excess of 17.6 g/day may cause harmful effects, but these are only likely to occur with supplement use.

Potassium in the Diet

The daily intakes of potassium in the United Kingdom are reported as 3.28 g (DEFRA, 2011). The main contributors of potassium in the British diet (DEFRA, 2001) are vegetables and potatoes (29%), and moderate levels are obtained from cereals (15%), dairy products (18%), meat (13%) and fruit (11%). Foods that are rich in potassium include dried fruits and nuts, chocolate, treacle, meat and raw vegetables.

FLUIDS: KEEPING THE BODY HYDRATED

Humans can survive for long periods of time without food; several weeks' survival has been reported. However, if fluids are withheld, there is a rapid deterioration and death may result within 10 days.

This is not surprising when we recognize that water is the single largest component of body composition, comprising 50–60% of the total body weight in an average adult. Water content is somewhat higher in males than in females, as the higher percentage of body fat in females is associated with less water than is muscle.

Water is an essential component of the body because of the following:

- The process of ingestion, digestion and absorption is facilitated by the presence of water, including the various secretions along the digestive tract containing digestive enzymes.
- Elimination of an unabsorbed material via the colon requires water to facilitate its passage.
- Metabolic reactions occur in an aqueous environment.
- Nutrients and metabolites are transported in solution within extracellular or intracellular fluids.
- Mucous membranes must be kept moist for normal functioning, including the exchange of gases during respiration in the lungs.
- The excretion of waste products via the kidney occurs with the help of water.
- Regulation of body temperature by transfer of heat within the circulation and the production of sweat.

See Chapter 10 for more detail on fluid balance, pp. 211–212.

What to Drink?

It is not necessary to consume only water.

As has been discussed earlier, it is only alcohol that, in practice, has a diuretic effect and may not contribute to hydration. However, low-alcohol beers can be used to help towards hydration. Most other commonly consumed beverages can be counted towards the fluid intake allowance. However, it is important to consider some of the other attributes of common drinks when selecting what to consume.

Water

This is often the easiest and cheapest fluid to drink. Consumption of water has increased in recent years, with the popularity of bottled waters. The habit of carrying a bottle of water during the day has become widespread and is a useful reminder to drink.

Soft Drinks

These include carbonated drinks, dilutables (squash/cordial) and fruit juice drinks. These are of varying nutritional quality. Some may be of 'low calorie' but others may provide up to four teaspoons of sugar per portion. Levels of phosphoric acid are often high in the carbonated drinks, and this has cariogenic potential. Some fruit juice drinks have added nutrients, such as vitamin C, but may also be high in sugar.

Fruit Juices

These are useful as they provide both vitamin C and possibly phytochemicals that may have additional health benefits. Juices are, however, rich in sugar. Juice consumption is especially problematic in young children in terms of oral health.

Milk

Despite a decreased consumption of milk in the last two decades, there is a growing market in flavoured milks and probiotic products based on milk. These may, however, contain added sugar. Milk provides a useful range of nutrients, especially calcium and riboflavin. In addition, it is a useful source of vitamin B_{12}, vitamin A, iodine, magnesium, phosphorus, potassium and zinc. It is a nutrient-dense food, in relation to its energy intake, especially if reduced fat milk is drunk.

Tea and Coffee

Both of these are popular beverages. They can make a useful contribution to hydration. If drunk with milk, additional nutritional value may be gained.

How Much to Drink?

Fluid intake is essential for our survival, and we require a regular intake. Yet, despite these key roles, there is no recommendation made on the intake of water in the Dietary Reference Values Report in the United Kingdom (DoH, 1991).

The optimal way of avoiding dehydration is to develop a habit of regular fluid intakes without waiting for thirst to intervene. The quantities needed depend on the factors discussed earlier that affect fluid losses and vary between individuals. As a general rule, however, most sedentary adults in a temperate environment require to drink between 1.2 and 1.5 L each day. This assumes that a further 1 L of fluid is obtained from the food consumed. In this way, a fluid intake of 35 mL/kg body weight per day would be achieved. The revised Eatwell Guide (Public Health England, 2016) now recommends six to eight glasses of fluids, which can include water, low fat milk, sugar-free drinks including tea and coffee (with up to 150ml per day for fruit juices, smoothies).

Water in Foods

Water is also obtained from the food consumed. Almost all food contains some associated water. Semi-liquid foods, such as soups, yogurts and ice cream, are obvious examples; fruits and vegetables contain a high percentage of water. Even foods that appear to be relatively 'solid', such as bread, cereal foods, cakes, meats and dairy products, contain some water. Some examples are shown in Table 5.2.

TABLE 5.2
Water Content of Some Foods (as a Percentage)

Food	Water
Lettuce	95
Tomato	93
Carrots	90
Orange	86
Apple	85
Boiled potatoes	80
Peas	78
Lentil soup	78
Fruit yogurt	77
Baked white fish	76
Banana	75
Boiled rice	68
Grilled oily fish	65
Ice cream	62
Cooked meat	60
Potato chips	52
White bread	37
Cheddar-type cheese	36
White flour	14
Sponge cake	15
Cornflakes	3
Semi-sweet biscuits	2.5

It follows that a person who has a small appetite or is unwell and, therefore eating very little will gain small amounts of water by this route and will need to make up for this by increasing their fluid intake. A normal mixed diet, however, will provide up to 1 L of water from the food consumed.

Overall, it is sensible to consume a range of drinks, according to the taste. Care should be taken that drinks do not cause damage to teeth or provide unnecessary additional energy, if there is concern about weight management. Most importantly, fluid intake should be frequent and adequate to maintain hydration.

Dehydration

Although there is no doubt about the essential nature of water in the body, the signs and symptoms of dehydration are less well described.

Mild dehydration (a deficit of 500 mL to 1 L or 1%–2% of body weight) will cause thirst to be triggered. There is no clear evidence whether this level of dehydration has a detrimental effect on cognitive function. Mild to moderate dehydration (a deficit of 1–3.5 L or 2%–5% of body weight) will lead to headaches, early fatigue, loss of precision in tasks, inability to concentrate, irritability and nausea. Progressively, greater dehydration will cause an elevation of body temperature, increased heart rate and respiration, dizziness, weakness and raised blood pressure. Ultimately, renal function will be impaired and the person may become comatose. Death can follow if fluid balance is not restored.

The prevalence of mild dehydration is not known, although it is likely that a substantial proportion of the population of all ages have inadequate fluid intake. Concern has been voiced about the need to ensure that schoolchildren have access to fluids during the day to prevent loss of concentration owing to dehydration. Among older persons who are admitted to hospital, dehydration and confusion are common findings.

Some long-term studies have indicated that chronic hypohydration may be associated with higher incidence of colon and breast cancer, although further research in these areas is needed.

SUMMARY

1. The minerals constitute a diverse group. Their roles may be structural, protective or regulatory.
2. Many of the minerals function as cofactors for enzymes involved in metabolic processes. These range from energy transformation to synthesis of essential biological materials in the body.
3. Intakes of the minerals in the United Kingdom are generally adequate, with the exception of iron and zinc, where there is evidence of inadequate intake and the absence of stores in a significant proportion of the population.
4. Fluid intakes may be marginal in some people and represent a significant risk of dehydration. Developing a habit to drink regular amounts of fluids is important.

STUDY QUESTIONS

1. List those groups in the population who are at risk of poor iron status and provide a discussion of the causes for each group.
2. The Scientific Advisory Committee on Nutrition (2003) recommended that the population as a whole would benefit from reducing their intake of salt to a maximum of 6 g/day. Discuss the recommendation in the context of current UK intakes, the importance of salt and the evidence behind this target.
3. Critically appraise the barriers and opportunities for adequate intake of iron in the general population.

ACTIVITIES

5.1 If you have previously kept a record of your daily food intake, you can return to this for the activity. If not, first, make a list of all the things you have eaten in the last 24 hours.

- Identify the main sources of salt/sodium in this intake (you may need to check food labels to do this accurately).
- What sort of foods are contributing to this salt intake? Are there lower salt alternatives available?
- Plan a modified diet that contains less salt.
- What problems would you have in achieving this? Are there some foods you could avoid straight away?

5.2 Map the main food sources of iodine and selenium in the Western diet, and consider the following:

- Identify the barriers in achieving a sufficient intake, for a healthy adult.
- What are the opportunities to modify the food chain in order to enhance the population intake?

BIBLIOGRAPHY AND FURTHER READING

Bates, B., Lennox, A., Prentice, A., Bates, C., Page, P., Nicholson, S. and Swan, G. 2014. National Diet and Nutrition Survey results from years 1, 2, 3 and 4 (combined) of the Rolling Programme (2008/2009–2011/2012). London, UK: Public Health England.

British Nutrition Foundation. 1995. Iron: Nutritional and physiological significance. The Report of the British Nutrition Foundation Task Force. London, UK: Chapman & Hall.

British Nutrition Foundation. 2001. Selenium and health. Briefing paper. London, UK: British Nutrition Foundation.

British Nutrition Foundation/Theobald, H.E. 2005. Briefing paper: Dietary calcium and health. *Nutrition Bulletin* 30, 237–277.

Broadley, M.R., White, P.J., Bryson, R.J. et al. 2006. Biofortification of UK food crops with selenium. *Proceedings of the Nutrition Society* 65, 169–181.

Colhoun, H. and Prescott-Clarke, P. (eds.). 1996. *Health Survey for England 1994*. London, UK: HMSO.

Combet, E. and Buckton, C. 2015. Micronutrient deficiencies, vitamin pills and nutritional supplements. *Medicine* 43(2), 66–72.

DEFRA. 2001. National food survey 2000. Annual report on food expenditure, consumption and nutrient intakes. London, UK: The Stationery Office.

DEFRA (UK Department for Environment, Food and Rural Affairs). 2011. *Family Food 2010*. London, UK: National Statistics Publication.

DoH (UK Department of Health). 1991. Dietary reference values for food energy and nutrients for the United Kingdom. Report on Health and Social Subjects No. 41. Report of the Panel on Dietary Reference Values of the Committee on Medical Aspects of Food Policy. London, UK: HMSO.

EURODIET Working Party: Final Report. 2001. European diet and public health: The continuing challenge. *Public Health Nutrition* 4(2A), 275–292.

Fairweather-Tait, S.J., Bao, Y., Broadley, M.R., Collings, R., Ford, D., Hesketh, J.E. and Hurst, R. 2011. Selenium in human health and disease. *Antioxidant Redox Signaling* 14, 1337–1383.

Jeejeebhoy, K.N. 1999. The role of chromium in nutrition and therapeutics and as a potential toxin. *Nutrition Reviews* 57(11), 329–335.

National Center for Social Research/MRC Human Nutrition Research. 2008. An assessment of dietary sodium levels among adults (aged 19–64) in the UK general population in 2008, based on analysis of dietary sodium in 24 hour urine samples. Available at: http://tna.europarchive.org/20110116113217/http://www.food.gov.uk/multimedia/pdfs/08sodiumreport.pdf.

Popkin, B.M., D'Anci, K.E. and Rosenberg, I.H. 2010. Water, hydration, and health. *Nutrition Reviews* 68, 439–458.

Public Health England. 2016. The Eatwell Guide - How does it differ to the eatwell plate and why? London, UK.

Rayman, M.P. 2002. The argument for increasing selenium intake. *Proceedings of the Nutrition Society* 61, 203–215.

Scientific Advisory Committee on Nutrition. 2010. *Iron and Health*. London, UK: The Stationery Office.

Serra-Majem, L., Pfrimer, K., Doreste-Alonso, J. et al. 2009. Dietary assessment methods for intakes of iron, calcium, selenium, zinc and iodine. *British Journal of Nutrition* 102, S38–S55.

Vanderpump, M.P., Lazarus, J.H., Smyth, P.P., Laurberg, P., Holder, R.L., Boelaert, K. and Franklyn, J.A. 2011. Iodine status of UK schoolgirls: A cross-sectional survey. *Lancet* 377, 2007–2012.

WHO, Food and Agriculture Organisation, International Atomic Energy Expert Group. 1996. *Trace Elements in Human Nutrition and Health*. Geneva, Switzerland: WHO.

WHO, UNICEF. ICCIDD (2001) Assessment of iodine deficiency disorders and monitoring their elimination. A guide for programme managers. 2007. Geneva, Switzerland: WHO.

Section II

Nutrition through the Life Cycle

6 Nutrition during Pregnancy and Lactation

AIMS

The aims of this chapter are to

- Establish the importance of nutrition in preparation for and throughout pregnancy.
- Discuss the nutritional needs during pregnancy and identify specific groups in the population who may be at particular risk in pregnancy.
- Describe the possible links between pregnancy outcome and long-term health.
- Discuss the nutritional needs in lactation.
- Identify some of the influences on the mother in choice of feeding method.

Pregnancy is a critical period of development for the fetus, a time when organs are formed and susceptible to injury from a range of dietary stimuli. It is also a vulnerable time for the mother, whose dietary requirement is increased in order to support the needs of the unborn child both in utero and during infancy through lactation.

Based on studies of well-fed pregnant women in the 1950s in the United Kingdom, the physiological norm for weight gain in a 40-week pregnancy was set at 12.5 kg. This appeared to be associated with optimal outcome of pregnancy. Since then, the Institute of Medicine (IoM) and the National Research Council in the United States initiated a re-examination of the guidelines for weight gain in pregnancy, describing adequate total pregnancy weight gain as a function of pre-pregnancy body mass index (BMI):

12.5–18 kg	BMI < 18.5
11.5–16 kg	BMI 18.5–24.9
7–11.5 kg	BMI 25–29.9
5–9 kg	BMI $\geq$ 30

There is, however, no formal, evidence-based guideline in the United Kingdom setting a specific weight target during pregnancy, and the Public Health Interventions Advisory Committee could not recommend endorsement of the U.S. IoM pregnancy weight gain guidelines for the United Kingdom (see the National Institute for Health and Care Excellence (NICE) Public Health Guidance number 27).

A 12.5 kg total weight gain comprises of the following:

Fetus	3.5 kg
Increased maternal tissues (including uterus, mammary glands and blood volume)	5.0 kg
Stored fat	4.0 kg

These increases were also believed to prepare the mother's body for lactation, in the form of stored energy for milk production.

On the basis of such figures, it would seem reasonable to conclude that the mother needs to consume a significantly greater amount of food during the pregnancy in order to provide sufficient nutrients and energy to build these extra tissues. The corollary of this is that pregnancy outcome, both in terms of the mother's health and the well-being of the baby, would be adversely affected if her nutritional intake were not increased.

In recent years, a better understanding has emerged of the relationship between nutrition of the mother and pregnancy outcome. This has shown it to be very much more complex than stated here, as well as far from fully understood.

This chapter considers the importance of nutritional status before pregnancy, at the time of conception and in the presence of major physiological changes, which occur during pregnancy. The indicator of outcome of pregnancy that is widely used is the birthweight of the baby. A favourable outcome is the delivery of a healthy full-term infant, weighing between 3.5 and 4 kg (in the United Kingdom, some countries use 4.5 kg as the upper end of the range). This is associated with the lowest risk of infant and perinatal morbidity and mortality. Above this birthweight, there is an increased likelihood of obstetric complications as well as neonatal mortality and morbidity. Babies born weighing less than 2.5 kg (termed 'low birthweight') have a 40-fold greater risk of neonatal mortality than those born at optimal weight, and the survivors have an increased risk of neurological disorders and handicap, as well as infection.

A recent review by Langley-Evans (2014) provides an overview of the evidence associating nutritional deficit in the womb and early life with a greater risk of disease in later life, for example, type 2 diabetes and cardiovascular disease. These permanent changes in physiological and metabolic states have become known as fetal programming. The evidence also suggests that the timing of the fetal insult in the womb can affect the type of disease risk. Greatest sensitivity will occur during periods of most rapid growth and maturation, and longer periods of exposure may be expected to impact on a larger range of organs, tissues and systems. This is covered in further detail later on in this chapter.

It is therefore important to ensure that women receive the optimal levels of nutrition both before and during pregnancy. Not only to ensure that the mother herself arrives at the end of pregnancy in a healthy state, well enough to be able to care for her newly born infant, but also to protect the baby from future disease risk.

NUTRITION BEFORE PREGNANCY

The nutritional status of a woman at the time of conception reflects her diet and lifestyle over a number of years, even perhaps going back to her own infancy and childhood. These are dependent on many environmental and social factors, which must be taken into account.

Several features of the pre-pregnancy diet may affect the chances of conception or the success of pregnancy, such as the following:

1. Vitamin D deficiency in adolescence may have resulted in rickets with pelvic malformations, making a normal delivery impossible. This is rare nowadays.
2. Folic acid deficiency has been shown to increase the risk of neural tube defects (NTDs) in babies.
3. A dietary deficiency of vitamin B_{12} may cause infertility.
4. A history of dieting, or in its extreme form anorexia nervosa, can result in poor nutritional status, with low reserves of many nutrients.

Research on underweight women has found that low body fat stores are associated with amenorrhoea and infertility. Evidence of this association comes from records obtained in wartime from places where food supplies were critical, such as Holland and Leningrad, as well as from more recent studies in infertility clinics and on women with anorexia. These indicate that a BMI of

20.8 appears to be a threshold for normal pregnancy and that there is a minimum ratio of fat/lean body mass needed to support pregnancy.

Women who are obese (BMI above 30) may also experience infertility, as the associated changes in insulin activity and sex hormones may reduce the viability of the ovum.

It would, therefore, appear to be desirable that a woman planning to become pregnant should aim to achieve a BMI within the range of 20–26. If this is achieved by adopting healthy nutritional practices, the reserves of micronutrients will also be maximized.

Research on primates and human volunteers suggests that the most crucial phase is the 14 days prior to conception, when the follicle in the ovary is growing rapidly before it extrudes the ovum at ovulation. The environment for the developing ovum in the ovary requires appropriate hormone levels. These are crucially dependent on the maternal state of nutrition both in terms of protein and other nutrients. These may include iodine to ensure normal thyroid hormone function, magnesium and zinc for the binding of hormones at their receptor sites and folic acid for the normal growth of the follicle.

It is clear that nutrition prior to pregnancy has long-term implications and that, for an optimum outcome, diet should be adequate and well balanced before conception.

NUTRITION AT THE TIME OF CONCEPTION

The embryo at conception and in the first weeks afterwards is extremely vulnerable. The majority of the organs and systems develop in the first 8 weeks after conception. The essential energy and nutrients for this are derived from the mother's circulation and from the lining of the womb. It is, therefore, critical that these can provide the necessary nutrients in appropriate amounts. At this stage of pregnancy, the placenta has not yet formed, so there is no mechanism to protect the embryo from deficiencies in the maternal circulation. It is, therefore, not surprising that nutritional status and nutritional reserves at this time are vital. Studies from the Dutch hunger winter (1944–1945) showed that, among the women who did bear children, they were the ones who had experienced the full duration of hunger (8 months) prior to conception who had the most severely affected infants with respect to malformations.

The Folic Acid Campaign is further discussed in Chapter 19, pp. 377–379.

Trials on the prevention of NTDs have shown that supplementing the diet of 'at-risk' women with folic acid (4 mg/day) for 3 months before conception and up to the 12th week of pregnancy significantly reduced the risk of NTD in the fetus. Since folate is needed for cell division, it is suggested that these levels override a metabolic abnormality linked to neural tube closure. In the majority of cases, it is impossible to predict which women might be at risk and only those who have already had one affected fetus can be identified as requiring particular supplementation. As a result of these studies, women who might become pregnant are now advised in the United Kingdom by the Department of Health (HEA, 1996) to increase their intake of folate by at least 400 μg daily. This is more than the typical diet provides, and therefore, foods fortified with folic acid or folic acid supplements are needed. Retinol has also received particular attention in recent years. Reports have suggested that extreme intakes of retinol (doses from 8,000 to 10,000 μg/day) are teratogenic (i.e. cause fetal malformations). Such a level of intake is likely to be taken regularly only in the form of supplements. The main dietary source of retinol that might contain these levels is liver. A 100 g serving of liver might contain up to 10,000 μg of retinol; it is unlikely, however, that this would be eaten on a daily basis. Nevertheless, women who may be trying to become pregnant are advised to avoid liver and liver products as well as supplements that contain megadoses of retinol, as there is a very small risk of harm. No cases of fetal damage attributable to liver intakes have been reported in Britain.

Alcohol is also a potential teratogenic agent, particularly if taken in large amounts, for example, in binge drinking. Women who are considering becoming pregnant should, therefore, avoid consuming large amounts of alcohol. This is important in view of the likelihood that damage may be done in the first weeks after conception before the woman realizes she is pregnant. In men who drink heavily, there is likely to be a reduced sperm count, which may be a contributory factor in reproductive failure in a couple.

The weight of the woman and, in particular, her body fat content at the time of conception is also an important determinant of the metabolic changes that occur during pregnancy. Research suggests that a low fat content at conception is a signal to the body to conserve energy so that the metabolism during the pregnancy becomes very efficient and the total energy costs of the pregnancy are low. This is mediated by altered leptin levels. Conversely, in women with high fat stores at conception, there is little energy conservation and the cost of pregnancy is high. Nevertheless, even with this adaptability, mothers with low fat stores give birth to lower-birthweight babies than do those with higher fat stores.

NUTRITION DURING PREGNANCY

Considerable changes occur in the mother's body during pregnancy. In addition to the developing fetus, there are changes in her own tissues, with an expansion of the plasma volume and red cell mass, increase in the size of the uterus and mammary glands and deposition of fat.

In the 1970s, incremental calculations of the amount of extra protein and fat laid down during pregnancy were performed, which gave an estimate of the energy and protein needs of these 'capital gains'. In addition, an allowance was added for the extra 'running costs' of the heavier maternal body. Such calculations produced a figure for the total additional energy cost of pregnancy of about 335 MJ (80,000 cal). These figures were used in many countries as the basis for setting recommended intake levels for pregnant women.

Recent findings have shown that energy metabolism exhibits considerable variation, with pregnancy being maintained successfully at an additional energy cost of 523 MJ (125,000 cal) in well-nourished women in Sweden and with an energy deficit of 30 MJ (7,150 cal) in women in the Gambia not receiving nutritional supplementation. A woman's adaptive mechanisms to pregnancy can include the following:

1. An increase in food intake to meet energy needs
2. Laying down of fat stores/mobilizing fat stores
3. An increase or reduction in the basal metabolic rate (including the costs of synthesis and maintenance of new tissues)
4. A reduction in physical activity costs

In this way, the energy costs of supporting a developing fetus can be maintained at very different levels of energy intake.

In addition to metabolic adaptations in terms of energy, the body also undergoes other physiological changes to increase the efficiency of nutrient utilization and to optimize the supply to the fetus. Many of these changes commence in the early weeks of pregnancy, while the fetus is still very small and its nutritional demands low. At this time, the mother may conserve nutrients in her tissues. Evidence suggests that this applies to protein in particular, with reduced amino acid oxidation occurring in the liver. In the later stages of pregnancy, as the fetus enters a rapid growth phase, this protein can be made available from the mother's tissues to supplement that consumed in the diet. In this way, the needs can be met without a major increase in intake being necessary.

The mother also makes greater use of lipids as a source of energy for her own needs, thus sparing glucose for the needs of the fetus. This change is brought about by alterations in hormone levels, particularly insulin. There are also adaptations in the muscular activity of the intestines, so that food spends a longer time being digested and absorbed. This increases the efficiency of absorption, particularly for minerals such as calcium and iron. In addition, both of these may be better absorbed in response to the physiological regulation, which occurs as a result of the increased need for the minerals.

The slowed activity of the intestines may cause heartburn (gastro-oesophageal reflux) and constipation. Heartburn arises because the lower oesophageal sphincter is more relaxed, which in combination with slower gastric emptying allows reflux of the acidic stomach contents into the lower part of the oesophagus, causing irritation and pain.

Constipation occurs because of the reduced gut motility and longer time available for absorption of water from the digestive tract. Increasing both fluid and non-starch polysaccharide (NSP) intakes can help to relieve this problem, as will maintain a moderate level of activity.

WHAT ARE THE DIETARY GOALS IN PREGNANCY?

Generally, pregnant women do not eat a diet substantially different from that eaten by the rest of the female population. Studies around the world of pregnant women in different cultures and at different levels of income show that pregnancy can occur successfully at varying levels of nutritional intake, although there are limits to the protection afforded the fetus at low intake levels. Whether the baby that is born is as healthy as possible may not necessarily be apparent in the first instance, since current research suggests that the intrauterine environment is crucial to long-term health (this is discussed later in the chapter).

Birthweights are lower in babies born to women who have lower energy and nutrient intakes, with particularly strong relationships seen with intakes of the minerals magnesium, iron, phosphorus, zinc and potassium and the vitamins thiamin, niacin, pantothenic acid, riboflavin, folic acid, pyridoxine and biotin. Increasing the food intake does not result in progressively larger and larger infants. Studies by Doyle et al. (1990) show that there is a threshold birthweight (of 3.27 kg) above which extra food intake makes little difference, but below which there is a progressively lower birthweight as intakes are reduced.

For optimal outcome measured in terms of lowest perinatal mortality, women who are underweight before pregnancy need to increase their food intake more and gain more weight than those of normal weight. The converse is true of overweight women. Various guidelines are now available outside the UK for the recommended weight to be gained in relation to pre-pregnancy BMI (see Table 6.1 for figures recommended in the United States).

TABLE 6.1

Guidelines on Weight Gain in Pregnancy

Pre-Pregnancy BMI (Weight/Height^2)	Recommended Weight Gain (kg)
<18.5	12.5–18
18.5–24.9	11.5–16
25–29.9	7–11.5
≥30.0	5–9

Source: Reproduced from Institute of Medicine (US) and National Research Council (US), *Weight Gain During Pregnancy: Reexamining the Guidelines*, Rasmussen, K.M. and Yaktine, A.L. (eds.), Committee to Reexamine IOM Pregnancy Weight Guidelines, National Academy Press, Washington, DC, 2009. With permission.

DIET IN PREGNANCY

APPETITE

The pregnant woman does not need to 'eat for two'. Instead, the mother's appetite should be a good guide to her overall needs for energy.

In the first 3 months of pregnancy, up to 70% of women suffer from nausea and vomiting. Although this is commonly termed 'morning sickness', probably only 10%–15% of women experience sickness in the morning. In the remainder, it can actually occur at any time of day or night and in some women occurs continuously. Nausea and vomiting of pregnancy (NVP) is a better name for this syndrome. It may range from a mild nausea to quite severe, frequent vomiting (hyperemesis gravidarum). The condition appears to be more prevalent in societies that consume animal products, and it has been suggested that NVP is a protective mechanism against potential parasites and pathogens that may be ingested at a critical time in early pregnancy and threaten the embryo. Paradoxically, NVP appears to be associated with a favourable outcome of pregnancy, including higher birthweight and longer gestation. It has been proposed that this may be the result of the adaptation of the placenta to a reduced food intake in the first trimester, which then favours fetal growth once NVP resolves. Frequent meals or snacks are recommended, even if the woman has little appetite for them. It is important that the food eaten is as nutritious as possible and often it is high-carbohydrate foods that are best tolerated. Dehydration is also a risk and salty foods that trigger thirst mechanisms may also be useful. An improved quality of the diet may be important to compensate for the period when food intake is low.

ENERGY

Appetite is usually good in the middle part of pregnancy, so that food intake is at or a little above normal pre-pregnancy levels. This ensures an adequate provision of energy and nutrients to form a reserve for the greater needs of the last months.

In the last 3 months, the needs of the fetus are high and the mother's appetite may increase. She is limited in her capacity for food, however, because of the pressure of the enlarged womb on her stomach. The diet chosen should contain a variety of foods to supply the necessary nutrients. Report 41 (DoH, 1991) recommends a small increase in energy intake of 0.8 MJ (200 cal) per day during the last trimester of pregnancy. This should be provided by increasing total food intake. Together with the adaptations to absorption efficiency and the metabolic changes already mentioned, this will ensure that the additional needs for many other nutrients will be covered.

NUTRIENTS

Particular attention should be paid to certain nutrients for which the increase recommended is greater than can be achieved from a diet designed to just meet the energy requirement. These nutrients are vitamins A and C, riboflavin, folate and vitamin D.

Although there is no increment recommended by the Scientific Advisory Committee for Nutrition (SACN) for iodine during pregnancy, a recent European Food Safety Authority report suggested that there was sufficient evidence to recommend an adequate intake of 200 μg/day for pregnant women. This additional requirement is 60 μg/day more than the SACN recommendation of 140 μg/day.

Increasing fruit and vegetable intake should provide extra amounts of folate and vitamins A and C. Taking extra milk or dairy products, which can contribute to the extra energy intake and also supplies protein and calcium, will also contribute to meeting the riboflavin needs. Vitamin D requirements may be a problem, especially in women who are pregnant through the winter and are, therefore, unable to synthesize skin vitamin D. If stores have not been accumulated during the

TABLE 6.2
Summary of Dietary Reference Values for Pregnancy

Nutrient	Recommendation
Energy	Increase by 200 kcal (0.8 MJ)/day in last trimester only.
Protein	Extra 6 g/day; total recommended 51 g/day.
Thiamin	Increase in line with energy: extra 0.1 mg/day; total recommended 0.9 mg/day.
Riboflavin	Needed for tissue growth: extra 0.3 mg/day; total recommended 1.4 mg/day.
Nicotinic acid	Metabolism becomes more efficient: no increase needed.
Pyridoxine	No evidence that increase needed.
Vitamin B_{12}	Little information available about needs: no increase.
Folate	Increased usage in pregnancy, maintain plasma levels with extra 100 μg/day; total recommended 300 μg/day.
Vitamin C	Drain on maternal stores in late pregnancy: extra 10 mg/day; total recommended 50 mg/day.
Vitamin D	Seasonal variation in plasma levels of vitamin; 10 μg/day as supplement.
Calcium	Maternal store drawn upon in early pregnancy and enhanced absorption: no increase.
Iron	Iron stores, cessation of menstruation and increased absorption should cover needs: no increase.
Magnesium, zinc and copper	Increased needs, but assumed to be met from increased absorption.

Source: Reproduced from DoH (UK Department of Health), Dietary reference values for food energy and nutrients for the United Kingdom, Report on Health and Social Subjects No. 41, Report of the Panel on Dietary Reference Values of the Committee on Medical Aspects of Food Policy, HMSO, London, UK, 1991. With permission.

previous summer, a supplement of vitamin D is advisable to ensure adequate calcium metabolism. A particular problem may arise in strictly vegetarian women of Asian origin, whose vitamin D status may be precarious and in whom supplementation with vitamin D has been shown to be of positive benefit for the birthweight and subsequent growth of the baby.

The NSP content of the diet is important in pregnancy because of the tendency for constipation. Including fruit and vegetables and cereal fibre in bread or breakfast cereals can provide sufficient NSP to relieve problems of constipation.

A summary of the dietary reference values for pregnancy is given in Table 6.2.

It should be noted that many of the recommendations made by the UK Department of Health (DoH, 1991) assume an adequate pre-pregnancy diet, resulting in good nutritional status and stores at the outset of pregnancy. Where these are not present, extra intakes will be necessary during pregnancy.

This is a particular problem with iron because it is recognized that a substantial proportion of women have a chronically low intake resulting in poor stores. An early check on haemoglobin and circulating ferritin will confirm if iron status is adequate or whether supplementation is required.

Moreover, where there is a short interval between pregnancies, levels of some nutrients, such as calcium, iron and folate, may be insufficiently restored. It may take 2 years to return levels to their original values. Attention to a nutrient-rich diet is, therefore, important in this situation.

Teenage girls who become pregnant are also particularly at risk, as their own growth needs are high and stores may be insufficient.

Food Safety

Other advice on dietary intake includes food safety issues. The presence of *Listeria monocytogenes* can cause a series of symptoms from mild to severe, but can also result in premature birth or miscarriage and meningitis in a newborn baby. This is a relatively rare condition (estimates are 1 in 30,000 in the United Kingdom), but pregnant women are advised to avoid potentially contaminated foods. These include certain cheeses, such as Brie, Camembert and blue-veined cheeses, and meat-based pates. Cooked chilled meats and ready to eat poultry may also be a source of contamination. Other microbiological contaminants include *Salmonella* and toxoplasmosis (mainly from cat litter).

However, there is little evidence to show that education of pregnant women to improve their diet has significant effects. Targeted interventions may make some impact in specific groups, and these are considered in the following text. In general, encouragement of healthy eating and increase in nutritional knowledge for the future benefit of the family are useful targets.

Throughout pregnancy, alcohol taken in moderate to large amounts may result in growth retardation or more seriously in fetal alcohol syndrome. This includes a series of characteristic malformations and defects affecting the face, heart, brain and nervous system and is generally associated with reduced mental capacity. In the United Kingdom, the new alcohol guidelines (2016) state that no level of alcohol is safe to drink in pregnancy.

SHOULD SUPPLEMENTS BE GIVEN?

There have been many studies of the effects of various supplements on pregnancy outcome. In general, the effects of supplementation (other than with folic acid) during pregnancy are small.

The provision of a balanced energy and protein supplement to undernourished women results in birthweight increases of less than 100 g. High-protein supplements may actually result in reductions in birthweight, possibly associated with development of a larger placenta rather than increasing the size of the fetus. A better understanding of the metabolic adaptations that occur in pregnant women suggests that the result of supplementation is a decrease in the efficiency of energy saving by the mother, with a resulting higher cost of the pregnancy. It is also unclear how much of the supplement the women consume; it may be used to replace intakes rather than add to existing nutrient levels.

Evidence suggests that the greatest effects of supplementation occur when this is given either in the first 3 months of pregnancy or, preferably, before conception. In the latter case, identifying mothers who have already given birth to a low-weight baby and providing supplements in the inter-pregnancy period has proved to be effective in avoiding a subsequent low birthweight. The Women, Infants, and Children program in the United States, which provides food or voucher support to women in low-income groups, has demonstrated a consistent benefit in terms of better health of the baby and reduced need for health and welfare support in the future. This is a cost-effective scheme with greater savings than costs.

In London, supplementation with multivitamins and minerals, of women who had borne a low-birthweight infant and who were found to have a poor diet (not meeting the majority of dietary reference values), resulted in a favourable improvement in folate and iron levels up to 9 months after delivery. Control subjects who did not receive the supplements continued to have low blood levels of these nutrients. This would be an unfavourable start for a subsequent pregnancy and indicates how poor nutrient intakes can be insufficient to restore blood levels of nutrients in the inter-pregnancy period.

Similarly, supplementation with specific nutrients, such as folate or iron, may be most effective if given pre-conceptionally or in the very early weeks of pregnancy. Although it occurs routinely in much obstetric care, there is controversy about the desirability of supplementation with iron during pregnancy. Some evidence suggests that pregnancy outcome is optimal at haemoglobin concentrations between 96 and 105 g/L, indicating that this level may be the most desirable. Haemoglobin levels above this value can be achieved by supplementation, but this may be counterproductive.

It could be argued that a low iron status is merely a marker of a generally inadequate diet, which may be low in other, less frequently measured nutrients. It would, therefore, appear to be preferable to improve the whole diet, rather than to focus on specific nutrients, which might result in an unbalanced intake.

The need to supplement with long-chain fatty acids has also been debated, particularly for women whose diet is low in dietary sources. Infant growth and development, especially of the brain and retina, is dependent on an adequate supply of docosahexaenoic acid. Poor status in the mother will mean low levels in the infant. Supplementation of the mother in late pregnancy with fish oil has been shown to increase levels of *n*-3 fatty acids in cord blood of the newborn infant. Supplementation can also increase concentrations of *n*-3 acids in breast milk.

Supplementation with calcium has been used effectively to reduce blood pressure in women at risk of hypertension in pregnancy. The greatest benefits have been seen in women with low dietary calcium levels. The amount used is at least 1 g of calcium per day. Longer-term studies of the offspring from these pregnancies have shown lower blood pressures in the children.

WHO IS MOST AT RISK IN PREGNANCY?

A number of groups in the population are particularly vulnerable to poor pregnancy outcome.

Teenage Mothers

Nutritional status at conception may be poor for a number of reasons. Adolescents are less likely to be eating a well-balanced diet. This applies particularly to girls who may be chronic dieters as a result of the current fashion for slimness. National data show that high proportions of young women aged 19–24 years in the United Kingdom have low intakes and biochemical status for several micronutrients. Low intakes of vitamins A and C, folic acid, calcium, iron, iodine and zinc have been reported with significant percentages of this population below the Lower Reference Nutrient Intake (LRNI) for vitamin A (19%), riboflavin (15%), iron (42%) and iodine (12%) (SACN, 2011).

Furthermore, if the girl is still growing, her own nutritional needs may be high and, if she continues to grow during the pregnancy, the baby's development will be compromised. A teenage mother may have social problems, including eating very little to conceal the pregnancy, having little money, perhaps smoking and living in poor-quality housing. All of these factors will contribute to a poorer pregnancy outcome with a higher incidence of low birthweight, perinatal mortality, premature delivery and maternal problems of difficult labour, anaemia and hypertension.

Low Income

Women of lower educational attainment and those who are from deprived social backgrounds are more likely to exhibit poor dietary patterns at conception. There is evidence that women living in the most deprived areas consumed diets poorer in protein, fibre and vitamins and minerals (SACN, 2011).

The cost of a diet appropriate to meet the needs of a pregnant woman has been calculated to be between 40 and 65% of the state benefits payable in the United Kingdom. For most women in this situation, it is unrealistic to spend this amount on food for themselves, and a nutritionally inferior diet is eaten, containing insufficient amounts of nutrients to meet the needs. This leads to a high incidence of low birthweight. Of particular concern is the fatty acid profile of the diet, which may include few long-chain polyunsaturated fatty acids (such as arachidonic and docosahexaenoic acids) that are crucial for the development of the neural and vascular systems and are particularly important in the last 3 months of pregnancy when brain growth is at its most rapid. These essential fatty acids are found in vegetable oils, green vegetables and oily fish, which occur less frequently in the diets of the poor. This deficit may have long-term consequences for the growth and development of their children.

The UK Government has introduced the Healthy Start programme, a UK-wide government scheme, which aims to improve the health of pregnant women and families on benefits or low incomes. Healthy Start supports low-income families in eating healthily, by providing them with vouchers to spend on cow's milk, plain fresh or frozen fruit and vegetables and infant formula milk, underpinned by ongoing advice and information on subjects such as breastfeeding and healthy eating. It also provides pregnant women, new mothers and young children on the scheme with

TABLE 6.3
Possible Indicators of Nutritional Vulnerability in Pregnancy

Indicator	Possible Causes
Low nutrient stores at conception	Adolescent growth spurt
	Closely spaced pregnancies
	Low BMI
	Intake affected by poverty
	History of dieting/disordered eating
Poor intake during pregnancy (evidenced by poor weight gain)	Poor-quality diet due to poverty, lack of interest in food, smoking, use of drugs or alcohol
	Previous low-weight birth
	Illness/sickness of pregnancy
	Negative attitude to pregnancy
	Cultural taboos on diet in pregnancy
Pre-existing or gestational disease/condition	Requires special diet/monitoring of food and drug balance during pregnancy
	Weight gain/weight loss

free Healthy Start vitamins. Women supported by Healthy Start are entitled to free vitamin tablets during pregnancy and until their child is 1 year old. Children aged from 6 months to their fourth birthday are entitled to free vitamin drops (UK Government, 2014).

Underweight and Overweight Women

The importance of adequate but not excessive weight gain has already been discussed. Infants born to underweight women may exhibit inadequate patterns of growth at 12 months, suggesting delays in development. Overweight women also have increased pregnancy risks, both for themselves and the outcome for the baby. In overweight women, dieting during pregnancy is never recommended; a low energy intake during pregnancy may result in ketosis and pose a threat for the developing fetus. However, maintaining a reasonable level of activity during pregnancy is desirable to avoid excessive weight gain and benefit the mother's physiological fitness. Aerobic exercise may be particularly beneficial for women with a predisposition to gestational diabetes, as it enhances insulin sensitivity.

Other Situations

Other at-risk situations that may occur are summarized in Table 6.3.

LONG-TERM CONSEQUENCES OF INTRAUTERINE EVENTS

Studies on animals have over many years shown that the tissues and organs of the fetus go through critical periods in their development, at specific times in uterine life. It has also been cleared that a positive or negative stimulus occurring during a critical period can have permanent and lifelong consequences, even after that stimulus has been removed or cancelled. This phenomenon is known as 'programming', and in evolutionary terms is probably an adaptation to improve the chances of short-term survival, while having longer-term consequences that may be detrimental. These are less important from the evolutionary perspective, if the consequence is delayed until post-reproductive life. The relevance of programming to humans has only been recognized from the mid-1980s, and since then an enormous amount of research has been published that shows the fundamental impact of events in fetal life on subsequent health of individuals.

Early clues to the need for this research came from observations that the distribution of coronary heart disease in the 1970s in the United Kingdom mirrored patterns of infant mortality at the start of the twentieth century. This suggested that events in early life that caused a high rate of infant deaths might in some way contribute to a higher risk of coronary heart disease in survivors. Following improvements in living standards in the middle of the twentieth century, coronary heart disease rates began to show a decrease in the later decades of the century. This fall could not be attributed to any major changes in adult lifestyle factors. Furthermore, as developing countries are becoming more Westernized, prevalence of coronary heart disease and other Western diseases is rising there, in much the same way as they did in the United Kingdom in the middle of the twentieth century.

Evidence in support of a link came initially from data contained in birth and development records of babies born in the early decades of the twentieth century, together with mortality records of those who have since died and measurements made on the survivors. A strong negative correlation between weight at birth and the incidence of coronary heart disease later in life was found (Barker, 1998). This did not apply only to babies that could be classified as 'low birthweight', but was true across the whole range of normal birthweights at full term. This negative association between weight at birth and coronary heart disease has since been demonstrated in several different study cohorts, in the United States, India and Norway.

Furthermore, relationships have been demonstrated between weight at birth and the presence of some of the accepted risk factors for coronary heart disease. The evidence suggests that restricted growth during uterine life programmes the fetus in a way that increases subsequent risk of coronary heart disease and other degenerative diseases. As the mechanisms underlying these findings are explored, it has become clear that birthweight alone is a crude indicator of changes that have occurred during uterine life. Changes in body proportions, including thinness, length, head and abdominal circumference are able to give more information about possible organs that may have been advantaged or disadvantaged in utero. The ratio of the placental weight to birthweight has also shown to be a useful indicator. At either extreme, an imbalance between these suggests that either the placenta was too small to provide adequate nutrients for the fetus or it was excessively large and, therefore, took a greater share of nutrients for its own development.

At the cellular level, it is understood that programming may

1. Alter gene expression, for example, resulting in different levels of enzyme activity, potential mechanism may be epigenetic (such as gene methylation and histone acetylation)
2. Affect cell division, resulting in fewer cell numbers within a particular organ
3. Influence levels of hormone secretion or sensitivity of receptor sites to hormones

Examples of these changes have been demonstrated in animal studies, but application of modern experimental techniques will allow more to be studied in humans to further the understanding of processes that happened in the womb.

Lower birthweight has been associated with the following conditions:

Higher Blood Pressure

A recent systematic review and meta-analysis of 31 studies explored the possible effects of high birthweight (HBW) on blood pressure and hypertension (Zhang et al., 2013). The mean difference in blood pressure and the relative risk of hypertension between individuals with HBW and individuals with normal birthweight was inversely associated with age. Systolic blood pressure (SBP) and diastolic blood pressure (DBP), as well as the prevalence of hypertension, were higher in younger children with HBW but lower in older adults with HBW compared with individuals with normal birthweight. The findings suggested that an individual with HBW is prone to hypertension and higher blood pressure during childhood. However, a 'catch-down' effect in the elevation of blood pressure is observed in subjects with HBW as they grow older. Thus, older individuals with HBW are less susceptible to hypertension than those with normal birthweight.

The relationship with blood pressure is also found when the ratio of placental weight to birthweight is considered. A disproportion between these weights, in either direction from the normal ratio of 1:6, is associated with a higher blood pressure. A number of mechanisms have been postulated to explain these findings. Poor nutrient supply may compromise renal development, with reduced numbers of nephrons that become more susceptible to raised glomerular pressure, leading to hypertension. The involvement of the hypothalamus, pituitary and adrenals is considered as a probable mechanism. The model proposes that the fetus is exposed to higher levels of cortisol. These may originate from the mother, as a result of physiological stress, and are insufficiently blocked by low activity of 11-beta-hydroxysteroid dehydrogenase in the placenta and thus reach the fetus. Down-regulation of this enzyme has been demonstrated in the placenta in the animal model. Alternatively, the fetus itself experiences stress and generates high levels of cortisol. The raised cortisol levels have multiple effects on the development and sensitivity of blood vessels as well as the response of the hypothalamus to signals from blood pressure receptors.

Insulin Resistance and Diabetes Mellitus

Many studies have confirmed the relationship between low weight and thinness at birth with a greater risk of impaired glucose tolerance, insulin resistance or type 2 diabetes in the adult. A systematic review of the evidence for this association was conducted in 2008. Of the 31 studies reviewed, inverse birthweight–type 2 diabetes associations were observed in 23 populations (9 of which were statistically significant) and positive associations were found in 8 (2 of which were statistically significant) (Whincup et al., 2008).

Raised plasma insulin concentrations and slower glucose clearance after challenge with glucose have both been demonstrated in children who were thin at birth. In adults who were thin at birth, lower rates of energy production from glucose in skeletal muscle during exercise have been shown. These findings have led to the hypothesis that the fetal metabolism responds to a reduced nutrient supply by reducing its utilization of glucose. This is achieved by a reduction in levels of insulin and insulin-like growth factor I and increased cortisol levels. Skeletal muscle growth and glucose uptake are both reduced, and amino acids and lactate are used for energy. Thus, there is reduced muscle bulk, resulting in a thinner baby and a relatively lower glucose utilization accompanied by less responsiveness to insulin. If this metabolic pattern persists into adulthood, it predisposes to the insulin resistance syndrome and type 2 diabetes.

A further consequence of programming that may determine glucose metabolism affects the size and function of the pancreatic cells that secrete insulin. Animal studies have shown that rats fed protein-deficient diets produced offspring with fewer pancreatic islet cells and a reduced ability to regulate glucose. Such a situation will result in insulin deficiency in adult life.

Cholesterol Metabolism and Blood Clotting

Animal studies have demonstrated that impaired nutrient supply to the fetus in the latter stages of gestation results in diversion of more oxygenated blood flow to the cranial region to protect development there. As a result, the trunk, and particularly the liver, becomes relatively deprived of nutrients, with the potential for permanent changes to be programmed at this stage. Studies on rats fed low-protein diets have identified changes in levels of enzymes associated with lipid metabolism and blood clotting in the liver. Studies in humans have indicated that infants born with a relatively larger head and either a shorter trunk or smaller abdominal circumference have raised levels of factors produced by the liver. These include blood-clotting factors, such as fibrinogen, and cholesterol fractions. Both of these may contribute to a higher risk of coronary heart disease in later life.

Other Conditions

Other possible conditions that may have fetal origins have been investigated. For many, there is still only emerging evidence and more research is needed. These include associations of fetal development with various cancers, intelligence, obesity, atopy and food allergies, immune status, polycystic ovary syndrome and osteoporosis. In addition, ageing processes appear to be associated with growth and nutrition in early life; lower weight at 1 year has been found to be associated with increased lens opacity, thinner skin, poorer hearing and reduced muscle strength in old age. Figure 6.1 summarizes the fetal influences on later health.

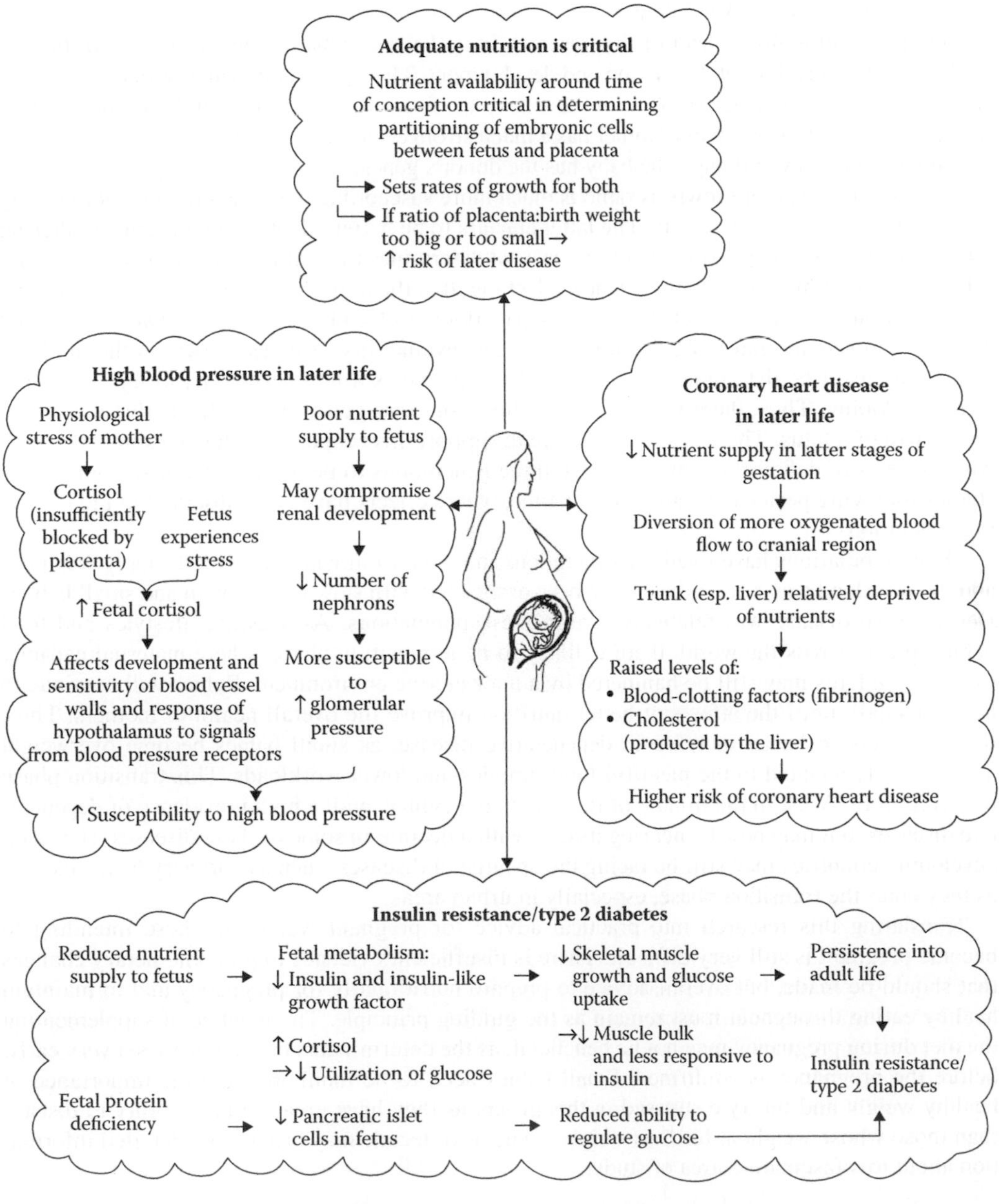

FIGURE 6.1 Summary of fetal influences on later health.

It should be stressed here that not every small baby is destined to have a lifetime of ill health. The effects of programming are inevitably modified by lifestyle factors. However, it is clear from the research to date that the greatest risk of developing degenerative diseases occurs in those who had been small at birth or small at 1 year of age and who are then exposed to adverse conditions in adult life (such as weight gain, smoking, a high saturated fat diet, lack of exercise). The largest babies, or the ones who had grown well in the first year of life, were found to have the lowest risk of developing these degenerative diseases.

These correlations are strong and show up to threefold differences in risk between those with the highest and lowest birthweights, for example, in the development of impaired glucose tolerance and diabetes. If adult BMI is taken into account, the risk increases to almost sevenfold in those who also become overweight.

The most tantalizing aspect of this research is to discover what aspects of maternal diet are the keys that determine fetal nutrition and development. There is strong evidence that the uterine environment is a major determinant of the size of the fetus. Research from embryo implantation studies shows that the recipient mother has a much stronger influence on the size of the baby than the donor mother, even though the baby has the donor's genes.

A fetus whose rate of growth is rapid is much more susceptible than one growing more slowly to a change in the nutrient supply. The latter appears to be better adapted to withstand a faltering nutrient supply. A key question, therefore, is what determines the setting of the growth trajectory. It is suggested, although human evidence is lacking, that the nutrient availability around the time of conception is critical in determining the partitioning of embryonic cells between fetus and placenta and sets the rates of growth for both. The availability of nutrients within the mother's womb may itself be determined by her own development as a fetus, when her ovary and uterus were developing. Thus, there is a strong possibility of cross-generational effects that determine the growth of a fetus. There is some evidence to support this proposal, both from studies on rats, where effects of deficiency may take up to three generations to be normalized, and from human studies following periods of famine in wartime, where effects have been observed in the following generation.

Many populations have lived for generations in an environment where food supply was poor and the workload was heavy; these have been associated with slow fetal growth and small babies. Degenerative disease was relatively rare in these populations. As Western lifestyles and food habits spread across the world, there is likely to be a transition phase, where maternal capacity to nourish a fetus may still be hampered by a poor uterine environment. Babies will continue to be born small, until the effects of better nutrition improve the overall health of mothers. Thus, there is likely to be an increase in degenerative disease, as small babies become overweight adults, poorly adapted to the plentiful food supplies and lower workloads. This transition phase occurred in the West in the middle of the twentieth century, with a high prevalence of degenerative diseases, but may now be nearing its end, with a decline in some of these diseases. However, developing countries may still be facing the upsurge of diseases, such as coronary heart disease, as they enter the transition phase, especially in urban areas.

Translating this research into practical advice for pregnant women or those intending to become pregnant is still very difficult. There is insufficient evidence to pinpoint dietary changes that should be made, but overall advice to prepare nutritionally for pregnancy and to maintain healthy eating throughout must remain as the guiding principle. The practice of supplementing the diet during pregnancy may not be beneficial, as the determinants of growth are set very early, before the pregnancy is confirmed. Small babies need to be monitored and the importance of healthy weight and lifestyle stressed in this group, as they have greater vulnerability to disease than those whose weight at birth was higher. The next decade may bring more detailed information about this fascinating area of study.

NURSING OR LACTATING MOTHER

Breastfeeding a newborn infant is the natural sequel to pregnancy. The process of lactation (or milk production) does not occur in isolation since the mother's breasts become prepared for lactation throughout pregnancy. By no means, all mothers choose to breastfeed their babies. In the United Kingdom, prevalence of breastfeeding at birth increased from 76% in 2005 to 81% in 2010, although there are great differences between middle-class mothers, of whom almost 89% may start breastfeeding, and lower-social-class mothers, where the prevalence at birth is in the order of 73% (McAndrew et al., 2012). However, the prevalence of breastfeeding fell from 81% at birth to 55% at 6 weeks and 34% at 6 months. For mothers who choose to breastfeed, it is usually a special and enjoyable experience. Those mothers who decide not to breastfeed can provide adequate nutrition for their babies using the many formula feeds available. However, certain aspects of human milk will not be present in the formula.

If a woman decides not to breastfeed her child, the breasts return to their normal pre-pregnant size within a fairly short period of time.

PROCESS OF LACTATION

There are two stages involved in lactation: milk production and milk ejection (see Figure 6.2).

Milk Production or Lactogenesis

Milk is made in the mammary glands of the breast, which contain cells arranged in lobules. The synthesis of milk is stimulated by the hormone prolactin released from the anterior pituitary gland, which in turn is stimulated by the process of suckling by the infant at the breast. Thus, the more the infant suckles, the more milk is synthesized, and milk production parallels demand.

Some proteins found in milk, such as the immune factors, enter from the maternal circulation, but the majority of the protein content is synthesized by the mammary glands. The fats that contain short-chain fatty acids are synthesized in the breast, but the long-chain fats are derived from the maternal diet. A mother who consumes a high level of long-chain fats will, therefore, have higher levels of them in her milk. The galactose part of the lactose molecule is synthesized in the breast and the glucose part is derived from the maternal circulation.

Milk Ejection or Let Down

The milk that is formed is not released from the breast until the baby suckles. This initiates a reflex in the mother, involving signals to the hypothalamus, which in turn cause the release of the hormone oxytocin from the posterior pituitary gland. It is this hormone that causes the specialized cells in the mammary gland to contract and eject the milk into the mouth of the infant. The reflex can be inhibited by the mother's mental state: if she is apprehensive, tense or tired, the reflex can fail and milk is not released. An understanding of the nature of the reflex, which allows sufficient relaxation and preparation for feeding, can prevent a great deal of frustration. After about 2 weeks of breastfeeding, the reflex becomes automatic and can be triggered simply by hearing the baby crying.

DIET IN LACTATION

As with pregnancy, no special diet is needed in lactation. It must be remembered, however, that the food eaten by the mother in the first 4–6 months of breastfeeding (before weaning takes place) has to meet all of her own needs as well as those of the baby, which are considerably greater than its

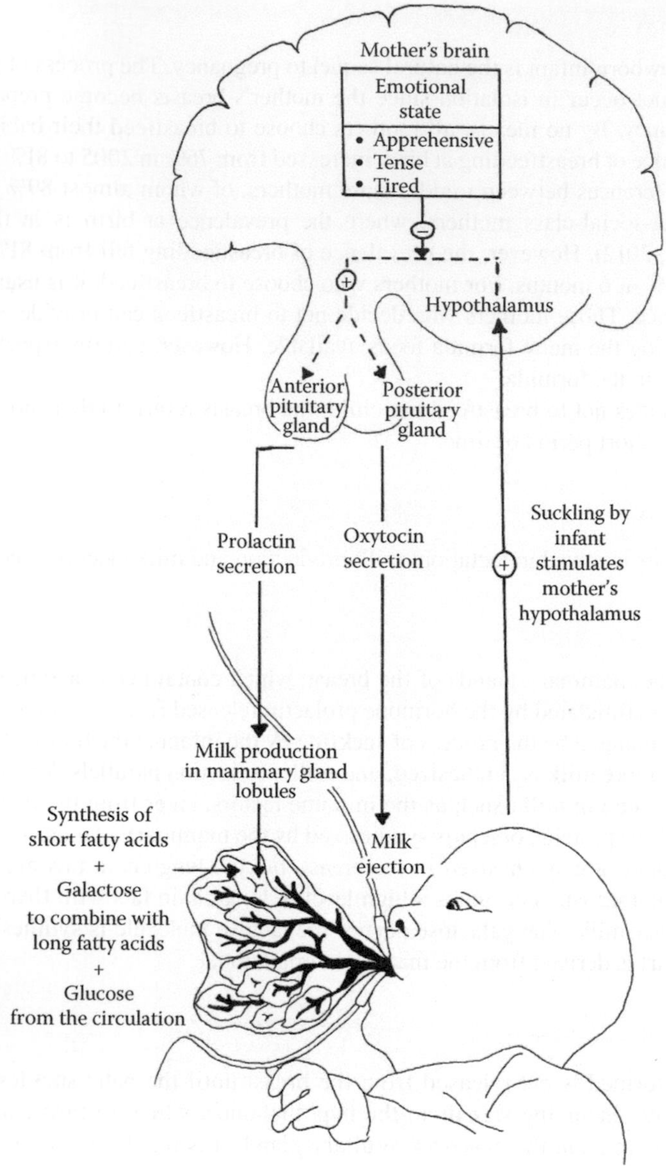

FIGURE 6.2 Process of lactation.

needs while in the womb. These increased requirements are reflected in the higher dietary reference values published by the UK Department of Health (DoH, 1991) and summarized in Table 6.4.

Energy

The average daily volume of milk produced varies from mother to mother. Data from the United Kingdom and Sweden indicate that the average volume of milk produced in the first 3 months of lactation ranges from 680 to 820 mL/day. The energy cost of producing this milk, assuming an 80% efficiency of energy conversion, has been calculated as 2.38–2.87 MJ (570–690 cal) per day in the first 3 months. After 3 months, and assuming that weaning begins at around 4 months, the output of milk falls to 700 mL/day, with an energy cost to the mother of 2.45 MJ (590 cal) per day.

TABLE 6.4

Dietary Reference Values for Lactation

Nutrient	Recommended Level
Energy	Additional 450–570 kcal (1.9–2.4 MJ)/day at 1–3 months Additional 480 kcal (2.0 MJ)/day between 3 and 6 months
Protein	To cover protein content of milk, increase by 11 g/day; total recommended 56 g/day
Vitamin A	To cover content in milk, increase by 350 μg/day; total recommended 950 μg/day
Thiamin	Increase only in line with increased energy requirement
Riboflavin	To cover extra content in milk, and its secretion, increase by 0.5 mg/day; total recommended 1.6 mg/day
Niacin	To cover extra content in milk, increase by 2.3 mg/day; total recommended 8.9 mg/day
Pyridoxine	No evidence exists of a need to increase intake
Vitamin B_{12}	To cover the content in milk, increase by 0.5 mg/day; total recommended 2.0 mg/day
Folate	To cover the content in milk, and absorption and utilization by the mother, increase by 60 μg/day; total recommended 260 μg/day
Vitamin C	To cover content in milk and maintain maternal stores, increase by 30 mg/day; total recommended 70 mg/day
Vitamin D	To maintain plasma vitamin D levels: recommend a supplement of 10 μg/day
Calcium	To cover content in milk and allow for efficiency of absorption by mother, increase by 550 mg/day; total recommended 1250 mg/day
Magnesium	To cover content in milk, and allow for absorption, increase by 50 mg/day; total recommended 320 mg/day
Iron	Extra content in milk can be met by lactational amenorrhoea; thus, no extra increment
Zinc	To cover zinc content of milk; no information about enhanced absorption is available; thus increase by 6 mg/day; total recommended 13 mg/day

Source: Reproduced from DoH (UK Department of Health), Dietary reference values for food energy and nutrients for the United Kingdom, Report on Health and Social Subjects No. 41, Report of the Panel on Dietary Reference Values of the Committee on Medical Aspects of Food Policy, HMSO, London, UK, 1991. With permission.

Some of this extra energy can be met from fat stores laid down in pregnancy, although the extent to which this is mobilized appears to vary between women. It is assumed that, on average, 0.5 kg of stored fat is used per month, although women have been recorded as losing between 0.6 and 0.8 kg/month during the first 4–6 months after delivery. In overweight women, a loss of 2 kg/month may be possible, but feeding on demand should continue to ensure that adequate milk production is maintained. Undertaking intense exercise to speed up weight loss can raise lactic acid levels in the blood, which will pass into the milk and affect the taste. However, moderate exercise is beneficial and should be encouraged, as long as energy needs continue to be met.

Dietary energy restriction may affect milk output, particularly in the first weeks before lactation is fully established. However, it is also possible that milk output is only compromised when body fat stores are below a particular threshold level. It is also important to recognize that restricting energy intake to a low level will have consequences for the quality of the diet and may result in other nutrient requirements not being met. There is a concern that toxic chemical residues, which may be present in maternal body fat, will be mobilized and secreted in the milk, if fat stores are used as a source of energy. There is little evidence, however, on which a judgement can be based.

In women who are chronically undernourished and, therefore, have very low body fat reserves, lactation can still occur satisfactorily even in these apparently adverse circumstances. Studies suggest that the greater efficiency of metabolism seen in pregnancy carries through into lactation, so that costs of maintaining the mother's body remain low, thus providing extra energy for milk production. However, the nutritional content of the milk probably starts to fall from the third or fourth month of lactation.

Protein

The protein content of milk supplies the amino acids necessary for the growth of the baby and the additional amount should be provided in the mother's diet. If the diet contains sufficient extra energy to satisfy those needs, then the protein content will also be adequate. On a poor diet, where the total food supply is inadequate, it is not possible to provide additional protein, but protein levels in the milk are maintained for several months even under these circumstances.

GENERAL CONSIDERATIONS

It can be seen from Table 8.4 that nutritional needs in lactation are greater than those in pregnancy. However, if a mother satisfies her need for additional energy, then the increased needs for all the other nutrients should be met, assuming the extra food eaten is well balanced.

Nutrients that warrant special attention are calcium and vitamins A and D. If it is not possible to increase food intake, then the nutritional quality of the milk may suffer. The water-soluble vitamins, B complex and C, will be present in smaller amounts. The other constituents, namely fats, lactose, protein and fat-soluble vitamins, may remain at an adequate level for 3–4 months, but will then decline. The weight gain of the baby may slow down or stop at this point, and alternative sources of food will be needed for the baby.

DECISION TO BREASTFEED

Human milk is ideally suited to the needs of the human infant. Nevertheless, a significant number of mothers do not take advantage of the process of lactation for a number of reasons. The arguments for and against breastfeeding from the mother's perspective are briefly reviewed and summarized in Figure 6.3. An additional

The benefits of breastfeeding are discussed further with respect to the infant in Chapter 7, pp. 129–133.

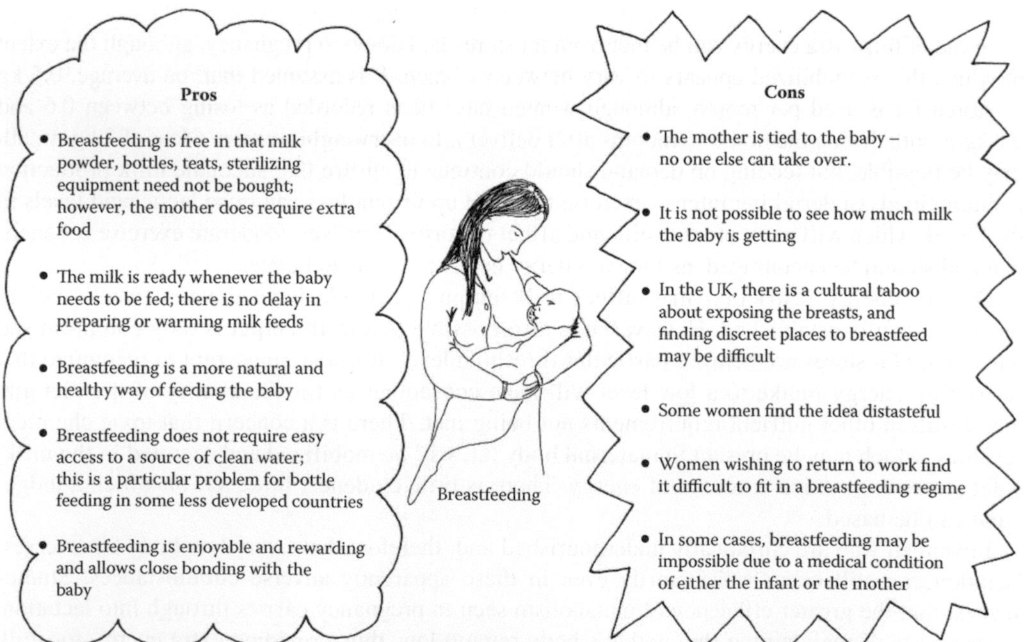
Pros
• Breastfeeding is free in that milk powder, bottles, teats, sterilizing equipment need not be bought; however, the mother does require extra food
• The milk is ready whenever the baby needs to be fed; there is no delay in preparing or warming milk feeds
• Breastfeeding is a more natural and healthy way of feeding the baby
• Breastfeeding does not require easy access to a source of clean water; this is a particular problem for bottle feeding in some less developed countries
• Breastfeeding is enjoyable and rewarding and allows close bonding with the baby
Breastfeeding
Cons
• The mother is tied to the baby – no one else can take over.
• It is not possible to see how much milk the baby is getting
• In the UK, there is a cultural taboo about exposing the breasts, and finding discreet places to breastfeed may be difficult
• Some women find the idea distasteful
• Women wishing to return to work find it difficult to fit in a breastfeeding regime
• In some cases, breastfeeding may be impossible due to a medical condition of either the infant or the mother

FIGURE 6.3 Arguments for and against breastfeeding.

advantage of breastfeeding is that it has been shown to protect women against breast cancer; this may explain the higher rates of breast cancer in developed than in the less developed countries.

Because the decision to breastfeed or not is based on so many deeply held beliefs, it should be respected, and mothers who choose not to breastfeed should not be made to feel that they are failing their baby in any way. What matters for the mother and infant is that the mother is confident with what she is doing and can provide all of the nutritional needs that her child requires. She can achieve this with formula milk or by ensuring that her own nutrition is adequate to provide good-quality milk for as long as she wishes to feed her infant.

SUMMARY

1. The outcome of pregnancy for both the mother and infant depends on nutritional status of the mother.
2. Nutritional status prior to pregnancy may determine fertility and the early development of the embryo.
3. During pregnancy, the first 3 months are the most critical from the nutritional perspective, as the placenta is not fully developed and the fetus depends entirely on the concentrations of nutrients in the mother's circulation.
4. The needs for some nutrients increase more than others. All nutritional needs can be met from a balanced diet, eaten in sufficient amounts. Many adaptations occur in the mother's body to ensure adequate nutrient supplies.
5. The nutrient supply to the fetus may not only determine the birthweight but also set up the programme for potential health in future years.
6. Lactation is a sequel to pregnancy and also requires adequate nutrition.
7. The quality of the milk is largely protected from shortcomings in the mother's diet for the first 3 months of lactation by increased efficiency in maternal metabolism.

STUDY QUESTIONS

1. Why is it important for a woman to be nutritionally fit at the time of conception?
2. Metabolic adjustments occur in a woman during pregnancy. In the following cases, state what the adjustments are and their consequences for nutritional intake or needs:
   a. Appetite
   b. Digestive tract function
   c. Metabolic rate
3. Design a poster or leaflet giving practical dietary advice for pregnancy.
4. Why might the following groups be particularly nutritionally vulnerable during pregnancy?
   a. Vegetarians
   b. Women on a low income
   c. Young adolescent girls (aged 13–15)
5. Identify five reasons commonly cited by women against breastfeeding and consider how you might offer a positive view to counter each reason.

ACTIVITIES

6.1 Think about what you have just read, and answer the following question:
How would the following cases cope with the metabolic demands of pregnancy?
1. A normal-weight woman in a food-deficient, poor country, who commutes to work daily, on foot (total distance 30 km).
2. A normal-weight woman living in an industrialized Western country

3. An overweight woman, living in a Western country.
4. A 14-year-old girl, living in a Western country, but in a low-income household.

6.2 1. Carry out a small survey among your colleagues. Ask whether they have opinions about breastfeeding and try to relate these to their own experience of breastfeeding. This may include seeing siblings breastfed, having breastfed an infant themselves or having seen friends breastfeeding.
Is there a gender difference in opinion?
Is there an age difference?
Do the opinions you collect match those given in Figure 6.3?
Can you add others to the list?
2. In what ways do you think health promotion could persuade people to breastfeed their children?

BIBLIOGRAPHY AND FURTHER READING

Anderson, A.S. 2001. Pregnancy as a time for dietary change? *Proceedings of the Nutrition Society* 60, 497–504.

Barker, D.J.P. 1998. *Mothers, Babies and Health in Later Life*. Edinburgh, Scotland: Churchill Livingstone.

Czeizel, A.E. 1993. Prevention of congenital abnormalities by periconceptional multivitamin supplementation. *British Medical Journal* 306, 1645–1648.

DoH (UK Department of Health). 1991. Dietary reference values for food energy and nutrients for the United Kingdom. Report on Health and Social Subjects No. 41. Report of the Panel on Dietary Reference Values of the Committee on Medical Aspects of Food Policy. London, UK: HMSO.

Doyle, W., Crawford, M.A., Wynn, A.H.A. et al. 1990. The association between maternal diet and birth dimensions. *Journal of Nutritional Medicine* 1, 9–17.

European Food Safety Authority (EFSA). 2014. Scientific opinion on dietary reference values for iodine. *EFSA Journal* 12(5), 3660.

Food Standards Agency. 2002a. *Food Portion Sizes*, 3rd edn. London, UK: The Stationery Office.

Food Standards Agency. 2002b. *McCance and Widdowson's The Composition of Foods*, 6th summary edn. Cambridge, UK: The Royal Society of Chemistry.

Frisch, R.E. 1994. The right weight: Body fat, menarche and fertility. *Proceedings of the Nutrition Society* 53, 113–129.

Godfrey, K.M. and Barker, D.J.P. 2001. Fetal programming and adult health. *Public Health Nutrition* 4(2B), 611–624.

HEA (Health Education Authority). 1996. *Folic Acid – What All Women Should Know* (Leaflet). London, UK: HEA.

Institute of Medicine (US) and National Research Council (US). 2009. *Weight Gain during Pregnancy: Reexamining the Guidelines*. Rasmussen, K.M. and Yaktine, A.L. (eds.). Committee to Reexamine IOM Pregnancy Weight Guidelines. Washington, DC: National Academies Press (US).

Jackson, A.A. and Robinson, S.M. 2000. Dietary guidelines for pregnancy: A review of current evidence. *Public Health Nutrition* 4(2B), 625–630.

Langley-Evans, S.C. 2015. Nutrition in early and the programming of adult disease: A review. *Journal of Human Nutrition and Dietetics*. 28(s1): pp 1–14.

Law, C.M. and Shiell, A.W. 1996. Is blood pressure inversely related to birth weight? The strength of evidence from a systematic review of the literature. *Journal of Hypertension* 14, 935–941.

Livingstone, V. 1995. Breastfeeding kinetics: A problem-solving approach to breastfeeding difficulties. *World Review of Nutrition and Dietetics* 78, 28–54.

McAndrew, F., Thompson, J. Fellows, L. et al. 2012. *Infant Feeding Survey 2010*. Health and Social Care Information Centre. Available on line at: http://www.hscic.gov.uk/catalogue/PUB08694 (last accessed 30 October 2014).

Rasmussen, K.M. 1992. The influence of maternal nutrition on lactation. *Annual Review of Nutrition* 12, 103–117.

Sayer, A.A. and Cooper, C. 2002. Early diet and growth: Impact on ageing. *Proceedings of the Nutrition Society* 61, 79–85.

Scientific Advisory Committee on Nutrition. 2011. *The Influence of Maternal, Fetal and Child Nutrition on the Development of Chronic Disease in Later Life*. London, UK: The Stationery Office.

UK Government. 2014. *Healthy Start*. London, UK: HMSO.

Whincup, P.H., Kaye, S.J., Owen, C.G. et al. 2008. Birth weight and risk of type 2 diabetes: A systematic review. *Journal of the American Medical Association* 300, 2886–2897.

Wolff, T., Witkop, C.T., Miller, T. et al. 2009. Folic acid supplementation for the prevention of neural tube defects: An update of the evidence for the U.S. Preventive Services Task Force. *Annals of Internal Medicine* 150(9), 632–639.

Yajnik, C. 2000. Interactions of perturbations in intrauterine growth and growth during childhood on the risk of adult-onset disease. *Proceedings of the Nutrition Society* 59, 257–265.

Zhang, Y., Li, H., Liu, S.J. et al. 2013. The associations of high birth weight with blood pressure and hypertension in later life: A systematic review and meta-analysis. *Hypertension Research* 36, 725–735.

7 Nutrition during Infancy, Childhood and Adolescence

AIMS

The aims of this chapter are to

- Describe the nutritional needs of the infant and how these are met by human and formula milks.
- Discuss the process and objectives of weaning and consider the problems that might arise.
- Consider the diets of preschool children and the key nutritional principles to be addressed in this group.
- Discuss the diets of school-age children, including adolescents.
- Consider the special nutritional dilemmas encountered by teenagers.

Adequate dietary intake and nutritional status among children are important for their own growth, development and function. However, there is clear evidence that childhood nutrition influences adult health. Research has shown that intrauterine nutrition influences adult morbidity and mortality, but childhood diet and nutritional status can modify the consequences of being born small. Diet in all the stages of childhood needs to be taken seriously because of its potential for producing normally developed children as well as determining their lifelong health and thus having an impact on a nation's health. With many diets in transition owing to changing social, economic and environmental conditions, consideration of the impact of these changes on the diets of children is important. Particular issues of concern include the establishment of good dietary habits, together with adequate physical activity to prevent the development of overweight, adequate intakes of calcium to promote bone health and sufficient intakes of minerals and vitamins in the face of a culture often centred on fast food. There are many gaps in our current understanding of children's food habits and influences on these. It is difficult to obtain good-quality information about these and, therefore, health promotion inputs may be missing their target.

INFANTS

Infants are totally dependent on other people for their food supply. During the first year of life, there is very rapid growth, so for its age and size, the infant has very high nutritional needs. Neither of these situations normally occurs again in a healthy individual. The main aim of infant feeding is to satisfy nutritional needs in the best possible way and to achieve a healthy infant who is growing at the appropriate rate and is developing normally. Although the main emphasis here is on the principles of feeding normal infants, it must be remembered that infants who are premature, ill, disabled or with any other special needs can also be fed successfully, often by only minor adjustment of the normal practice.

GROWTH

Babies grow faster in their early months and more slowly in the latter part of the first year. An infant's birthweight is doubled within 4–6 months and trebles within the first year.

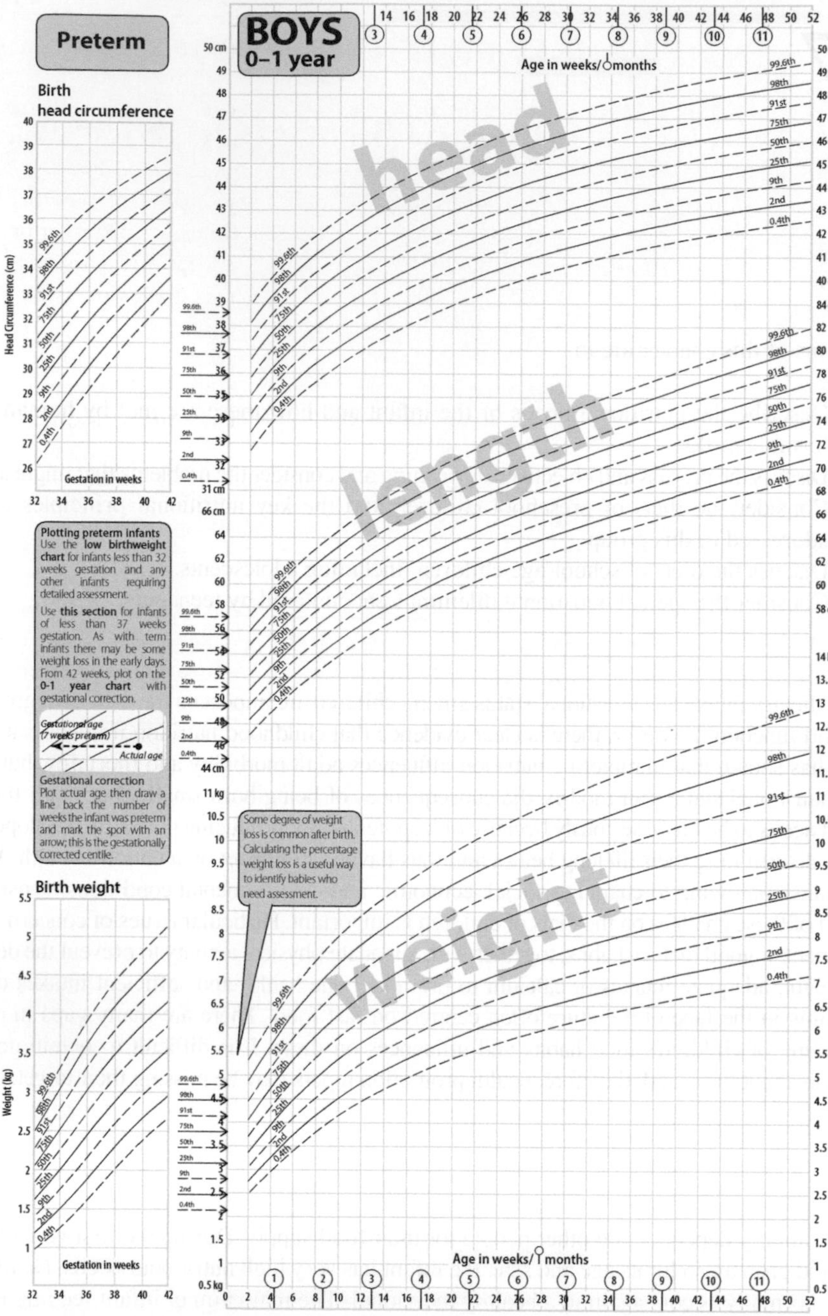

FIGURE 7.1 Example of a standard growth curve used to monitor child development.

Growth is slower thereafter, and the weight at 5 years is on average twice that of the weight at 1 year. Standard growth curves (see Figure 7.1) are used to monitor a child's development in terms of height and weight. They are based on percentiles, which represent the range of expected normal results in a group of children. The position of any one child represents their rank if 100 children had been measured. Monitoring weight and height at intervals allows a child's progress to be followed. Deviations over time from the child's usual curve may indicate inadequate nutrition, perhaps as a result of concurrent illness. This may be seen frequently in children in developing countries, who may experience periods of infection, possibly often in addition to chronic poor nutrition, resulting in slowed growth.

As in uterine life, postnatal growth may be slowed owing to insufficient cell multiplication or cell growth. The timing of poor nutrition will determine which aspect of growth is affected more. If fewer cells are made, then it is impossible for this to be remedied later by better nutrition. However, failure of cells to grow may be compensated by 'catch-up' growth, if nutrition improves. Key periods of cell multiplication occur at different times for different organs. Brain development, for example, occurs very rapidly in the first months after birth, and cell multiplication stops by the age of 12–15 months. Although growth continues, the brain is almost at adult size by the age of 5 years. Thus, infancy and childhood are critical periods for nutrient supply to the brain. There has been considerable debate about critical periods for fat cell formation, and some evidence suggests that overfeeding in infancy may encourage multiplication of fat cells. These may be associated with higher leptin levels and possible leptin resistance in later life. However, this requires further study.

Nutrition and Development

An infant born at full term is able to suck but is not able to bite or chew pieces of food, so that its diet must be a liquid one. The liquid designed by nature as food for the newborn is milk produced by its mother. This provides not only nourishment but also immune protection and developmental stimuli.

Alternative milks have been developed; these are highly modified to make them suitable for infants. In Britain, two types of milks derived from cows' milk are available: whey-dominant types based on the dialyzed whey protein and casein-dominant types based on the entire protein fraction. Modern milks are as similar in composition to human milk as possible; however, they lack the immunological and hormonal factors. Modified soya milks and other hydrolyzed protein formulas have also been developed to meet the needs of children with diagnosed allergies.

The ability to bite and chew lumps of food begins at 5–6 months, and it is at this stage that an increasing variety of tastes and textures can begin to be introduced into the baby's diet. An ability to chew lumpy food by 6–7 months is an important developmental step, and chewing is best learned at this age. If it is delayed, the child may have difficulty in learning to chew later. The ability to chew is also related to early speech development. Early feeding is thus an important preparation for verbal communication.

By the age of 1 year, the infant has progressed from a newborn only able to suck liquids from a nipple or teat to increasing independence of eating and attempting to feed itself. By this age, a child may have up to eight teeth, which help in the biting and tearing of food. Molar teeth for proper grinding of food develop late in the second year, when chewing ability becomes more fully developed.

Development of the Digestive Tract

In the young infant, digestive enzymes are not fully developed and certain dietary components may not be readily digested. Only small amounts of lipase are produced by the pancreas during the first 3 months (lingual lipase is therefore the primary enzyme for dietary fat digestion in the neonate), and pancreatic amylase increases only after 6 months. Breastfeeding is believed to promote the release of gastrin and cholecystokinin in the infant and may promote both the digestive process and the development of the gut. A young infant has the ability to absorb some undigested protein. This is particularly important for the absorption of antibodies present in maternal milk or colostrum during the first days of breastfeeding. However, it may also result in the absorption of proteins, such as egg albumen or lactoglobulin from cows' milk, if these are consumed in the early part of infancy. These proteins will generate antibodies within the infant and may lay the foundations of future allergic reactions. There has been a long-standing concern about early exposure of infants and children to peanuts in some weaning foods. The 'Learning Early about Peanut' (LEAP) study was the first randomized trial to show prevention of peanut allergy in a large cohort of high-risk infants, when infants were exposed to the allergen early.

Food allergy and atopy are covered in more detail in Chapter 21, pp. 408–410.

Nutritional Needs

It must be assumed that the nutritional needs of the infant are ideally met by breast milk, when this is produced in sufficient quantity by a fully breastfeeding mother. For this reason, the UK Department of Health (DoH, 1991) took the view that no dietary reference values (DRVs) were required for breastfed infants. Values were, therefore, set for formula-fed infants, which are based on the nutritional composition of breast milk and the average amounts consumed. In addition, some allowance is made in certain cases for poorer efficiency of digestion and absorption of the nutrients in formula milks. DRVs for infants are shown in Table 7.1.

Energy

Energy needs are determined primarily by body size and composition, physical activity and rate of growth. Infants have a high basal metabolic rate owing to the large proportion of metabolically active tissue and the large loss of body heat over a relatively great surface area. In the second half of the first year, the growth rate slows, but the level of activity increases as the child starts to crawl and then learns to walk around the age of 1 year. The total energy expenditure in infants has recently been measured using the doubly labelled water (DLW) technique, which has produced lower results than had been previously reported. Results from studies of energy intakes confirm these results.

Table 7.2 shows the gradual reduction in the energy requirement per kilogram of body weight as growth rates slow down; however, as body size increases, the total energy needs become greater. The energy requirement for children is up to four times greater than that of the adult, when expressed per unit of body weight. This emphasizes the special need for adequate energy and explains why a shortfall of energy may have such serious consequences for growth.

TABLE 7.1

Reference Nutrient Intakes for Selected Nutrients for Infants

Nutrient	0–3 Months	4–6 Months	7–9 Months	10–12 Months
Protein (g/day)	12.5	12.7	13.7	14.9
Thiamin (mg/day)	0.2	0.2	0.2	0.3
Riboflavin (mg/day)	0.4	0.4	0.4	0.4
Niacin (nicotinic acid equivalents) (mg/day)	3	3	4	5
Folate (μg/day)	50	50	50	50
Vitamin C (mg/day)	25	25	25	25
Vitamin A (μg/day)	350	350	350	350
Vitamin D (μg/day)	8.5	8.5	7	7
Calcium (mg/day)	525	525	525	525
Iron (mg/day)	1.7	4.3	7.8	7.8
Zinc (mg/day)	4.0	4.0	5.0	5.0

Source: Reproduced from DoH (UK Department of Health), Dietary reference values for food energy and nutrients for the United Kingdom, Report on Health and Social Subjects No. 41, Report of the Panel on Dietary Reference Values of the Committee on Medical Aspects of Food Policy, HMSO, London, UK, 1991. With permission.

TABLE 7.2

Estimated Average Requirement for Energy for Children up to the Age of 12 Months

	Average Weight (kg)		Requirement/kg	EAR [kJ (cal)]	
Age (Months)	Boys	Girls	Body Weight (kJ (cal))	Boys	Girls
1	4.15	4.00	480 (115)	1990 (480)	1920 (460)
3	6.12	5.70	420 (100)	2570 (610)	2390 (570)
6	8.00	7.44	400 (95)	3200 (760)	2980 (710)
9	9.20	8.55	400 (95)	3680 (880)	3420 (820)
12	10.04	9.50	400 (95)	4020 (960)	3800 (910)

Source: Reproduced from DoH (UK Department of Health), Dietary reference values for food energy and nutrients for the United Kingdom, Report on Health and Social Subjects No. 41, Report of the Panel on Dietary Reference Values of the Committee on Medical Aspects of Food Policy, HMSO, London, UK, 1991. With permission.

Protein

In infants, the role of protein is almost entirely to support growth. The infant requires more protein per unit weight than the adult and has a particular requirement for the essential amino acids histidine and taurine. Human milk provides a relative excess of some of the amino acids (glutamine, leucine and isoleucine) needed for tissue synthesis and relatively lower levels of others (arginine, alanine and glycine). This means that the neonate has to be very efficient in transforming some amino acids into others to fulfil needs for tissue synthesis. Adequate amounts of feed should be provided to allow the protein to be used for growth rather than to meet energy needs. Excessive amounts of protein are undesirable and may be harmful to the infant, as they increase the amounts of waste material to be excreted in the urine and might result in dehydration. In addition, immature kidneys cannot adequately filter high-molecular-weight proteins.

Fats

Fat should comprise 30%–50% of an infant's energy intake; above this level, it may be poorly digested. In breast milk, fats supply 50% of the energy. Fats are an important part of an infant's diet because of their energy density, that is, they provide a substantial amount of energy in a relatively small volume. The essential fatty acids found in milk, and particularly the long-chain *n*-3 fatty acids, are important for the development of the brain, vascular systems and retina in early months of life. In particular, docosahexaenoic acid may not be synthesized in sufficient amounts by the infant from precursors in the diet to meet the needs of tissue development.

Carbohydrates

Carbohydrate, predominantly in the form of lactose, supplies 40% of the energy in an infant's diet. Lactose yields glucose and galactose on digestion; the latter is essential in the development of the brain and nervous system. Undigested lactose is fermented in the digestive tract to lactic acid and lowers the pH. This is beneficial as many of the pathogenic organisms that can cause gastroenteritis do not thrive in an acidic environment. Infants can also digest and utilize sucrose, although this sugar is sweeter tasting than lactose and can induce a preference for sweet foods in the infant. The ability to digest starch is limited.

Fluid

Because of their relatively small total body water content, babies have a vital need for fluids. Their small body weight/surface area ratio makes them susceptible to dehydration, for example, in hot weather and illness. As an absolute minimum, the normal infant requires between 75 and 100 mL of fluid per kilogram body weight daily and should be provided with 150 mL/kg, to ensure that all needs are met. Under normal circumstances, this amount of fluid is provided by the milk feed and no additional water is required.

The infant loses water through the skin and respiratory tract, through sweating in warm environments and through the urine and faeces. The volume of urine produced is dependent on the fluid intake and on the amount of solutes to be excreted. An adult kidney is able to concentrate solutes and reduce water loss, if fluid intake is low, but a baby's kidneys initially lack this ability. Thus, feeding a diet with a high 'solute load', in particular with high protein and sodium contents, results in increased water loss via the kidney. Under normal circumstances, fluid intake should be sufficient to cope with this. However, difficulties may arise if

- A baby is given an over concentrated feed (unmodified cows' milk is inappropriate for this reason)
- Amounts of feed are very small (due to illness)
- There is fluid loss via other routes (vomiting, diarrhoea, sweating)
- Solids are given at a very young age (below 2 months)

In each of these cases, additional water should be given to avoid dehydration.

Minerals

Babies require a wide range of minerals in their diet. These include calcium, phosphorus and magnesium for bone development, iron and copper for red blood cell formation and zinc for cell division and growth, together with other trace elements. The iron content present at birth has usually been used in red blood cell formation by 4–6 months, and an additional source of iron is needed at this stage. Calcium and phosphorus are present in equimolar quantities in human milk, which matches the ratio in the body. An excessive intake of phosphorus can dangerously lower calcium levels. This is a particular problem in premature infants and those fed on unmodified formula. The minerals in human milk are associated with the protein or fat fractions of the milk, which probably facilitates their availability.

Vitamins

The vitamin content of milk is generally adequate, with the exception of vitamins D and K. Human milk is low in vitamin D, and the UK Department of Health (DoH, 1991) recommends that breastfeeding mothers should take a vitamin D supplement of 10 µg/day to ensure adequate levels in their milk, especially in the winter months. Formula-fed infants receive adequate levels of the vitamin.

Breastfed infants are also at risk of low vitamin K intakes. It has been a routine practice to give newborn infants a dose of the vitamin in the first days of life by intramuscular injection or oral dose.

Meeting Nutritional Needs

A baby's nutritional needs are generally met either by the use of human milk from the breast or formula derived from cows' milk, modified to a composition resembling that of human milk. The continued development of formula milks ensures that they come closer to the content of human milk than ever before. In Western societies, mothers are free to make the choice between breastfeeding and bottle-feeding, without fear that their baby will be disadvantaged in any way as a result of their decision. The professional consensus is that breastfeeding is better for the baby and possibly confers benefits to the mother. In many poor areas of the world, the use of infant formula may increase health problems rather than solving them. Where standards of hygiene are poor, with inadequate water supplies and non-existent or poor sanitary facilities, it is almost impossible to prepare artificial feeds with the degree of cleanliness necessary to prevent infection. In addition, poverty may tempt the mother to prepare excessively dilute feeds in an attempt to extend the supply of the milk powder. This can and does lead to serious malnutrition in the infant. In such a situation, the only safe choice for infant feeding is with human milk from the breast. The spread of formula milk throughout poor regions of the world not only has resulted in greatly increased deaths from infection in infants but has also removed the birth-spacing benefits of breastfeeding.

BREASTFEEDING OR BOTTLE-FEEDING?

Across the world, there are programmes and activities to promote breastfeeding, since it is recognized as nutritionally the best way of feeding the newborn infant. The World Health Organisation (WHO) and the United Nations Children's Fund jointly promote the Baby-Friendly Hospital Initiative, which encourages hospitals to put in place a number of measures that will facilitate the initiation and continuation of breastfeeding. At least 21,000 hospitals (approximately 27% of maternities worldwide, and 8.5% of maternities in industrialised countries) have been certified as baby friendly around the world (Labbok, 2012).

In the United Kingdom, the Infant Feeding Survey (IFS) has been conducted every 5 years since 1975. The 2010 IFS was the eighth national survey of infant feeding practices to be conducted. The main aim of the survey was to provide estimates on the incidence, prevalence and duration of breastfeeding and other feeding practices adopted by mothers in the first 8–10 months after their baby was born. Previous surveys identified the reasons given by mothers for the choice of infant feeding method. Most women decide before the birth how they will feed their baby. The decision is based on the mother's own attitude to the idea of breastfeeding but is also influenced by the views of her own mother, friends and partner. Previous experience of feeding is also a strong influence. The key changes in 2010 were the following:

- The initial breastfeeding rate increased from 76% in 2005 to 81% in 2010 in the United Kingdom. This includes all babies who were put to the breast at all, even if this was on one occasion only, and also includes giving expressed breast milk.
- The highest incidences of breastfeeding were found among mothers aged 30 or over (87%), those from minority ethnic groups (97% for Chinese or other ethnic group, 96% for Black and 95% for Asian ethnic group), those who left education aged over 18 (91%), those in managerial and professional occupations (90%) and those living in the least-deprived areas (89%).
- The prevalence of breastfeeding fell from 81% at birth to 69% at 1 week and to 55% at 6 weeks. At 6 months, just over a third of mothers (34%) were still breastfeeding.
- Mothers continued to breastfeed for longer in 2010 than was the case in 2005. The gap in breastfeeding levels at birth between 2005 and 2010 was five percentage points (76% in 2005 compared with 81% in 2010), and by 6 months, the gap became nine percentage points (25% in 2005 compared to 34% in 2010). This suggests that policy developments to improve support and information provided to mothers to encourage them to continue breastfeeding may have had an impact.
- Across the United Kingdom, 69% of mothers were exclusively breastfeeding at birth in 2010. At 1 week, less than half of all mothers (46%) were exclusively breastfeeding, while this had fallen to around a quarter (23%) by 6 weeks. By 6 months, levels of exclusive breastfeeding had decreased to 1%, indicating that very few mothers were following the UK health departments' recommendation that babies should be exclusively breastfed until around the age of 6 months.

The rates presented above are lower than in most other north European countries. The reasons cited for choosing breastfeeding are generally very positive, including that it is the best and most natural way of feeding the baby and that it is convenient. Other reasons mentioned included that it develops a closer bond with the baby, is cheaper and more natural. Those who choose to bottle-feed have more negative views about breastfeeding, considering that they would be tied to the baby and wanted others to be able to feed it, worrying about how much milk the baby receives and generally finding the idea distasteful.

The attitude of society in general is important in helping women make the choice and in supporting and helping breastfeeding mothers. Unfortunately, many people have negative attitudes to breastfeeding, considering it inappropriate and even shameful behaviour, especially if carried out, however, discreetly, in public; this can affect the new mother. The ambivalent view of society about the function of breasts can make it difficult for some women to consider feeding their baby themselves.

The most common reasons for stopping in the early weeks were given as rejection of the breast by the baby and painful nipples. However, when feeding continued for more than a week but had stopped by 4 months, insufficient milk was the most commonly cited reason for stopping. In reality, this should rarely be a reason for failure to breastfeed and probably represents inadequate support and information being made available in the first days of breastfeeding while the process is becoming established. More help for new breastfeeding mothers could increase success rates. An additional reason for stopping breastfeeding between 4 and 6 months was that the mother was returning to work (mentioned by 39% of respondents).

Overall, this survey shows an encouraging improvement in incidence and prevalence of breastfeeding. In particular, improvements have occurred in those groups where previous levels of breastfeeding had been lowest.

Formula Milk and Breast Milk Compared

The composition of formula milks available in Britain is governed by a directive from the European Commission (EEC, 1991) and Statutory Instrument 77 (MAFF, 1995). Derived from cows' milk, they are classified as 'casein dominant', based on the entire protein fraction, or 'whey dominant', containing the dialyzed whey protein. Modifications include the addition of lactose, maltodextrins, vegetable oils, various vitamins and trace elements and reductions in the level of protein, electrolytes and some minerals, such as calcium.

Bottle-feeding, if carried out correctly, with due attention to hygiene, appropriate concentrations and closeness during the feeding, can provide most of what the infant needs. However, the unique composition of human milk, with more than 200 constituents and with a varying content, will probably never be matched by a manufactured formula feed. The composition of breast milk is not constant between women and within the same woman for different lactations and even during the day. The milk secreted towards the end of a feed (hind milk) is richer in fat and, therefore, higher in energy value than the fore milk, at the start of the feed. This may play a part in appetite control, with the richer hind milk providing a feeling of satiety. Obviously, this cannot happen with a formula feed.

Proteins in Milk

The proteins in human milk are predominantly whey proteins, including alpha-lactalbumin, lactoferrin and various immunoglobulins; casein forms only 30%–40% of the total protein. Although the lactalbumin is a major source of amino acids, the other whey proteins have a non-nutritional role, in particular, as protective agents (see below for their role in immunity).

In cows' milk, casein comprises 80% of total protein, which can form tough, leathery curds in the stomach and be more difficult to digest. In the formula milks based on whey, the casein content is reduced (from 27 g/L in cows' milk to 6.0 g/L). Beta-lactoglobulin, which is normally found in cows' milk and is a potential allergen, is also absent from these formula milks.

Human milk also contains non-protein nitrogen compounds, including taurine, urea and a number of hormones and growth factors. Their functions are still uncertain but may well help with the normal development of the infant. Until their function is clearly defined, it is unlikely that these substances will be included in formula milks.

Carbohydrates in Milk

Lactose concentrations in human milk are greater than in cows' milk, although levels in formula are similar. Formula milks may also contain maltodextrin as a source of carbohydrate. Lactose enhances the absorption of calcium as a result of the lower pH resulting from fermentation to lactic acid, which makes the calcium more soluble.

Fats in Milk

Although the total fat contents of human and cows' milks are similar, the fatty acid compositions are quite different. Modified milks contain added oils to increase the unsaturated fatty acid content towards that of human milk. Nevertheless, there remains a much greater diversity of lipids in human milk, which contains cholesterol, phospholipids and essential fatty acids. Digestion and absorption of fat from human milk is aided by the presence of lipase within the milk secretion, which starts the process of digestion before the small intestine is reached. Some milks have been reformulated to include more essential and long-chain fatty acids.

Vitamins

The levels of the water-soluble vitamins in milk reflect the maternal levels and thus rely on a sufficient intake by the mother. In the West, it is rare for vitamin levels to be deficient in milk due to maternal undernutrition. Human milk also contains binding factors for folate and vitamin B_{12}, which facilitate their absorption. Most formula milks contain levels of the vitamins greater than those found in human milk. However, apart from vitamins D and K, for which intake may be too low from human milk, there appears to be no advantage in this.

Minerals

Levels of many minerals are modified in the manufacture of formula from cows' milk. This is because their concentrations would generally be too high for the human infant to cope with. In particular, this applies to calcium, phosphorus and the electrolytes. Many of the minerals are associated either with proteins or fat globules, and this appears to facilitate their absorption. Specific binding factors have been identified for iron and zinc, which make the absorption of these minerals from human milk much greater than that from formula.

Immunological Factors

Apart from the nutrients and water, human milk contains a number of other constituents. Most importantly, it contains a range of substances that enhance the immune system of the baby. Among these are the following:

- White blood cells – T and B lymphocytes, neutrophils and macrophages
- Immunoglobulins, which are the circulating antibodies
- Lysozyme, which has specific antibacterial action
- Lactoferrin, which binds iron to prevent its uptake by bacteria that need it for growth and replication and promotes growth of *Lactobacillus* sp.

- Bifidus factor, which promotes growth of bifidobacteria that prevent the growth of potentially pathogenic bacteria
- Cytokines and growth factors

The overall effect of these constituents is to promote the development of the baby's own immune system and reduce the risk of infection, while it is still immature. Immune factors specific to the environment are produced by the mother's gastrointestinal and respiratory tracts, which then stimulate the mammary glands to synthesize similar compounds. Thus, the immunity provided is 'tailor made'. Evidence from around the world, including both industrialized and developing countries, indicates that there are lower infection rates in breastfed compared with bottle-fed infants.

Other Factors

Human milk may also contain substances passed through the mother, such as drugs, alcohol, nicotine and pollutants. This causes some concern to mothers, and, where possible, such agents should be avoided when feeding the baby. However, environmental pollutants may be stored in maternal body fat and can be released during the lactation process. At present, there is insufficient evidence to determine the risk from these.

HIV infection may be transmitted through breastfeeding. However, whether a woman who is infected chooses to breastfeed is largely dependent on the alternatives available to her and her baby. If these are safe, it is probably better to feed with formula; if not, then the recommendation of the WHO is that breastfeeding is the better option. The advantages of breastfeeding in these situations still outweigh the risk of infection from HIV.

Other Milks Available

Alternative milks are available for infants who are allergic to cows' milk or lactose. The most widely available are those based on modified soya protein. These milks contain glucose and carry a possible risk to teeth. Their use should be carefully monitored. Hydrolyzed protein formulas are available for highly allergic children, and these should be used under supervision.

Special milks for babies born preterm are also available, although their use is still controversial. It has been recognized that mothers, giving birth to preterm infants, produce milk that has a higher content of fat, protein and sodium and less carbohydrate. This would appear to be necessary to sustain the rapid growth of the baby and to compensate for the lack of reserves with which it is born. A combination of breast milk and preterm formula is considered the best compromise for these infants.

Future Health

It has been claimed that breastfeeding confers advantages in terms of the later health of the baby. Some studies have shown more advanced development during childhood in those children who received breast milk, even for a short period in infancy. A meta-analysis by Anderson et al. (1999) showed that breastfeeding conferred an advantage of 3.2 point increments in cognitive function by adolescence. A study of adults aged 53 (from the British 1946 birth cohort) confirmed that breastfeeding was significantly and positively associated with educational attainment, but this was largely accounted for by the cognitive effect at 15 years.

Other possible benefits include less allergic disease, lower cholesterol levels, and lower incidence of obesity (Oddy, 2012), heart disease and multiple sclerosis. Breastfed infants have higher levels of low-density lipoprotein and very-low-density lipoprotein as infants; this may be linked to lower cholesterol levels in later life, through adaptation of enzyme levels.

Some of these benefits are difficult to demonstrate and require long-term studies. However, using records from the early years of the twentieth century, Barker (1994) showed that men who were breastfed beyond the age of 1 year actually experienced higher mortality rates. It is suggested that

See Chapter 6 for a detailed account of the early life origine of diseases, pp. 110–114.

this is a reflection of inadequate nutrition and possibly restricted growth, since breast milk is not a complete food beyond about 5–6 months. On the other hand, other work by Barker shows that infants who gained weight well and had highest weights at the age of 1 year had the lowest incidence of impaired glucose tolerance and cardiovascular disease. Clearly, nutrition in the first year of life has to be good enough to promote growth and development for long-term health. However, more specific research is required to dissect the key parameters at play.

WEANING

The process of weaning an infant literally means 'to accustom' the baby to new foods and in so doing to diversify the diet from milk to one containing solid foods. The age at which this occurs and the foods used vary between different cultures and communities and may be as early as 2 months or as late as 12 months. Neither of these extremes is nutritionally ideal. The optimal age of weaning is between 4 and 6 months, with recommendations, in the United Kingdom, to start weaning at 6 months of age.

In the United Kingdom, the 2010 IFS has shown that there had been a move to slightly later introduction of solids. Only 5% of mothers had introduced solids by the age of 3 months, compared to 10% in 2005 and close to 70% in 1990. By the age of 4 months, 30% had introduced solids and only 5% of the babies in the survey were not receiving solid foods by the age of 6 months.

Why Should a Baby Be Weaned?

Developmental advantages ensuing from weaning have already been mentioned. Further, from the age of 4 months onwards, the physiological development of the baby allows more varied foods to be ingested and digested and their waste products to be excreted. Early weaning tends to result in faster weight gain, but, by the age of 1 year, differences between infants weaned before 8 weeks and those weaned after 12 weeks have disappeared. In addition, there is a small tendency for infants weaned early to experience more respiratory illnesses and cough in the first year of life. Early weaning may precipitate an allergic response, and in infants who are at high risk of developing allergies, weaning as late as possible is advised.

Weaning has important developmental advantages. The ability to manipulate a bolus of food in the mouth and swallow it, to coordinate a utensil and bring food to the mouth and to drink from a cup all help in the development of muscles in the face. These are important in the acquisition of speech.

From the nutritional point of view, weaning is required to provide certain nutrients that can no longer be supplied in sufficient amounts by breast or formula milk. In particular, this applies to energy, protein, iron, zinc and vitamins A and D.

There is particular concern about iron status in infants, with low stores and the possibility of anaemia in 12% of young children. The low iron status may result in delayed psychomotor development and defects in cellular immunity.

An infant's stomach capacity is considerably smaller than an adult's, which makes it very important to ensure that the foods offered contain enough energy in a compact form. Commonly, the first food introduced to the infant is the local staple cereal. In the West, this may be specially formulated, designed for weaning and enriched with a number of nutrients. Rice (or other non-wheat cereals) is preferred to wheat, which may cause gluten allergy to develop. In developing countries, the local staple is used, prepared as a gruel or porridge.

Other purées may then be introduced, for example, potato, vegetable, pulse or fruit purées and dairy products such as custard or yoghurt. These are all smooth with a relatively bland taste, with which the infant can gradually become familiar. As the child becomes accustomed to the novelty of solid foods, minced meat, fish and other sources of protein, such as sieved soft

TABLE 7.3

Suggested Food Groups to Be Included in the Diet at 6–9 Months and 12 Months

	Number of Servings/Day	
Food Group	**6–9 Months**	**12 Months**
Bread, cereals, potatoes	2–3	At least 4
Fruits and vegetables	2	At least 4
Milk and dairy products	500–600 mL milk	2–3 servings + 350 mL milk
Meat, fish and alternatives	1	1–2
Fatty, salty and sugary foods	Avoid	Limit

cheese, can be included, together with vegetables and fruit that have been minced or mashed to retain more texture.

As chewing ability develops, the pieces of food offered become more distinct, allowing chewing to be practised. *Finger foods* held in the hand allow the child some independence and help to develop coordination as well as provide some nutritional value. These can include rusks, fingers of toast or pieces of hard cheese.

The diet should aim to provide a variety of different food groups, to ensure that a range of nutrients is consumed (Table 7.3). Particular attention may need to be paid to iron and vitamin D sources; vitamin C will help the absorption of iron and should also be provided. Some examples of suitable foods to provide these nutrients are shown in Table 7.4.

Milk should remain the cornerstone of the infant's diet, as it contains important amounts of protein, calcium and vitamins as well as provide energy. Amounts of milk offered should be 600 mL at 4 months when weaning starts but still 350 mL in the 1 year old. The type of milk offered to the infant is also important. The UK Department of Health (DoH, 1994) recommends that infants should continue to receive breast milk, formula or a 'follow-on' milk up to the age of 1 year. *Follow-on* milks have been introduced in recent years, as suitable for infants from 6 months of age. They are less modified than infant formula but still contain added nutrients to provide a valuable source of nutrition. Special 'infant drinks' may contain large amounts of sugar and should be avoided or only used rarely and with care. Drinks should be offered in a cup, and the practice of leaving a child with a bottle or 'trainer' cup (one with a feeding spout)

TABLE 7.4

Sources of Iron, Vitamin C and Vitamin D Suitable for Weaning

Sources of Iron	**Sources of Vitamin C**	**Sources of Vitamin D**
Red meat (beef, lamb), pork poultry	Citrus fruits, e.g. oranges, satsumas	Oily fish, for example, sardines
Liver, liver sausage	*Summer fruits*: strawberries, peaches, nectarines	Eggs and egg dishes
Oily fish, e.g. sardines	Green leafy vegetables	Fortified margarine
Eggs and egg dishes	Tomatoes, green pepper, peas	Breakfast cereals fortified with vitamin D
Beans and lentils	Potatoes	Baby cereals fortified with vitamin D
Baby foods fortified with iron	*Unsweetened fruit juice*: diluted	Evaporated milk
Breakfast cereals with added iron		Some yogurts
Green leafy vegetables		
Dried fruits, e.g. apricots, prunes		
Fish fingers		

for periods of time is discouraged as it can lead to pooling of drink in the mouth. This can cause decay of newly erupted milk teeth.

Pasteurized cows' milk should not become the major milk drink until after the age of 1 year. This is because it contains low levels of iron and vitamin D and may contribute to deficient intakes if taken as the main milk in the diet. The high concentration of proteins and minerals may also harm the infant's immature kidneys. However, cows' milk may be used to make dishes containing milk, such as custards and sauces. Infants should not be given low-fat milks, such as skimmed milk or semi-skimmed milk, as these contain insufficient fat and, therefore, have a low energy density.

Throughout the weaning process, the following are recommended:

- The child is always supervised during mealtimes.
- Sugar and salt are not added to the infant's food.
- Foods should not be heavily spiced.
- Nuts should not be included in the diet.
- Soft-boiled eggs should be avoided because of possible contamination with *Salmonella*; hard-boiled eggs are safe.
- Pâté and mould-ripened soft cheeses (such as Brie) should be avoided because of the risk of *Listeria* contamination.
- Drinks other than milk should be offered from a cup from the age of 6 months; they should be diluted and unsweetened.

Special 'infant drinks' may contain large amounts of sugar and should be avoided or only used rarely and with care.

Commercial weaning products are of value. They are often fortified with additional nutrients, which are especially useful when the child has a very small intake, or when home-prepared foods may provide very few nutrients. Commercial weaning foods are however limited in term of taste range (mostly sweet), and do not always offer an enhanced energy density over breastmilk (Garcia, 2013).

Infants cannot cope with large amounts of foods rich in non-starch polysaccharides (NSPs), such as whole grain cereals and pulses, and these should not be an important part of the weaning diet. However, small amounts can be included, and quantities increased when appetite is bigger.

By the age of 1 year, the infant should be eating solids several times per day and be included in family meals. The complete process of weaning may take longer than this, however, and full chewing ability will not be attained until the molar teeth have erupted towards the end of the second year.

Supplements of vitamins A, C and D are available; these are recommended for all infants from the age of 1 to 5 years and for breastfed infants from the age of 6 months. The daily dose of supplement provides 200 μg of vitamin A, 20 mg of vitamin C and 7 μg of vitamin D.

It should be remembered throughout that the infant is undergoing a process of learning about food, and, to develop a child with a broad appetite for foods, many different tastes should be offered. Variety in the diet helps to ensure an adequate nutritional intake. Nutrients that need attention remain iron, zinc and vitamin D. Refusal of a specific food need not eliminate it completely from the diet. It can be reintroduced later. Important foundations are being laid down at this time, and it is essential that the caregiver makes this a pleasurable learning experience for the infant. Sometimes the weaning process falters and a child that has been gaining weight may stop doing so. This has been called 'failure to thrive' and is of multifactorial origin. There is no evidence that it is associated with deprivation and neglect. There appears to be an underlying lack of interest in food in the child, slower eating and diminished appetite. Delayed progression on to solids and a limited variety of foods eaten have also been described. Intervention with dietary advice and practical management of mealtimes can result in rapid improvement, if there is no underlying organic cause.

CHILD FROM 1 TO 5 YEARS OF AGE

These years provide a time to move from the milk-centred diet of the first year of life to the typical diet of the family. In nutritional terms, this represents a change from a diet which contains approximately 50% fat, no NSP and simple sugars rather than starches (as seen in the milk-fed infant), to one meeting or approaching the dietary guidelines, with 35% fat, 5% added sugar (the previous guideline stated 11% non-milk extrinsic sugars (NMES)) and plenty of starch and NSPs. Clearly, there needs to be a gradual transition from one to the other.

The food habits developed at this time will be the foundation for the approach to diet and nutrition for the rest of the individual's life. During this period, the child will also develop some independence in relation to food, and this may lead to conflict with the parents. Infants more readily accept new foods and tastes. During early childhood, there may be an increasing reluctance to try new foods. This served a protective function in the past, as a young child began to wander off and might have been tempted to try a hazardous food. Exposing children to new foods is, however, important. Perseverance, which may necessitate up to 5 or 10 exposures to the food, can pay off. Modelling on others who are eating the food is a helpful way of persuading a young child to accept it. Finally, presenting a novel food together with a familiar taste can be useful, for example, as part of a liked dish. Parents have an important role in determining what food is available for the child in the home. The attitude of parents to food is central, and conscious or subconscious preferences for foods or attributes attached to a food will be passed on to the child. Foods used as a positive reward (chocolate or sweets for good behaviour) or a hurdle to be overcome to achieve something pleasurable (having to eat up all the vegetables on the pate in order to play/watch television) can foster attitudes to these foods that were not necessarily intended. Children need guidance, and family food rules are beneficial to provide a framework in which their own food habits can develop. Ideally, these should focus on healthy foods and eating patterns.

Growth is slower than in the first year of life but tends to occur in spurts, often accompanied by surges of appetite. Activity also increases markedly during the second year, as the child becomes increasingly mobile. Full dentition by about the age of 2 also increases the dietary repertoire. Because capacity remains relatively small, between-meal snacks are likely to be needed in addition to the three main meals of the day. It is important to maintain healthy eating guidelines in mind when selecting snack foods, since these should be contributing to total nutritional intake rather than being additional to it. Unfortunately, poorly selected snacks, often comprising little more than sugar, in drink or solid form, can seriously compromise nutritional intake, as they dull the appetite at mealtimes. Snacks can include the following:

- Fresh or dried fruit (although the latter may stick to the teeth and be cariogenic)
- Wholemeal sandwiches with nutritious fillings
- Raw vegetables as 'finger food' to chew
- Dry breakfast cereal
- Low-sugar or savoury biscuits
- Yoghurt or milk
- Popcorn (plain, rather than sugar coated)
- Scones or similar plain cakes

Meals should consist of nutrient-dense foods, with at least 250 mL of milk daily, and cereal and bread used to fill up to appetite. Appetite remains the best guide to overall food needs at this age.

Food refusal can be a major problem and can cause a great deal of stress to parents. The child needs a consistent and firm response from the parent, so that the association of eating with mealtimes is learned. If the child does not eat at table and is then allowed to snack between meals, disorganized eating habits may develop for the rest of their life. Experimentation with food within limits is important. Given a wide range of foods to experience, we all develop as individuals in our choice of foods with specific likes and dislikes. Ideally, our children should develop with few dislikes, if we give them the appropriate guidance and personal example.

A national study (Gregory et al., 1995) of children aged 1.5–4.5 years, as part of the National Diet and Nutrition Survey (NDNS) in Britain, found that, on the whole, children were eating large amounts of salt and sugar and insufficient fruit and vegetables. Although the mean intake of energy was found to be lower than the estimated average requirements (EARs), the children appeared to be growing well. As a result, it has been suggested that energy requirements may need to be decreased by 10%–12% from their current levels. Other findings included the following:

- Those who had the highest energy intakes also consumed the most NSP.
- Total sugar intakes represented 29% of total energy and starches 22%; the intake of NMES comprised 19% of total energy.
- There was a reciprocal relationship between fat and sugar intakes.
- Fat intakes were generally between 34% and 36% of total energy and, therefore, in line with Department of Health recommendations (DoH, 1991). It should be remembered that young children should not be rigorously put on low-fat diets, as this can compromise their total energy intake. Other studies show that low-fat/high-fibre diets are being given to this age group, reflecting confusion about healthy eating guidelines.
- Iron intakes were low in a proportion of children: 24% of those aged 1.5–2.5 years, and 16% of those under 4 years had intakes below the lower reference nutrient intake (LRNI), with low ferritin levels indicative of low stores of iron and low haemoglobin levels resulting in anaemia in 1 in 12 of the sample. Apart from help with iron-rich foods, parents may need advice about promoters and inhibitors of iron absorption.
- Dental caries was found in 17% of this age group.

In a secondary analysis of these data, it was found that only 1% of children met the reference nutrient intake (RNI) recommendations for iron, zinc and vitamins A and C and guidelines on NMES. Two or fewer of the targets were met by 76% of the children. Compliance with the recommended levels of intake was related to socio-economic status, with more children from lower social groups, with a head of household in a manual category and mothers with fewer educational qualifications meeting the least number of RNIs/recommendations.

Overall, it can be concluded that the quantity of the diet of this age group in the United Kingdom is currently adequate, although certain aspects of its quality probably need attention. In particular, there needs to be

- More attention given to iron-containing foods
- A reduction in both the amount and frequency of consumption of sugars, especially in the form of soft drinks (these could be replaced by milk or water)
- A reduction in the consumption of savoury snacks that are high in salt
- An increase in the consumption of fruit and vegetables
- More attention to the impact of socio-economic factors on food choice in families

SCHOOL-AGE CHILDREN

Influences on Nutritional Intakes

When children start school, their eating patterns begin to be increasingly influenced by factors other than the home environment. However, it should be remembered that parents remain the 'gatekeepers' of what is consumed at home and can still have a considerable influence by determining what is provided at mealtimes and what snack foods are available for children to help themselves. They also continue to serve as important role models.

Autonomy

A study of 9-year-old children in the United Kingdom reported that this group felt that parents had a great deal of control over their food choices. However, the greatest number (90%) reported control over the content of breakfast, with 2/3 reporting control over snacks and only 1/3 reporting control over the amount of food eaten (Robinson, 2000). This appears to leave children with a reasonable amount of autonomy in various aspects of their diet.

Adolescence itself is a time of transition, associated with progress towards autonomy. This is reflected in all aspects of the teenager's life but inevitably impacts on food choice and nutritional intake.

Rejection of food selected or prepared by parents is a normal aspect of this developing autonomy. Foods chosen as alternatives may be less healthy, as a gesture of independence and, perhaps, peer solidarity. There is also likely to be experimentation with foods and adoption of novel dietary practices. At other times, the adolescent may still want to be part of the family and eat what is provided at home.

Growth

Growth rates are relatively slow during the preadolescent years, but growth still occurs nonlinearly with surges accompanied by increases of appetite. Periods of slow growth may be accompanied by a relatively small appetite, and, at such times, particular attention must be paid to the nutrient density of the diet. In adolescence, periods of rapid growth take place that have profound effects on appetite.

School may also be emotionally taxing for children, which may affect their food intake. In addition, beginning school is often accompanied by exposure to many childhood infections and periods of (often minor) illness. These can have an impact on food intake and, if numerous, may affect growth.

Activity

Apart from growth, activity is the other main influence on appetite in this age group. Starting school may significantly alter a child's activity pattern; the direction of the change depending on how active the child was during preschool years. Children of primary school age tend to be relatively more active in their play, and levels of activity have been shown to decline in a large proportion of adolescents, especially girls. Following the *Health of the nation* report (DoH, 1992), physical activity in children has become a focus of policy in the United Kingdom. In its 2010 report on physical activity guidelines, the DoH makes three recommendations for children and young people aged 5–18 years (DoH, 2010):

1. All children and young people should engage in moderate to vigorous intensity physical activity for at least 60 minutes and up to several hours every day.
2. Vigorous intensity activities, including those that strengthen muscle and bone, should be incorporated at least 3 days a week.
3. All children and young people should minimize the amount of time spent being sedentary (sitting) for extended periods.

There is concern that many hours are being spent watching television, playing computer games and staying in the house rather than being involved in physical activity or even just walking. Estimates from studies in Scotland suggest that teenagers may now expend between 2 and 3 MJ (500–700 cal) per day less than their peers did 60 years ago. Average time spent watching television has been shown to be positively associated with increased body weight, skinfold, fat mass and prevalence of overweight in prepubertal children. The reasons for this association are complex.

Societal Pressures

Pressures from friends will increasingly influence food intakes as a child goes through school, and this becomes most notable in adolescence. In addition, societal pressures linked to body image have a major impact on the food intake of some individuals, especially girls at this age. Adolescence is the peak age for dissatisfaction with body image and attempts at dieting being prevalent, more so in girls than boys at this age. Changing food trends are particular influences. In recent years, there has been a major shift from traditional meals, and many children and teenagers consume a series of snacks during the day rather than eating 'normal' meals. The choice of foods available in fast-food outlets can be a limiting factor for making healthy selections.

There is also widespread concern about the impact of advertising on food choices in this group. Food advertising is the single largest category of advertisement shown during children's television programmes. The majority of these are for products that are high in sugar and fat and low in fibre and include confectionery, snack foods and breakfast cereals. This trend is also seen in other countries, such as the United States and Australia. The advertisements for these foods are often humorous, animated and easy to follow, so that they are memorable to children. In contrast, there are no advertisements for foods that should form a substantial part of a healthy diet, such as fruit and vegetables. Although advertisements by themselves do not change food habits, there is concern that the balance of those shown is in conflict with health promotion messages.

Nutritional Needs

Steady growth during childhood up to adolescence, increasing per year by 10 cm in height and 2.5 kg in weight, is reflected by a gradual increase in the need for nutrients. There is a certain amount of accumulation of stores during this time, most notably of body fat, which then becomes available to contribute to the fuel required for the pubertal growth spurt. Calcium is also laid down and provides some of the needs for bone growth.

At adolescence, growth rates are greater than at any other time of life, except early infancy. In most girls, the growth spurt begins between the age of 10 and 13 and in boys between 12 and 15 years. In both cases, rapid growth takes place over a period of 3 years. Girls gain lean tissue and fat and increase by 20 cm in height and 20 kg in weight. In boys, there is a loss of fat and a gain in lean tissue, with increases of 30 cm in height and 30 kg in weight. These increases account for approximately 40% of adult weight. It is to be expected, therefore, that the nutritional requirements at this time will reflect this growth.

The timing of the need for additional nutrients varies with the individual and depends on the onset of growth. In the West, peak appetite occurs around the age of 12 in girls and 14 in boys, apparently corresponding to the most rapid growth period. The demand for new tissue synthesis results in increased nutrient requirements for

- Calcium, phosphorus, magnesium and vitamin D for bone
- Protein, zinc and iron for muscle
- Iron, folate, vitamin B_{12} and copper for the synthesis of extra blood cells to supply it with oxygen
- Adequate energy to sustain this synthesis and the B vitamins to release it

If energy needs are not met, the growth spurt may be delayed or reduced. However, energy needs for growth probably do not exceed 10% of total energy requirements at this time.

Once the growth spurt is over, nutrient requirements settle down to adult levels.

TABLE 7.5

Dietary Reference Values for Children from 4 to 18 Years

Nutrient	Age 4–6 M	Age 4–6 F	Age 7–10 M	Age 7–10 F	Age 11–14 M	Age 11–14 F	Age 15–18 M	Age 15–18 F
Energy								
(MJ/day)	7.16	6.46	8.24	7.28	9.27	7.92	11.51	8.83
(cal/day)	1715	1545	1970	1740	2220	1845	2755	2110
Protein (g/day)	19.7	19.7	28.3	28.3	42.1	41.2	55.2	45.0
Thiamin (mg/day)	0.7	0.7	0.7	0.7	0.9	0.7	1.1	0.8
Riboflavin (mg/day)	0.8	0.8	1.0	1.0	1.2	1.1	1.3	1.1
Niacin (nicotinic acid equiv.) (mg/day)	11	11	12	12	15	12	18	14
Folate (µg/day)	100	100	150	150	200	200	200	200
Vitamin C (mg/day)	30	30	30	30	35	35	40	40
Vitamin A (µg/day)	500	500	500	500	600	600	700	600
Calcium (mg/day)	450	450	550	550	1000	800	1000	800
Iron (mg/day)	6.1	6.1	8.7	8.7	11.3	14.8	11.3	14.8
Zinc (mg/day)	6.5	6.5	7.0	7.0	9.0	9.0	9.5	7.0

Source: Reproduced from DoH (UK Department of Health), Dietary reference values for food energy and nutrients for the United Kingdom, Report on Health and Social Subjects No. 41, Report of the Panel on Dietary Reference Values of the Committee on Medical Aspects of Food Policy, HMSO, London, UK, 1991. With permission.

Selected DRVs are shown in Table 7.5 for the age groups from 4 to 18 years. In addition to these specific guidelines, children's diets should approach the general recommendations on fat and carbohydrates (shown in Table 7.6).

No distinction is made between genders for the majority of nutrient requirements for children up to the age of 10 years. After this age, with the onset of the pubertal growth spurt, different figures are set for male and female adolescents. In part, these reflect the different body weights at these ages. However, special needs for menstrual losses are incorporated in the iron requirement calculations.

There are no DRVs given for vitamin D, as it is assumed that sufficient will be synthesized in the skin during everyday activity. However, some children of Asian origin may require a dietary supplement.

These dietary guidelines should be met in the same way as for adults, by eating a diet in line with the Eatwell Guide, which provides an appropriate balance between the five main groups shown. Thus, the diet should provide mainly starchy carbohydrate sources and fruit and vegetables (five servings per day

TABLE 7.6

General Recommendations on Fat and Carbohydrates

Total fat	35% of food energy
Saturated fatty acids	11%
Polyunsaturated fatty acids	6.5%
Total carbohydrate	50% of food energy
Non-milk extrinsic sugars	11%
Intrinsic and milk sugars + starch	39%
Non-starch polysaccharides	18 g/day

of each of the two groups). In addition, there should be three servings of milk and dairy products and two servings of meat and alternatives. Intakes of fatty and sugary foods should be limited; they may be included in the diet when the needs for the other four groups have been met.

It is helpful if meals are planned to include items from each of the food groups wherever possible.

WHAT DO CHILDREN AND ADOLESCENTS EAT?

Studies of children's attitudes to healthy eating in recent years have shown that in general children understand the concept of a balanced diet as described in the 'Eatwell Guide' model. They are also aware of the relationship between diet and health, both now and for the future. Children also demonstrate an awareness of the potential risk for heart health of excessive fat intakes and the desirability of a normal body weight. The health implications of being too thin and the dangers of eating disorders are also recognized. For this age group, however, social pressures are important, and knowledge does not necessarily translate into behaviour.

A number of studies took place during the 1980s and early 1990s on groups of children from 5 to 17 years of age. In general, these studies showed that the health of schoolchildren in Britain is good. There was no widespread evidence of dietary deficiency, and no biochemical or functional improvements were seen with the use of supplementation. However, a European study has reported that the diet of UK children is among the worst in Europe, being high in fat and sugar and low in fibre, iron, calcium and possibly folate.

The UK NDNS began in 1992 as a series of cross-sectional surveys, each covering a different age group: preschool children (1.5–4.5 years), young people (4–18 years), adults (19–64 years) and older adults (65 years and over). In 2008, the NDNS became a rolling programme with a more detailed breakdown by age subgroups. There were 3378 children aged 1.5–18 years who participated in the latest survey, which involved completion of a 4-day food and drink diary and an interview to collect background information on dietary habits, socio-demographic status, lifestyle and physical activity. Those who agreed also provided a blood sample to allow assessment of biochemical indices of nutritional status and a 24-hour urine collection to assess salt intake, and physical measurement data were collected.

The latest findings from this study, covering the 4-year period from September 2008 to December 2011 (Bates et al., 2014), are summarized here.

Health-Related Aspects

- Similar proportions of boys and girls were overweight (14% and 15%, respectively); overweight, including obese (31% and 33%, respectively); and obese (17% and 19%, respectively).
- Boys are more physically active than girls. Activity levels tend to fall with age, particularly among girls. The median 'counts per minute' (cpm) in those aged 4–10 years were 577 cpm and 541 cpm in boys and girls, respectively. Equivalent figures for those aged 11–15 years were 473 and 335 cpm.
- The proportion of children who reported ever having had a proper alcoholic drink (not just a taste) increased with age, from 11% of boys and 7% of girls aged 8–10 years to 55% of boys and 53% of girls aged 13–15 years. Three per cent of boys aged 13–15 years and 4% of girls of the same age reported usually drinking once a week or more.

Dietary Patterns

- Children aged 10 years and under consumed similar quantities of bread (all types combined) and 'pasta, rice, pizza and other miscellaneous cereals', as did adults. Children aged 11–18 years consumed more 'pasta, rice, pizza and other miscellaneous cereals' than bread. *Biscuits* were also consumed by more than 70% of those aged 10 years and under.

- For most age groups, 'semi-skimmed milk' had the highest mean consumption and was the most commonly consumed type of milk. The exception was those aged 1.5–3 years for whom 'whole milk' was the most commonly consumed milk. For all age groups, 'cheddar cheese' had the highest mean consumption compared with other types of cheese.
- *Chicken and turkey* were the most commonly consumed type of meat for all age groups.
- Only 12% of children consumed oily fish over the 4-day recording period. *White fish coated or fried including fish fingers* was the most commonly consumed type of fish for children aged 10 years and under.
- Children aged 1.5–3 years were the highest per cent consumers of 'fruit' over the 4-day recording period (93%), followed by children aged 4–10 years (90%). Children aged 11–18 years were the lowest per cent consumers of 'fruit' (67%).
- *Vegetables (not raw) including vegetable dishes* were consumed by 80% or more participants in all age groups. *Salad and other raw vegetables* were less commonly consumed by children; about 50% of whom ate this type of food over the 4-day recording period.
- The highest percentage of consumers of 'chips, fried and roast potatoes and potato products' was in the 4–10 years age group (79%).
- Consumption of fruit and vegetables for children aged 11–18 years was 3 portions per day for boys and 2.7 portions per day for girls. The proportions of children that met the 'five-a-day' recommendation were 10% of boys and 7% of girls in this age group.
- The mean consumption of 'sugar confectionery' and 'chocolate confectionery' combined was highest in the 11–18 years age group (19 g per day) and the 4–10 years age group (18 g per day). *Chocolate confectionery* was consumed by 56%–59% of children aged 4–18 years and 'sugar confectionery' by 49% of those aged 4–10 years and 35% of those aged 11–18 years.
- Children aged 4–10 years were the highest consumers of 'fruit juice' over the 4-day recording period (62%). Highest mean consumption of 'soft drinks, not low calorie' was seen in children aged 11–18 years (261 g per day), while the highest mean consumption of 'soft drinks, low calorie' was seen in children aged 10 years and under (183–185 g per day).

Nutritional Intakes

- Reported total energy intake was 4.75 MJ/day (1126 kcal/day) for children aged 1.5–3 years and 6.46 MJ/day (1532 kcal/day) for children aged 4–10 years. For children aged 11–18 years, mean total energy intake was 8.30 MJ/day (1972 kcal/day) for boys and 6.60 MJ/day (1569 kcal/day) for girls.
- Mean energy intakes were below the EAR for children aged 11 years and over (75.1% and 68.5% for boys and girls, respectively). However, it should be borne in mind that the DLW sub-study showed evidence of under-reporting of energy intakes in this age group.
- *Cereals and cereal products* was the main contributor to energy intake in all age groups. *Meat and meat products* and *milk and milk products* were the other major contributors with 'milk and milk products' making a larger contribution in younger children. The contributions to the total food energy intake of the main macronutrient groups are shown in Table 7.7.
- Intake of saturated fat exceeded the DRV (no more than 11% food energy) in all age/sex groups and was higher in the 4–10 age group than the 11–18 age group for both sexes (13.1% and 12.7%, respectively, for boys; 13.3% and 12.4%, respectively, for girls). *Milk and milk products, cereals and cereal products* and *meat and meat products* made similar contributions to saturated fat intake in older children, while in younger children, 'milk and milk products' was the largest contributor.

TABLE 7.7
Contributions of the Main Macronutrient Groups to Total Energy Intake for Young People Aged 4–18

Macronutrient	Contribution to Food Energy	Main Contributing Food Groups
Protein	14.9% (boys)	Meat and meat products
	14.6% (girls)	Cereals and cereal products
Carbohydrate	51.5% (boys)	Cereals and cereal products
	51.5% (girls)	Sugar and preserves
Total fat	33.6% (boys)	Cereals and cereal products (biscuits, buns, cakes and pastries)
	33.9% (girls)	Meat and meat products
Saturated fatty acids	12.8% (boys)	
	12.8% (girls)	
Non-starch polysaccharides	12.2 g (boys)	Vegetables, potatoes and savoury snacks
	10.7 g (girls)	Cereals and cereal products

- NMES intake exceeded the DRV (no more than 11% food energy at the time, decreased to 5% in 2016) for all age/sex groups, most notably for children aged 4–10 years and 11–18 years where mean intake provided 14.7% and 15.6% of food energy, respectively. For children, the main source of NMES was 'non-alcoholic beverages' (soft drinks and 'fruit juice' – soft drinks alone provided 30% of NMES intake in the 11–18 years age group). *Cereals and cereal products* was the other major contributor in children mainly from cakes, biscuits and breakfast cereals.

Micronutrient intakes were generally above the RNI for most nutrients, for most age groups. However, some intakes were below the LRNI, and the prevalence of this increased with increasing age and was more likely in girls than boys.

- Mean intake of vitamin D was below the RNI for children aged 1.5–3 years both with and without the contribution of supplements. For children aged 11–18 years, 13% and 15% had vitamin A and riboflavin intake below the LRNI, respectively; 8% of girls aged 11–18 years had folate intake below the LRNI.
- Intakes of minerals from food sources were below the RNI for some age/sex groups, in particular children aged 11–18 years. A substantial proportion of this age group, especially girls, had intakes of some minerals below the LRNI. For example, mean iron intakes were below the RNI for girls aged 11–18 years and 46% of girls had iron intake below the LRNI. Mean intakes of calcium and zinc (and iodine for girls only) were also below the RNI in the 11–18 years age group, and about a fifth of girls aged 11–18 years fell below the LRNI.
- Intakes of potassium, magnesium and selenium were below the RNI in all age groups except children aged under 11 years, and substantial proportions fell below the LRNI. It should be noted that the DRVs for these minerals are based on limited data, so caution should be used when assessing adequacy of intake using the LRNI.
- Mean intakes of all minerals were close to or above the RNI for children aged under 11 years, and few children in this age group had intakes below the LRNI.

Other smaller studies confirm these findings. In general, the transition from primary to secondary school is associated with the beginning of greater independence in food choice and is accompanied by an increased consumption of less desirable foods and a reduction in desirable foods, most notably fruit and vegetables.

In addition, socio-economic status results in differences in the nutritional quality of children's diets, with lower intakes of total energy and lower intakes of nutrients when energy intakes had been taken into account. This trend corresponds to that reported in adults.

School Meals

A meal in the middle of the school day is important nutritionally, socially and educationally. In terms of academic performance, it is important that children eat in the middle of the day to maximize their learning opportunities.

The nutritional guidelines for school meals that had existed since the 1944 Education Act were abolished in the United Kingdom in 1980. Prior to this date, the meal offered at school had to provide one-third of a child's daily requirements of protein, energy and some minerals and vitamins. From 1980, the only obligation that remained was to provide a meal for those who were entitled to free school meals, by reason of low income. Since this date, considerable concern has been expressed about the nutritional adequacy of the diets of schoolchildren.

Following a period of consultation, nutritional standards in UK schools have been established, taking effect from July 2009. There is once more a duty to provide a paid meals service in schools, and guidance documents have been produced by the Parliamentary Office of Science and Technology. Schools have more autonomy than in the past and, at secondary level, hold budgets for the provision of meals. This means that many schools are able to adopt whole school policies on food and nutrition. The School Nutrition Action Group initiative has provided a framework for the formation of school-based alliances between teachers, pupils and caterers together with help from appropriate health professionals. Many of these are in place, and they allow the consumers to be involved in the decision-making process and thereby increase their sense of ownership of the school meal provision. School management also needs to be involved to ensure there is an adequate provision for a lunch break in the timetable and that a suitable environment exists to enable meals to be taken in comfortable surroundings.

When aspects of healthy eating are part of the school curriculum, the food service can provide the practical illustration in a positive way, contributing to the pastoral welfare of the children.

Some issues about the provision of meals in school remain to be resolved. These include the following:

- Ensuring that cultural diversity is recognized in the meals provided.
- Improving the uptake of free school meals – reports suggest that to achieve this, a number of factors, for example, insensitive administration that results in an associated stigma, the quality of the food, eating environment and service, all need to be addressed. Some local education authorities have introduced swipe cards for all children, so that there is no distinction made at the point of purchase between the children receiving free lunches and those who are paying.
- Provision of drinking water to accompany the meals.
- Monitoring of the provision of the meals and maintenance of standards. This is a role for the appropriate government agency.

Minimum Nutritional Standards

The national nutrition standards are based on the food groups in the Eatwell Guide (see Table 7.8). In terms of defining a healthy diet, they incorporate the following principles:

- A balanced diet with plenty of variety and enough energy for growth and development
- Plenty of fibre-rich starchy foods, such as bread, rice, pasta, potatoes and yams

TABLE 7.8
Minimum Nutritional Standards for School Meals

Food Groups	Primary School	Secondary School
Starchy foods such as bread, potatoes, rice and pasta	Provide at least one from this group daily. Items cooked in oil or fat should not be served more than three times a week.	Provide at least two from this group daily. At least one of these should not be cooked in oil or fat.
Fruit and a vegetable	One item of both must be available every day. Fruit-based desserts must be available twice a week.	Two items of both should be available daily.
Milk and dairy foods	Provide at least one from this group daily.	Provide at least two from this group daily.
Meat, fish and alternative sources of protein (cheese may be provided as an alternative for primary school children only)	Provide at least one from this group daily. Red meat must be served twice a week; fish must be served once a week.	Provide at least two from this group daily. Red meat must be served at least three times a week; fish must be served at least twice a week.

Source: DfES (UK Department for Education and Skills), *Healthy School Lunches for Students in Secondary Schools*, DfSE, London, UK, 2001.

- Plenty of fruit and vegetables
- Not eating too many foods containing a lot of fat, especially saturated fat
- Moderate amounts of dairy products
- Moderate amounts of meat, fish or alternatives
- Not having sugary foods and drinks too often

In addition to these general principles, specific nutrients have been identified as important for children of school age. These are

- *Calcium* – Important for bone health
- *Iron* – Important for preventing anaemia
- *Folate* – Important for adolescent girls and young women, but establishing a good intake in early years forms a sound base
- *Zinc* – For normal growth and development

Slightly different nutritional standards have been established for children in primary and secondary schools. In addition, there are separate standards for children of nursery school age.

These standards apply to all lunches (hot or cold) provided during term time. There are additional recommendations for the provision of water, free of charge. Milk to drink should also be available every day. It is recommended that some hot food be offered daily, especially in the winter months.

Caterers are also given guidance on good practice, which includes the following key points:

- Reflect the likes and dislikes of children.
- Work with the school to check that healthy eating principles are being reinforced by both the curriculum and the lunch service.
- Actively encourage children to have a balanced diet.
- Aim to offer a selection of foods, which, over the week, reflects the proportions in the Eatwell Guide, and make changes gradually.
- Offer a variety of foods.
- Use a variety of cooking methods that lead to minimum destruction of nutrients.

TABLE 7.9
Summary of Caroline Walker Trust Nutritional Guidelines for School Meals

Nutrient	Guideline
Energy	30% of the estimated average requirement
Fat	Not more than 35% of food energy
Saturated fatty acids	Not more than 11% of food energy
Carbohydrate	Not less than 50% of food energy
Non-milk extrinsic sugars	Not more than 11% of food energy
NSP (fibre)	Not less than 30% of the calculated reference value
Protein	Not less than 30% of the RNI
Iron	Not less than 40% of the RNI
Calcium	Not less than 40% of the RNI
Vitamin A	Not less than 40% of the RNI
Folate	Not less than 40% of the RNI
Vitamin C	Not less than 40% of the RNI
Sodium	Not more than 30% of the SACN recommendation

Source: The Caroline Walker Trust 2005. With permission.
Notes: NSP, non-starch polysaccharide; RNI, reference nutrient intake; SACN, Scientific Advisory Committee on Nutrition.

In addition to the aforementioned, guidance is provided on various foods within each food group, portion sizes, special dietary requirements and monitoring of the nutritional standards. Even though the new minimum standards have been expressed in terms of food groups and servings from these, caterers are encouraged to use the Caroline Walker Trust Guidelines on School Meals to check the nutritional value of the meal provided. These are shown in Table 7.9. This is particularly important where children have a free choice in a cash-cafeteria selection. Throughout, caterers are encouraged to promote healthy eating and encourage children in a variety of ways to eat the food provided.

Where children can leave school at lunchtime, caterers have to compete effectively with local food outlets. Attractive packaging, advertising and promotions can all help keep children in school for lunch.

Alternatives to School Lunch

Packed lunches brought in to school may be of variable nutritional content. Confectionery and soft drinks may also be available in school, often as a fund-raising activity, and may tempt the children to eat these items rather than more nutritious foods. In some schools, children can go out of school at lunchtime, and foods purchased away from school may include pizzas, chips, burgers or cakes and soft drinks. The UK DoH survey (DoH, 1989) found that foods eaten out of school were generally of lower nutrient density, especially among the older schoolchildren. In particular, these meals contained less protein, iron, calcium, retinol, thiamin, riboflavin and vitamin D. A small section of the teenage population has no lunch, with 11% of girls and 5% of boys aged 14–16 reporting this.

Overall, a well-balanced lunch can provide between 30% and 40% of the nutrients required in the day. If no food is taken or a very poor-quality snack is eaten, then the likelihood of daily nutritional needs not being met increases because it becomes more difficult to achieve adequate intakes from the remaining meals. Eating is a social activity, and having lunch with one's peers can provide an important socialization activity, teaching the individual about food habits and learning from others. A proportion of children come to school without having eaten breakfast or a snack on the way to school. In some schools, breakfast clubs have been established that provide food before the school day begins. The School Fruit Initiative aims to provide all primary schoolchildren with a piece of fruit in school each day. This is still being developed, but pilot schemes report a fair measure of success. School milk is also being reintroduced into some primary schools, to try to address some of the potential nutritional problems in this age group.

However, it must be recognized that providing healthier choices for children in school does not necessarily lead to changes in behaviour. One study reports the outcomes of a 2-year programme in secondary schools (Parker and Fox, 2001). This had a number of dietary targets, including increasing intakes of high-fibre bread, fruit and vegetables, non-fried potatoes and non-cream cakes. After 2 years, there was some change in consumption of high-fibre bread, but other changes were not sustained. This study demonstrates the challenge of improving dietary intakes of children in school.

SOME POTENTIAL NUTRITIONAL PROBLEMS

As part of the development of increasing independence, children, and particularly teenagers, may encounter difficulties with their diet, or may make challenging choices, which might result in nutritional problems:

- Vegetarianism and veganism
- Teenage athletes
- Pregnancy
- Dieting
- Smoking and alcohol consumption

VEGETARIANISM

An increasingly common finding among children and teenagers in the United Kingdom is the rejection of the omnivorous diet in favour of a vegetarian (non-meat) diet. The NDNS survey results (2014) stated that 2% of children reported that they were vegetarian and less than 1% of participants reported following a vegan diet. In addition to the reasons for choosing to be vegetarian that are discussed in Chapter 10, this age group may be subject to peer pressure or initially make the decision as a bid for independence from parental control.

Unfortunately, many young vegetarians may have an inadequate understanding of the principles of nutrition, so that the traditional 'meat and vegetables' becomes just 'vegetables' or cheese omelette or baked beans on toast. There may be little attempt to introduce other dietary items, such as pulses, cereals or grains, into the diet to replace the animal foods being avoided. In this way, iron, zinc and niacin may become inadequate, as well as calcium, if dairy products are omitted. It has already been mentioned that iron intakes are low in teenagers, particularly girls. A small study in London found that anaemia was three times more common among vegetarian 12–14 years olds, with an incidence of 25%, compared to 9% in omnivores.

There is also concern about low calcium intakes and future health. The majority of bone mass is accrued during the teenage years, with high assimilation rates of dietary calcium. DRVs are high to allow for this. If calcium intakes are low, it is likely that less bone will be made. This may have repercussions in later life, with an increased risk of osteoporosis.

Many vegetarian meal replacements are now available, based on soya or Quorn, which are acceptable and which can help to maintain an adequate nutritional intake, although they can be expensive as an everyday item. It should be remembered that a well-planned vegetarian diet can be nutritionally adequate and may be advantageous in terms of long-term health benefits.

Teenage Athletes

Teenage athletes are particularly vulnerable, if they spend a lot of time training and participating in their chosen sport. This is because the energy needs for their physical activity must be met in addition to their needs for growth. Most schoolchildren participate in some sport, which involves no more than 2–3 hours per week; playing in school teams may occupy a further 3–4 hours a week. This amount of extra physical activity increases nutritional needs slightly but probably not beyond the limits of the usual recommended levels for nutrients with the exception of energy. As with adult athletes, there is a particular need for carbohydrate, preferably in its starchy form, to sustain muscle glycogen levels. School sports teachers should be aware of this.

See Chapter 22 for an introduction to sport nutrition, pp. 421–430.

Where a teenager aspires to be of national class standard, training may take up much more time, often from a very young age. This imposes considerable nutritional needs both for energy and associated nutrients in line with the increase in energy. Energy needs may be 50% greater than those for an average teenager. Meeting these necessitates eating an enormous amount of extra food, which can be quite daunting for a teenager. There may be reluctance to do this for fear of becoming overweight or appearing greedy. However, full athletic potential and normal growth cannot be achieved without the appropriate nutritional input.

Pregnant Teenagers

Pregnancy is associated with changing nutritional requirements. When these are additional to the high needs of adolescence, there is a risk that the intake may not be adequate to meet both. In the United States, the pregnancy rate is approximately 71 per 1000 teenage girls, with a third terminated (aborted). The United Kingdom has the highest pregnancy rate in Western Europe, but a gradual decrease has been observed (1998–2008) from approximately 48 to 40 per 1000 females aged below 18.

In addition to the nutritional needs, there may be social and emotional factors that compound the nutritional difficulties. Dietary habits of pregnant teenagers have been shown to be more erratic than those of pregnant adults, and low levels of vitamins A and C, folate, calcium, iron and zinc have been recorded. If the pregnancy is unwanted, as is often the case, the girl may try to limit weight gain or even diet to lose weight. There may be parental rejection and she may leave home, which can reduce her opportunities to obtain a healthy diet.

See Chapter 6 for a detailed account of pregnancy and increased nutritional requirements, pp. 101–122.

Attendance at antenatal clinics may be erratic or non-existent, so monitoring of the pregnancy to anticipate problems and obtain advice about diet may be missed. Unsurprisingly, there is an increased risk to both mother and fetus in teenage pregnancies. Maternal mortality may be 2.5 times greater at the age of 15 than between 20 and 24; the infant is likely to be of low birthweight and is at higher risk of morbidity and mortality from a number of causes.

A teenager who becomes pregnant needs to increase her nutrient intakes and gain sufficient weight to allow the normal development of her baby. She requires foods with high nutrient density and cannot afford to include foods with low nutrient density in her diet. She may also require supplements.

Dieting

Dissatisfaction with body image is a prevalent phenomenon in Western societies, affecting more females than males. This is transmitted to children from their parents and inevitably influences attitudes and behaviours in children. The preference for slimness is strongly related to the child's current body weight, but a desire to be thinner is found among those with a normal body weight and also those that are underweight. The desire for a thinner body has increasingly been reported in preadolescent children. Over half of teenage girls questioned reported feeling fat and wanting to be thinner; the figure for boys in this study was approximately 20%.

Dieting is a natural corollary to this dissatisfaction, with over 40% of teenage girls reporting past attempts at dieting, 23% reporting being on a diet at the time of study and a further 6% claiming to be dieting all the time. The intensity and duration of dieting are also variable, with some diets lasting only a few days, but other girls reporting continuing their diets for more than 4 weeks.

Dieting practices may be variable. Some may reduce fat, snack or total energy intake and increase fruit and vegetable intake. However, up to 15% are reported to use extreme weight loss measures, such as fasting, skipping meals (usually breakfast), vomiting and using diet pills. Filling up on diet drinks to prevent hunger is also reported. Dieting can become a habit, establishing a pattern of chaotic eating. The food intake is continually restrained; if the restraint slips, a binge may occur, with large amounts of 'forbidden' foods being eaten. However, restraint is very soon re-established. Changing to a vegetarian diet may be part of a dieting strategy and be perceived as a means of weight management.

This type of dietary intake pattern can lead to inadequate energy and nutrient consumption, with subclinical deficiencies developing and implications for future health. In particular, poor nutritional status at the beginning of pregnancy may harm the fetus. Low iron status may lead to poorer cognitive abilities, and low zinc status may depress immune function and lead to higher rates of infection. Finally, poor status of antioxidant nutrients may facilitate damage at cellular level, which may in years to come result in degenerative diseases. In its most severe form, disordered eating can develop into bulimia nervosa or anorexia nervosa, both of which carry serious health risks. In the extreme, anorexia may result in death. Adolescent girls tending towards thinness should be counselled about the dangers for their future health. A body mass index of 18 or less is a useful criterion for the need to intervene.

Dieting is less of a problem among boys, although anorexia has been reported in up to 5%. In some, an obsessional preoccupation with sport as a means of weight control may replace the vomiting and purging used by girls. Usually, adolescent boys are more concerned about becoming taller and stronger and concentrate more on body building than restricting their body size.

Smoking and Alcohol Use

Both smoking and the use of alcohol are becoming more common among older children and teenagers in the United Kingdom. Alcohol interferes with the absorption and metabolism of a number of nutrients including amino acids, calcium, folate, thiamin and vitamin C. If the intake is modest, these effects are probably of little concern. However, binge drinking may have a more serious impact on nutrient levels. In the latest NDNS report, 3% of boys aged 13–15 years and 4% of girls of the same age reported usually drinking once a week or more. This sort of drinking may also be accompanied by vomiting, which removes nutrients from the body. Ultimately, nutritional status may be affected. In addition, alcohol itself will have damaging effects on the organs of the body, just as in an adult.

Smoking increases the free-radical load in the body and, therefore, the requirement for vitamin C. This should be provided in greater amounts to those teenagers who smoke. In the United Kingdom, 22% boys and 26% girls aged 13–15 years have experienced smoking. A particularly vulnerable situation exists in those teenagers who are dieting and smoking, to help control their hunger and their weight. In this case, nutrient intakes may be inadequate to offer protection against the harmful free radicals in cigarette smoke.

SUMMARY

1. The transition from infant to teenager and young adult involves enormous changes in body size and composition. The constituents of the new tissues must be obtained from the diet. Thus, at all stages of this process, nutritional requirements are high.
2. Human and formula milk can provide the nutritional needs of the infant, although human milk confers some immunological and developmental advantages.
3. The process of weaning should start at 6 months. It parallels stages of development but is nutritionally important.
4. Between the years of 1 and 5, the child consolidates the early experience with food and becomes more independent. Growth rates are slower but, because appetite can be small, the nutrient density of the diet is of great importance.
5. The diet of the school-age child is increasingly affected by external influences. It is important that well-balanced diets are provided at home. It must be recognized that children need to exercise choice in their food intake, as part of development. However, a sound foundation of education about food can make these choices healthier.
6. Teenagers are more vulnerable than the other age groups to peer pressure and may pass through phases of experimentation with food. Again, a core of well-balanced food provided at home can ensure that good nutrient intakes are maintained.

STUDY QUESTIONS

1. Describe and discuss the nutritional and non-nutritional differences between human milk and formula milk.
2. a. What are the main nutritional principles underlying the balance of the diet suitable for children aged between 5 and 10 years?
   b. What problems might be encountered?
   c. Which nutrients might be most at risk?
3. At what ages are teenage boys and girls most nutritionally vulnerable and for what reasons?
4. Discuss the physiological factors that influence feeding in infancy.
5. What are the current UK and worldwide guidelines for weaning (complementary feeding), and what evidence is this guidance based on? Discuss the potential consequences of not adhering to these guidelines.
6. Suggest some ways in which teenagers could be targeted for nutritional advice.

ACTIVITY

7.1 Perform a short survey of weaning and baby foods available on the supermarket shelf.

- Review the label for age suitability – Is this in accordance with the weaning age recommendation?
- What are the main ingredients on the product label? Is this in accordance with the list of ingredients?
- Have you tasted one of these products? Which flavour is the most discernible?
- How are ingredients selected to enhance sweetness? Why?
- Are there drawbacks to the prevalence of sweet baby foods on the market?

BIBLIOGRAPHY AND FURTHER READING

Anderson, J.A., Johnstone, B.M. and Remley, D.T. 1999. Breast feeding and cognitive development: A meta-analysis. *American Journal of Clinical Nutrition* 70, 525–535.

Barker, D.J.P. 1994. *Mothers, Babies and Diseases in Later Life*. London, UK: British Medical Journal.

Bates, B., Lennox, A., Prentice, A., Bates, C., Page, P., Nicholson, S. and Swan, G. 2014. *National Diet and Nutrition Survey: Results from Years 1–4 (Combined) of the Rolling Programme (2008/2009–2011/12).* London, UK: Public Health England, and Food Standards Agency.
Buttriss, J. L. The Eatwell Guide refreshed. *Nutrition Bulletin* 41(2), 135–141.
Crawley, H. 2005. *Eating Well at School: Nutritional and Practical Guidelines.* Caroline Walker Trust and National Heart Forum.
Crawley, H. 2006. *Eating Well for under-5s in Child Care.* St Austell: Caroline Walker Trust.
DfES (UK Department for Education and Skills). 2001. *Healthy School Lunches for Students in Secondary Schools.* London, UK: DfSE.
DoH (UK Department of Health). 1989. Dthe diet of British schoolchildren. Report on health and social subjects 36. London, UK: HMSO.
DoH (UK Department of Health). 1991. Dietary reference values for food energy and nutrients for the United Kingdom. Report on Health and Social Subjects No. 41. Report of the Panel on Dietary Reference Values of the Committee on Medical Aspects of Food Policy. London, UK: HMSO.
DoH (UK Department of Health). 1991. The health of the nation: a strategy for health in England. London, UK: HMSO.
DoH (UK Department of Health). 1994. Weaning and the weaning diet. Report on Health and Social Subjects 45. Report of the Working Group on the Weaning Diet of the Committee on Medical Aspects of Food Policy. London, UK: HMSO.
DoH (UK Department of Health). 2011. *UK Physical Activity Guidelines. Fact Sheet 3: Children and Young People (5–18 Years).* London, UK: HMSO.
Du Toit, G., Roberts, G., Sayre, P.H. et al. 2015. Randomized trial of peanut consumption in infants at risk for peanut allergy. *New England Journal of Medicine* 372(9), 803–813.
EEC. 1991. Commission directive on infant formulae and follow-on formulae. *Official Journal of the European Communities* L175, 35–49.
García, A. L., Raza, S., Parrett, A., and Wright, C. M. 2013. Nutritional content of infant commercial weaning foods in the UK. *Archives of Disease in Childhood*, 98(10), 793–797.
Garcia, A.L., McLean, K., and Wright, C.M. 2015. Types of fruits and vegetables used in commercial baby foods and their contribution to sugar content. *Maternal & Child Nutrition.* In press. doi: 10.1111/mcn.12208.
Gregory, J.R., Collins, D.L., Davies, P.S.W., Hughes, J.M., and Clarke, P.C. 1995. *National diet and Nutrition Survey: Children Aged 1.5 to 4.5 years. Volume 1: Report of the Diet and Nutrition Survey.* London, UK: HMSO.
Gregory, J.R., Lowe, S., Bates, C.J. et al. 2000. *National Diet and Nutrition Survey: Young People Aged 4–18 Years. Volume 1: Report of the Diet and Nutrition Survey.* London, UK: The Stationery Office.
Hill, A.J. 2002. Developmental issues in attitudes to food and diet. *Proceedings of the Nutrition Society* 61, 259–266.
Jackson, A.A. 2015. Feeding the normal infant, child and adolescent. *Medicine* 43(2), 127–131.
Labbok, M.H. 2012. Global baby-friendly hospital initiative monitoring data: Update and discussion. *Breastfeeding Medicine* 7, 210–222.
MAFF (Ministry of Agriculture, Fisheries and Food). 1995. *The Infant Formula and Follow-on Formula Regulations. Statutory Instrument 77.* London, UK: HMSO.
Mcandrew, F., Thompson, J., Fellows, L., Large, A., Speed, M. and Renfrew, M.J. 2012. Infant feeding survey 2010 [Online]. Health and Social Care Information Centre. Available at: http://www.hscic.gov.uk/catalogue/PUB08694 (accessed 30 October 2014).
Oddy, W.H. 2012. Infant feeding and obesity risk in the child. *Breastfeeding Review* 20, 7–12.
Parker, L. and Fox, A. 2001. The Peterborough Schools Nutrition Project: A multiple intervention programme to improve school-based eating in secondary schools. *Public Health Nutrition* 4(6), 1221–1228.
Robinson, S. 2000. Children's perceptions of who controls their food. *Journal of Human Nutrition and Dietetics* 13, 163–171.
Scottish Executive. 2003. Hungry for Success. A Whole School Approach to School Meals in Scotland. Edinburgh: Scottish Executive. Accessed from: www.scotland.gov.uk/hungryforsuccess
Smithers, L. and McIntyre, E. 2010. The impact of breastfeeding – Translating recent evidence for practice. *Australian Family Physician* 39(10), 757–760.

8 Nutrition during Adulthood and Ageing

AIMS

The aims of this chapter are to

- Review the dietary guidelines that have been made for adults in the United Kingdom and identify the particular needs of men and of women.
- Review the nutritional aspects of a vegetarian diet.
- Consider the effects of alcohol consumption on the achievement of dietary goals.
- Discuss why women may be considered a nutritionally vulnerable group at certain stages of their life and whether the dietary guidelines address their problems.
- Discuss some human situations that may influence diet and so affect the attainment of the guidelines, including belonging to an ethnic minority group, having a low income, retirement and ageing.

Dietary reference values (DRVs) and nutritional guidelines have, of necessity, been devised for the population as a whole. It would be both impractical and confusing to set a great number of different recommendations for various subgroups in the population. The guidelines current in the United Kingdom are very much in line with those in other Western countries and are the result of a wide consensus.

The progress towards achieving these guidelines is slow, and in some cases, trends in consumption appear to be moving contrary to the desired direction. It has been suggested that the guidelines are too ambitious as they set goals that only a very small amount of the population currently meet. An intermediate set of guidelines, closer to the actual patterns of consumption in the population, may be a more realistic target.

Nutrient requirements and the basics of a nutritionally balanced diet are covered in Chapter 2, pp. 11–29.

It is also important that a 'whole-diet' approach is adopted. Many people at present mistakenly believe that, if they change just one aspect of their diet, they are already eating more healthily. For example, there has been an increase in use of low-fat spread and semi-skimmed milk. These changes are desirable, but they do not go far enough towards a healthier diet. Such changes may result in a lower energy intake from dairy fat, which is then replaced by fats contained in biscuits or processed convenience foods. More extensive changes to the diet, for example, becoming vegetarian may have a number of positive health effects but, at the same time, increase risks from unforeseen consequences in the diet.

In addition, it should be recognized that there are many groups within the population who, for a diverse number of reasons, cannot achieve the targets. All of these groups will be considered in this chapter, exploring the reasons why they may have different needs, and considering some of the barriers that prevent them achieving dietary guidelines.

ADULT MEN

Many dietary guidelines around the world originated from a concern about morbidity and mortality from coronary heart disease. Consequently, they were based largely on findings from studies of men, since almost all the early studies targeted groups of men. In addition, their primary focus was related to intakes of fat, which for many years has been the major dietary factor linked to coronary heart disease development. Only in more recent years have dietary guidelines widened to include other dietary components, such as starchy carbohydrates, alcohol, salt and other micronutrients, including the antioxidant vitamins.

Do Men Have Problems Achieving These Guidelines and Are They Appropriate?

Most men understand that they are at risk of heart disease, although many adopt the attitude that '*it will not happen to me*'. Consequently, motivation to change dietary habits may not be very great. This may be sustained by social norms, which, in some cultural subgroups, expect men to have a traditional diet that contains plenty of meat and not to eat the more 'feminine' salad, fruit and vegetables.

There is also a lower attendance rates to health services by men than by women and a lower uptake of screening services. Exposure to information about healthy eating is generally less among men, as women gain this information from magazines (often in association with articles on cookery or weight loss), from information at health centres and supermarkets. In all cases, men have less access to these sources.

Further, traditional education philosophy excluded boys from learning about food and nutrition at school; the National Curriculum in the United Kingdom has introduced some teaching about health and diet to all children, regardless of gender.

Concern about body weight is much less among men, although current trends in the United Kingdom show that more men than women are overweight. In addition, the distribution of body fat in men, with a greater tendency to deposit abdominal fat means that overweight is a greater health risk.

Traditionally, more men have been smokers and heavy drinkers; however, in both cases, rates in women have increased in the last two decades. These are lifestyle factors, which may compound risk in several chronic diseases that also have nutritional risk factors. Men, therefore, are at nutritional risk, and it is important that attempts to change to a healthier diet are made, encompassing whole diet changes.

Studies show that, when changes are made, results are better in the younger age group than in older men. In addition, men in the higher social classes are more likely to make changes. Therefore, greatest benefits are seen here. There is a need to target men to increase their awareness of the importance of dietary change as well as exercise and other lifestyle factors, such as drinking and smoking, in a more active approach to disease prevention. This will be easier to achieve in some groups than others; regrettably, those with the greatest need for change are often the ones who are most difficult to reach. Imaginative approaches on the part of primary healthcare teams and health promoters are needed. These can include health promotion in the workplace or through social clubs, perhaps related to support of sporting activities.

ADULT WOMEN

There is a dilemma in trying to devise an optimal diet for women, as different stages in a woman's life may require different nutritional priorities.

Women generally have a smaller food intake than men, related to their lower energy needs. Within this smaller intake, however, they still need to obtain all of the nutrients essential for good health. Consequently, they have a lower margin for error in their diet – most of what they eat has to be nutrient rich. Eating too much 'empty energy' will result in an insufficient intake of micronutrients and possible health risks.

Most of the specific health issues for women have been discussed in other parts of this book; they are highlighted here to remind the reader of the vulnerability of the female to poor nutrition at various ages.

A female adolescent requires a certain amount of body fat to be present for normal reproductive activity to begin. Yet, during this time of life, many adolescent girls feel an enormous pressure from society to restrict their weight gain and achieve a slim body shape. These two goals are difficult to reconcile, with the result that some girls do not start to menstruate or, having started, stop again, as their body weight falls. This has implications for bone health in later life, in particular, because adolescence is also the time when the bone assimilates its minerals and achieves most of its final mass. Once into her early twenties, a woman is no longer able to add significant amounts of calcium to her bones, with the result that, if the bone mass is not optimal, she may develop osteoporosis in her early old age.

In early adult years, a woman may want to have children. Research dating back to the Dutch hunger winter in 1944–1945 (when the population of Holland suffered severe food shortages for a period of 8 months), but replicated in many studies since then, has shown that an adequate amount of body fat is needed for normal fertility. The normal development of the fetus is threatened if the woman is underweight. More recent work shows that various vitamins and minerals must be present in sufficient amounts from the beginning of the pregnancy to avoid low birthweight and associated risks to the child, both in its early and later life.

Certain diseases are also a particular threat for women. Women experience anaemia much more commonly than men, principally because the iron lost in blood during menstruation is not replaced adequately from the diet. Both cancer of the breast and heart disease cause a large number of deaths and are believed to have a dietary component. In addition, osteoporosis is a condition that causes disability in many more elderly women than men.

Physical activity, which is beneficial in promoting health, has for many years been more socially acceptable for men than for women. There is now an increase in women taking part in sport, but problems of time and access to sports facilities still bar many women from being more active. There may be a reluctance also to expose a less than perfect body in the gym.

Social research shows that a woman's food choices tend to be dictated more by the likes and dislikes of her partner and children than by her own preferences, even when she is the one with the major responsibility for food provision within the household. Thus, even if a woman might want to eat a healthier diet, she may experience pressure from her family to minimize change.

Finally, it must be recognized that women represent the majority of those living in poverty. In the United Kingdom, women are 5% more likely to be living in poverty than men and are daily faced with the associated effects on nutrition, discussed in "Low Income and Nutrition" section of this chapter (Women's Budget Group, 2005). As a result of these conflicts and dilemmas, women generally have more nutritional problems than men.

VEGETARIANS

There has been a steady increase in the United Kingdom in the number of people who reject meat from their diet and follow some variant of the vegetarian diet. Surveys suggest that between 5% and 10% of the population may be following some form of vegetarian diet. Numbers tend to be greatest in females and among teenagers and young adults, although people of all ages are represented. The move to vegetarianism may initially include the rejection only of red meat, but might further also exclude white meats, fish and, occasionally, other animal products such as eggs and cheese. Thus, the diet is based on cereals, pulses, nuts, vegetables and fruit. Many vegetarians, but not vegans, also include dairy products and eggs. Various categories of vegetarianism have been defined according to the foods of animal origin that are included in the diet (e.g. a lacto-ovo-vegetarian will eat cheese and eggs, a pescarian will eat fish).

The reasons for adopting a vegetarian diet vary, but may include the following:

- Compassion for animals and concerns about animal welfare
- Rejection on ethical grounds of the intensive production methods used in animal husbandry and food production
- Concern over Western overindulgence in food and exploitation of poorer countries and world resources
- Dislike of the taste, texture or smell of meat
- Concern over the safety of meat and animal products in the light of 'food scares', such as *Salmonella*, bovine spongiform encephalopathy and the use of antibiotics
- Religious or cultural reasons

From a nutritional perspective, an ideal diet is one that contains a wide variety of foods, providing maximum opportunities to meet nutritional requirements. However, it cannot be said that foods of animal origin are an essential part of such a diet, and there are many populations around the world who exist on diets that are exclusively plant based. Problems of deficiency may arise when there is over-reliance on a limited number of foods or foods of limited nutritional value, for example, cassava, yam and maize. Where the quantity of food supplied by such a diet is sufficient and the diet contains a variety of plant foods, then nutritional adequacy is not a problem. This is generally the case in Western societies and a well-planned vegetarian diet may provide a greater diversity of foods than one based around meat, including more vegetables, pulses and nuts. As a result, many nutrients may be present in greater amounts than in an omnivorous diet. However, meat and animal products are rich in a number of minerals and vitamins that may not be sufficiently replaced in a vegetarian diet.

In general, a well-balanced vegetarian diet containing grains, vegetables and nuts is likely to provide more of the following nutrients: folate, vitamin C, carotene, thiamin, vitamin E and potassium.

Nutrients about which there may be some concern, especially if the diet lacks dairy products, include the following: protein, iron, calcium, iodine and zinc, vitamin B_{12}, vitamins A and D and *n*-3 fatty acids.

Vegetarians are probably more prone to iron deficiency anaemia because of the poorer bioavailability of iron from plant-based diets. Attention should be paid to maximizing absorption by including enhancing factors, such as foods containing vitamin C in the diet. Vitamin B_{12} occurs only in foods of animal origin and therefore, their strict exclusion will be a risk factor for deficiency. Many foods designed for vegetarian diets, such as meat substitutes, are fortified with the vitamin, but vigilance is needed to ensure an adequate intake.

It is particularly important that attention is paid to these nutrients in the diets of vegetarian infants, children and adolescents as covered in Chapter 7, p. 147.

Vitamin D status may be compromised when the vegetarian diet is also very high in phytate and low in calcium, as has been reported in some macrobiotic diets and among people of Asian origin in the United Kingdom.

Lower intakes of the long-chain *n*-3 fatty acids are also a feature of vegetarian diets that exclude fish. Levels of these fatty acids are lower in plasma of adult vegetarians and also in the milk during lactation. These fatty acids have a role in the development of the retina and central nervous system in the infant, and the significance of these lower levels for infant development is being studied.

More interest has been focused on the positive aspects of a vegetarian diet, in relation to some of the chronic diseases prevailing in Western societies. Studies of adult vegetarians show that they have similar energy intakes compared with omnivores. However, the body mass index (BMI) of vegetarians is on average 1 kg/m^2 lower than in matched omnivores. The reasons for this are unclear, but may be attributable to lower fat or alcohol intakes. One of the reported consequences of the lower body weight is a lower blood pressure, which may confer advantages in terms of stroke and coronary heart disease.

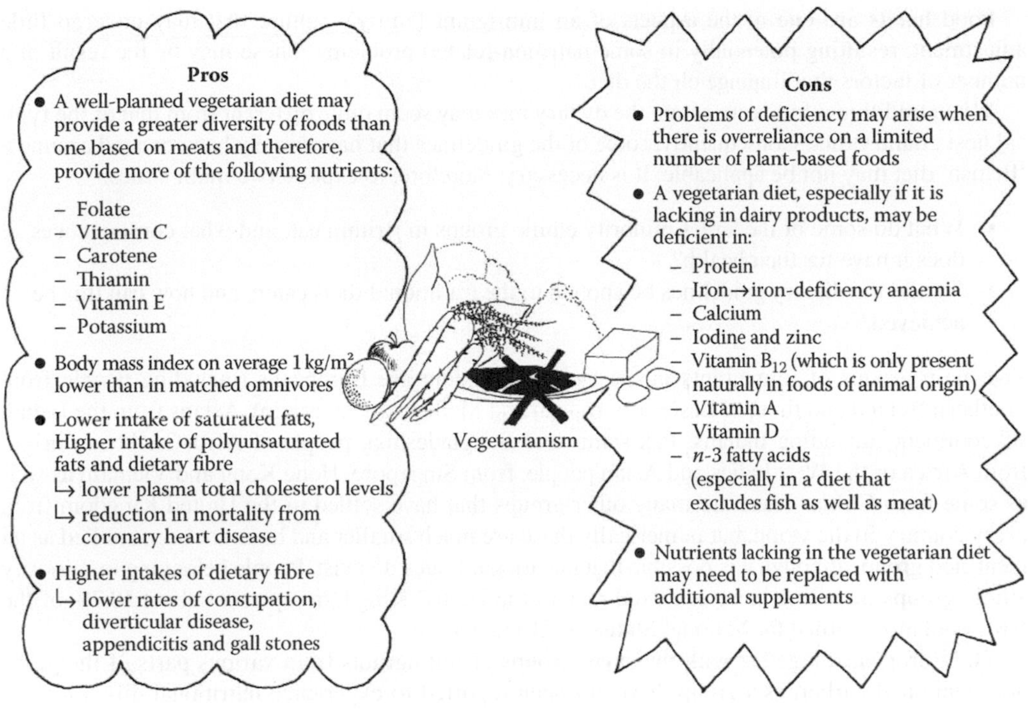
Pros
• A well-planned vegetarian diet may provide a greater diversity of foods than one based on meats and therefore, provide more of the following nutrients:
– Folate
– Vitamin C
– Carotene
– Thiamin
– Vitamin E
– Potassium
• Body mass index on average 1 kg/m² lower than in matched omnivores
• Lower intake of saturated fats, Higher intake of polyunsaturated fats and dietary fibre
↳ lower plasma total cholesterol levels
↳ reduction in mortality from coronary heart disease
• Higher intakes of dietary fibre
↳ lower rates of constipation, diverticular disease, appendicitis and gall stones
Vegetarianism
Cons
• Problems of deficiency may arise when there is overreliance on a limited number of plant-based foods
• A vegetarian diet, especially if it is lacking in dairy products, may be deficient in:
– Protein
– Iron→iron-deficiency anaemia
– Calcium
– Iodine and zinc
– Vitamin B12 (which is only present naturally in foods of animal origin)
– Vitamin A
– Vitamin D
– n-3 fatty acids (especially in a diet that excludes fish as well as meat)
• Nutrients lacking in the vegetarian diet may need to be replaced with additional supplements

FIGURE 8.1 The possible advantages and disadvantages of a vegetarian diet.

Data from five cohort studies (Key et al., 1998), including 76,000 subjects, have shown that vegetarians had a 24% reduction in mortality from coronary heart disease. Mortality in semi-vegetarians, who ate fish only or meat less than once per week, was intermediate between meat eaters and vegetarians. It is proposed that these differences can be attributed to lower intakes of saturated fat in vegetarians and related lower plasma total cholesterol concentrations. In addition, vegetarians tend to have higher intakes of polyunsaturated fatty acids, especially linoleic acid and dietary fibre. Both of these will also affect cholesterol levels and decrease the risk of coronary heart disease.

Higher intakes of dietary fibre are also possibly responsible for lower rates of constipation, diverticular disease, appendicitis and gallstones that have been reported among vegetarians. At present, there is no firm evidence that vegetarian diets protect against cancers.

Overall, a planned vegetarian diet can meet many of the dietary guidelines and contribute to better health. There are a number of possible shortcomings from the exclusion of meat and dairy products, and these nutrients should be replaced from other foods. A badly constructed vegetarian diet will, however, carry no health advantages and may be hazardous to long-term health. The possible advantages and disadvantages of a vegetarian diet are summarized in Figure 8.1.

MINORITY ETHNIC GROUPS

Many people around the world for a variety of political or economic reasons move to and settle in a foreign country, becoming immigrants. If the culture of the host country is similar to that of the immigrant's own mother country, settlement is relatively easy. If there are many cultural, religious and language difficulties, the immigrant may experience alienation in the host country. If the immigrant is a refugee forced to leave the home country, the psychological challenges of adjustment may also create difficulties with the diet.

Food habits are one of the aspects of an immigrant family's culture that may undergo little adjustment, resulting potentially in some nutrition-related problems. These may be the result of a number of factors that impinge on the diet.

When traditional foods are eaten, the dietary mix may seem quite different from that of the typical host country diet. Consequently, some of the guidelines that have largely been created around a 'British' diet may not be applicable. It is necessary, therefore, to explore two main issues:

- What do some of the larger minority ethnic groups in Britain eat, and what consequences does it have for their health?
- Should the dietary guidelines be applied to the traditional diets eaten, and how can this be achieved?

The main groups of immigrants in the United Kingdom are Europeans (including people from Southern Ireland and those of Eastern European and Mediterranean origin), Asians from the Indian subcontinent (including Indians, Pakistanis and Bangladeshis), people of Afro-Caribbean origin from Africa or the West Indies and Asian people, from Singapore, Hong Kong and Vietnam as well as some from China. There are many other groups that have settled in the United Kingdom from every country in the world, but numerically these are much smaller and have not been studied as an identified group, although it is possible that nutritional issues do exist. People belonging to minority ethnic groups including those of mixed race in the United Kingdom represent about 10.7% of the UK population (Office for National Statistics, 2013a and b).

The Europeans, together with the small groups of immigrants from various parts of the globe not mentioned earlier, as a group, have not been reported to experience nutritional difficulties or possible deficiencies in Britain. It is possible that, like any other individual, they may experience personal dietary problems, which may be exacerbated by factors related to their ethnic origin.

LOW INCOME AND NUTRITION

People on a low income may be living in poverty. This is a relative term: it can be taken to mean an absolute lack of material possessions but, in Western society, it is more commonly used to reflect disadvantage in relation to the rest of society. In practice, the definition varies between different organizations. Two definitions that are used are the following:

- People receiving less than half of the average income (whether from employment or state benefits)
- People having to spend more than 30% of income on food

Numbers of people in poverty have been increasing in Europe throughout the last decades. It is documented that people in these situations have poorer health in almost every measure used to assess health, with excess morbidity and mortality at all ages. Various groups are particularly vulnerable to poverty. These include the following:

- Families with children, in particular, where there is a lone parent or where neither parent is in employment.
- Women, owing to the traditional dependence of women on a male breadwinner, their traditional role as carers of children and their poorer pension rights as a result of incomplete employment records. In two-adult households where the woman is the sole wage earner, the income is usually lower than in those with a male wage earner.
- People with a disability, owing to poorer employment prospects and higher than average living costs.
- Members of minority ethnic groups, owing to a higher unemployment rate and a greater representation among the low paid. In addition, there are now many refugees and asylum

seekers throughout Europe who are often in severe financial hardship, which also reflects on their nutritional intakes.

- Young people who have left school but have not been able to find work. They have very low entitlements to benefits and may not be supported by their families, leading perhaps to homelessness and a life in poverty.
- Homeless people have major problems in achieving an adequate food intake. They may have additional problems that compromise nutritional status, such as alcohol or drug abuse. Alcohol may provide a substantial proportion of the energy intake. Studies on this group find that they are up to four times more likely to be underweight and have a diet that is low in a wide range of nutrients. Shelters for the homeless and soup kitchens are an important source of nutritional provision, and attention to the quality of the food could make a difference to the status of this group.

Income is not the only factor contributing to poorer health experienced by people in these groups. One of the main factors is likely to be their diet, but poorer housing, low self-esteem, poorer educational opportunity and lifestyle habits detrimental to health, such as smoking, all make a contribution.

Characteristics of the Diet

Expenditure on food is described as elastic, which means that when income is limited and other, fixed, expenses have to be met, the food budget can be trimmed accordingly. However, those on a limited income may spend up to three times more, proportionately, on food compared with the average UK family.

The expenditure on food is cost efficient; the annual National Food Survey consistently shows that the lowest income groups obtain more nutrients per unit of money spent. Table 8.1 shows some of the foods typically bought by the low-income and high-income groups, and in Table 8.2, the amount bought per 1 pence of expenditure is shown.

Studies such as these of the foods eaten typically show that low-income families rely more heavily on white bread, whole milk, sugar, eggs, meat products and margarine, and consume less reduced fat milk, poultry, carcass meat, fish, fresh vegetables (excluding potatoes), fruit, brown and wholemeal bread. Vegetables and potatoes are more likely to be processed rather than fresh. There

TABLE 8.1

Types of Foods Eaten by the Highest (Q5) and Lowest (Q1) Income Groups Studied by the National Diet and Nutrition Survey 2008/2009–2011/2012 (Consumption in g/Person per Week)

	Income Group	
Food	**Q5**	**Q1**
Fruit	121	73
Vegetables (not inc. potatoes)	205	162
Total fruit and vegetables (not inc. fruit juice)	326	235
Fruit juice	78	68
Meat	109	103
Red meat	70	66
Fish	27	18
Oily fish	10	4
5-a-day (portions/day)	4.7	3.5
Percentage achieving 5-a-day	38%	24%

Source: Bates (2014).

TABLE 8.2

'Value for Money' of Foods Bought by High-Income (A) and Low-Income Groups (D) (Amount Purchased in Grams per 1 Pence Spent)

	Income Group	
Food	**A**	**D**
Milk, cream and cheese	9.3	13.8
Meat and meat products	1.9	2.8
Fish	1.3	2.0
Fats and oils	3.8	6.0
Sugar and preserves	7.0	12.9
Vegetables and potatoes	6.3	10.4
Fruit	6.8	9.0
Bread	7.8	11.5
Cereals	4.2	6.3
Soft drinks	22.1	31.3
Alcoholic drinks	2.3	3.8
Confectionery	1.6	2.0

Source: Calculated from DEFRA, *National Food Survey 2000: Annual Report on Food Expenditure, Consumption and Nutrient Intakes*, The Stationery Office, London, UK, 2001.

is also less variety of foods eaten; for example, among pregnant women in Edinburgh and London, the poorest had only half the number of different foods in their diet compared with the richer women. The diet is, therefore, more likely to be monotonous, with few new additions.

Table 8.2 shows that, for every food group, those households with a lower income buy more (by weight) for their money. This applies to even simple products, such as confectionery or soft drinks. Overall, expenditure is also less, with a mean expenditure of £22.03 by group A and £14.07 by group D recorded by DEFRA (2001). Overall, the lowest income households spend a greater proportion of their weekly budget on food. In 2011, the lowest income households spent 16.6% of their household budget on food compared with 11.3% for all households (DEFRA, 2012).

This cost efficiency often necessitates shopping around to find the best value for money, which may be time-consuming. Some poorer residential areas may have limited shopping facilities, and the term 'food deserts' has been coined to describe this situation. Access to the wider choice of foods in larger supermarkets may be limited by lack of transport or insufficient resources to make the trip worthwhile. In general, about 30% of the British population have no access to a car and are, therefore, dependent on public transport for their access to more distant shops. In addition, the temptation of a large variety of foods on offer makes a stark contrast with the amount of money available. Consequently, local and often smaller shops may be used, where both choice and value for money are likely to be less. There may also be a problem of a lack of storage facilities, necessitating frequent purchases of perishable items. Shopping becomes a chore, with little scope for enjoyment. It should also be noted that 'value for money' in terms of quantity of food purchased does not necessarily equate to nutritional value. The cheaper foods bought may have poorer nutritional content; for example, cheaper meat products contain more fat and salt, and cheaper vegetables may be less fresh and have lower vitamin contents.

Nevertheless, families try to maintain conventional eating patterns to lessen the impact of low income, often eating cheaper versions of 'mainstream' meals. Also, parents endeavour to protect their children against the effects on the diet of poverty, buying foods that the children prefer. As a consequence, children in low-income families may actually receive more of their favourite foods

TABLE 8.3
Cost of Common Snack Foods, in Pence, to Supply 420 kJ (100 cal)

Food	Costs to Provide 420 kJ (100 cal) (pence)
Orange	45.0
Apple	44.0
Kit Kat (chocolate wafer)	24.4
Chocolate bar (cadburys)	23.1
Crisps (walkers ready salted)	21.3
Fruit yogurt[a]	14.7
Extra strong mints[a]	12.2
Banana	8.9
Sponge cake[a]	7.2
Cola[a]	7.1
Whole milk	6.8
Wholemeal bread[a]	2.4
Digestive biscuits[a]	1.6

Note: Values calculated from Food Standards Agency (FSA, 2002b) and at 2014 supermarket economy prices (based on Tesco supermarket online prices).
[a] Tescos Everyday Value own brand range.

than children from better-off households. To achieve this, parents in several studies record missing meals. Protecting the children also means that the family meal is focused on what the children prefer and will eat, rather than the likes and dislikes of other family members. Eating may cease to be a pleasure and becomes simply a means to ward off hunger.

Food selection is made from a rational perspective, with a view to the meal it can produce in the most economical way. Therefore, foods that may require preparation and addition of several other ingredients to constitute a meal are less attractive. A ready-made product, such as a meat pie, needs few additional items to make it into a complete meal, in contrast to a leaner meat, which itself contains less energy and requires vegetables, pasta, potatoes, bread, etc. to make a meal. Predictability of portion size and number also helps in meal planning.

As one of the primary concerns is to feel satiated after a meal, foods that provide a large amount of energy for a small financial outlay may be preferred. Consequently, foods high in fat and sugars will be more satisfying than a low-fat, low-sugar food and will provide a cost-efficient source of energy. The cost to supply 420 kJ (100 cal) from a variety of snack foods is shown in Table 8.3. Not all are nutritionally poor; for example, bread and milk can provide a cheap nutritious snack.

Nutritional Implications

Current dietary advice (discussed in Chapter 2) is to eat more fruit, vegetables and starchy carbohydrate, and to reduce the intake of fats, particularly from whole fat dairy products and meats rich in saturated fats. In addition, the consumption of fish is encouraged. The National Food Surveys show that the trend towards a healthier pattern in the diet is more marked in the higher-income groups surveyed and, in many cases, is moving in the opposite direction in the poorer groups. Thus, although there is a small downwards trend in fat intake in poorer families, more of that fat is still saturated, and fruit and green vegetable consumption in one study was found to be equivalent to two apples and ten Brussels sprouts per person per week.

Evidence collected in many centres around the United Kingdom has shown that the costs of a 'healthier basket' of foods are greater than for a 'less healthy' basket. The difference in price varies between regions of the country, but may represent an excess cost of 20% for the 'healthier' basket. In addition, the access to many of the healthier items may be more limited in the areas where the poorer families may shop.

The stresses of living on a low income mean that health concerns are not one of the highest priorities, even though evidence suggests that the desire to eat more healthily exists. Knowledge about what constitutes a healthier diet is also present among poorer families, although it may be fragmentary. Reports have shown that, if there was more money to spend, then this would be used to buy more fruit, vegetables and leaner meats. At present, for such families, the cost of the food takes precedence over issues of taste, cultural acceptability and healthy eating.

Members of these families run the risk of having lower intakes of many of the micronutrients. In particular, these include iron, zinc, calcium, magnesium and potassium, as well as the vitamins, especially vitamin C, folate, riboflavin, niacin, beta-carotene and vitamin E. Many of these are the 'antioxidant nutrients', which are believed to be especially important to health. At the same time, the diet may be low in non-starch polysaccharides (NSPs) and polyunsaturated fats, but contain excessive amounts of saturated fat and sugars. The consequences for health are likely at all ages. Links with nutrition have been discussed also in the relevant sections of the book; a summary is provided here:

- Infants are less likely to be breastfed, although there has been an increase in prevalence reported in the Infant Feeding 2010 Survey. Breastfeeding is protective against infection in early life, enhances gut development, and may protect against allergy and eczema. It is also associated with better school performance in childhood and a higher IQ for children born pre-term.
- Infants in low-income families have a higher consumption of infant formulae, potatoes, confectionery, squashes and soft drinks and a lower consumption of milk products and fruit. Nutrient intakes are higher in saturated fats and cholesterol and lower in carotene and vitamin C.
- Toddlers have slower growth and slower recovery from infection, but also more have a high BMI, more dental caries and higher blood lipids. Their diets are higher in saturated fatty acids, sugars, starch and sodium (present in higher amounts in processed foods that form a larger part of the diet). There are lower intakes of NSPs, beta-carotene, vitamin C, iron, zinc, calcium and iodine.
- Older schoolchildren have lower intakes of most vitamins and minerals, lower levels of activity and poorer bone accretion. There are higher rates of anaemia among teenage girls and lower iron status, which probably impacts on cognitive ability. If the poor iron status continues into pregnancy, there are higher risks of stillbirth and low birthweight and increased risk of hypertension and heart disease in the offspring later in their lives.
- Lone parents have a greater likelihood of falling below the lower reference nutrient intake (LRNI) for many nutrients, and they have also greater 'poverty index' (this was assessed on a number of lifestyle factors associated with low income). Pregnant women have generally lower intakes of energy and nutrients, poorer weight gain and higher occurrence of low birthweight babies. This has implications for their future health and perpetuates the intergenerational effects of deprivation.
- Older adults have lower nutrient intakes, poorer immune status and higher risk from all diet-related diseases.
- Special dietary requirements are more difficult to follow.

Practical Help

Attempts have been made to devise sample diets that would be nutritionally sound, and at the same time, cost no more than a low-income budget could afford. One such was the 'ten pound diet' produced by Ministry of Agriculture, Fisheries and Food (MAFF; see Leather, 1992), which gave precise amounts of 26 different food groups/items, which could be used to plan meals for 1 week within this budget. Many people felt that this diet was socially unacceptable, as it expected people on a low income to eat differently from the rest of society.

More practical help is reported by the National Food Alliance, which brings together many local projects engaged in empowering people on low income and enabling them to work together in low-cost cafes, food cooperatives and other support groups. In this way, access to and education about food are improved, the feelings of isolation are reduced and self-esteem can be enhanced. In association with these more social improvements, there can be a better diet and a greater interest in food and eating healthily.

Further work was undertaken on a strategy on food and low income by the Low Income Project Team (DoH, 1996). This aimed to bring about a better understanding of the costs of healthy eating and facilitate access to healthier foods by involving policy makers and providers of the food. As part of this initiative, ways of mapping price and availability of healthy food have been developed. This can then be used to identify areas that serve their local community poorly in terms of healthy food and attempt to address this. Local projects as part of the Governments initiative on Social Exclusion in the United Kingdom are helping local groups around the country to improve their access to better quality food; this may be through, for example, local street markets, 'Get Cooking' clubs or community cafes.

OLDER ADULTS

In this discussion, the term 'elderly' is used to refer to men and women of pensionable age. In the United Kingdom, this generally means 65 years or over for men and over 60 years for women. The upper end of this age spectrum is not defined, but there are increasing numbers of people over 100 years old in the United Kingdom (the majority are women).

The population of the UK aged 65 and over was 11.1 million (17.4% of the total population) in 2013, up by 290,800 from 2012. The number of people in this age group has increased by 17.3% in the last 10 years (Office for National Statistics, 2013b). The total numbers of the elderly are increasing in most Western countries: by 2030, it is estimated that one in four of the adult population will be aged over 65 years. In the United Kingdom, the greatest increase in the early part of the twenty-first century will be particularly in the over-85 age group, with a smaller relative increase in the over-75s. The numbers between 60/65 and 74 will fall slightly, reflecting the lower birth rates in the 1930s and during the Second World War. The over-85 group are the most vulnerable sector of the retired population and the most likely to experience nutritional problems. However, it is anticipated that the increased knowledge of nutrition among younger adults, and the consumption by some of a healthier diet, will reduce the occurrence of nutritional problems as they get older. The 2010 Global Burden of Disease study suggests disability-adjusted life-years (the number of years someone can expect to live with a disability at the end of their life) are around 13 and 16 years for men and women, respectively, and that this has not changed significantly from 1990 to 2010 (Murray et al., 2013). What has increased is the number of people living to an age when this comes into effect, and therefore, the importance of chronic disability is rising. The proposals of the 'Health of the nation' white paper of adding 'years to life and life to years' are particularly relevant in this group.

In making general statements about the vulnerability of the elderly population, it is important to remember that there is considerable variation between individuals, as at any age. Preparation for retirement and a healthy old age should have begun earlier in life, with the acquisition of good eating habits and a healthy lifestyle, involving both physical and mental stimulation. Several studies confirm that health and good nutrition coexist in the elderly, and when one begins to deteriorate, often so does the other.

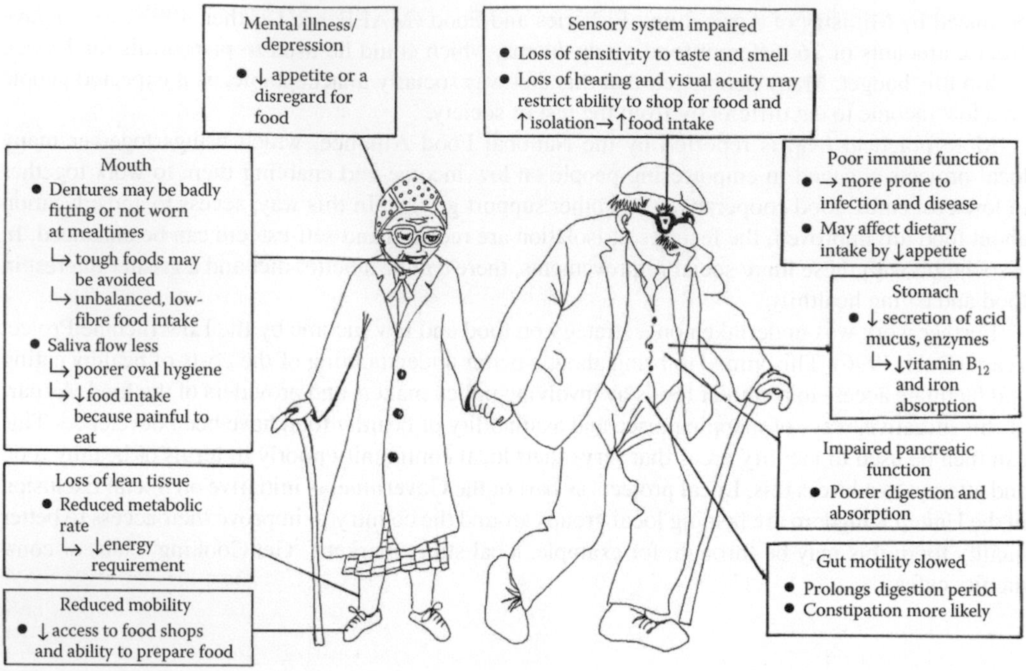

Mental illness/ depression
● ↓ appetite or a disregard for food
Sensory system impaired
● Loss of sensitivity to taste and smell
● Loss of hearing and visual acuity may restrict ability to shop for food and ↑isolation→↑food intake
Mouth
● Dentures may be badly fitting or not worn at mealtimes
↳ tough foods may be avoided
↳ unbalanced, low-fibre food intake
● Saliva flow less
↳ poorer oval hygiene
↳ ↓food intake because painful to eat
Poor immune function
● → more prone to infection and disease
● May affect dietary intake by ↓appetite
Stomach
● ↓ secretion of acid mucus, enzymes
↳ ↓vitamin B12 and iron absorption
Loss of lean tissue
● Reduced metabolic rate
↳ ↓energy requirement
Impaired pancreatic function
● Poorer digestion and absorption
Gut motility slowed
● Prolongs digestion period
● Constipation more likely
Reduced mobility
● ↓ access to food shops and ability to prepare food

FIGURE 8.2 Factors resulting in increased risk in older adults.

Why Are Some Elderly Persons at Risk?

Elderly people are at increasing risk of having marginal nutrition resulting from the ageing process itself and its impact on social factors, as well as an increased incidence of disease. These factors are summarized in Figure 8.2. Ageing is believed to be the result of a gradual dysregulation of cellular function over time. The free-radical theory of ageing is still extensively researched, with mixed outcomes so far. For example, the supplementation with several antioxidants, most notably vitamins E and C has been associated with a reduced risk of age-associated chronic diseases as well as maintenance of cognitive function.

It is helpful to consider how ageing affects some of the body's systems, which may in turn contribute to poor nutritional status.

Sensory System

Changes to the sensory system will have an impact on both the ability to obtain food and its enjoyment. Loss of hearing or visual acuity may restrict shopping as well as social contacts, leading to isolation. Loss of sensitivity to taste and smell, which is a normal feature of ageing, can reduce the attractiveness of food. Elderly people may actually complain that food does not taste 'as it used to'. This is more likely to be a reflection of their failing sense of taste, rather than a change in the food itself. Enhancing flavours with herbs and spices can overcome some of these problems. However, it should also be recognized that a zinc deficiency can contribute to loss of taste acuity.

Gastrointestinal System

The loss of teeth should not have a major impact on food intake, assuming dentures are properly fitted. The adult dental health survey in 2009 reported that 23% of the 65–74 age group have none of their own teeth, down from 42% in 1998. Although more elderly people are keeping their teeth for longer, there is still a substantial proportion of this group dependent on dentures. If the dentures are badly fitting, not checked regularly or even not worn at mealtimes because of discomfort, the dietary intake may suffer. Foods that are coarse, tough or require prolonged chewing may be avoided, possibly resulting in unbalanced intakes. Saliva flow is less in an older person, which may result in poorer oral hygiene and associated infections adding to oral discomfort.

There is a reduced secretion of acid, mucus and enzymes in the stomach in old age, and a decrease in pancreatic function. Gut motility is slowed, and this may prolong the digestion period to compensate for the poorer enzyme secretions, but a more likely result is constipation. An adequate intake of dietary fibre (NSPs) as well as sufficient fluids is, therefore, desirable. The use of laxatives is to be discouraged, especially those based on mineral oils, which can deplete the body of fat-soluble vitamins. The reduced gastric secretion may produce a lower level of intrinsic factor for vitamin B_{12} absorption, as well as reduced solubilisation of iron and its consequent absorption.

Kidney Function

The amount of active renal mass declines with age and is on average 30% less at 80 than at 30 years. Consequently, the kidneys may have a poorer ability to concentrate the urine as well as eliminate waste products more slowly. Therefore, fluid balance will be under less precise control. In addition, thirst mechanisms are less sensitive. Thus, an elderly person runs the risk of dehydration, if fluid intake is not consciously maintained. Sometimes, the added problem of incontinence or even a reluctance to have to get up in the night to empty the bladder may discourage an individual from drinking enough. Consequences of dehydration include confusion, dry lips, sunken eyes, increased body temperature, dizziness and low blood pressure. An intake of eight cups (1.5–2 L) of drink per day is recommended.

Lean Tissue

There is a progressive loss of lean tissue throughout life, although the actual extent depends on lifestyle factors. On average, 40% of the peak tissue mass may be lost by the age of 70 years. This results in reduced basal metabolism and, consequently, a reduced energy requirement. The loss of lean tissue also results in a loss of strength, and this may discourage an elderly person from engaging in even gentle physical activity. Thus, it is clearly important to minimize the loss of lean tissue by maintaining physical activity throughout life. This also maintains appetite and promotes an adequate nutritional intake. There may be little change in total body weight associated with losses of lean tissue because of an increase in the amount of body fat with age. The loss of lean tissue also represents a reduction in both total body water and potassium in the overall composition of the body.

Mobility

The prevalence of disability rises with age, and in 2011/2012, it was estimated that around 45% of adults over the age of 65 years suffer from some form of disability. Arthritis, hypertension, heart disease, hearing and visual impairments, orthopaedic impairments and diabetes are the most frequent problems that pose difficulties for this age group in carrying out daily activities. Loss of muscle mass and increase frailty mean that falls and fractures are more frequent in older age. This is compounded by bone health and osteoporosis, as discussed in the following text.

Bone Health and Osteoporosis

Bone loss is a normal component of ageing, and in many people, the progressive bone loss causes no clinical problems, whereas in others the bone is sufficiently weak to fracture even under a minor impact.

Osteoporosis is thus the loss of bone mass and microarchitecture with age resulting in fragile bones, which are susceptible to fractures. The most vulnerable sites for fracture are the radius at the wrist, the vertebrae of the spine and the neck of the femur in the pelvis. All of these fractures cause pain and disability and represent a significant cause of morbidity and mortality, resulting in immense costs to the health services. According to the International Osteoporosis Foundation,

1 in 3 women and 1 in 5 men over the age of 50 will experience an osteoporotic fracture – or 8.9 millions fractures annually. This more common occurrence in women is because of the accelerated loss of bone at the time of the menopause, linked to the withdrawal of the female hormones. Hip fracture has the highest costs in terms of morbidity and mortality. It nearly always necessitates hospital admission, with an average length of stay of 30 days. Only about one-third of these patients regain their former mobility. Deaths within the first 6 months after a hip fracture are approximately 20%. There are many factors that interact to increase susceptibility to osteoporosis that results in a fracture. Genetic factors play a role, and these interact with environmental and dietary factors. Prevention of fracture depends on attention to long-term diet as well as maintenance of muscle strength and balance in old age to reduce the risk of falling. Supplementation of elderly people with calcium and vitamin D has been effective in reducing fracture risk and is a well-tolerated treatment. The use of drugs that slow bone resorption may also be preventative. It is important for the nutritional well-being of this age group to maintain mobility as long as possible.

Adult bone health is determined by the 'peak bone mass' (PBM) achieved at the end of bone accretion, and the later rate of bone loss. Current evidence suggests that the most desirable method of prevention is to achieve a high PBM by the age of 20–25, so that the critical point for fracture is not reached when bone is lost in later life. Figure 8.3 shows the average rate of bone accretion up to PBM and the decline in bone mass with ageing. Bone mineral is lost from about the age of 35–40, at the rate of 0.3%–0.4% of the bone mass per year. Bone accretion is most efficient and rapid during the teenage years, with 90% of PBM achieved by a mean age of 16.9 years and 95% by 19.8 years. Both endogenous and exogenous factors play a part in determining bone mass. It has been estimated that genetic components may account for 75% of the variation in mass. However, exogenous factors have an important role to play. It is evident that several factors needed for optimal bone formation should be in place at this critical time. The raw materials for bone formation must be supplied in sufficient amounts. This includes principally calcium, but also other minerals and vitamins. Rates of calcium deposition have been reported to peak during puberty, reaching levels up to 1960 mg/day. In comparison, daily turnover in an adult is between 300 and 600 mg/day. It has been proposed that intakes as high as 1300 mg/day may be needed for maximum calcium retention. Calcium sources need to feature at all meals during the day for teenagers to ensure this level of intake. Unfortunately, data about calcium intakes in teenagers show that these are often below the reference levels of 800 mg for females and 1000 mg for males.

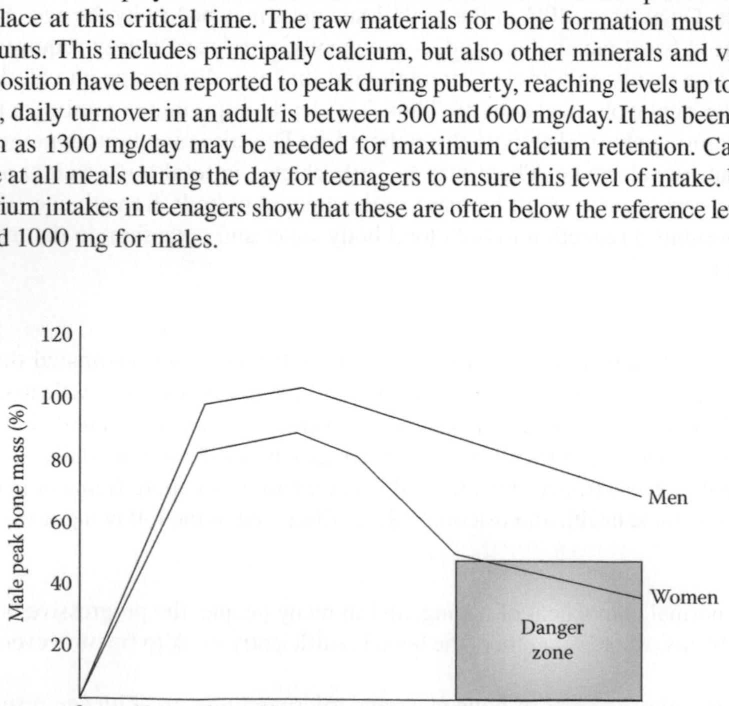

FIGURE 8.3 Changes in bone mass with age. (Reproduced from British Nutrition Foundation, 1991. With permission.)

Other factors that may help in the development of a high PBM in young adults are the following.

- *Exercise:* Weight-bearing exercise in particular promotes bone metabolism. In addition, exercise promotes food intake, ensuring higher intakes of calcium as well as helping to maintain a normal body weight.
- *Body weight:* Excessively thin females (with a BMI below 20) may be amenorrhoeic. The absence of normal menstrual cycles and lack of oestrogen will prevent normal bone accretion. This may be a problem both in girls suffering from eating disorders and those who train excessively and try to reduce their body weight. Body size is generally a good indicator of bone mass. Increased muscular development requires stronger bones to support movement, thus promoting greater bone density. The larger frame of the male is also associated with a greater bone mass than the smaller female.
- *Alcohol and smoking:* These both reduce bone accretion and are, therefore, detrimental to bone health.
- *Vitamin D:* Adequate exposure to sunlight for the synthesis of vitamin D is important, because of the critical need for vitamin D in calcium absorption.
- *Vitamin K:* Osteocalcin and matrix gla-protein are both vitamin K-dependent factors involved in bone mineralization. An adequate intake of this vitamin is, therefore, important to facilitate bone development.
- *Vitamin C:* This is an essential factor for the synthesis of collagen that forms part of the structural framework for bones.
- *Other dietary factors:* Inclusion of phytate, NSP, high protein, sodium or phosphorus intakes in the diet may play a part. They may hinder calcium absorption or promote increased urinary excretion.

Once PBM has been achieved, weight-bearing exercise and a healthy dietary intake are required to maintain it. Any period of immobilization will have a detrimental effect on the bones. All of the factors listed earlier continue to be important for bone health. The bones are a major source of alkaline buffering capacity in the body, consequent on their content of citrate, carbonate and sodium ions. In general, the Western diet is rich in foods that produce acid residues on metabolism, which, therefore, need to be buffered, drawing ions out of the bones. Such foods include protein sources (both animal and plant) and cereals. Osteoclasts are stimulated by a more acidic pH and thus resorb more calcium from the bones. This is excreted in greater amounts in acidic urine, perhaps contributing to osteoporosis.

Some foods, such as milk, produce a relatively neutral residue, whereas fruit and vegetables produce an alkaline residue. Evidence to support the beneficial effects of milk, fruit and vegetables on bone was provided by the Dietary Approaches to Stop Hypertension (DASH) study (Sacks et al., 2001), in which an increase in the number of servings of fruit and vegetables resulted in a substantial reduction in urinary calcium excretion.

Vegetarianism and high-fluoride intakes have been linked to lower incidence of osteoporosis, although the mechanisms are not clear.

At the menopause, the use of hormone replacement therapy for a period of about 5 years is recognized as an important means of preventing bone loss. Women who are overweight at this time of life appear to have a lower risk of the condition; it is believed that naturally occurring oestrogens produced by metabolism in the adipose tissue offer some protection to the bones. Smoking accelerates the normal rate of bone loss after the menopause. Male smokers also have an increased risk of bone loss. Exercise can promote bone health even in the elderly and can minimize the progressive reduction in bone mass. Exercise is also important in helping to maintain mobility and balance which reduces the risk of falls that could result in a fracture. Supplementation with calcium and vitamin D after the menopause has been shown to delay bone loss and reduce the risk of fractures in some studies, but there is still debate about the general application of this measure and the doses needed.

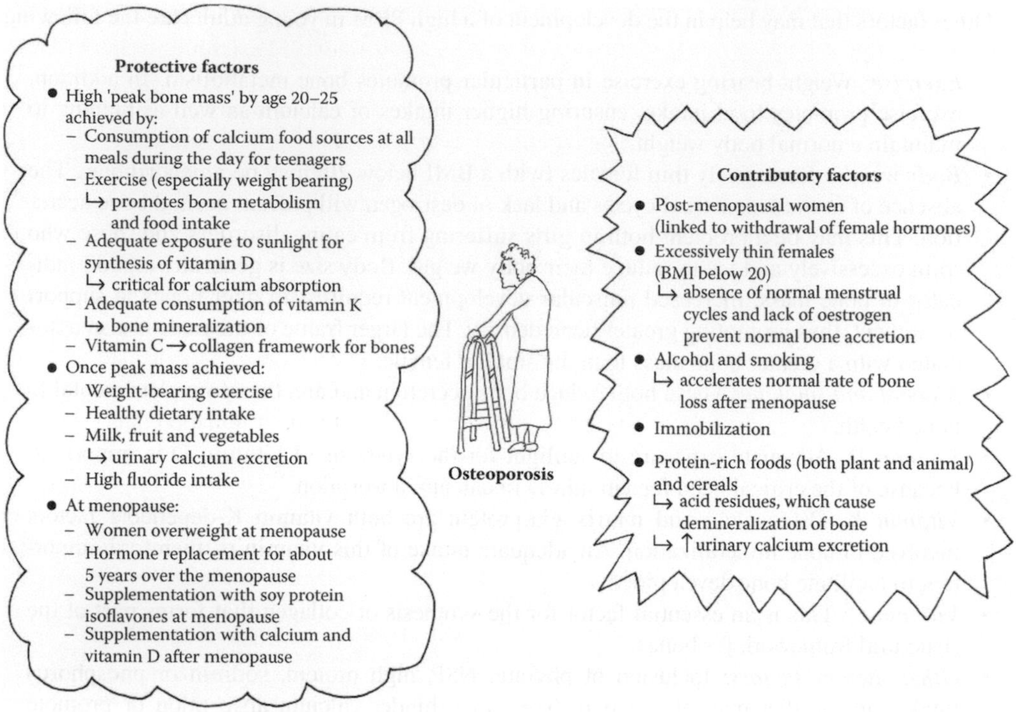

FIGURE 8.4 Factors influencing bone health.

Soy protein and isoflavones have also been shown to reduce the loss of bone density around the time of the menopause, although more research is needed. These factors are summarized in Figure 8.4.

General screening for osteoporosis is not currently a public health recommendation in the United Kingdom, although those at high risk would benefit from early diagnosis. Risk of osteoporosis is greater in people with coeliac disease and inflammatory bowel disease and on prolonged steroid therapy. Individuals with a family history of (maternal) osteoporotic fracture may be at greater risk. Dual x-ray adsorptiometry is the most widely used method, although new techniques include biochemical markers of bone resorption, such as urinary pyridinium crosslink excretion and quantitative ultrasound. Overall, there are many unanswered questions on the subject of osteoporosis. It seems clear, however, that achieving a high PBM in early adulthood is probably one of the best ways of preventing the development of the condition.

Immune System

This becomes less efficient with age, with the result that there is a higher risk of infection. In particular, there are lower levels of T-lymphocytes, as well as an increased production of autoantibodies. A poor nutritional status, in particular, with relation to protein, zinc and vitamin levels can contribute to poor immune function. This may expose the individual to more minor infections, but also increase the risk of more serious problems, such as pneumonia or wound infections. The immune system of very old cohort of adults are increasingly studied to better understand the trajectories of healthy ageing, with immune senescence and inflammaging two core concepts studied.

Brain and Nervous System

Cognitive function may decline with age, and this is another factor that hinders independent living. Dementia is the most common cause of cognitive impairment and is defined as a significant memory impairment and loss of intellectual functions. Increased oxidative stress and an imbalance in antioxidant status may both contribute to the decline in cognitive function. A study in the United States found that plasma levels of vitamin C, E and A, carotenoids and selenium were correlated with memory function among people aged over 60 years (Perkins et al., 1999). The same survey found that 7% of elderly Americans suffered from poor memory. Antioxidants protect the integrity of blood vessels in the brain and, therefore, maintain circulation. This may also be effective in protection against stroke, which is the most common cause of vascular dementia. Other studies have shown that oxidative injury is present in the brains of patients with Alzheimer's disease and may play a role in its development. Various components of brain tissue appear to be affected, including lipids, proteins and DNA, and it is likely that several different antioxidants may be needed to protect the whole range of molecules. In addition, a number of B vitamins especially vitamins B_6, B_{12} and folate may play a role in the development of dementia through their involvement in the metabolism of homocysteine. Elevated levels of homocysteine have been implicated in development of cognitive impairment. Therefore, maintenance of an adequate diet before old age may be protective against some of the degenerative changes in the brain, and in turn facilitate better nutrition in old age.

Other Factors

In addition, an elderly person is more vulnerable to many degenerative diseases, which often develop over a considerable number of years. These may include atherosclerosis, arthritis, lung diseases and cancers. All of these may directly affect dietary intake. Drug treatment for the disease may have an effect on appetite, digestion, absorption, excretion or metabolism of nutrients. Patients suffering from a number of chronic conditions may be taking several drugs, which can interact with one another and produce side-effects, such as nausea, diarrhoea, constipation or confusion.

Factors Affecting Nutritional Status

In addition to ageing and its consequences, social and environmental factors may affect the nutritional status of an elderly person.

Inadequate Intake

There are many contributory factors influencing a poor food intake. These are summarized in Table 8.4.

Physical/Medical Factors

- Reduced mobility, from rheumatism, arthritis or as a consequence of a stroke or lung disease, may be sufficiently severe to make the individual housebound or even bedfast. Similarly, lack of strength may render the opening of food packaging difficult.
- Dentition and the state of the mouth play an important part in the food intake.

TABLE 8.4

Factors Contributing to Poor Food Intake in the Elderly

Physical/Medical Factors	Social Factors	Psychological Factors
Mobility	Money available	Depression
Selection of foods bought	Food storage/preparation facilities	Bereavement
Food preparation	Education/knowledge of nutrition	Mental illness
Dentition	Social isolation	Alcoholism
Appetite		
Disease		
Drugs		
Ability to open food cans and packages		

- Appetite may be reduced by coexisting disease or by its treatment, for example, disease of the gastrointestinal tract, associated with nausea and vomiting or discomfort after eating, will severely limit appetite.
- Various drugs used in the treatment of a variety of illnesses may also have a depressing effect on the appetite.
- Mental illness and depression are also likely to affect food intake; there may be a complete disregard for eating with a loss of time sense so that mealtimes are ignored.

Social Factors

- Availability of money: Many of the retired population live on a fixed income. They may spend in excess of 30% of their income on food – considerably more than the United Kingdom average of 9.5%.
- Lack of education about the importance of nutrition and the existence of out of date beliefs about food may prevent the elderly individual having a healthy diet and may render them vulnerable to cranky notions that they see in the media.
- Social isolation may be the result of retirement, re-housing, death of friends and relatives, breakdown of the nuclear family or illness. Several studies have shown that food intake was less and nutritional status poorer among those living alone and experiencing isolation. In particular, the widowed and men were more acutely affected than the long-term single and women. Conversely, where an effort was made to share food and eat in company, the food intake was better.

Psychological Factors

- Depression, often the result of bereavement, is probably one of the major causes of inadequate food intake in an otherwise healthy person and may persist for many years, resulting in malnutrition.
- Altered mental function, with memory loss and unusual behaviour, may also occur and result in erratic eating. There is an increase in the numbers of people cared for in the community rather than in institutions. It is important that the nutritional needs of these individuals are addressed. Severely demented patients are cared for in nursing homes and hospitals, where food and care are provided. It is still important, however, that nutritional intakes are monitored and checked for adequacy.
- Consumption of large amounts of alcohol may be a coping mechanism for depression or bereavement. The problems associated with excessive drinking may worsen other consequences of ageing.

Less Efficient Digestion and Absorption

Relatively, little is known about the effects of ageing on the functioning of the digestive tract. Reduced secretion of stomach acid and pancreatic enzymes may result in poorer digestion and absorption. There may also be minor malabsorption syndromes, associated with a decrease in the intestinal mucosal surface and broader, shorter villi. Absorption may also be reduced as a result of chronic use of laxatives. The extent of these changes in a normal elderly person is, however, unknown.

Altered Needs

Many bodily functions become less efficient with ageing.

- There is decreased nutrient uptake by cells, so that an apparently adequate intake for a younger person may not produce the same levels in the cells in an elderly person.
- Energy needs decrease with ageing because of the reduction in basal metabolic rate consequent on reduction in lean tissue mass as well as reduced activity. The latter is a cultural phenomenon and attempts are being made to change perceptions about the importance of

physical activity in older people. In many societies, people remain active to a very old age, yet in Britain activity levels are generally very low in this age group. A reasonable level of activity will ensure adequate energy intake to cover the expenditure and incidentally provide sufficient other nutrients in the diet to meet requirements. Conversely, a low activity level may result in such low intakes of energy that basic nutritional requirements cannot be met. Thus, there is an important nutritional argument for maintaining activity levels. In addition, activity will help to promote cardiovascular fitness and maintain muscle mass.
- Protein needs may be higher as protein synthesis, turnover and breakdown all decrease with advancing age. Homeostatic mechanisms regulating protein levels in the body may be less efficient in elderly people. In addition, ill health, trauma and disease states may upset the equilibrium. Insufficient energy intake may also compromise protein balance, as protein will be used to meet energy needs.
- The presence of disease and its treatment by drugs may affect nutritional needs and the effects may be exacerbated by drug interactions. Further problems may arise in a confused patient who fails to take drugs at prescribed times. Up to 60% of drugs taken by the elderly are obtained without prescription. One of the most common is aspirin, which interferes with the absorption of vitamin C and may cause bleeding along the gut. It may thus cause a vitamin C deficiency or anaemia. Laxatives are also frequently obtained without prescription and can deplete the body of potassium, causing depression and affecting cardiac function.

What Is the Nutritional State of Older Adults?

A major survey of diet and nutrition in people aged over 65 was carried out in Britain between 2008/2009 and 2011/2012 as part of the National Diet and Nutrition Survey (NDNS) programme. The study covered free-living individuals as well as a sample living in institutions. Some of the main findings are summarized:

- The foods and drinks consumed by the largest proportion of the sample were tea, coffee and water (100%); cooked vegetables (including vegetable dishes) (93%); fruit (86%); potatoes (80%); savoury sauces, pickles, gravies and condiments (77%); buns, cakes, pastries and fruit pies (69%); white bread (68%); and biscuits (72%). Whole grain breakfast cereals were eaten by 61% of the sample, and the most commonly used type of milk was semi-skimmed milk (used by 72%). Butter was the most popular fat used (45%) followed by reduced fat spread, not polyunsaturated fat (35%). The most commonly consumed meats were ham and bacon (60%), followed by chicken and turkey (52%) and beef and veal dishes (47%). Fish was eaten by 39% of the sample. Sugar was used by 73% of the sample. Alcoholic beverages were consumed by 32% of the sample. In general, these findings suggest a dietary pattern that is quite traditional and shows relatively low uptake of foods such as skimmed milk, low-fat or polyunsaturated spreads or salads. The eating pattern of the older subjects and those living in institutions was even more traditional.
- More people are retaining their teeth into old age than was the case in the past. The state of dentition has an impact on the foods chosen and limits intakes of fruit and uncooked vegetables. The quality of the diet was strongly related to the oral health of the subjects, with higher nutrient intakes in those subjects with some natural teeth. The difference in nutrient intake with dental state was not significant in the group in institutions. However, these subjects had more dental plaque and caries and consumed more sugar than the free-living subjects.

The mean BMI in the over 65 age group is 27.9 for men and 27.8 for women. While there is little difference between the genders with regard to obesity (28% for men compared with 26% for women), more men are overweight (55% compared with 35% for women), and only women fell into the underweight and morbidly obese categories (2% and 4%, respectively).

The following can also be considered:

- Energy intakes were generally below the estimated average requirements (EAR) for this age group. Reported average energy intakes were only 82% of EAR. However, with 83% of men and 66% of women being overweight or obese, it can be assumed that energy intakes are adequate for most people's requirements. In general, energy intakes decreased with age for both men and women.
- Proportions of macronutrients in the diet were in line with intakes across the adult population and did not comply with dietary guidelines. Percentage contributions to energy intakes were protein 17.4%, total fat 35.4%, saturated fatty acids 13.8%, carbohydrate 47.2% and non-milk extrinsic sugars (NMES) 11.5%. Average intakes of NSP were 13.9 g/day, well below the DRV, and there was a positive correlation between NSP intake and number of bowel movements.
- Average intakes for minerals and vitamins exceeded the reference nutrient intake (RNI). However, in both groups, there were numbers of individuals in whom the intakes fell below the LRNI. In general, subjects in institutions were less likely to have such low intakes. This could be linked to the use of milk and fortified foods in the menus. The findings are summarized in Table 8.5.
- Intakes of sodium and chloride were above the RNI in both groups of subjects. In the free-living group, systolic blood pressure levels were positively associated with urinary sodium/potassium ratio.

TABLE 8.5

Percentages of Elderly Subjects (over 65) with Nutrient Intakes from Food Sources below the Lower Reference Nutrient Intake

Nutrient	Men	Women
Vitamins		
Vitamin A	4	2
Thiamin	0	0
Riboflavin	5	4
Niacin equiv.	0	0
Vitamin B_6	0	0
Vitamin B_{12}	0	1
Folate	1	1
Vitamin C	1	1
Minerals		
Iron	2	2
Calcium	3	4
Magnesium	19	13
Potassium	13	14
Zinc	10	5
Selenium	30	42
Iodine	1	2

Source: Bates, B. et al., *National Diet and Nutrition Survey: Results from Years 1–4 (Combined) of the Rolling Programme (2008/2009–2011/12)*, Public Health England, and Food Standards Agency, HMSO, London, UK, 2014.

TABLE 8.6
Prevalence of Suboptimal Biochemical Indices for Nutrients in Elderly Subjects (Over 65 Years)

Nutrient	Men	Women
Vitamins		
Vitamin A (plasma retinol)	0	0
Vitamin D (plasma 25(OH)D)	17	24
Vitamin E (plasma alpha tocopherol)	0	0
Vitamin C (plasma vit. C)	4	4
Vitamin B_{12} (serum B_{12})	6	6
Minerals		
Iron (haemoglobin)	15	12
Iron (haemoglobin and plasma ferritin)	2	3

Source: Bates, B. et al., *National Diet and Nutrition Survey: Results from Years 1–4 (Combined) of the Rolling Programme (2008/2009–2011/12)*, Public Health England, and Food Standards Agency, HMSO, London, UK, 2014.

- In those subjects whose intake of NMES was within the normal population range of 8%–15% of total energy, there was no evidence that micronutrient intakes were compromised. Micronutrient intakes were however marginally lower at NMES intakes outside this range. In general, micronutrient intakes reflected energy intake.
- Biochemical assessments showed suboptimal indices for a number of nutrients, particularly vitamins D, C, and B_{12} and iron. These are summarized in Table 8.6.
- Subjects from the community who were in manual social groups had lower average intakes of nutrients per unit of energy, but higher intakes of sodium.
- Lower intakes of energy were seen in both men and women who lived alone, compared to those who lived with others. In men living alone, this also resulted in lower intakes per unit energy of some nutrients. This was not the case in women.

Overall, these findings demonstrate that the diet of older adults in Britain is largely comparable to that of younger adults. However, dietary choice may be affected by factors such as social class, household composition and dentition, as well as state of health and age. Changes in dietary intake will lead to poorer indices of nutrients and may lead to poorer health. Institutional care can help to maintain nutrient intakes.

What Are the Nutritional Requirements for the Elderly?

There is still a lack of reliable data about the specific nutritional needs of elderly people and research is needed. In part, this is related to the heterogeneity of the group, which makes generalized recommendations difficult. In practice, most recommendations for nutrients are extrapolated from those for younger adults and, as such, may be inappropriate.

The principal guidelines for a healthy diet apply equally in those past retirement age. In many ways, it becomes even more important that nutrient-dense foods are eaten, since a smaller food intake increases the risk of nutrient needs not being met.

It should also be remembered that DRVs (DoH, 1991) and comparable figures published in other countries apply to healthy individuals. It may be that the presence of disease in certain older people may alter their nutritional needs. Therefore, it can be concluded that nutritional requirements are probably similar in the elderly to those in younger adults, but individual differences may occur, owing to particular circumstances. These may include health problems, decreased physical capacity, presence of drug–nutrient interactions, possible depression and economic constraints.

Advice about diet and health to people who have retired could include the following:

- Enjoy food.
- Follow basic healthy eating guidelines relating to fat, fibre, salt and sugar by using the Eatwell Guide.
- Recognize that snacks can be an important part of the diet.
- Make sure that fluid intakes are adequate.
- Keep some food stocks in the house for emergencies.
- Try to spend some time outdoors, especially in the spring and summer.
- If alone, try to arrange to share meals with friends/neighbours.
- Ask for help with shopping when necessary.
- Try to keep active.
- Remember that food provides warmth.

In planning diets for an elderly person, particular attention should be paid to nutrients that have been identified as being 'at risk' in studies of this age group. These include vitamin D, vitamin E, thiamin, pyridoxine, folate, vitamin C and vitamin B_{12}, as well as iron, zinc and calcium. Energy and protein intakes must be adequate to allow protein to be used for wound healing and tissue repair rather than for energy needs. In patients receiving diuretic therapy, potassium or magnesium levels may be at risk. A diet containing a variety of foods fitting in with the Eatwell Guide, and a sufficient intake of fluids and a moderate activity level will ensure good nutritional status in an elderly person.

It should be recognized, however, that probably the most common nutritional disorder among the elderly in Western society is obesity. As at any other age, this is multifactorial in origin and is detrimental to health. If the overweight is very longstanding, the likelihood of successful, significant weight loss in an elderly person is small. Nonetheless, in cases of diabetes, hypertension and arthritis, weight loss is desirable and should be actively encouraged.

The most vulnerable elderly people are those who are ill and frail. It is necessary to identify those at risk as rapidly and efficiently as possible, before they enter a spiral of deficiency and inadequate intake, leading to further deficiency. Ten major risk factors have been identified:

1. Depression/loneliness
2. Fewer than eight protein-containing meals/week
3. Long periods without food
4. Little milk drunk
5. High level of food wastage
6. Disease/disability
7. Low income
8. Inability to shop
9. Sudden weight change
10. Fruit and vegetables rarely in the diet

The presence of several of these factors points to increased nutritional vulnerability and the need for intervention.

Community services available for the elderly in the United Kingdom include the provision of luncheon clubs and day centres for those who are reasonably mobile and 'meals on wheels' and home helps for those elderly who cannot get out or are incapable of fully looking after themselves. They provide social contact as well as helping the nutritional status.

In the United Kingdom, approximately 5% of people aged 65 and over, and 20% of people aged 85 and over live in communal care establishments. These are the most vulnerable subgroup, since it is largely because they are ill, infirm and incapable of caring for themselves that they live in these settings. The diet provided by the institution may be nutritionally incomplete, particularly with respect to vitamins C and D, although other nutrients have also been shown to be low. There may be problems for the individual with appetite, eating and swallowing. Many disease processes may make an adequate nutritional status difficult to achieve or assess. However, every effort should be made to ensure that the elderly in institutions are properly fed. National Care Standards, including nutritional standards, were introduced in 2002 in the United Kingdom and more recently the Food Standards Agency published guidance for caterers on food served to older people in residential care. The aim is to provide guidance on general healthy eating for older people (aged 75 years and above) who do not have specific nutritional requirements due to illness or disease. It is based on the DRV recommendations of the Scientific Advisory Committee on Nutrition (SACN), previously known as the Committee on Medical Aspects of Food and Nutrition Policy, COMA) and the Eatwell Guide. It also takes into account the likely excesses and insufficiencies identified in the NDNS and provides example menus (FSA, 2007).

Finally, it should be remembered that, although some of the retired population do encounter nutritional problems, the great majority live a reasonably healthy life and succeed in caring adequately for themselves. A positive outlook and a continued interest in life are important prerequisites. When interest in food wanes, decline in health follows.

SUMMARY

1. The principles of the balanced diet apply to all adults; however, particular emphasis may be needed on some aspects rather than others in certain situations.
2. Men may have less access to information and be less prepared to make changes for a variety of reasons.
3. For women, nutritional needs differ at stages of the life cycle. Pressures from society, demands of pregnancy and their own health may provide conflicting messages about how to interpret the dietary guidelines.
4. Ethnic minority group members may have a traditional diet that is healthy but, by becoming Westernized, there is a reduction in nutritional quality of the diet.
5. A vegetarian diet can be a positive contributor to health but may lack some nutrients if not well planned.
6. Low income may be a major barrier to consuming a healthy diet.
7. A nutrient-dense diet is important with increasing age, as nutritional needs remain high but appetite decreases. Maintaining physical activity can help to promote appetite.

STUDY QUESTIONS

1. a. Female body can experience several major biological changes during the life cycle. In what ways might these affect the dietary advice given to women?
   b. Do you believe that dietary advice given to men should vary with their life stage?
2. a. What are the main threats to health affecting members of the Asian community in the United Kingdom?
   b. What changes to diet and/or lifestyle could be of benefit?

3. For what reasons does living on a low income pose a threat to eating healthily and/or having a healthy lifestyle?
4. Prepare a leaflet designed for those who care for the elderly, summarizing the main principles of eating healthily at this age.
5. a. Discuss with a group of fellow students, or your tutor, some of the reasons why people generally appear to have difficulty achieving the dietary goals. What sources might you use to check how well goals are being achieved to help you in this discussion?
   b. Identify ways in which meeting goals could be made easier.
   c. Who might need to be involved in (b)?

ACTIVITIES

8.1 Refer back to Chapter 2 to remind yourself of the basics of a healthy diet. What are the DRVs – what are they based on?
- Are they to be used for assessing the diets of individuals?
- Why are healthy eating guidelines produced?
- What is the difference between DRVs and healthy eating guidelines?
- What were the nutritional targets set in the 'Health of the nation' report?
- How are these converted into a practical way of planning diets?
- How does the Eatwell Guide help consumers to achieve a healthy diet?

8.2 Work with a partner on this activity. Imagine you are given the brief of tackling one aspect of health promotion for a group of men (it could be reducing alcohol intake, losing weight, taking more exercise or altering the diet). Make some suggestions about:
- Which group of men you would like to use as your client group?
- Which aspect of health promotion you would like to tackle?
- How you might go about identifying the problem and trying to suggest solutions?

What do you think are going to be the main barriers to success?

8.3 Keep a record of your expenditure on food for a period of 1 week. Use the Eatwell Guide to break down this expenditure into the main food groups.
- Which of the groups costs you the most and which the least?
- Is it possible for you to change your expenditure on food?
- Could you spend less during the following week?

Prepare a plan of which food groups you could buy less and which more during the next week. How easy do you find this exercise?

Make a list of the constraints that operate for you in trying to be more economical in your food expenditure. Which could you overcome, and which are beyond your control?

BIBLIOGRAPHY AND FURTHER READING

Appleby, P.N., Key, T.J., Thorogood, M. et al. 2002. Mortality in British vegetarians. *Public Health Nutrition* 5(1), 29–36.

Bates, B., Lennox, A., Prentice, A. et al. 2014. *National Diet and Nutrition Survey: Results from Years 1–4 (Combined) of the Rolling Programme (2008/2009–2011/12)*. Public Health England, and Food Standards Agency. London, UK: HMSO.

British Nutrition Foundation. 1991. Calcium. Briefing paper no. 24. London, UK: British Nutrition Foundation.

Davies, L. and Knutson, C.K. 1991. Warning signals for malnutrition in the elderly. *Journal of the American Dietetic Association* 91, 1413–1417.

DEFRA. 2001. *National Food Survey 2000: Annual Report on Food Expenditure, Consumption and Nutrient Intakes*. London, UK: The Stationery Office.

DEFRA. 2012. *Family Food Survey 2011*. London, UK: HMSO.

DoH (UK Department of Health). 1991. Dietary reference values for food energy and nutrients for the United Kingdom. Report on health and social subjects no. 41. Report of the Panel on Dietary Reference Values of the Committee on Medical Aspects of Food Policy. London, UK: HMSO.

DoH (UK Department of Health). 1996. Low income, food, nutrition and health: Strategies for improvement. A report by the Low Income Project Team for the Nutrition Task Force. Wetherby, UK: Department of Health.

DoH (UK Department of Health). 2001. *Health Survey for England. The Health of Minority Ethnic Groups.* London, UK: The Stationery Office.

Dowler, E.S., Turner, S. and Dobson, B. 2001. *Poverty Bites; Food Health and Poor Families.* London, UK: Child Poverty Action Group.

Finch, S., Doyle, W. and Lowe, C. 1998. *National Diet and Nutrition Survey: People Aged 65 Years and Older.* Volume 1. Report of the diet and nutrition survey. London, UK: The Stationery Office.

Food Standards Agency. 2002a. *Food Portion Sizes*, 3rd edn. London, UK: The Stationery Office.

Food Standards Agency. 2002b. *McCance & Widdowson's The Composition of Foods*, 6th summary edn. Cambridge, UK: Royal Society of Chemistry.

Food Standards Agency. 2007. *Guidance on Food Served to Older People in Residential Care.* London, UK: TSO.

Gonzalez-Gross, M., Marcos, A. and Pietrzik, K. 2001. Nutrition and cognitive impairment in the elderly. *British Journal of Nutrition* 86, 313–321.

Hamlyn, B., Brooker, S., Oleinikova, K. et al. 2002. *Infant Feeding 2000.* London, UK: The Stationery Office.

Hill, S.E. 1990. *More than Rice and Peas. Guidelines to Improve Food Provision for Black and Ethnic Minorities in Britain.* London, UK: Food Commission.

Key, T.J., Fraser, G.E., Thorogood, M. et al. 1998. Mortality in vegetarians and non-vegetarians: A collaborative analysis of 8300 deaths among 76000 men and women in 5 prospective studies. *Public Health Nutrition* 1, 33–41.

Leather, S. 1992. Less money, less choice: Poverty and diet in the UK today. In National Consumer Council (ed.), *Your Food: Whose Choice?* London, UK: HMSO, pp. 72–94.

Murray, C., Richards, A., Newton, J. et al. 2013. UK health performance: Findings from the Global Burden of Disease Study 2010. *The Lancet* 381(9871), 997–1020.

National Food Alliance. 1994. *Food and Low Income: A Practical Guide for Advisers and Supporters Working with Families and Young People on Low Incomes.* London, UK: National Food Alliance.

NHS Information Centre for Health and Social Care. 2011. *Executive Summary: Adult Dental Health Survey 2009.* London, UK: The Health and Social Care Information Centre, Dental and Eye Care Team.

Office for National Statistics (ONS). 2013a. *2011 Census, Local Characteristics on Ethnicity, Identity and Religion.* London, UK: HMSO.

Office for National Statistics (ONS). 2013b. UK population estimates 2013. Available at: http://ons.gov.uk/ons/rel/pop-estimate/population-estimates-for-uk--england-and-wales--scotland-and-northern-ireland/2013/sty-population-estimates.html.

Papworth Trust. 2013. Disability in the United Kingdom 2013: Facts and figures. Available at: http://www.papworthtrust.org.uk/sites/default/files/Facts%20and%20Figures%202013%20web_0.pdf.

Perkins, A., Hendrie, H.C., Callahan, C.M. et al. 1999. Association of antioxidants with memory in a multiethnic elderly sample using the Third National Health and Nutrition Examination Survey. *American Journal of Epidemiology* 150, 37–44.

Ritz, P. 2001. Factors affecting energy and macronutrient requirements in elderly people. *Public Health Nutrition* 4(2B), 563–568.

Sacks, F. M., Svetkey, L. P., Vollmer, W. M., et al. 2001. Effects on blood pressure of reduced dietary sodium and the Dietary Approaches to Stop Hypertension (DASH) diet. *New England Journal of Medicine*, 344(1), 3–10.

Sellen, D.W., Tedstone, A.E. and Frize, J. 2002. Food insecurity among refugee families in East London: Results of a pilot assessment. *Public Health Nutrition* 5(5), 637–644.

Sharma, S. and Cruickshank, J.K. 2001. Cultural differences in assessing dietary intake and providing relevant dietary information to British African-Caribbean populations. *Journal of Human Nutrition and Dietetics* 14, 449–456.

Van Staveren, W.A., de Groot, L.C., Burema, L. et al. 1995. Energy balance and health in SENECA participants. *Proceedings of the Nutrition Society* 54(3), 617–629.

Women's Budget Group (WBG). 2005. *Women's and Children's Poverty: Making the Links.* London, UK: WBG.

Section III

Digestion, Absorption and Nutrient Metabolism

9 Gut Structures, Functions and Control of Digestion

AIMS

The aims of this chapter are to

- Describe the anatomical structures and physiological requirement for digestion and absorption of nutrients.
- Describe the main functions of the gastrointestinal (GI) tract.
- Describe how digestion and absorption are controlled.

BASIC ANATOMY AND PHYSIOLOGY

The gastrointestinal (GI) tract extends from the mouth to the anus over 7–10 m. It includes the mouth and salivary glands, the oesophagus, the stomach, the small intestine, the pancreas, the liver and the gall bladder, and the colon, rectum and anus (Figure 9.1). Each anatomical site performs a specific set of tasks enabling digestion and/or absorption of food components and nutrients. The wall of the GI tract comprises (inward to outward) the mucosa, either squamous or columnar, the submucosa (connective tissues), the muscularis, smooth muscle fibres responsible for waves of contractions, peristalsis and motility along the GI tract, and the serosa, another layer of connective tissues. Glands, blood vessels and nerves are present in the GI tract wall, enabling lubrication, digestion, sensing, control and transport of nutrients.

The oral cavity (mouth) plays an important role as the first anatomical site involved in the digestion of food, mainly through chewing, grinding the food down to smaller particles (teeth), lubrication (saliva) as well as digestion thanks to digestive enzymes secreted in the saliva (lipase and alpha-amylase). There is, however, very limited absorption taking place at this site. Dental health is an important factor for nutrition, as it will influence the food which can be eaten (in the infant and elderly, in particular).

The food bolus is then swallowed, passing through the pharynx, following the relaxation of the upper oesophageal sphincter and peristalsis (motility) pushing it down the oesophagus. The oesophagus is not a site of digestion or absorption. Upon relaxation of the lower oesophageal sphincter, the food enters the stomach.

The stomach is divided into several regions comprising the fundus, cardia, body, antrum and pylorus. The presence of folds (rugae) enables the stomach pouch to extend following a meal. The stomach plays an important role in the liquefaction of food, the churning and homogenizing of the food to smaller particles, via action of three set of muscles (circular, longitudinal and diagonal) and acid which is secreted by the parietal cells. Gastric acid also enables the killing of most bacteria ingested. The content of the stomach is slowly delivered to the small intestine via the pyloric sphincter, under tight control of gastric emptying rates, which depend on the nutrient composition of the meal, as well as satiety messages relayed to the stomach. The absorption in the stomach is negligible.

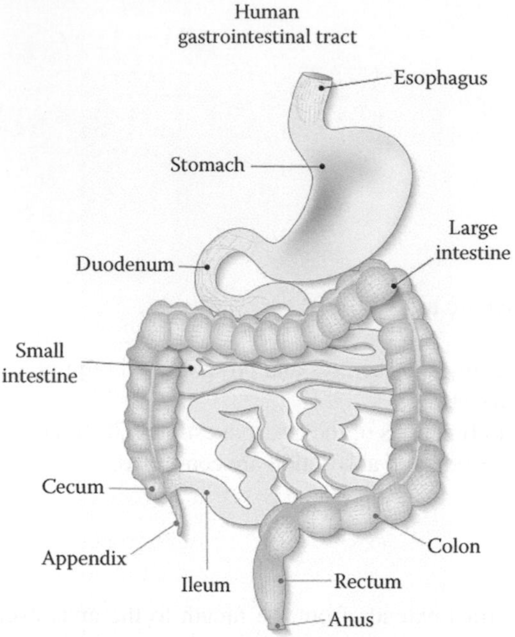

FIGURE 9.1 The gastrointestinal tract.

The small intestine is divided into three sections: the duodenum, the jejunum and the ileum. The bile and pancreatic juice are delivered to the duodenum at a site called the ampulla of Vater, with their release regulated by the sphincter of Oddi.

The bile and pancreatic juice aid digestion of major nutrients. When the food enters the duodenum, the acidic pH is neutralized by the secretion from the pancreas, rich in bicarbonate. The chyme passes through the small intestine to the jejunum, which is the longest section of the small intestine, characterized by its long villi, and finally to the ileum, the final part. The small intestine mucosa is columnar, and lined with villi, finger-like projections which increase the intestinal surface area. The villi themselves are three-dimensional structures covered by mucosal cells, a large majority of which are absorptive: they are covered in microvilli, which contribute even further to the enhanced surface area dedicated to absorption. This anatomical site is responsible for the absorption of most of the main nutrients and electrolytes.

The small intestine connects to the colon via the ileocaecal valve, which prevents reflux from the colon to the small intestine. The small intestine is characterized by the presence of villi and microvilli, which increases its surface area, primarily to enhance nutrient absorption. The colon is composed of the caecum, transverse and distal colon, rectum and anus. Undigested foods (including dietary fibre) are fermented by colonic bacteria, and the products of bacterial metabolism, including the short chain fatty acids, are absorbed at this site. The presence of folds (rugae and pits) allows for mixing of the luminal content to optimize water and electrolyte reabsorption.

FUNCTIONS OF THE GI TRACT

The main functions of the GI tract are digestion, secretion, motility and absorption. The GI tract mucosa is also the first barrier between foods and pathogens present in the lumen and the human body. It is associated with a dense and complex array of immune cells [the gut-associated lymphoid tissue (GALT)] which help maintain a steady state, healthy gut environment.

Digestion

Foods and nutrients are subject to both mechanical and chemical digestion.

Mechanical digestion mechanisms include chewing and grinding in the oral cavity, churning in the stomach, and peristalsis and segmentation in the small and large intestines. Mechanical digestion reduces the size of food particles and enables release of nutrients from the food matrix. It also enhances the action of enzyme by mixing and solubilizing food component, and increasing the surface area.

Chemical digestion is carried out in the presence of GI tract secretions, which contain enzymes and digestive juices which contribute to the hydrolysis of nutrients. While some enzymes are secreted and present in digestive juices (including amylase), others may remain bound to the gut mucosa and act in situ (e.g. sucrase). Chemical digestion ranges from the non-specific (i.e. the action of gastric juice) to the very specific (the enzyme alpha-amylase, present in saliva and pancreatic juice, only cleaves specific bonds in specific carbohydrate molecules). The combination of chemical and mechanical digestion enables the reduction of food particles (to less than 1.2 mm in the stomach), to facilitate their passage through the GI tract (via several sphincters), and cleavage of nutrient molecules into their building block, to facilitate their absorption.

Secretion

The main GI tract secretions include the saliva, the gastric juice, the bile and pancreatic juice, and mucous. Water and electrolytes are also secreted in the large intestine, along with immunoglobulins (sIgA) secreted by the GALT. The approximate daily volumes of the GI tract secretions are summarized in Table 9.1, along with the pH of each secretion. pH is a key attribute of a secretion function.

The salivary glands (submandibular, sublingual and parotid glands) secrete saliva in the oral cavity, at a daily output of approximately 1.5 L. The saliva contains immune factors including sIgA, lysozyme and lactoferrin, bicarbonate (pH regulation), digestive enzymes (salivary lipase and alpha-amylase) and mucous secretions (containing mucin). The saliva carries and enables lubrication of the food bolus, facilitates swallowing, contributes to the first steps of digestion and assists in maintaining a healthy oral environment.

The gastric mucosa contains four main cell types, including cells secreting hydrochloric acid (the parietal cells, also known as oxyntic, which also secrete the intrinsic factor required for vitamin B_{12} absorption), cells secreting the proteolytic enzyme zymogen pepsinogen (chief cells), mucous-producing cells (mucous neck cells) and cells secreting the hormone gastrin (the G cells). The main component of gastric juice is acid (HCl); hence, the pH of stomach contents is typically 1–2, although this is partially buffered following a meal (pH 5). Nonetheless, the acidity of stomach contents creates a harsh environment for the surrounding mucosa, which is thick and covered in

TABLE 9.1

Approximate Daily Volume and pH of the Key Secretions of the Gastrointestinal Tract

	Daily Volume (mL)	pH
Saliva	1000	6.0–7.0
Gastric secretion	1500	1.0–3.5
Pancreatic secretion	1000	8.0–8.3
Bile	1000	7.8
Small intestine	2000	7.5–8.0
Brunner gland secretion	200	7.5–8.9
Large intestine (mucous)	200	7.5–8.0

TABLE 9.2

Composition of the Bile Originating from the Liver and Bile Stored in the Gall Bladder

	Unit	Liver Bile	Gall Bladder Bile
Bile salts	g/L	11	60
Bilirubin	g/L	0.5	3
Cholesterol	g/L	1	3–9
Fatty acids	g/L	1.2	3–12
Lecithin	g/L	0.4	3
Water	g/L	975	920
Ca^{++}	mmol/L	2.5	11.5
Cl^-	mmol/L	100	25
HCO_3^-	mmol/L	29	10
K^+	mmol/L	5	12
Na^+	mmol/L	145	130

protective mucous. The mucous protects against both acid damage and proteolytic damage, carried out by pepsin (converted from the inactive pepsinogen in the presence of acid). The gastric acid denatures most proteins (relaxes their three-dimensional structure) and, therefore, stops the action of salivary amylase and lipase. However, further (gastric) lipase is secreted in the gastric juice, enabling further digestion of fats (triacylglycerides) in a process most efficient in the presence of large quantities of substrate. The enzyme pepsin cleaves protein semi-specifically: there are several forms of pepsin, and their active site can accommodate a range of amino acids. The action of pepsin on proteins yields large oligopeptides and free amino acids (which are important in stimulating further gastrin secretion).

The key exocrine secretion of the liver is the bile, which is essential for the digestion and absorption of fat (bile composition is summarized in Table 9.2). Bile acids are derivatives of cholesterol with glycine or taurine (such as glycocholic acid) and are amphipathic – they have an affinity to both aqueous and lipid environment, which is essential for fat digestion and absorption, as they are used to form micelles. An active reabsorption mechanism is at play: 95% of the bile acids delivered to the duodenum are absorbed back into the blood within the ileum. A secondary function of the file is its excretory function, for

- Toxins (such as steroid hormones, antibiotics) which are reabsorbed in the small intestine and excreted via the kidney.
- Bilirubin, a product of breakdown of haemoglobin. The senescent red blood cell is despatched into its various components. The heme is converted to bilirubin in the Kupffer cell, a specialized macrophage, and later is conjugated to glucuronic acid in the liver prior to excretion via the bile. This conjugated bilirubin reaches the colon, where it is metabolized by colonic bacteria. Derivatives of this reaction give faeces their brown colour.

The pancreas secretes pancreatic juice, rich in bicarbonate (essential for the neutralization of the acid pH of chyme exiting the stomach) and proteases, which are mostly secreted as zymogens (an inactive version of the enzyme, in a bid to spare the host tissue). The major anions are chloride and bicarbonate, and the major cations are potassium and sodium. The proteases secreted by the pancreas acinar cells include trypsin, chymotrypsin, carboxypeptidase and elastase. Trypsinogen is the zymogen version of trypsin, and it is activated by the membrane-bound enterokinase. Non-protease enzymes are released in their active forms (amylase, lipase, ribonuclease and deoxyribonuclease).

TABLE 9.3

Key Functions and (Exocrine) Secretions of the Gastrointestinal Tract Organs

Organ	Key Functions	Secretions
Mouth	Chewing, swallowing (early stage)	Saliva, which lubricates food contents and protects the mucosa
	Digestion (early stages)	*Saliva* – contains alpha-amylase and lipase, which contribute to starch and lipid digestion.
Oesophagus	Swallowing	Mucus for protection of the mucosa against food abrasion and acid reflux from the stomach
Stomach	Mechanical and chemical digestion	HCl (solubilize foods)
		Pepsin (proteolytic activity)
		Mucus (lubricate and protect gastric mucosa from damage)
Pancreas	Secretion of digestive enzymes	Proteolytic enzymes, secreted as zymogen (require activation)
		Other non-proteolytic enzymes for the chemical digestion of fats (lipases), starch (amylase) and nucleic acids (ribonucleases)
	Neutralize the acid pH of the chyme	Bicarbonate
Liver	Neutralize the acid pH of the chyme	Bicarbonate
	Eliminate toxins	Bile, which contains bilirubin, as well as other toxins for excretion
	Contribute towards digestion of fats	Bile, which contains bile acids, amphipathic molecules enabling micelles formation
Gall bladder	Storage of bile	Concentrated bile, which is rehydrated when required
Small intestine	Mixing and movement of luminal content	Mucous and water
	Further digestion	Digestive enzymes, some membrane bound
Colon	Storage and movement of undigested meal components	Mucous (lubrication)

The small intestine secretes mucous (Brunner glands and goblet cells), bicarbonate (Brunner glands), water and electrolytes as well as digestive enzymes (crypt of Lieberkuhn). In the large intestine, the crypt of Lieberkuhn secretes mucous, water and electrolytes.

The key functions of the GI tracts are summarized alongside the relevant secretions at each site in Table 9.3.

Motility

Motility occurs in the GI tract via smooth muscle contractions. The various steps include the following:

- Chewing, which lubricates and subdivides the food in smaller particles.
- Swallowing, a reflex in three phases (oral, pharyngeal and oesophageal).
- Gastric motility, which mixes luminal content, and is responsible for gastric emptying via the pyloric sphincter. It is regulated by the amount, type of nutrients in the stomach and the size of the food particle (if larger than 2 mm, the food particles will be subject to further liquidize until small enough to go through the pyloric sphincter). When lipids reach the ileum, this is sensed by chemoreceptors and sends a signal to the stomach to "slow" gastric emptying. Gastric emptying is also slowed by high blood glucose.

- Intestinal motility, with forward motion (propulsing the chime down the gut lumen through ring of muscle contractions) and segmentation (mixing the chime, via contraction of longitudinal muscle). In the large intestine, anti-peristaltic movement increases absorption. In the fasted state, the intestine does not rest but instead is subject to strong motions that "clears" the lumen of excess bacteria and food remnants. This is known as the migrating motor complex.

The control of both peristalsis and segmentation is via humoral (hormones) and neural networks.

ABSORPTION

Nutrients must cross several barriers before getting absorbed; they include the following:

Digestion and absorption of specific nutrients is covered further in Chapter 10, pp. 193–214.

- The mucous barrier (present to protect mucosa from the contents of the gut lumen).
- The apical membrane of the enterocyte – this is the cell membrane facing the gut lumen; it is a lipid bilayer which presents a challenge to non-lipid soluble nutrients.
- The enterocyte (the actual cell, with structure which may be involved in the metabolism of the nutrient in situ).
- The basal membrane, a second lipid bilayer.

There are two main types of transport: passive (which does not require energy) and active (which requires ATP, often to change the conformation of a transporter).

Passive transporters include the ion channels and the facilitated transporters. Simple diffusion usually occurs 'down a concentration gradient', from a high concentration (in the lumen) to a low concentration (in the enterocyte), for example. Diffusion does not require any carrier and applies to very small molecules, such as glycerol, for example. In comparison, facilitated diffusion requires special carriers embedded in the cell membrane. These form channels which the nutrient can take to go across the cell membrane. The process still requires a concentration gradient, without requirement for energy.

In comparison, active transport requires specialized transporters, to move nutrients often against a concentration gradient.

Primary active transport directly requires ATP in order to move the nutrient. The sodium–potassium pump is involved in primary active transport since it requires ATP (it is a transmembrane ATPase) which moves sodium and potassium against the concentration gradient (sodium towards the outside, potassium towards the inside of the cell) and enables the maintenance of the cell potential (potassium is always at higher concentration inside the cell and low concentration outside, while sodium and chloride extracellular concentrations are high and low inside the cell).

Secondary active transport does not directly involve ATP but instead relies on an electrochemical gradient, which is itself generated via primary active transport (such as glucose transportation by the sodium-dependent glucose transporter SGLT1 alongside sodium, which is 'pumped' in the gut lumen via primary active transport, against a concentration gradient).

CONTROL OF EATING AND DIGESTIVE FUNCTIONS

Signals relating to all of the processes involved in the initiation and cessation of eating are integrated and organized by the brain. These controlling mechanisms have been studied mainly in experimental animals. This is because humans are more complicated, with many cultural and social conventions, which influence food intake and which can override the physiological mechanisms.

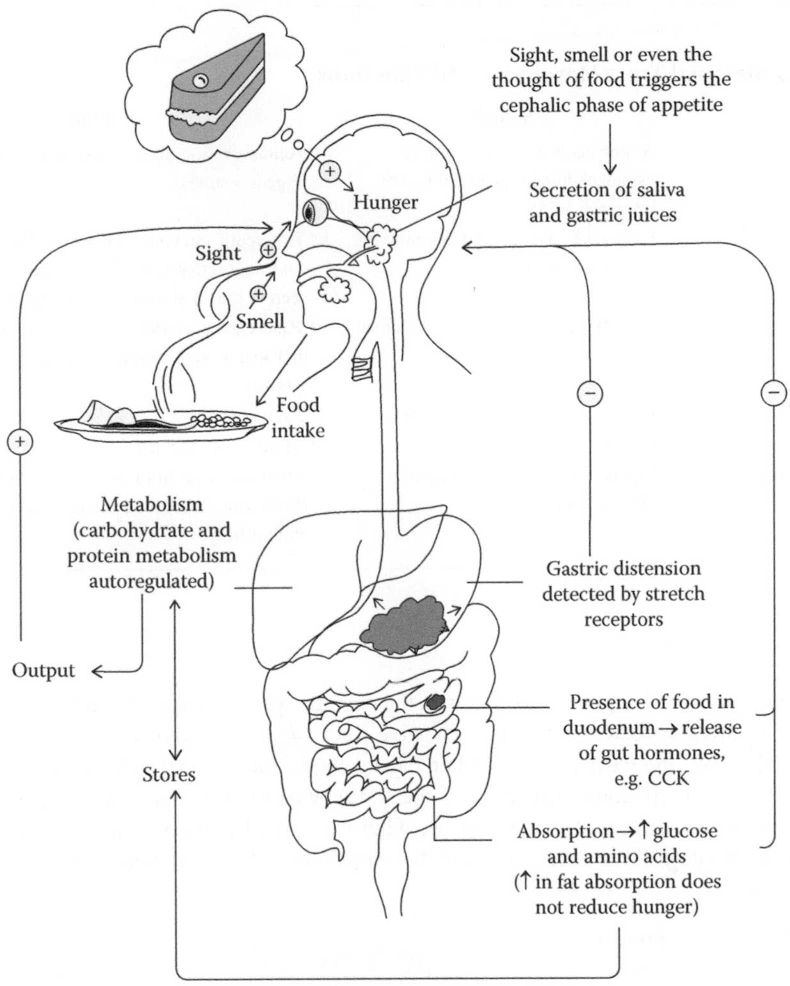

FIGURE 9.2 Physiological factors controlling hunger and food intake.

A schematic diagram of the various components of the control mechanism integrated by the brain is given in Figure 9.2.

In an individual whose weight remains constant, there is evidently a balance between the input of food and its metabolism and energy output. Consideration of the various stages of the process helps to identify where control mechanisms could be operating.

The enteric endocrine system is the collective set of hormones synthesized by the GI tract (see Table 9.4 for a summary). These hormones are crucial to regulate the GI tract function. The enteric nervous system plays a particular role in sensing and closely interacts with the central nervous system via the vagus nerve and sacral nerves (parasympathetic system) and the sympathetic chain. The enteric nervous system includes the following:

- The myenteric plexus (a network of nerves) is embedded in the smooth muscles lining the GI tracts and exerts controls mainly over motility. It will therefore influence peristalsis and segmentation, as well as the rate of gastric emptying.
- The submucous plexus is embedded in the submucosa. Its most important role is to sense the luminal environment, to regulate the blood flow to the GI tract and to control epithelial cell function.

TABLE 9.4

Key Gastrointestinal Tract Hormones and Functions

Hormone	Stimuli	Actions
Gastrin	Amino acids and peptides in the stomach lumen (and inhibited by stomach acid)	↑ Acid secretion, motility (stomach, small and large intestine)
Cholecystokinin	Fatty acids and amino acids entering the small intestine	↑ Pancreatic enzyme secretion, gall bladder contraction to release bile, liver function to secrete bile, ↓ stomach acid secretion and motility
Secretin	Acid pH in the small intestine lumen	↑ Pancreatic secretion of water and bicarbonate, bile secretion, ↓ stomach acid secretion and motility
Ghrelin	Unclear – related to gastric filling	↑ Appetite
Motilin	Unclear – related to fasting	↑ Motility of stomach and small intestine
Gastric inhibitory peptide	Lipids and glucose in the small intestine lumen	↑ Insulin release from beta cells of the pancreas (endocrine function) ↓ stomach acid secretion and motility

Sensory Signals

The sight, smell or even thought of food triggers the cephalic phase of appetite, during which hunger is stimulated by insulin secretion and the digestive tract is/gets prepared for the ingestion of food by secretion of saliva and gastric juices. When eating starts, the food stimulates the senses of taste and touch (via the texture and consistency of the food). Variety in the sensory properties of foods offered in a meal can further stimulate eating, whereas a meal that contains only one item more rapidly leads to satiation. This is the sensation that stops food intake at a meal and is associated with a feeling of fullness.

Pre-Absorptive Information

Ingested food causes gastric distension (the stretching of the stomach). This is detected by stretch receptors, which send signals to the brain. The presence of food and early digestion products in the duodenum causes the release of a large number of gut hormones, some of which have been shown to inhibit food intake. The most extensively studied of these is cholecystokinin (CCK), which has been shown to produce satiety in many animal species, including humans. CCK is stimulated particularly by the presence of protein and fat digestion products in the duodenum. The presence of residual protein in the stomach at the start of a meal has a restraining effect on food intake and particularly on the intake of protein. Peptides, such as PYY and ghrelin, signal to the brain that the stomach is full (Wilding, 2002). Satiety is described as the sensation that delays the next food intake, thus affecting the interval between meals.

Ingestion of liquids, even those containing macronutrients, is less well regulated by these mechanisms than ingestion of solids.

Post-Absorptive Signals

All of the digestion products have been proposed as regulators of food intake. Fluctuations in blood glucose level and, therefore, its availability to the cells of the nervous system and brain were originally believed to be the cornerstone of feeding behaviour regulation. Carbohydrate-rich meals suppress further intake for between 1 and 3 hours after eating. This may be associated with the period during which insulin levels are raised after a meal. This is the glucostatic theory of food intake. However, it cannot satisfactorily explain control of eating in all situations.

A further theory, the lipostatic theory, proposes a relationship between body fat reserves and eating behaviour, such that an increase in stored fat would reduce intake. It is only recently, however, that a mechanism to support this has been identified.

Leptin is a relatively recently discovered (in 1994) protein, released principally from adipose tissue as well as other tissues. Because it is released at one site and acts at a distant site, it fulfils the criteria of a hormone. The amounts produced reflect the size of the fat store in both humans and animals. Leptin release from adipose tissue is also influenced by levels of feeding, such that fasting results in a rapid fall in leptin secretion and levels rise again on refeeding. In addition, exposure to cold inhibits leptin release. Leptin secretion from adipose tissue is also influenced by several other hormones. Its release is stimulated by insulin, glucocorticoids, oestrogens and cytokines (released as part of immune reactions). The major inhibitors of leptin release are adrenaline and noradrenaline, mediated by the sympathetic nervous system. One of the functions of leptin is to act in the hypothalamus, where it causes the release of a number of neuropeptides, including neuropeptide Y. This has a potent action to inhibit food intake in opposition to ghrelin. In obese humans and animals, leptin receptors have a low sensitivity, resulting in poor recognition of the size of fat stores and, therefore, dysregulation of food intake. The primary function of leptin in humans is to respond to undernutrition, when falling levels of leptin remove a relative inhibition to eating, and also inhibit reproductive function.

Amino acid levels also have an effect on feeding behaviour, with shifts in plasma and brain concentrations of particular amino acids causing changes in intake. There is competition between different amino acids for uptake across the blood–brain barrier; consequently, an elevation of one amino acid may inhibit the uptake of others. The importance of some amino acids lies in their role as precursors for brain neurotransmitter substances; these may be the effectors of changes in feeding behaviour.

METABOLISM

The blood levels of metabolites are regulated by the liver and peripheral tissues, which remove them from the circulation and may also have an effect on feeding behaviour.

It is becoming clear that metabolism of the energy-providing nutrients is regulated with different levels of precision. Alcohol, as a potential toxin, must be oxidized completely and removed as quickly as possible. Its metabolic regulation is perfect, and all alcohol is completely metabolized.

The metabolism and function of specific nutrients is covered further in Chapters 11 and 12, pp. 215–252.

The capacity of the body to store carbohydrate and protein is limited, and the blood levels of glucose and amino acids are carefully controlled. Under normal circumstances in overall energy balance, very little carbohydrate is actually converted to fat. If carbohydrate is overfed for a long period, it has to be converted to fat and can of course contribute to obesity. However, the conversion of carbohydrate to fat is very inefficient, with approximately 25% of the potential energy wasted as heat. Metabolism of both glucose and amino acids is thought to 'autoregulate' to match the intake level.

Fat metabolism, however, exhibits no such 'autoregulation', probably because of the large capacity for fat storage in the body. Therefore, fat metabolism does not correlate well with fat intake, and there is no evidence that fat oxidation adjusts when intake increases. Consequently, one can conclude that fat intake plays a smaller role in the control of food intake than do either carbohydrates or proteins. This may provide an explanation for the 'fattening' effects of high-fat diets, which can be consumed without any consequent change to fat oxidation. Also, evidence from feeding studies of diets where fat content has been covertly increased shows that a change in fat levels has no effect on satiety and subsequent food intakes. This means that such diets are easy to consume, leading to 'passive overconsumption', and may be a significant contributory factor in obesity.

There are interesting questions about the short-term partitioning of nutrients between meals. If, as is usual, the absorption of macronutrients after a meal exceeds the rate at which they are oxidized, they must be stored temporarily. For fat that is not an issue: it can be stored at no cost and then used as needed. For carbohydrates (and the carbohydrate generated by dietary proteins), the absorbed glucose can either be stored as glycogen in muscular liver (at lowest) or converted to fat (with energy wastage) for storage prior to utilization.

Although this is no net lipogenesis, there may, for some people, be episodic, cyclical lipogenesis between meals with low efficiency energy wastage.

Integration by the Brain

Early research identified hunger and satiety centres in the hypothalamus; these could be artificially stimulated or destroyed, resulting in starvation or overeating. The function of these centres was thought to be the maintenance of adequate levels of energy-providing nutrients in the blood. The dietary macronutrients (carbohydrates, fats and proteins) were the primary candidates for these regulatory factors. It is now clear that this is an oversimplified picture. The brain receives information from receptors and metabolites about the whole feeding process, from an initial thought about food to the final metabolism of its breakdown products. Changes in plasma concentrations of nutrients resulting from metabolism in the liver and peripheral tissues are also detected. In particular, leptin levels are believed to be important, through their action on neuropeptide Y, causing inhibition of food intake. Low levels of leptin are thought to cause a number of adaptive changes to minimize weight loss, including increased food intake. In addition, levels of serotonin, which promotes feelings of satiety, are influenced by the amounts of tryptophan crossing the blood–brain barrier. By these means, food intake and metabolic processes can be regulated to match the body's needs. This complex integration occurs in the brain, probably by appropriate changes in the levels of neurotransmitters.

In addition, it has been proposed that unconscious reflex pathways are established, particularly during childhood, whereby the body 'learns' the metabolic consequences of particular eating patterns and responds accordingly. If such reflexes are not established, perhaps due to erratic eating behaviour in childhood, then control mechanisms remain less efficient. Much remains to be learned about the complex control of eating.

SUMMARY

1. The main functions of the GI tract are secretion, motility, digestion and absorption.
2. The GI functions are controlled by a complex set of humoral and neural interactions – the neural and humoral system play a key role in sensing the gut lumen content to trigger the relevant physiological reaction.
3. There are three key phases of regulation of GI function: cephalic, gastric and intestinal, which prime the GI tract to receive and handle foods for optimal nutrient absorption.
4. A wide range of secretions are released in the GI tract. Some are very specialized, some not. They include proteolytic and non-proteolytic enzymes, as well as electrolytes, bicarbonate water, bile and hormones.

STUDY QUESTIONS

1. What secretions in the GI tract are essential to the digestion and absorption of the following foods, and why?
   a. A bowl of ice cream
   b. A plate of pasta
   c. A slice of cold meat

2. Describe the different types of motility involved in the digestion of a single meal, from mouth to rectum.
3. Why are the stomach and intestines not digested by the stomach acid and digestive enzymes secreted in the lumen?

ACTIVITY

9.1 Draw the timeline of the journey of your last meal through the gastrointestinal tract.
- Which factors could slow or accelerate transit?
- Would transit change for the same meal in an elderly person?

BIBLIOGRAPHY AND FURTHER READING

Blundell, J.E. and Halford, J.C.G. 1994. Regulation of nutrient supply: The brain and appetite control. *Proceedings of the Nutrition Society* 53, 407–418.

Cotton, J.R., Burley, V.J., Weststrate, J.A. et al. 1994. Dietary fat and appetite: Similarities and differences in the satiating effect of meals supplemented with either fat or carbohydrate. *Journal of Human Nutrition and Dietetics* 7, 11–24.

Cryan, J.F. and Dinan, T.G. 2012. Mind-altering microorganisms: The impact of the gut microbiota on brain and behaviour. *Nature Reviews Neuroscience* 13(10), 701–712.

Laforenza, U. 2012. Water channel proteins in the gastrointestinal tract. *Molecular Aspects of Medicine* 33(5), 642–650.

Lamichhane, A., Kiyono, H. and Kunisawa, J. 2013. Nutritional components regulate the gut immune system and its association with intestinal immune disease development. *Journal of Gastroenterology and Hepatology* 28(S4), 18–24.

Moss, C., Dhillo, W.S., Frost, G. and Hickson, M. 2012. Gastrointestinal hormones: The regulation of appetite and the anorexia of ageing. *Journal of Human Nutrition and Dietetics* 25(1), 3–15.

Wilding, J.P. 2002. Neuropeptides and appetite control. *Diabetic Medicine* 19, 519–527.

10 Digestion and Absorption of Nutrients

AIMS

The aims of this chapter are to

- Describe and discuss how proteins, carbohydrates and fats are digested and absorbed.
- Outline how vitamins, minerals, electrolyte and phytochemicals are absorbed.

DIGESTION AND ABSORPTION OF MACRONUTRIENTS

PROTEINS

Digestion of Proteins

Proteins must be digested in order to release the amino acids of which they are composed so they can enter the body pool and be used for cell growth, repair or protein synthesis. The chemical linkages between amino acids are all peptide bonds, yet a number of different, specific, peptidases are needed to cleave these bonds because of the differing nature of the side chains on the amino acids adjacent to the bonds. Therefore, a single type of peptidase could not split a protein chain into its constituent amino acids in the same way that a single lipase or amylase can split fat into fatty acids or starch to glucose. Several different peptidases act on the proteins of our foods, each attacking bonds adjacent to particular side chains on the amino acids (endopeptidases). Other enzymes attack bonds at the ends of the peptide chain, taking off single amino acids, one after the other (exopeptidases).

In the stomach, hydrolysis of the protein takes place by the action of the hydrochloric acid secreted there. This denatures the protein and allows the peptides to be attacked. In addition, the acid also activates the enzyme pepsinogen (a zymogen) into its active form of pepsin. This enzyme attacks a range of peptide bonds and, therefore, is able to split the long protein chain into a series of shorter, polypeptide chains.

On passing from the stomach, the polypeptides are further digested by enzymes secreted from the pancreas and activated in the duodenum. These include trypsin, chymotrypsin, collagenase, elastase and carboxypeptidase. These enzymes are able to split the chain at specific peptide bonds, as well as remove end amino acids. Final digestion is completed by enzymes located in the brush border of the small intestine, including aminopeptidases and tripeptidases. These split the remaining peptides into single amino acids or pairs of amino acids, which are absorbed and finally hydrolyzed to amino acids in the intestinal mucosal cells.

Absorption of the Products of Protein Digestion

There are a number of specific carrier molecules that transport the products of protein digestion across the intestinal mucosa into the bloodstream. Separate carrier systems have been identified for the basic, neutral and dicarboxylic amino acids, and there is competition between the individual amino acids for the carrier. In addition, there are carriers for small peptides. The process is summarized in Figure 10.1.

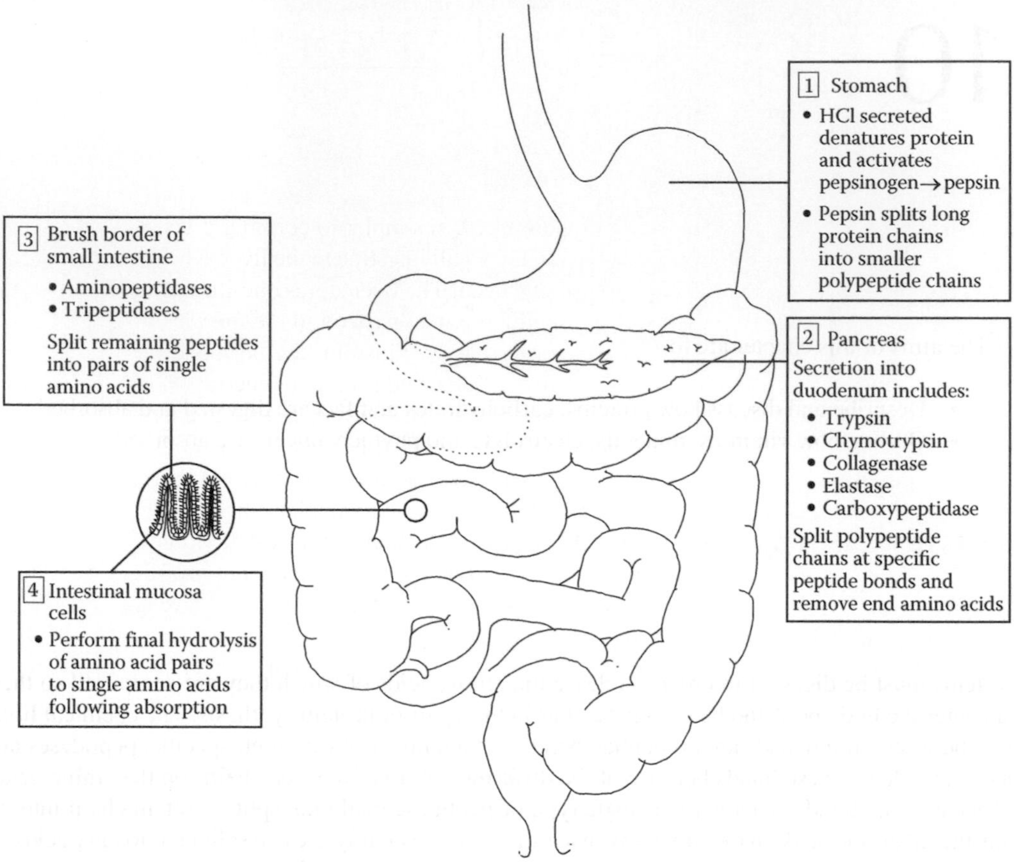

FIGURE 10.1 Digestion of proteins.

It is worth pointing out that ingestion of supplements, which may contain several amino acids of the same chemical type, will result in competition for absorption. Thus, the amino acid present in greatest concentration will be absorbed preferentially, but the absorption of the others may be impaired. This may result in unbalanced amino acid absorption. Further, absorption of amino acids and peptides from natural, protein-containing foods occurs more quickly and efficiently than that from an equivalent mixture of free amino acids.

In general, protein digestion is extremely efficient, and up to 99% of ingested protein is absorbed as amino acids. In very young infants, however, whole antibody proteins secreted in maternal milk are absorbed from the gut, in a process known as pinocytosis. This absorption of whole immunoglobulins confers protection against infections, particularly during the first days of life, when colostrum is secreted by the mother's mammary glands. Colostrum is rich in immunoglobulins, which confer immunity to the child. It is also possible that proteins from cows' milk or wheat flour may, if given at this time of life, set up antibody production in the infant. This occasionally causes subsequent 'food intolerance' or 'food allergy'.

Most of the amino acids pass into the bloodstream from the intestines and travel to the liver in the hepatic portal vein. Some pass into the liver cells, others go into the general circulation. The liver is thought to monitor the absorbed amino acids and to adjust their rate of metabolism according to the needs of the body. A small number of amino acids remain in the cells of the intestinal mucosa, for synthesis of protein and other nitrogen-containing compounds. Glutamine is thought to promote cell division in the gastrointestinal mucosa and is used by the intestinal cells as a primary source of energy. It is particularly important in times of trauma to maintain gut integrity.

FATS

Digestion of Fats

Fat digestion is uncomplicated. One type of lipase (a fat-splitting enzyme) can split the link between glycerol and any fatty acid. A small amount of lipase, called lingual lipase, is produced in the mouth. This is probably of greatest importance in infants, as it is particularly active in the breakdown of milk fats. Milk digestion is also facilitated in breast-fed infants by the presence of a lipase in the milk itself.

The main process of fat digestion starts in the stomach, where the churning action breaks it down into a coarse emulsion. The emptying of fats from the stomach into the duodenum causes the release of several hormones called enterogastrones, which inhibit further stomach emptying. In this way, the release of fats for digestion in the intestine is slowed down, and a fat-rich meal stays in the stomach for longer, creating satiation. The main lipase is that from the pancreas, which splits fats in the jejunum into a mixture of fatty acids and glycerol, together with some monoglycerides.

However, fats are not soluble in the watery mixture of the small intestine and would normally aggregate into large droplets. These need to be split up into tiny droplets by emulsifying agents, which are both fat and water soluble. In the gut, this is carried out by the bile acids, which emulsify the fat and enable lipase to act. Bile acids are made in the liver from cholesterol, concentrated and stored in the bile ducts and gall bladder, and then secreted into the duodenum when the food enters from the stomach. Partly split fats and free fatty acids aid the bile salts in emulsifying the neutral fats. The bile acids that have been used in fat digestion are reabsorbed in the ileum, and pass in the blood to the liver, where they act as a stimulus for their resecretion into the bile. They, thus, undergo what is termed an enterohepatic circulation. Interference with this circulation will alter the level of bile acids and their precursor – cholesterol. The bile salts that return to the liver act as an inhibitor to further synthesis from cholesterol. If fewer return to the liver, then more synthesis of bile salts from cholesterol can occur, thus lowering the level of cholesterol in the blood.

Phospholipids are also broken down by removal of their fatty acids, by the action of the enzyme phospholipase. Cholesterol esters in the diet are hydrolyzed by esterases to remove the fatty acid and so release cholesterol for absorption.

Absorption of the Products of Fat Digestion

Once the fats have been split into their constituents, they merge into tiny spherical complexes, known as micelles, which diffuse easily into the intestinal cell (or enterocyte). Once inside the enterocyte, the fat digestion products are reassembled into triglycerides, although not the same as the original ones in the diet. These are then coated with phospholipids and apolipoproteins to produce chylomicrons. This 'envelope' provides a means of stabilizing lipids in an aqueous environment, such as the circulation. In addition to the triglycerides, the chylomicrons also contain other fat digestion products, such as cholesterol and fat-soluble vitamins. Too large to diffuse into the blood capillaries of the gut wall, the chylomicrons pass into the lacteals of the lymphatic system, and eventually enter the bloodstream at the thoracic duct in the neck, where the lymphatic system drains into the blood. Fat digestion is summarized in Figure 10.2.

Some smaller fatty acids, containing 4–10 carbon atoms, are able to pass into the blood capillaries in the gut and so are absorbed directly into the hepatic portal vein, where they attach to plasma albumin and are transported to the liver. These types of fatty acids have the advantage of being a little more water soluble; they are, therefore, not so dependent on emulsification by the bile for their digestion. In some patients, where there is a fat digestion problem owing to a lack of bile, introducing short-chain

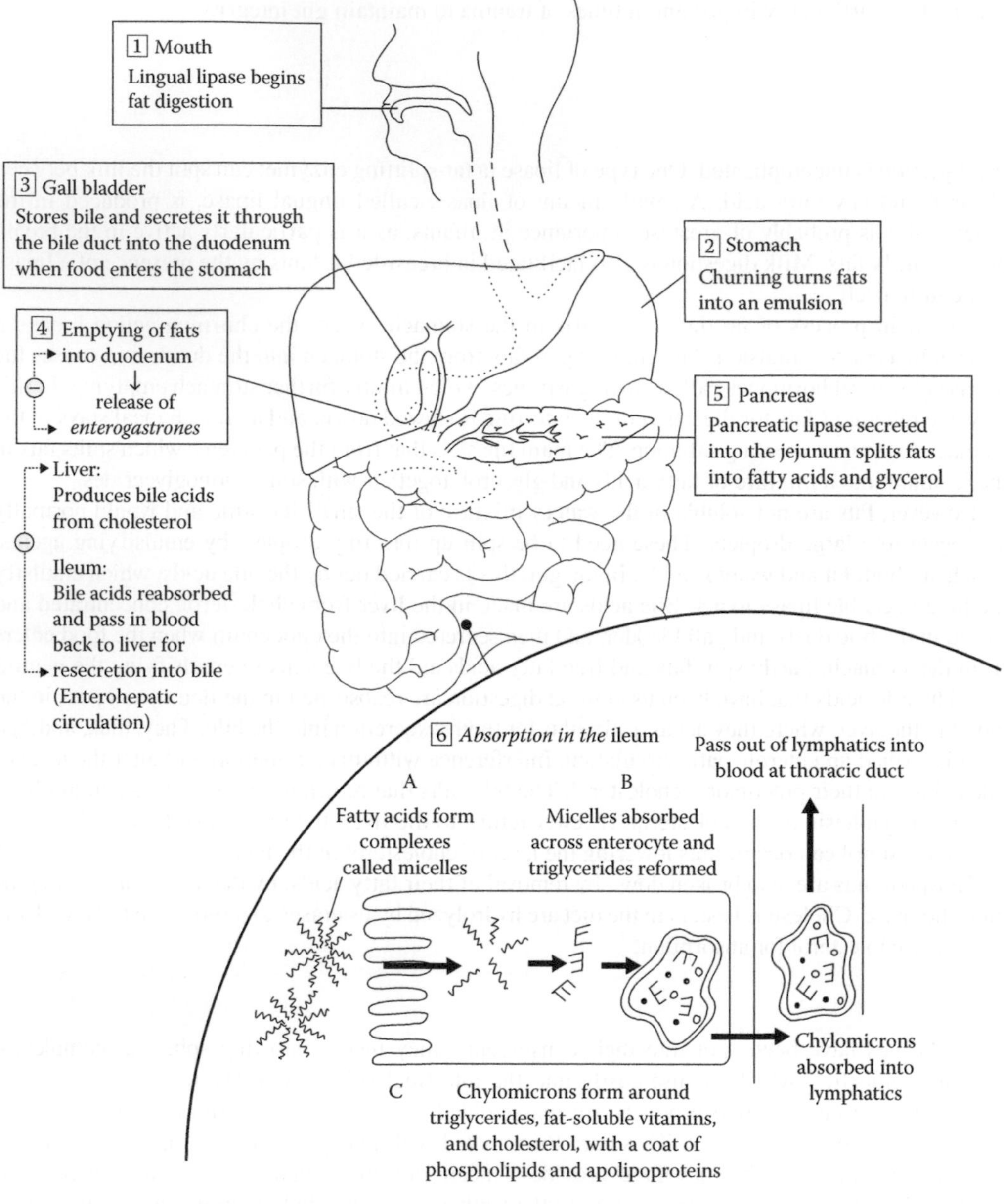

FIGURE 10.2 Digestion and absorption of fats.

fats into the diet may be a temporary way of adding dietary fat, which would otherwise not be tolerated. The two ways in which fat digestion products enter the body are summarized in Table 10.1.

Fat digestion is normally very efficient, with 95% of ingested fat being absorbed. However, in some instances, digestion and/or absorption will be defective. If fat is undigested or unabsorbed, it will appear in the faeces. This produces a characteristic faecal appearance, with waxy stools, which tend to be foul smelling and, because they float, are difficult to flush away. This condition is called steatorrhoea. Unabsorbed fats will remove other fat-soluble components from the body, in particular, the fat-soluble vitamins, and chronic steatorrhoea may be associated with a specific vitamin deficiency.

TABLE 10.1
Summary of Fate of Fat Digestion Products

Short-chain fatty acids Medium-chain fatty acids Glycerol	Absorbed directly into the hepatic portal vein
Triglycerides (reconstituted from long-chain fatty acids and monoglycerides) Cholesterol Phospholipids Fat-soluble vitamins	Made into chylomicrons; absorbed into lacteals, carried via the lymphatic system into the blood

Causes of steatorrhoea may include the following:

- Failure to produce lipase as a result of pancreatic insufficiency or problems with the production or secretion of bile
- Gallstones, which can block the secretion of bile into the gut
- Inefficient absorption of fat due to defects in the surface of the small intestine, which may be flattened or inflamed
- Ingestion of mineral oils, such as liquid paraffin, as a laxative

Carbohydrates

The purpose of digestion is to make all dietary carbohydrates into small units (mostly of glucose), which can be absorbed across the mucosal wall of the digestive tract and used by the cells in metabolism. Digestion is brought about by both physical and chemical means. Biting and chewing in the mouth, and churning by the stomach, ensure that pieces of food are broken down into a semi-liquid chyme, so that enzyme action can occur.

Digestion of Carbohydrates

Sugars

The diet contains simple sugars not only of different sizes but also in different physical states. Some are consumed in their natural state, contained within the cells of the food plant. These include all the simple sugars found in fruits and vegetables. We eat them with the cell walls and other plant material with which they are associated. Eating them often requires a certain amount of effort in biting, chewing and digestion. These sugars have been termed 'intrinsic' and are generally considered to have little or no undesirable effects on our health.

In addition, the diet also contains sugars which are free, that is, extracellular or not contained within cells. These come from milk, where the lactose is free in solution, from honey, which contains free fructose and glucose, and from the large number of foods that contain added sugars. These sugars are 'unpackaged' and readily available both for bacterial action in the mouth and for rapid absorption and metabolism. The name 'extrinsic sugars' has been given to this group. Those present in milk are not considered to cause detrimental effects to health. However, the 'non-milk extrinsic sugars', which include sucrose, corn syrup and synthetic fructose in recipes and manufactured foods and drinks, have potentially damaging effects for health.

Whether sugars are intrinsic or extrinsic will determine how much cellular breakdown has to take place before they are released. Apart from this, the simple monosaccharides require no digestion before being absorbed. Disaccharides, such as lactose and sucrose, require to be split by their specific enzymes, lactase and sucrase, into monosaccharides before they can be absorbed. These enzymes are to be found in the brush border of the mucosal cells of the duodenum and upper jejunum. Studies of the process of digestion show that the digestion of sucrose and lactose is virtually complete in the small intestine.

However, some individuals lack the enzyme lactase and are thus unable to complete the digestion of this sugar. This may arise for two different reasons. The most common is 'primary lactase non-persistence', which is a normal disappearance of lactase from the mucosal cells after infancy. This occurs in many ethnic groups around the world whose customs do not include the use of milk beyond infancy. Caucasians are one of the few groups who continue to produce lactase throughout life; even so, the ability to digest lactose declines with age. In the United Kingdom, lactase non-persistence has been recorded in 55% of ethnic Indians and 82% of ethnic Afro-Caribbeans. If milk is consumed by someone with lactase non-persistence, the lactose remains in the intestines, attracting water and causing a feeling of distension, abdominal discomfort and diarrhoea. These signs result from fermentation of the lactose by intestinal bacteria, producing large amounts of gas and acid. Milk derivatives such as yogurt, in which the lactose has been fermented, do not cause these problems. In addition, small amounts of milk may be tolerated if introduced gradually. The use of probiotic preparations that contain milk-fermenting bacteria can also facilitate tolerance to milk.

Lactase deficiency may also arise as a secondary condition, resulting from damage to the intestinal mucosa by some other disease process, such as malnutrition, HIV infection and parasitic infestations. Deficiencies of sucrase may also occur, but these are rare.

Starch

In the mouth, salivary amylase (ptyalin) acts on cooked starch granules. It is not clear how far this digestion progresses and whether there are differences between people who eat their food very quickly and those who chew each mouthful thoroughly. It is also possible that this early breakdown of starch in the mouth may make a significant difference to overall digestibility. The enzyme travels down to the stomach, mixed with chewed food. It is now thought likely that, protected by starch and some of its degradation products, salivary amylase continues to be active until the chyme reaches the small intestine.

Here, pancreatic amylase continues the breakdown of starch, acting on 1–4 linkages in both raw and cooked starch. Amylose in starch is degraded to mainly maltose and maltotriose, with small amounts of glucose produced; amylopectins are broken to oligosaccharides; by the time, the chyme reaches the distal part of the duodenum.

Digestion is completed by oligosaccharidases bound to the surface of the brush border cells; these are substrate specific and liberate glucose as the end product of the digestion process.

Some starch is resistant in varying degrees to digestion by amylases. A classification of the digestibility of starch has been proposed (see Table 10.2). It must be remembered, however, that digestibility is variable and probably dependent on the composition of the meal.

Also, the nature of starch granules varies from one food to another, some being more susceptible to the action of amylase than others. Most readily digested are the starches of most cereals, sweet potato and tapioca. Starch from raw potato and unripe banana is resistant, but cooking of the potato and ripening of the banana increases digestibility. Starch in peas, beans and yams is most resistant to digestion by amylase. Dietary oligosaccharides found in onions, garlic and leeks, artichokes, beans, peas and some cereals are not broken down or absorbed in the small intestine, and pass further along the bowel together with resistant starch (although they are not starch molecules).

Resistant starches that escape digestion in the small intestine become available for fermentation in the colon by the bacterial flora. The result of this process is an increase in faecal mass owing to the multiplication of the bacteria, production of short-chain fatty acids (acetic, propionic and butyric acids) and a decrease in colonic pH. In addition, CO_2, H_2 and some CH_4 are produced. These contribute to a sensation of bloating and flatulence. It has been estimated that between 20% and 30% of the potential energy contained in the resistant starch becomes available to the body in the form of short-chain fatty acids absorbed from the colon. Figure 10.3 summarizes the digestion of carbohydrates.

TABLE 10.2
Classification of Starch According to Digestibility

Type of Starch	Example of Occurrence	Probable Digestion in the Small Intestine
Rapidly digestible	Freshly cooked starchy food	Rapid
Slowly digestible	Mostly raw cereals	Slow but complete
Resistant		
Physically inaccessible	Partly milled grains and seeds	Resistant
Resistant granules	Raw banana and potato	Resistant
Retrograded	Cooled, cooked potato, bread and cornflakes, savoury snack foods	Resistant

Source: Reproduced from Englyst, H.N. and Kingman, S.M., Dietary fibre and resistant starch: A nutritional classification of plant polysaccharides, in Kritchevsky, D., Bonfield, C. and Anderson, J.W., eds., *Dietary Fibre*, Plenum Press Publishing Corporation, New York, 1990. With permission.

Non-Starch Polysaccharides

In the mouth, high-fibre foods generally require more chewing. This slows down the process of eating and stimulates an increased flow of saliva. The saliva contributes to the volume of the swallowed food bolus. Once in the stomach, the fibre-rich food tends to absorb water and the soluble component starts to become viscous. Both of these changes delay stomach emptying. In the small intestine, the soluble fibre travels slowly because of increased viscosity; this prolongs the period of time available for the absorption of nutrients. The fibre may also bind some divalent ions in the small intestine, making them unavailable for absorption at this point.

Once in the large intestine, the soluble fibre becomes a food source for the growth and multiplication of the bacterial flora. The consequences of this are exactly the same as described above for resistant starch. Thus, both resistant starch and soluble non-starch polysaccharides (NSPs) contribute to increasing bulk in the large intestine and the production of fatty acids and gases.

Insoluble fibre, which has reached the colon largely unchanged, swells by water holding and adds further to the volume of the colonic contents. The faeces, therefore, are both bulkier and softer because of increased water content.

Absorption of Carbohydrates

After digestion, the resulting monosaccharides are absorbed from the gut lumen across the mucosa into the blood by one of three mechanisms:

1. Simple diffusion
2. Facilitated diffusion
3. Active transport

The latter two processes allow faster absorption of the simple sugars than could be achieved by simple diffusion alone. This becomes particularly important in the later stages of absorption, as concentrations in the gut lumen fall. Active transport involves the breakdown of ATP and the presence of sodium (Na^+). Glucose and galactose are taken up by the same (secondary) active transporter, the sodium-linked glucose transporter SGLT1. Other monosaccharides are carried by passive transporters. Passive transporters have limited capacity, so not all monosaccharides, such as fructose, may be transported, with some remaining in the gut lumen (and accumulating in the colon where they may induce osmotic diarrhoea). Meanwhile, SGLT1 has low transport capacity, so some of the glucose is transported by GLUT2, a passive carrier, which is mobilized to the cell membrane in response to high glucose load that cannot be effectively removed from the lumen by SGLT1 only.

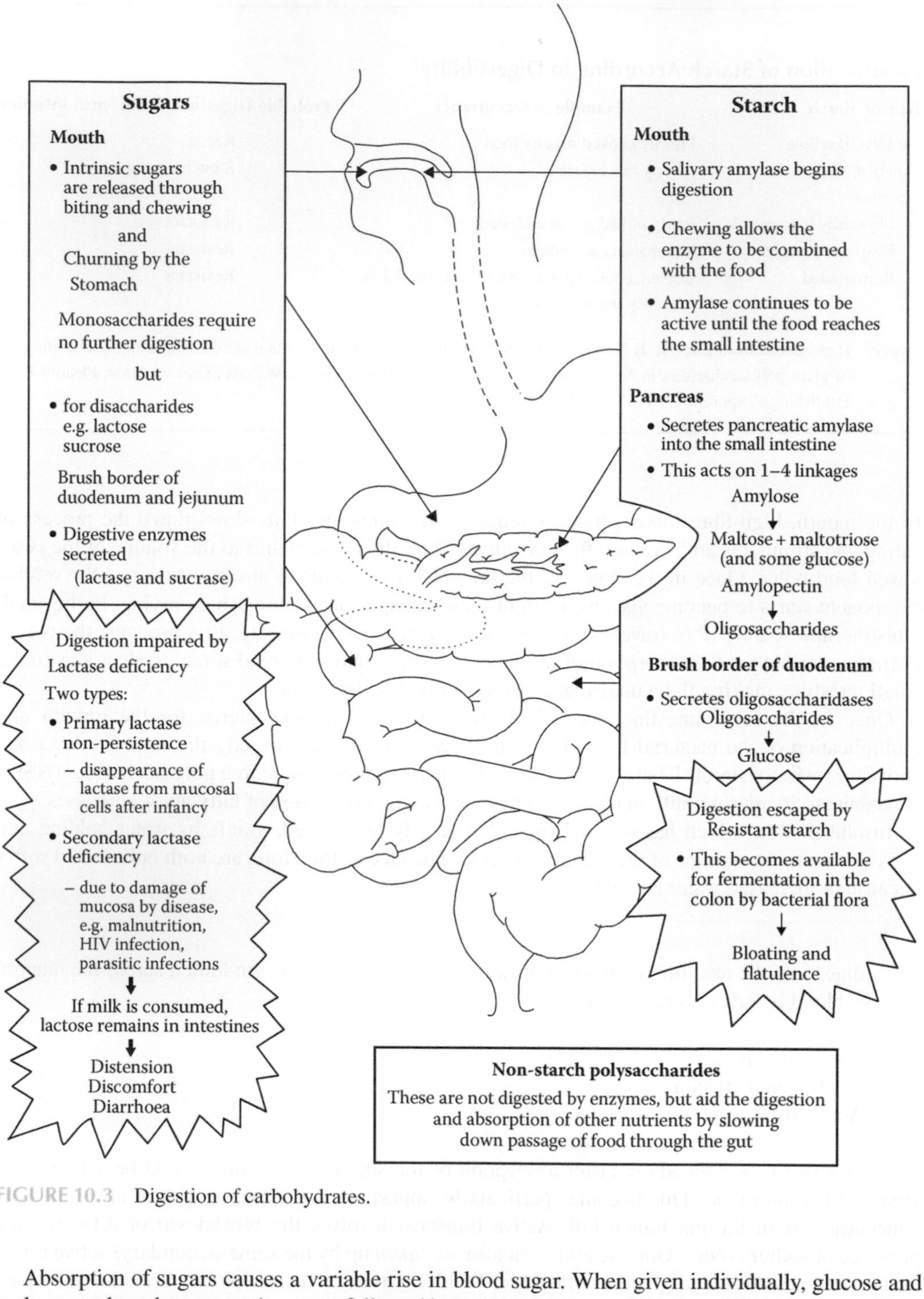
Sugars
Mouth
• Intrinsic sugars are released through biting and chewing
and
Churning by the Stomach
Monosaccharides require no further digestion
but
• for disaccharides e.g. lactose sucrose
Brush border of duodenum and jejunum
• Digestive enzymes secreted (lactase and sucrase)
Digestion impaired by Lactase deficiency
Two types:
• Primary lactase non-persistence
– disappearance of lactase from mucosal cells after infancy
• Secondary lactase deficiency
– due to damage of mucosa by disease, e.g. malnutrition, HIV infection, parasitic infections
If milk is consumed, lactose remains in intestines
Distension
Discomfort
Diarrhoea
Starch
Mouth
• Salivary amylase begins digestion
• Chewing allows the enzyme to be combined with the food
• Amylase continues to be active until the food reaches the small intestine
Pancreas
• Secretes pancreatic amylase into the small intestine
• This acts on 1–4 linkages
Amylose
Maltose + maltotriose (and some glucose)
Amylopectin
Oligosaccharides
Brush border of duodenum
• Secretes oligosaccharidases
Oligosaccharides
Glucose
Digestion escaped by Resistant starch
• This becomes available for fermentation in the colon by bacterial flora
Bloating and flatulence
Non-starch polysaccharides
These are not digested by enzymes, but aid the digestion and absorption of other nutrients by slowing down passage of food through the gut

FIGURE 10.3 Digestion of carbohydrates.

Absorption of sugars causes a variable rise in blood sugar. When given individually, glucose and maltose produce the greatest increase, followed by sucrose, lactose, galactose and fructose. The effects are not necessarily the same when these sugars are consumed as part of a meal. The level of glucose in the blood rises to a maximum in about 30 minutes and falls to fasting levels after 90–180 minutes. The rate of rise to the maximum and the rate of fall vary with the nature of the meal and are related to the digestion rates occurring in the small intestine and the speed of release of glucose.

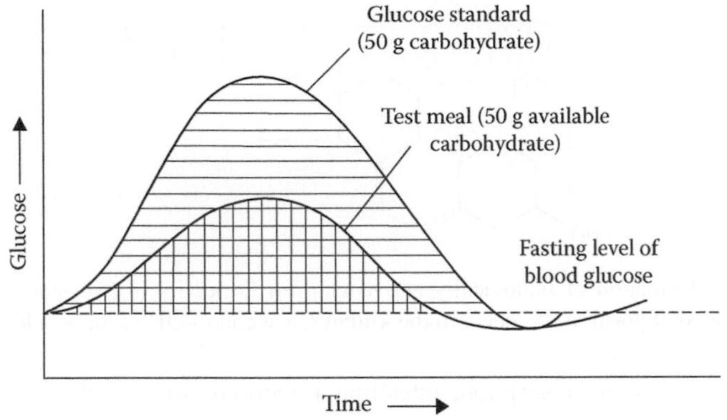

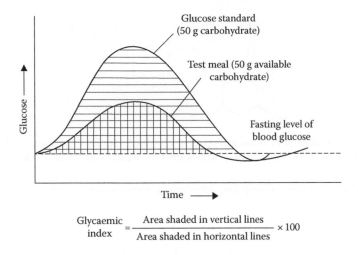

$$\text{Glycaemic index} = \frac{\text{Area shaded in vertical lines}}{\text{Area shaded in horizontal lines}} \times 100$$

FIGURE 10.4 Rise in blood glucose after eating, and the calculation of glycaemic index.

It is possible to measure the relative effects of different carbohydrate foods on the blood sugar level. The rise in blood glucose following ingestion of a portion of a test food containing 50 g of available carbohydrate is compared with the effect on blood glucose of a 50 g available carbohydrate portion of a standard, such as glucose or white bread. Comparison of the areas under the two glucose curves obtained produces a 'glycaemic index' (Figure 10.4).

The glycaemic index of a large number of foods has been determined. Glycaemic responses vary between individuals, but the ranking of response to different foods can be predicted from the standard results. Diets with a low glycaemic index have been shown to have various health benefits, including reduction of blood lipids and improved blood glucose control in diabetic subjects. They also enhance satiety and increase athletic endurance. More research is needed to increase the evidence base on relationships between glycaemic index and health, in specific conditions and for the general population. There are moves to introduce labelling of products with their glycaemic index, although there needs to be public education about the significance of this measure before any such initiative.

By definition, we would not expect the NSPs to be absorbed. However, these compounds do not travel through the digestive tract completely unchanged. Physical breakdown and bacterial fermentation are the main changes that alter both the soluble and insoluble fibres as they pass through the digestive tract. Some of the fatty acids released as a result of fermentation are absorbed and provide usable energy. They might also play an important role in cell signaling.

The impact of the metabolic product of NSP on gut health is covered in more detail in Chapter 11, p. 231.

DIGESTION AND ABSORPTION OF VITAMINS

Vitamin A

Both forms of vitamin A in the diet have to be released from complexes for absorption across the intestinal membrane, but the retinol is quickly re-esterified once inside the mucosal cell, and then incorporated into chylomicrons for transport. Carotenes are broken down to yield retinol. Although this conversion should theoretically yield two molecules of retinol from each beta-carotene, only one is thought to be produced normally. Some carotenoids remain unconverted and are absorbed as such. These include some hydroxy-carotenoids, such as lutein, alpha- and beta-cryptoxanthin. Absorption of retinol from pre-formed sources has an overall efficiency of 70%–90% if fat intakes are adequate, but only 15%–50% of carotenes are absorbed.

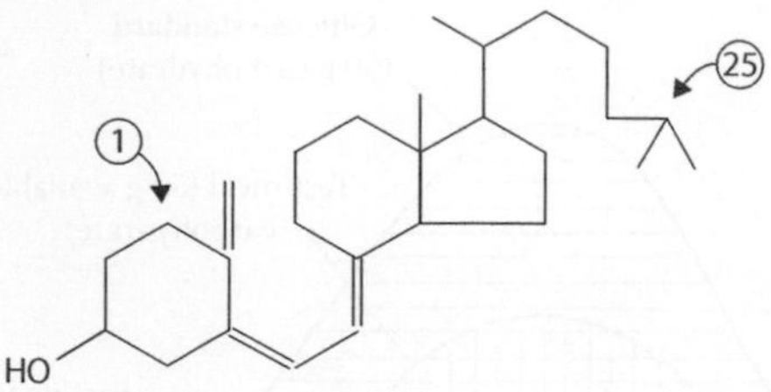

FIGURE 10.5 The formation of biologically active vitamin D occurs in two stages. First, in the liver, an —OH group is added at position 25. Then, in the kidneys, a second –OH group is added at position 1.

Protein deficiency, fat malabsorption, intestinal infections and diarrhoea will all reduce the efficiency of absorption.

Vitamin D

About 50% of the dietary vitamin is found in the chylomicrons leaving the digestive tract in the lymph; most of this vitamin finds its way to the liver with the remnants of the chylomicrons. Vitamin D synthesized in the skin diffuses into the blood and is picked up by a specific vitamin-D-binding protein, which transports it to the liver, although some may remain free and be deposited in the fat and muscle.

Before vitamin D can perform its functions in the body, two activation stages occur. In the liver, an —OH group is added at position 25 on the side chain (see Figure 10.5), to form 25 hydroxy-cholecalciferol (25-OH · D_3), which is secreted into the blood and circulates attached to the carrier protein. This first activation is controlled by levels of the biologically active product of the second activation in a feedback mechanism.

The next stage occurs in the kidneys, where a second hydroxyl group is added at position 1, to yield 1,25-dihydroxy vitamin D (1,25-$(OH)_2$ · D_3, or calcitriol). This is the biologically active form of the vitamin, and its levels are tightly controlled to maintain calcium homeostasis. The activity of the enzyme 1-alpha-hydroxylase, which catalyses this reaction, is determined by parathyroid hormone and low blood calcium levels, which increase its activity. High levels of phosphate inhibit calcitriol production. When the body does not require calcitriol to be produced, the kidneys perform an alternative hydroxylation at position 24, producing 24, 25-dihydroxy vitamin D. The role of this metabolite is unclear, but it may be a way of 'switching off' production of the active hormone.

Vitamin E

Tocopherols generally occur free in foods; tocotrienols are esterified and must be split from these before absorption. In the presence of fats, absorption rates of the vitamin are 20%–50%, with lower rates of absorption occurring as dosage increases. Thus, absorption from supplements may be as little as 10%.

In the plasma, the vitamin is transported in the low-density lipoprotein (LDL) fraction and concentrates in the cell membranes. Highest concentrations are found in the adipose tissue; levels increase here with increasing intakes. Other organs and tissues that contain the vitamin include liver, heart, skeletal muscle and adrenal glands. Levels in the plasma and liver are the first to decrease when intakes are inadequate to meet requirements.

Vitamin K

Between 40% and 80% of the ingested vitamin appears in the chylomicrons entering the lymph. When fat absorption is impaired, as little as 20% may be absorbed. The water-soluble synthetic form is absorbed directly into the hepatic portal vein and carried to the liver, where it is activated and then released along with the naturally occurring forms of vitamin K. These are carried in the LDL to target sites. Turnover of vitamin K is rapid and stores are small.

Thiamin

Thiamin is readily absorbed from the diet by both active and passive mechanisms. At high levels of intake, most absorption is passive. Absorption may be inhibited by alcohol and by the presence of thiaminases, which are found in some fish. However, because these are destroyed on cooking, the problem exists only where raw fish is eaten regularly, as in Japan and Scandinavia.

On absorption, thiamin is phosphorylated to thiamin pyrophosphate (also called thiamine diphosphate), especially in the liver. The major tissues that contain thiamin are the skeletal muscle (about 50% of all thiamin), heart, liver, kidneys and brain.

Riboflavin

Absorption occurs readily from the small intestine as riboflavin. It is believed that absorption is better from animal than plant sources. In the plasma, it is carried in association with albumin, which carries both the free vitamin and coenzyme forms.

Niacin

There is rapid absorption of dietary niacin, both by active and passive mechanisms.

Excess free niacin may be methylated and excreted in the urine. A low level of this metabolite in the urine (<3 mg/day) is indicative of a deficiency state and may be used as an assay method.

Vitamin B_6

The vitamin has to be released from its phosphorylated forms prior to absorption; once in its free form, absorption is rapid. The liver and muscles are the main sites for pyridoxal phosphate in the body; once it is phosphorylated, the vitamin is trapped in the cell.

Folate

Most folate in the diet is in the bound form and, for optimal absorption, glutamates have to be removed to produce the monoglutamate, 5-methyl tetrahydrofolate (5-methyl THF); this is achieved with conjugase enzymes found in the brush border and lysosomes of the duodenum and jejunum. These enzymes are zinc dependent and can also be inhibited by alcohol. There may also be conjugase inhibitors in some foods, such as beans, which prevent the freeing of folate. Overall, 50% of dietary folate is believed to be absorbed. The absorption of folic acid is more efficient, with up to 85% of intake being bioavailable (i.e. well absorbed or assimilated). In the United States, a dietary folate equivalent has been introduced to allow an overall folate provision to be estimated from a variety of sources with varying bioavailabilities.

Most folate is stored in the liver, which is, therefore, also a good dietary source of folate. Once taken up by target cells, folates are conjugated to produce polyglutamates.

Vitamin B_{12}

Ingested vitamin B_{12} has to be combined with intrinsic factor produced by the stomach before it can be absorbed. The binding occurs in the duodenum where the pH is less acid than in the stomach. The vitamin–intrinsic factor complex is then carried down to the terminal ileum (the last part of the small intestine), from where the vitamin is absorbed, leaving the intrinsic factor behind. The process is slow, although at low levels of intake, 80% of dietary vitamin may be absorbed. Absorption rates fall as intake increases. In the absence of intrinsic factor, there is only minimal absorption of the vitamin by passive diffusion and eventually a deficiency state will develop. Although some of the vitamin may be synthesized by bacteria in the bowel, it is not absorbed from here and does not form a useful source.

Vitamin C

Both forms of the vitamin are readily absorbed by active transport and passive diffusion mechanisms, although dehydroascorbic acid is believed to be absorbed better than ascorbic acid itself. The percentage of the ingested dose absorbed falls, as the amount consumed increases. Overall, at levels of vitamin C usually consumed, absorption rates are 80%–95%. In the plasma, vitamin C occurs principally as free ascorbate; plasma levels are a reflection of the size of the dietary intake and continue to increase until they reach a plateau at 1.4 mg/dL (100 μmol/L) at intakes of 70–100 mg/day.

The adrenal gland, pituitary and the lens of the eye have high concentrations of vitamin C. Among other tissues that have a significant content of the vitamin are the liver, lungs and white blood cells. The content of vitamin C in the white blood cells is used as an indicator of tissue levels of the vitamin.

The total content of vitamin C in the body is known as the body pool. Normal values for this are 2–3 g in the adult; when this falls to less than 300 mg, clinical signs of scurvy may appear. Vitamin C status, in other words the amount of vitamin C within body tissues and fluids, is dependent on many factors (see Figure 10.6). These include the following:

- *Intake*: This depends on the composition of the food, its length of storage, processing and cooking methods.
- *Absorption*: This is affected by the total dose of vitamin ingested, the speed of travel through the digestive tract and the presence of other factors in the tract, such as glucose levels, trace elements and nitrosamines.
- *Metabolism*: Rates of usage will vary with metabolic demand and the ability to recycle the vitamin; demand may be higher in smokers, pregnancy, exercise, inflammation, diabetes and in polluted environments. Plasma levels are lower with increasing age.
- *Excretion in urine*: This depends on the levels in the plasma, glomerular filtration rate and the renal threshold.

DIGESTION AND ABSORPTION OF MINERALS, TRACE ELEMENTS AND ELECTROLYTES

Calcium

Calcium salts are generally not highly soluble, which makes their absorption from the diet problematic. Several factors can enhance or inhibit the absorption of calcium.

Enhancing factors

The most important of these is vitamin D, which causes the synthesis of a calcium-binding protein in the intestinal cells that transports calcium into the plasma. The ability to synthesize this protein and the amounts made are regulated by homeostatic mechanisms involving parathyroid hormone and active vitamin D, in response to changes in circulating levels of plasma calcium. In this way, calcium absorption can be increased to meet increased needs in the body.

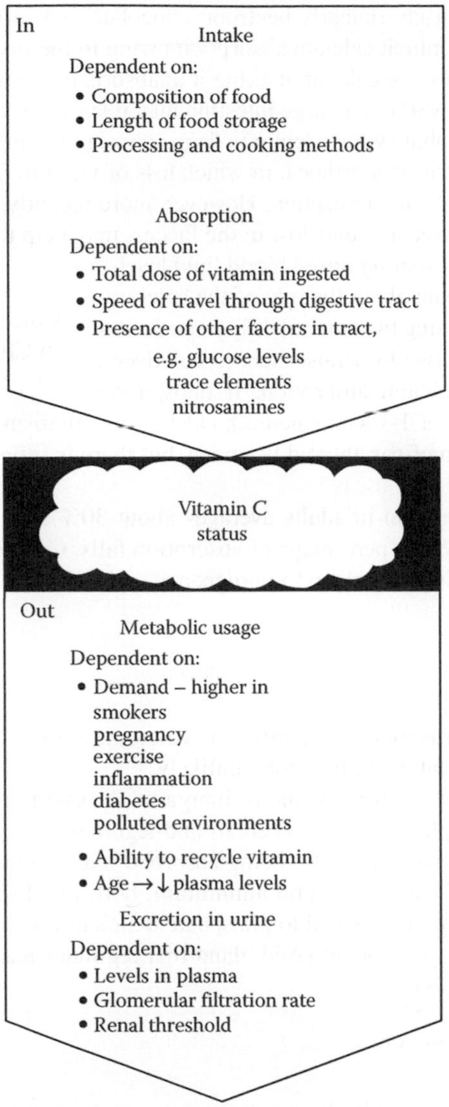

In
Intake
Dependent on:
• Composition of food
• Length of food storage
• Processing and cooking methods
Absorption
Dependent on:
• Total dose of vitamin ingested
• Speed of travel through digestive tract
• Presence of other factors in tract,
e.g. glucose levels
trace elements
nitrosamines
Vitamin C
status
Out
Metabolic usage
Dependent on:
• Demand – higher in
smokers
pregnancy
exercise
inflammation
diabetes
polluted environments
• Ability to recycle vitamin
• Age → ↓ plasma levels
Excretion in urine
Dependent on:
• Levels in plasma
• Glomerular filtration rate
• Renal threshold

FIGURE 10.6 Summary of factors influencing vitamin C status.

Lactose (present in milk) also enhances calcium absorption by keeping it in a soluble form. The presence of lactose and the large amounts of calcium found in milk make this an excellent source of the mineral. Other sugars and protein also enhance calcium absorption. The acidic environment of the upper digestive tract also facilitates the solubility of calcium. Therefore, taking large amounts of 'indigestion preparations' that lower acidity may compromise calcium absorption.

Inhibitory factors

Calcium absorption is reduced by phytic acid present in whole cereals, owing to the formation of insoluble calcium phytate. However, yeast fermentation probably breaks some of this down in the making of bread. It is also believed that people who regularly eat foods containing phytate develop a phytate-splitting enzyme, allowing them to make greater use of the calcium.

Oxalates (present in spinach, rhubarb, beetroot, chocolate, tea infusions, wheat bran, peanuts and strawberries) may also inhibit calcium absorption owing to the insoluble nature of the calcium oxalate salt. NSPs may trap some calcium making it unabsorbable in the small intestine. However, fermentation of the soluble NSP in the large intestine may release the calcium for absorption here.

Unabsorbed fats will combine with calcium to form soaps, removing the calcium from the body. This is a particular problem in steatorrhoea, in which loss of vitamin D, a fat-soluble vitamin, may aggravate the problem of calcium absorption. However, more recently, it has been suggested that a high calcium intake, with large amounts lost in the faeces, may help to remove some fats from the body and be of benefit in preventing raised blood lipid levels.

Calcium homeostasis is covered in Chapter 12, pp. 244–246.

There has been some doubt about the role of the calcium–phosphorus ratio in determining the bioavailability of calcium. At normal 1:1 ratios of the two minerals, there is no adverse effect of phosphorus on calcium absorption. If phosphorus intakes are very high (ratio of 1:3 with calcium), calcium metabolism may be altered, with hypocalcaemia and oversecretion of parathyroid hormone, but there is little evidence that absorption of calcium is affected.

Overall absorption of calcium in adults averages about 30% at a low-moderate intake (up to 500 mg); as intakes increase, the percentage of absorption falls. Generally, as the need for calcium increases, for example, during growth and in pregnancy and lactation, the efficiency of absorption improves.

Phosphorus

The body absorbs phosphorus more efficiently than calcium, at rates of 60%–90%, depending on body needs. An inadequate intake is, therefore, unlikely.

Dietary phosphorus can be either organic or inorganic in origin, most absorption taking place in the inorganic form. Phosphorus found in cereals and legumes as phytate is only partly liberated during digestion, with approximately 50% being absorbed. Absorption from the digestive tract is reduced by the presence of magnesium and aluminium, both of which may be found in indigestion preparations. This is unlikely to lead to phosphate deficiency, unless there is also a metabolic problem involving the kidneys or parathyroid gland that regulates phosphate levels. Calcium also reduces phosphorus absorption.

Magnesium

Absorption of magnesium occurs in the small intestine and appears to be more efficient when intakes are low. Absorption is improved by vitamin D and reduced by the presence of fatty acids and phytate. Plasma magnesium levels are kept constant by precise regulation of excretion via the kidney to match amounts absorbed.

There are many situations in which magnesium competes with or interferes with the action of calcium in the body. For example, magnesium inhibits the blood clotting process, and it may also inhibit smooth muscle contraction by blocking the calcium binding sites. However, the actions of vitamin D and parathyroid hormones, which regulate calcium, both require the presence of magnesium.

Iron

The two forms of iron in the diet are absorbed with different efficiency. Organic (haem) iron must be hydrolyzed from any protein to which it is attached and is then absorbed relatively easily, albeit slowly; the overall absorption of iron from meat may be 20%–25%. The absorption takes place most effectively in the duodenum and is inversely related to the level of iron stores.

Non-haem, inorganic iron must first be solubilized and hydrolyzed before absorption can occur. Hydrochloric acid in the stomach performs this function and also converts any ferric (Fe^{3+}) iron in food to its (absorbable) ferrous (Fe^{2+}) state. This reaction is also facilitated by ascorbic acid (vitamin C), which can dramatically improve inorganic iron absorption. Other factors that can enhance the absorption of inorganic iron include citric acid, lactic acid, fructose and peptides derived from meat; all of these form ligands with the ferrous iron, maintaining its solubility and thus facilitating absorption. Alcohol is also believed to enhance iron absorption.

There are, in addition, a number of factors that reduce absorption of inorganic iron. These generally bind with the iron, making it unavailable for absorption. Most notable are the following:

- Phytate (in whole cereal grains)
- Polyphenols (in tea, coffee and nuts)
- Oxalic acid (in tea, chocolate, spinach)
- Phosphates (in egg yolks)
- Calcium and zinc

These interactions make it extremely difficult to predict how much iron will be absorbed from a particular meal. For example, iron absorption from plant foods can be as little as 2%–5%, but can be enhanced tenfold by the presence of vitamin C. Tea will reduce iron absorption by as much as 60%. Overall, iron absorption from the diverse UK diet is estimated to be 15%. Under certain circumstances, for example, in pregnancy, absorption may be 90%. However, if the diet contains little or no meat, and substantial amounts of phytate-rich foods, absorption is likely to be less than 10%. Factors influencing iron absorption are summarized in Figure 10.7.

Advice to people who have marginal intakes of iron should, therefore, include simple guidelines about food combinations that may be beneficial. However, it is clear that there is often little relationship between dietary iron intake and iron status, and mechanisms exist in the body that regulate uptake in response to physiological circumstances in as yet incompletely understood ways.

Control of absorption

Once iron has been absorbed into the body, there is no means of eliminating a surplus, which can be toxic in excess, other than by loss of blood. In severe iron overload, the patient may be

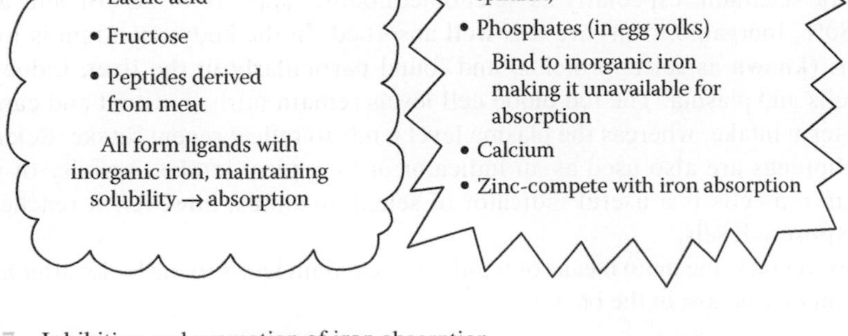

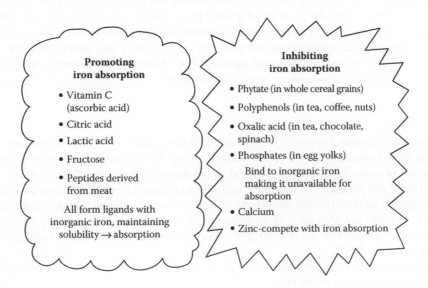

FIGURE 10.7 Inhibition and promotion of iron absorption.

bled to remove iron or is prescribed a chelating drug, which binds to the iron and allows it to be excreted. It is clearly preferable to have a mechanism that can prevent the entry of iron into the body when it is not needed. In a healthy individual, a 'mucosal block' operates, which regulates the amount of iron allowed into the circulation according to the level of stores present in the body. Thus, more is absorbed when the body stores are low or the needs are increased, for example, in pregnancy.

As it passes through the mucosal cell, the iron is oxidized back to the ferric state and attached to the transport protein transferrin for circulation around the body. Iron not required by the body is trapped within the mucosal cell and is lost in the faeces when the lining cells of the gut are shed at the end of their life cycle.

Zinc

Both ingested zinc as well as that secreted in various digestive juices, such as bile and pancreatic juice, are available for absorption. Zinc is released from bound sources and attaches to amino acids, which facilitate its absorption. The amount absorbed is regulated to match the needs of the body, although the mechanisms are unclear. There is competition for the absorption mechanism from other divalent ions, such as calcium and iron, which may reduce zinc uptake. Stress has been shown to increase zinc uptake.

Inhibitors of zinc uptake include phytate (especially in the presence of calcium), oxalic acid, polyphenols and folic acid. Zinc taken into the mucosal cells may be bound to metallothionein and then lost from the body when the cells are shed. This is thought to provide an important mechanism for regulating body levels of zinc. Overall, rates of zinc absorption average 30%, although considerable variation may occur with different dietary combinations.

Copper

Copper is absorbed mainly in the duodenum and jejunum, at rates of 35%–70%. The efficiency of absorption appears to vary inversely with intake. The transfer of copper across the basolateral membrane of the enterocyte is energy dependent and carrier mediated, and there is competition for the pathway from other minerals, most notably zinc and iron. Other inhibitors include an alkaline pH, molybdenum, calcium and phosphorus, and possibly the presence of phytates and sulphides. Absorption is enhanced by the presence of animal protein, human milk and fructose. On absorption, copper is bound to plasma albumin, but becomes rapidly bound to caeruloplasmin in the liver, which then forms the major circulating source of copper. Copper is also secreted into the digestive tract, especially in bile, and this forms the main excretory route and is believed to be an important mechanism for maintaining a constant body pool of copper.

Selenium

Absorption of selenium, especially as selenomethionine, appears to be efficient and may be as high as 80%. Inorganic forms are less well absorbed. In the body, selenium is incorporated into proteins (known as selenoproteins) and found particularly in the liver, kidneys, muscle, red blood cells and plasma. The red blood cell levels remain fairly constant and can be used to assess long-term intake, whereas the plasma level tends to reflect recent intake. Selenium levels in toenail clippings are also used as an indicator of long-term intake. Activity of glutathione peroxidase in red cells is a useful indicator of selenium status; however, it reaches a plateau with high exposure levels.

Urinary excretion is the main means of regulating selenium levels in the body; after high intakes, some selenium may be lost in the breath.

Iodine

Iodide absorption is efficient (via sodium/iodine symporters), and the free iodide is concentrated by the thyroid gland, which takes it up actively against a concentration gradient. The gland contains 70%–80% of the body's iodide and uses it in the synthesis of thyroid hormones, combining it with the amino acid tyrosine in a stepwise process. The completed hormones contain three or four atoms of iodine. These are stored attached to a protein colloid until required. Release is regulated by the thyroid-stimulating hormone produced by the anterior pituitary gland. Any iodine that is not used in the final hormones is recycled. When iodine stores are replete, most (approximately 90%) of the iodine consumed is excreted in urine.

Fluoride

Fluoride in solution is very readily absorbed from the digestive tract; absorption of food sources ranges from 50% to 80%. After absorption, fluoride is taken up, particularly by the bones and teeth, where it becomes incorporated into the calcium phosphate crystal structure apatite, replacing the (—OH) group and forming fluorapatite. This is a harder material and more resistant to decay than apatite. The presence of fluoride also accelerates the remineralization process when teeth have started to demineralize in the presence of low oral pH. Finally, the presence of fluoride in saliva alters the bacterial flora in the mouth and reduces acid production. Thus, the pH fall after sugar consumption is less in the presence of fluoride. All of these mechanisms help to protect teeth.

Sodium and Chloride

Both sodium and chloride are readily absorbed. Sodium has been shown to be absorbed by a series of pathways that can function in both the small intestine and the colon.

In the West, intakes of sodium are generally much greater than the requirements, and thus, the sodium taken into the body must be regulated by excretion.

Chloride is absorbed passively, generally following electrochemical gradients established by the absorption of cations. It is also extensively secreted into the digestive tract, although most of this is subsequently reabsorbed.

The concentration of sodium in extracellular fluids is maintained at 3.1–3.3 g/L (135–145 mmol/L). If levels increase above this, water is retained to maintain osmolality and the extracellular fluid volume increases. This is subsequently lost by increased sodium and water excretion over 1–2 days. Conversely, a fall in sodium levels will result in conservation by the kidneys of both electrolytes and water. These mechanisms result from the interplay of a number of hormonal and nervous system factors; a full explanation will be found in physiology textbooks.

Sodium excretion occurs principally via the kidneys, which filter and then reabsorb large amounts of sodium in the course of a day. This provides a great deal of flexibility to adjust the plasma levels precisely. Significant losses may also occur in sweat, when physical work is performed in hot conditions. Acclimatization results in a lowering of the sodium losses in sweat; in the short term, exposure to conditions causing excessive sweating may necessitate an increased salt intake.

Excretion of chloride is primarily through the kidneys, where it accompanies sodium loss.

Potassium

Potassium absorption occurs readily in the upper small intestine and colon with 90% of ingested potassium absorbed, although the mechanisms are not fully understood. Potassium levels in the body are carefully regulated to maintain low levels in the plasma (3.5–5.5 mmol/L) and much

TABLE 10.3
Average Values for Daily Turnover of Body Water in a Temperate Climate

Input (mL)		Output (mL)	
Food	1000	Urine	1300
Drinks	1200	Faeces	100
Metabolism	350	Skin	750
		Lungs	400
Total	2550		2550

higher levels (150 mmol/L) in the intracellular fluid. The total amount of potassium in the body is related to the lean body mass.

Regulation occurs by means of hormonally controlled secretion into the glomerular filtrate in the kidneys. The kidneys are very efficient at removing surplus potassium from the body, but less precise at preventing loss when body levels are low. Small amounts of potassium may be lost in the faeces and sweat.

Fluid Balances

There is a daily turnover of body water equivalent to approximately 5% of our body weight. The actual amount depends on a variety of circumstances. The average values for a healthy individual who is sedentary and lives in a temperate climate are given in Table 10.3.

Water Loss

It can be seen from the aforementioned that water is lost from the body in a variety of ways.

Urine The amount of urine produced is under hormonal control and is adjusted to achieve fluid balance in the body. Therefore, the volume and concentration of urine will reflect the state of hydration of the individual. Following large intakes of fluid, the urine will be dilute and pale and straw-like in colour. Pale urine is an indicator of a good level of hydration in the body. As fluid intake decreases, or other losses of fluid increase, the colour of the urine becomes darker. Thus, dark yellow or even brownish urine is a sign of severe dehydration. This is a very simple guide that anyone can follow to monitor his or her state of hydration.

The volume of urine is affected by certain dietary items. Protein and sodium contents of the diet can both increase the volume of urine that needs to be excreted (known as obligatory loss). This is associated with the need to eliminate waste products (urea from protein metabolism, and sodium) and maintain homeostasis. Thus, both a high-protein and a high-salt diet will increase obligatory urine losses. In these cases, it is important to increase fluid intakes to ensure adequate levels to meet excretory needs.

Alcohol is a diuretic and, therefore, increases the loss of urine from the body. Whether this will have a dehydrating effect depends on the volume of fluid ingested with the alcohol. It is estimated that a 10 mL diuresis occurs for each gram of alcohol ingested. In practice, therefore, an 8 g intake of alcohol (equal to 1 unit) would cause 80 mL of diuresis. If this was taken as a half pint of beer, then more fluid would have been taken in than was being lost, and dehydration would not result. However, with stronger drinks, taken in a smaller volume, such as wine and spirits, alcohol ingestion will lead to diuresis, causing dehydration.

Caffeine-containing drinks, such as coffee, tea, chocolate and colas, together with some of the 'energy drinks' on the market also have the potential to act as diuretics. This also applies to related compounds, such as theophylline and theobromine, that are found in tea and chocolate. There has been considerable debate about this matter and widely repeated advice that all of these drinks are of no value for hydration because of their diuretic effects.

However, it has now been established that there is no evidence in the scientific literature to show that at normal intakes of caffeine, that is, less than 300 mg/day, there is any diuretic effect and the beverage can contribute fully to the hydration of the body. In the United Kingdom, the daily caffeine intake from tea and coffee has been found to be 239 mg/day, well within the limit stated earlier. Studies that have indicated a diuretic effect of caffeine have used higher doses than this (300–700 mg), in caffeine-depleted well-hydrated individuals. In this case, caffeine does have a diuretic action.

Faeces The fluid loss here is generally small. However, amounts can increase if there is diarrhoea when up to 2 L may be lost via this route each day. Diarrhoeal disease associated with contaminated water is a major cause of death in children in developing countries, and emphasizes the importance of aiming to maintain hydration in this situation.

Skin Losses through the skin occur continuously and are an essential part of the body's temperature control mechanism. They will, therefore, vary with the environmental temperature and the amount of physical activity. In a hot environment, the body loses heat by evaporation of large amounts of sweat, and the fluid balance may become disturbed. Amounts of sweat may increase to 2–3 L as a result. Physical activity compounds these losses. Any increase in physical activity generates body heat, which must be lost through sweating. Moderate exercise may increase sweat losses to 1 L/hour. If this occurs also in a warm environment, sweat losses may be as high as 2–3 L/hour. Individuals working in hot environments, such as steel workers, miners and catering workers also have high sweat losses that need regular replacement.

Children exposed to heat may lose proportionately more sweat because of a greater surface area to volume, and they will have a more critical need for water to replace this. Thirst mechanisms may not be very sensitive, so encouragement to drink may be needed.

In a person who has a raised body temperature, it is estimated that skin losses of water as part of thermoregulation are increased by 500 mL for each 1°C above normal.

Lungs Losses occur here continuously, as gaseous exchange in the lungs takes place in a moist environment. Losses increase when there is low humidity, for example, in dry climates or air-conditioned offices, as well as in aircraft and at high altitude. Increased respiratory rates during exercise also increase the hourly rate of water loss from the lungs. Water loss also increases via this route in patients who are attached to ventilators.

Water Gain

Water is produced in the body during metabolic reactions, and this contributes a small amount to the body's water economy. This is a continuous source of water for cellular needs.

Consumption of liquids is governed by thirst and habit, both of which can be overridden. When fluid volumes fall in the body, there is normally a rise in osmolality of body fluids, and an increase in sodium concentrations. These trigger the thirst mechanism. It can be seen that thirst does not prevent the fall in fluid volume, but follows on from it, by which time there is already some dehydration. Furthermore, the thirst mechanism is not a very sensitive trigger for fluid intake. Other triggers might include a dry mouth and reduced saliva production. Overall, it is much better to be in the habit of taking fluids regularly, without waiting to be thirsty. In people with a high fluid turnover, such as athletes, anticipating the need for fluid and keeping hydrated is a sensible precaution against dehydration. In unusual circumstances, if large amounts of salt have been lost through profuse sweating, an intake of a large volume of water may reduce plasma osmolality further and cause continued urine loss. This situation is potentially dangerous and requires an intake of salt with water to restore normal electrolyte balance. In the majority of circumstances, adequate salt is obtained from normal dietary intakes to prevent this happening.

Large intakes of fluid can also be taken voluntarily, for example, on social occasions. In this situation, there is rarely any thirst for the drinks, but the normal controlling mechanisms are overridden by conscious control.

Similarly, thirst sensations may be weak or can be ignored. The sense of thirst decreases with age, so the risk of dehydration is greater in older adults. Children may also not respond adequately to the sensation of thirst and become vulnerable to dehydration, especially if undertaking physical activity in which they become very involved. The urge to drink may also be ignored if it is inconvenient or difficult to empty the bladder. This may be for social reasons, or because of a lack of facilities, or incontinence or impaired mobility. All of these situations may present a risk of dehydration.

DIGESTION AND ABSORPTION OF PHYTOCHEMICALS

Phytochemicals are abundant non-nutrient compounds present in plant foods. They vary in structure, from small molecules to large, polymeric structures and can be classified as phenolics (flavonoids, tannins, lignans, coumarins, stilbenes and phenolic acids), carotenoids, phytosterols, alkaloids such as caffeine, nitrogen containing compounds and organosulphur compounds (sulphides and glucosinolates). More than 30,000 phytochemicals have been identified so far, and in many cases, there is incomplete knowledge of their mechanisms of digestion and absorption and general bioavailability, which varies widely, possibly due to their great structural diversity. Circulating concentrations of phytochemicals and their metabolites show wide variability among humans, even in feeding studies where intake is tightly controlled. The process of phytochemical disposition in the human body involves absorption, metabolism, distribution and excretion, similar to that for drugs and other xenobiotic compounds and involves overcoming several barriers both in the gastro-intestinal (GI) tract and in the liver. Individual variability at each stage of this process and genetic phenotype may contribute to the observed pharmacokinetic differences.

Aqueous solubility is recognized as a key factor for the bioaccessibility and thus bioavailability of many phytochemicals. They may also be subjected to metabolism and degradation by intestinal enzymes, such as the esterases, glycosidases, hydrolases and oxidases, originating from both the host and the microbiota that inhabit the gut. Phytochemicals often occur in plant foods bound to sugars as glycosides or other conjugates and must be hydrolyzed before they can be absorbed. This hydrolysis can be carried out by β-glucosidases bound to the brush border membrane of the small intestine (e.g. lactase phlorizin hydrolase) or gut bacterial β-glucosidases in the colon. The aglycones can then be absorbed by the enterocytes or colonocytes, possibly by diffusion or some other transport system such as the sodium-dependent glucose transporter, where they undergo first stage metabolism in the gut epithelium or liver resulting in conjugates that are excreted in urine and bile. Transcellular transport of these conjugates is dependent on various transporters including the solute carrier transporters and the ATP-binding cassette transport proteins, which are able to export compounds from intestinal cells.

Polyphenols are one of the largest families of phytochemicals, and their structural variation partly dictates their digestion and absorption. Breakdown of the food matrix by digestive secretions may release phytochemicals, making them available for absorption. However, plant polyphenols have low bioavailability due to naturally low aqueous solubility, poor gastrointestinal stability, passive diffusion and active efflux of phenolic phytochemicals in the gastrointestinal tract. The bioavailability of flavonoids shows great variation, for example, isoflavones have the highest levels (up to 30%), whereas intact anthocyanins have very low bioavailability (0.1%–1%).

Many polyphenols occur in plants bound to sugars as glycosides, with a few also occurring in the free unbound or aglycone form. The type of sugar attached to the polyphenol aglycone dictates absorption, since the small intestine is unable to hydrolyze sugars attached to polyphenols other than glucose. Therefore, polyphenol glycosides such as the rutinoside, for example, cannot be absorbed and instead accumulate in the colon, where they are hydrolyzed by colonic bacteria into smaller molecules (the phenolic acids) and can then be absorbed. Polyphenolic compounds accumulating in the colon may have a prebiotic mode of action, and their breakdown products may contribute significantly to the bioactivity originally attributed to the parent compound.

Tannins differ from other polyphenolic phytochemicals in that they have a high molecular weight and often form insoluble complexes with carbohydrates and proteins. The complex polymer structure of tannins makes them difficult to analyze and, therefore, to understand their bioavailability; however, they have been extensively recovered in faeces and their indigestibility may help explain their supposed health effects, as evidence suggests that colonic bacteria may break them down into more bioactive and bioavailable forms. Similarly, intestinal bacteria play a major role in lignan conversion, for instance, by producing the enterolignans enterodiol and enterolactone. Conversely, the oral absorption of stilbenes such as resveratrol in humans is about 75% and is thought to occur mainly by transepithelial diffusion; however, extensive metabolism in the intestine and liver results in an oral bioavailability considerably less than 1%.

Plant carotenoids, on the other hand, are more bioavailable. Their digestion and absorption rely on mechanisms relevant to fat digestion and absorption: emulsification and micellization. Uptake of carotenoids by the enterocyte was mainly thought to happen via simple diffusion. However, recent evidence indicates a receptor-mediated transport mechanism.

Phytosterols are structurally related to cholesterol and follow a similar digestion and absorption pathway. Phytosterols are known to reduce serum low-density lipoprotein cholesterol level without changing high-density lipoprotein cholesterol or triglyceride levels. The cholesterol-lowering action of phytosterols is thought to occur, at least in part, through competitive replacement of dietary and biliary cholesterol in mixed micelles, which undermines the absorption of cholesterol.

SUMMARY

1. Protein digestion is simple, and absorption requires specialized transporters. Some amino acids will compete with others for absorption
2. The simple sugars are readily digestible and are absorbed via specialized transporters.
3. Carbohydrates that are not susceptible to digestion in the small intestine are fermented by the colonic microflora and play a key role in colon health.
4. Starches may be digestible or resistant. The digestible starches release glucose more slowly than do simple sugars. In addition, food sources of starch generally contain other nutrients.
5. NSPs can be classified as soluble or insoluble. The soluble NSPs contribute to viscosity in gut contents, and slow the absorption of nutrients. The insoluble NSPs retain water and increase bulk in the large intestine. Both forms have beneficial effects for health, both within the digestive tract and for general metabolism.
6. Digestion of fats requires the presence of bile from the liver. Failure of fat digestion results in steatorrhoea.
7. Fat is transported in the circulation in the form of lipoproteins, which vary in their content of triglycerides and cholesterol.
8. Fat-soluble vitamins (A, D, E, C) require fat to be absorbed.
9. Levels of the minerals are generally closely regulated, either by control of absorption or by control of excretion, to prevent excessive amounts accumulating in the body.
10. Some of the minerals, especially calcium, zinc, copper and iron, may compete with one another for absorption.
11. Polyphenolics are poorly absorbed and accumulate mostly in the colon where they are broken down by bacteria.

STUDY QUESTIONS

1. Describe the factors influencing iron absorption, and how there will vary in different age groups.
2. Consider the key steps in the digestion and absorption of the following meals. Which macro and micronutrients are present to be digested and absorbed? How to the nutrient interfere with each other?
    a. A tomato soup
    b. A cheeseburger
    c. A bowl of bran flakes with skimmed milk and blueberries, and a cup of coffee

ACTIVITY

10.1 Construct a table to identify the key steps of digestion and absorption of dietary fat, protein and carbohydrate. Focus on the various gut structures which are involved, the role of enzymes and secretions.

BIBLIOGRAPHY AND FURTHER READING

Englyst, H.N. and Kingman, S.M. 1990. Dietary fibre and resistant starch: A nutritional classification of plant polysaccharides. In Kritchevsky, D., Bonfield, C. and Anderson, J.W. (eds.), *Dietary Fibre*. New York: Plenum Press Publishing Corporation, pp. 49–65.

Gallagher, J.C., Yalamanchili, V. and Smith, L.M. 2012. The effect of vitamin D on calcium absorption in older women. *The Journal of Clinical Endocrinology and Metabolism* 97(10), 3550–3556.

Goncalves, A., Roi, S., Nowicki, M., Dhaussy, A., Huertas, A., Amiot, M.J. and Reboul, E. 2015. Fat-soluble vitamin intestinal absorption: Absorption sites in the intestine and interactions for absorption. *Food Chemistry* 172, 155–160.

Gorissen, S.H., Burd, N.A., Hamer, H.M., Gijsen, A.P. and van Loon, L.J. 2013. Carbohydrate co-ingestion with protein delays dietary protein digestion and absorption but does not modulate postprandial muscle protein accretion. *The FASEB Journal* 27(1_MeetingAbstracts), 249–246.

Harrison, E.H. 2012. Mechanisms involved in the intestinal absorption of dietary vitamin A and provitamin A carotenoids. *Biochimica et Biophysica Acta (BBA)-Molecular and Cell Biology of Lipids* 1821(1), 70–77.

Lampe, J.W. and Chang, J.-L. 2007. Interindividual differences in phytochemical metabolism and disposition. *Seminars in Cancer Biology* 17, 347–353.

Nicola, J.P., Reyna-Neyra, A., Carrasco, N. and Masini-Repiso, A.M. 2012. Dietary iodide controls its own absorption through post-transcriptional regulation of the intestinal Na^+/I^- symporter. *The Journal of Physiology* 590(23), 6013–6026.

Schafer, A.L., Weaver, C.M., Black, D.M. et al. 2015. Intestinal calcium absorption decreases dramatically after gastric bypass surgery despite optimization of vitamin D status. *Journal of Bone and Mineral Research* 30(8), 1377–1385.

Sitrin, M.D. 2014. Digestion and absorption of dietary triglycerides. In Leung, P.S. (ed.), *The Gastrointestinal System*. Dordrecht, the Netherlands: Springer Netherlands, pp. 159–178.

van Duynhoven, J., Vaughan, E.E., Jacobs, D.M. et al. 2011. Metabolic fate of polyphenols in the human superoraganism. *Proceedings of the National Academy of Sciences of the Unites States of America* 108(Suppl. 1), 4531–4538.

Wilder-Smith, C.H., Materna, A., Wermelinger, C. and Schuler, J. 2013. Fructose and lactose intolerance and malabsorption testing: The relationship with symptoms in functional gastrointestinal disorders. *Alimentary Pharmacology and Therapeutics* 37(11), 1074–1083.

11 Metabolism and Function of Macronutrients

AIMS

The aims of this chapter are to

- Describe the roles of proteins, carbohydrates and fats as energy substrates and in other physiological processes.
- Describe the key aspect of amino acid metabolism, glucose homeostasis and fat transport in the body.
- Discuss the part played by adipose tissue in metabolism.

Macronutrients fulfil key functions beyond providing energy to the body. These functions are outlined in this chapter, alongside basic insight into their metabolism.

PROTEINS

Proteins serve a large number of functions in the body. Some are key components in structure, some are enzymes, hormones or buffers; others play a part in immunity, transport of substances around the body, blood clotting and many other roles (summarized in Figure 11.1).

The energy contribution of macronutrients is covered in Chapter 16 on energy intake and expenditure, pp. 317–318.

AMINO ACID METABOLISM

The cells of the body are able to synthesize the carbon skeleton and add the side chains of 12 of the 20 amino acids, using amino groups from other amino acids; these are the dispensable (or non-essential) amino acids. However, there are eight amino acids that cannot be made by the body in this way and, therefore, have to be supplied in the diet. These are called the indispensable (or essential) amino acids.

The dietary sources of macronutrients are covered in Chapter 3, pp. 31–58.

They are leucine, isoleucine, valine, lysine, tryptophan, threonine, methionine and phenylalanine. Histidine is also indispensable for children and also, in some circumstances, for adults. It has been proposed that this classification is too rigid, as it is recognized that some amino acids may become indispensable in certain circumstances (Table 11.1).

The body is able to convert many amino acids from one to another, by the process of transamination. This process involves moving an amino group from a donor amino acid to an acceptor acid (called a keto acid), which in turn becomes an amino acid (Figure 11.2). The remnants of the donor amino acid (the carbon skeleton) are then utilized in other metabolic pathways, usually to produce energy or in the synthesis of fatty acids. Alternatively, they may themselves receive an amino group and be reconverted to an amino acid.

Amino acids may also be broken down by the process of deamination, in which the amino group, having been removed, is incorporated into urea in the liver and eventually excreted via the kidneys

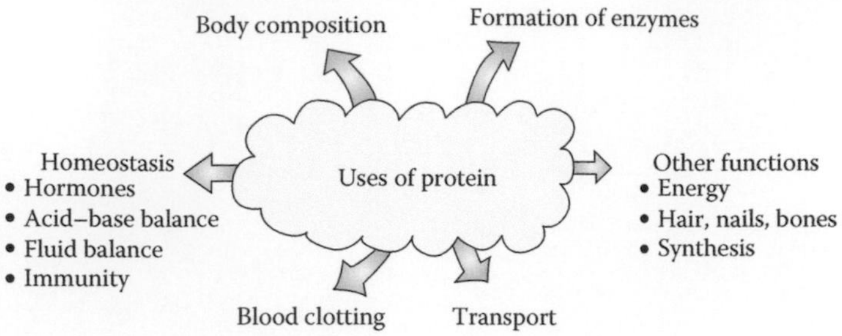

FIGURE 11.1 Summary of uses of protein.

TABLE 11.1
Amino Acids That May Become Indispensable under Certain Circumstances

Amino Acid	Situation When It May Become Indispensable
Cysteine and tyrosine	In the neonate May also spare methionine and phenylalanine
Arginine	In urea cycle disorders Metabolic stress
Taurine	In neonates and during growth Prolonged parenteral nutrition
Glutamine	May be needed in trauma, cancer and patients with immune deficiencies

in urine. The amount of urea excreted daily is a useful indicator of the rate at which protein turnover is taking place and can also be used to calculate the protein needs of an individual. The remaining carbon fragment can be converted to pyruvate and then glucose, in which case the amino acid is known as 'glucogenic'. Alternatively, if it leads to the formation of acetyl coenzyme A and then ketone bodies or fatty acids, the amino acid is called 'ketogenic'.

Several amino acids are both glucogenic and ketogenic, meaning that their carbon skeletons can give rise to both glucose and fats. Only the amino acids leucine and lysine are purely ketogenic and cannot be used to make glucose.

These exchanges allow the body to make maximum use of its protein supplies, both from the diet and from that which is recycled within the body.

Amino Acid Pool

The amino acid pool contains amino acids obtained from protein in the diet and amino acids released from breakdown of cells and general metabolic processes of renewal in the body. From this pool, the cells of the body can take the amino acids they need to produce the proteins they require. If the pool does not contain the appropriate amounts needed, a cell has two possible options:

1. It can simply make less of the protein it requires, limited by the amino acid present in least amounts.
2. It can break down some of its own protein to release the amino acids it requires for synthesis.

Obviously, neither of these alternatives is the ideal solution; in both cases, less protein than required is present in the cell, either because some was broken down to make new protein or because too little was synthesized. If this situation continues, there will be a deterioration of function. It is, therefore, important that the amino acid pool is adequate for the body's needs. This also means that

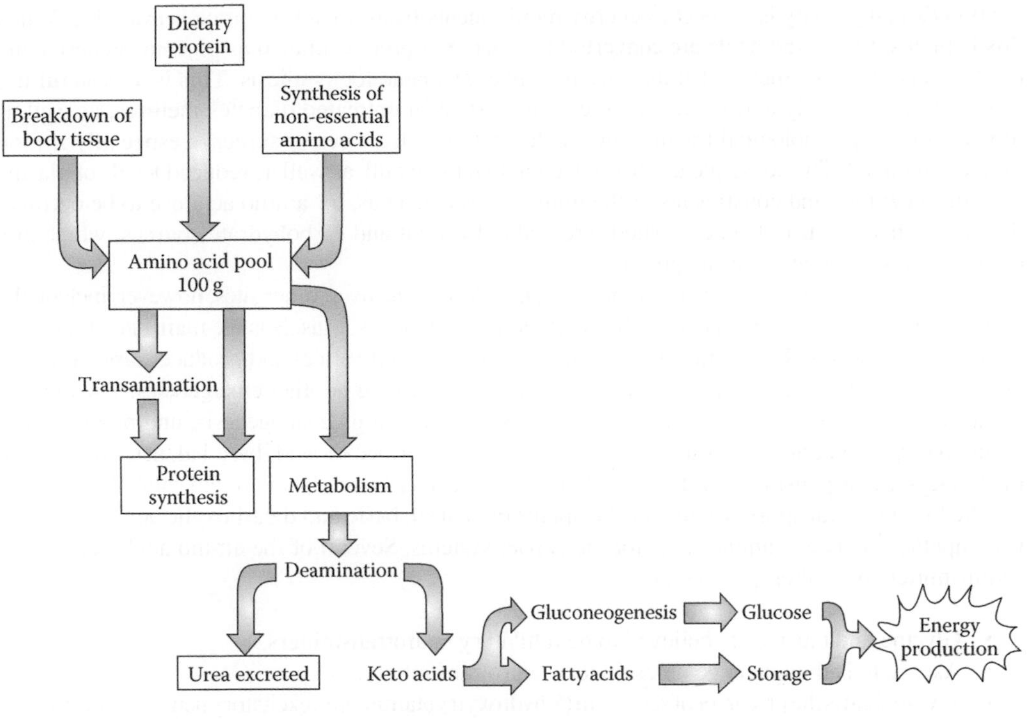

FIGURE 11.2 Summary of amino acid metabolism.

it must contain the indispensable amino acids in the right proportions, so that synthesis can take place. If one of these amino acids is in short supply at the time that it is needed, perhaps because the diet did not contain much, then synthetic reactions will be restricted to an extent determined by this amino acid. This is then termed the limiting amino acid, and this concept is used later in this chapter in the discussion of protein quality.

The total size of the amino acid pool has been estimated at 100 g, including the plasma and smaller amounts in the tissues. It principally contains dispensable (non-essential) amino acids, since the indispensable amino acids are used rapidly or, if present in excess, are deaminated. The pool represents the balance of the flux between the incoming amino acids (from diet and tissue breakdown) and the use of amino acids for synthesis of proteins or for deamination and energy production. It has been estimated that the total amount of protein turnover in a day is in the region of 250–300 g; this is greater in infants and less in the elderly. The balance is regulated by the needs of the body and the size of the pool. If the pool becomes too large, then more deaminating enzymes will be activated and amino acids will be broken down and their nitrogen excreted as urea. The carbon skeletons will be used for energy or to synthesize fat.

Since the body has no means of storing excess protein or amino acids, eating more protein than the body requires results in breakdown of amino acids, with the production of fatty acids, glucose, urea and heat. Since we generally live in warm houses and wear appropriate amounts of clothes, this excess heat is not used for maintaining body temperature but is largely dissipated as waste heat.

If insufficient protein is eaten, the body has to use its own 'endogenous' protein to provide the amino acids needed for the pool and, therefore, to maintain normal protein turnover. In time, the tissue proteins will be seen to waste, and the ability of the body to maintain all of the functions requiring protein will deteriorate. Eventually, a state of protein deficiency will occur.

If insufficient energy sources are being supplied to the body in the form of carbohydrate or fats (even if protein intake appears adequate), then protein will be degraded and used for energy, since the body's first priority is to meet its energy requirements from whatever source is available. When this happens, the amino acids are converted to glucose (a process known as gluconeogenesis) and used for energy. This means that they are no longer available for synthesis. This is a wasteful use of protein by the body and is seen to an extreme extent in untreated diabetes mellitus, as well as in situations of physiological trauma (such as fever, burns, fractures or surgery), especially if food intake is reduced. The consequences are a decline in muscle bulk as well as reduced levels of plasma proteins, enzymes and constituents of the immune system. Thus, for amino acid use to be optimal, the energy needs must also be satisfied, preferably from fat and carbohydrate sources, which are, therefore, described as 'sparing' protein.

The greatest part of amino acid metabolism takes place in the liver; other sites, however, include the skeletal muscle and, to a lesser extent, the heart, brain and kidneys. Muscle is the main site of metabolism of the branched-chain amino acids (leucine, isoleucine and valine) and produces large amounts of glutamine and alanine, which can be used for energy in fasting or other emergencies. The kidneys are also an important site of amino acid metabolism, including gluconeogenesis, and production of ammonia from glutamine, which is essential for the maintenance of acid–base balance. In addition, the kidneys are responsible for ridding the body of nitrogenous waste from protein catabolism.

The brain has transport systems for the uptake of neutral, basic and dicarboxylic acids, and there is competition between amino acids for the carrier systems. Several of the amino acids act as neurotransmitters or as their precursors:

- Glycine and taurine are believed to be inhibitory neurotransmitters.
- Aspartate is thought to be an excitatory neurotransmitter.
- Tryptophan is the precursor of serotonin (5-hydroxytryptamine), an excitatory neurotransmitter.
- Tyrosine is used in the synthesis of dopamine, noradrenaline and adrenaline (the catecholamines).
- A number of neuropeptides are found in the brain; these have a wide range of functions, including regulating hormone release, endocrine roles and effects on mood and behaviour.

Thus, changes in uptake of amino acids or varying levels in the brain can have diverse effects.

Control of Protein Metabolism

Amino acid and thus protein metabolism are under the control of the endocrine system. Recent evidence suggests that the body has a well-defended system for metabolic adaptation, which protects essential functions and internal homeostasis. This is necessary in the face of varying protein intakes and changing internal demands. Protein synthesis is promoted by insulin, which facilitates the uptake of amino acids into tissues. On the other hand, glucagon, catecholamines and glucocorticoids have the opposite effect and promote protein degradation. Growth hormone is an anabolic agent for protein. However, the exact effects of these hormones may vary between tissues and at different levels of nutrient intake.

For example, the effect of insulin on peripheral tissue uptake of amino acids is maximal for the branched-chain amino acids but minimal for tryptophan. Thus, after a carbohydrate-containing meal, which stimulates insulin release, the uptake of tryptophan into tissues, including the brain, is increased, as competing amino acids are no longer present. This is believed to stimulate serotonin synthesis in the brain and may be responsible for the drowsiness experienced after carbohydrate ingestion. It also contributes to a reduction in food intake.

Contribution of Protein to Body Composition

Protein is a key component of the structure of the body. Each cell contains protein as part of the cell membrane and within its cytoplasm. Muscles, bones, connective tissues, blood cells, glands and organs all contain protein. Proteins are synthesized during growth, repaired, maintained and replaced during life, and form a source of amino acids that can be drawn on in emergencies, although at the expense of the tissue it comes from. Only the brain is resistant to being used as a source of amino acids for emergency use. Thus, the protein in our body structure is not static but a dynamic constituent that is in a state of continuous flux.

Formation of Enzymes

Almost all enzymes are proteins and thus proteins are instrumental in facilitating most of the chemical reactions that occur in the body. This includes the digestion of nutrients (including protein), the regulation of energy production in cells and the synthesis of all the chemical substances found in the body. Enzymes are essential to normal life.

Homeostasis

The physiological mechanisms of the body aim to maintain a constant internal environment in the face of continued changes that might disturb it. This is achieved by the action of various proteins operating in specific ways.

Hormones

Many of these consist of amino acids. They act as the messengers carried in the circulation and control the internal environment, for example, by regulating metabolic rate (thyroid hormones), blood glucose levels (insulin, glucagon), blood calcium levels (parathyroid hormone, calcitonin), the digestion process (secretin, cholecystokinin [CCK]) and response to stress (adrenaline).

Acid–Base Balance

Proteins act as buffers in the circulation by accepting or donating H^+ ions and thereby maintaining a fairly constant pH in the blood and body fluids.

Fluid Balance

Because of their size and inability to leak through the walls of the blood vessels, proteins in the plasma exert an osmotic effect that holds fluid within the circulation. This prevents excess pooling of body fluids in the tissue spaces. A reduction in the levels of albumin and globulin causes oedema as a result of loss of fluid from the circulation into the tissue spaces.

Immunity

Proteins play a key role in the function of the immune system. They are needed for normal cell division to produce the cellular components. In addition, the antibodies and other humoral agents that are released are composed of amino acids. Thus, a protein deficiency will result in defective immune function. This is seen clearly in children suffering from protein–energy malnutrition, who have an increased susceptibility to infection as a result of poor immune function. There is good evidence that certain amino acids may have a more specific role in immunonutrition. Among those being studied, glutamine, which is a precursor for glutathione, improves gut barrier function and may be an essential nutrient for a number of immune system cells. Glutamine has been described as conditionally essential in critically ill patients, when there is trauma or physiological stress. Other amino acids that have been studied in similar situations include arginine and taurine.

Transport

Many of the substances that need to be carried around the body from either the digestive system or stores to sites of action cannot travel in the blood alone, usually because they are insoluble or potentially harmful. When these substances are attached to proteins, particularly albumin or globulins, transport is facilitated. The level of carrier protein present at any time may determine the availability of the particular substance to the tissues. Haemoglobin is a transporting protein, serving to carry oxygen in the body. In this case, it is the ability of the haemoglobin molecule to take up a large amount of oxygen that provides the advantage over oxygen transport simply in solution by the blood. Reduced availability of haemoglobin (either because of iron or protein deficiency) will affect the provision of oxygen to the tissues.

In addition, transport proteins also carry substances across cell membranes, for example, during absorption in the digestive tract. As well as facilitating transport, proteins may also bind with some constituents of the body to provide a safe method of storage; for example, iron is stored in association with ferritin.

Blood Clotting

Several proteins found in plasma play an essential role in blood clotting, including prothrombin and fibrinogen. Failure to synthesize these (e.g. in deficiency of vitamin K, which acts as a cofactor) will result in prolonged bleeding times.

Other Functions

Although not its primary role, protein can serve as a source of energy when insufficient carbohydrate and fat are available to meet the body's needs: 1 g provides 17 kJ (4 kcal). Dietary protein also plays a role in satiety, and consumption of protein-rich meals is followed by an enhanced sensation of fullness.

It is also important to note that non-protein nitrogenous compounds are produced from some of the amino acids. Glycine is used in haem, nucleic acid and bile acid synthesis. Other examples include the use of tryptophan to make nicotinic acid and tyrosine in catecholamine synthesis. Proteins also form the major components of the hair and nails, as well as the structural framework of bones.

FATS

Metabolic Roles

Meeting the Energy Needs: Fat Metabolism

Fat is a concentrated source of energy. It supplies 37 kJ/g (9 cal/g), which is more than any other macronutrient. It has the advantage that a large amount of energy can be consumed in a relatively small volume of food (energy dense). This may be important for people with a small appetite or those whose energy needs are very high, such as infants, athletes or those undertaking other strenuous activity. In addition, it can be helpful when patients are being fed by a tube, where a smaller volume of feed is an advantage.

However, the disadvantage of the high energy concentration is that it is easy to over-consume energy – a small amount of fat-rich food can provide unexpectedly high fat intakes. The converse of this is that, where people have very little fat in their diet, they have to consume large volumes of food to meet their energy needs. For children, in particular, this volume may be unobtainable and this may be one of the contributory factors to undernutrition in developing countries. Adding a small amount of oil to a traditional starchy rural diet can make a great deal of difference to overall energy intake.

As well as supplying energy in the diet, fats also provide a vehicle for other essential nutrients, in particular, the fat-soluble vitamins (vitamins A, D, E and K) and the essential fatty acids. The absorption of fat-soluble vitamins from the digestive tract depends on the presence and normal digestion/absorption of fats. Thus, people on low-fat diets may be at risk of insufficient intake of these vitamins.

The storage and release of energy from adipose tissue are under continuous hormonal control, mainly by insulin and noradrenaline. It has been proposed that the adipose tissue is an essential buffer in the body to regulate fats whose levels vary with intermittent food intake (see "Storage: The Adipose Tissue" section of this chapter).

Fat Requires Specialized Proteins for Transport around the Body

Because of their hydrophobic nature, fats have to be carried around the circulation in association with hydrophilic substances, otherwise they would separate out. Chylomicrons, which facilitate the entry of digested fats into the circulation, are one example of such an association. These are the largest and lightest of a group of aggregates collectively known as lipoproteins. Lipoproteins are classified according to their density and can be separated by ultracentrifugation of a blood sample. At one end of the range are the large light chylomicrons, then, arranged in decreasing size, are the very-low-density, low-density and high-density lipoproteins, usually referred to by their acronyms VLDL (very-low-density lipoprotein), LDL (low-density lipoprotein) and HDL (high-density lipoprotein).

Fats in the blood are carried in lipoproteins, irrespective of whether they have originated from the diet or have been synthesized in the body. In both cases, the triglyceride and cholesterol esters are coated with a shell of phospholipid and apolipoprotein. The apolipoprotein provides an 'identity tag' by which the body cells recognize the particular type. The lipoproteins are not constant in their composition: they are dynamic particles, which release and pick up their constituents as they travel around the body.

Chylomicrons contain predominantly triglycerides and are thus very low in density. The major constituents of VLDLs are also triglycerides. LDLs contain mostly cholesterol and are its major carriers in the body. HDLs are predominantly made up of protein, with smaller fat contents than the other types. This accounts for their high density. There is also a difference in size, with the chylomicrons being the largest and the HDL the smallest of the particles.

Chylomicrons start to appear in the blood within 30 minutes of eating a fat-containing meal, with a peak after approximately 3 hours. They cause an increase in plasma lipid levels, and serum samples taken during this time have a milky appearance because of this. Some chylomicrons may continue to enter into the blood after a fat-rich meal over a period of up to 14 hours.

As chylomicrons circulate in the blood, fats are removed from them by specific lipoprotein lipases (LPLs) in the blood vessel walls, especially in the liver, skeletal muscle and adipose tissue, and free fatty acids and glycerol are released. The body uses these products for particular metabolic processes needed at the time. This may involve fuelling muscle contraction or perhaps being stored in the adipose tissue for subsequent use. Chylomicrons may also pass some of their free cholesterol to HDLs.

The remnants of the chylomicrons are eventually broken down in the liver and used to make other lipoproteins. The liver cells synthesize fat (endogenous fats) brought in from fatty acids; cholesterol is also synthesized. Eventually, the fats made in the liver are packaged as VLDLs and exported into the rest of the body.

As the VLDLs travel through the body, LPL removes their triglycerides, in much the same way as for chylomicrons. Both chylomicrons and VLDLs contain the apolipoprotein CII, which activates LPL. As they lose triglycerides, the VLDLs become smaller and the proportion of cholesterol in them increases. Thus, they are transformed into LDLs.

One other transformation also occurs. This is the loss of some of the apolipoprotein, so that the remaining 'identity tag' is that of the LDLs. This is apolipoprotein B_{100} (apo-B_{100}) and is vital for the normal metabolic functioning of LDLs.

The function of LDL is to act as the major carrier of cholesterol, taking it to the tissues where it is needed in cell membranes or for synthesis of metabolites, such as steroid hormones. Specific receptors for apo-B_{100} are present on cell surfaces. These allow the LDLs to attach to the cell, and the whole LDL–receptor complex is taken into the cell, where it is broken down by enzymes. The activity and number of receptor sites can vary, thus controlling cholesterol uptake by cells. In the genetically determined condition familial hypercholesterolaemia, subjects lack the LDL receptor, resulting in high circulating levels of LDLs.

HDLs are responsible for the removal of spare or surplus cholesterol as well as apolipoproteins from cells and other lipoproteins; this is known as reverse cholesterol transport. When cholesterol

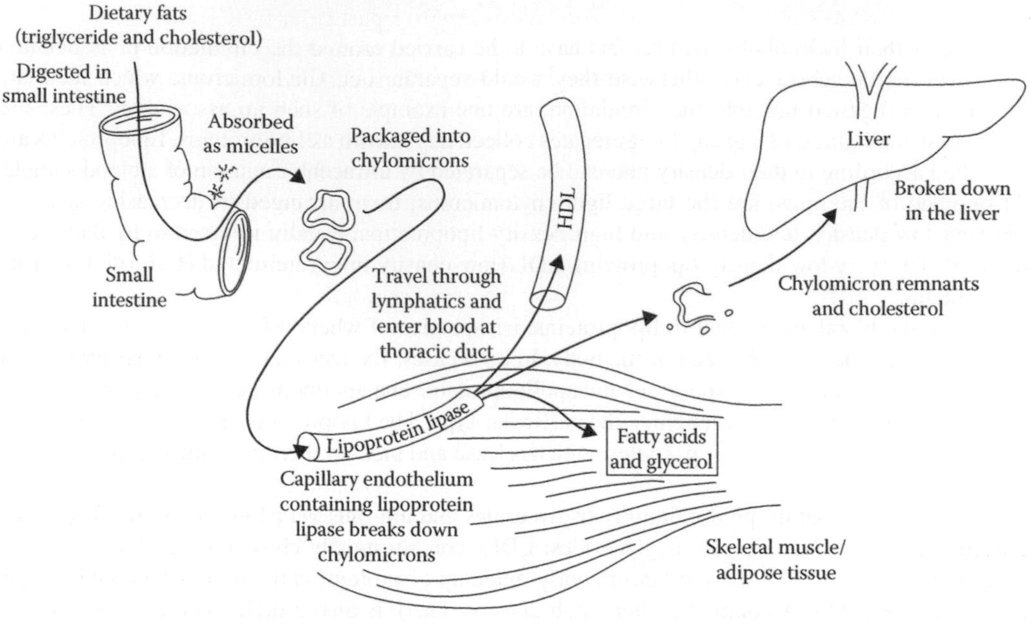

FIGURE 11.3 Exogenous lipid transport.

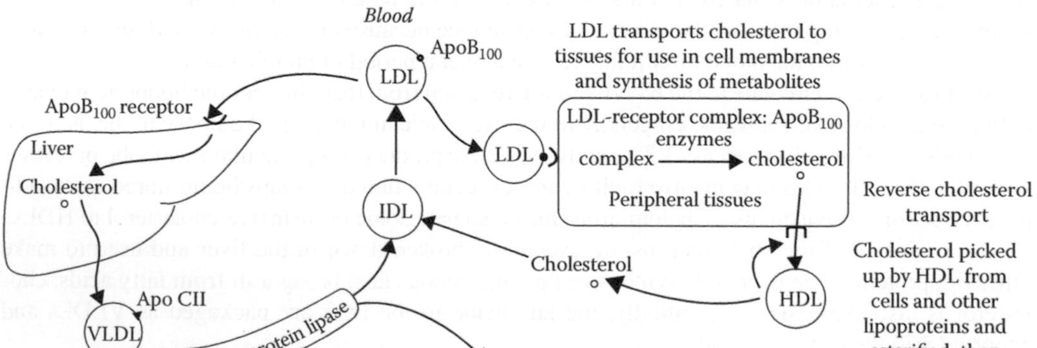

FIGURE 11.4 Endogenous lipid transport and metabolism.

is picked up by the HDLs, it quickly becomes esterified, which allows it to be taken into the hydrophobic core of the lipoprotein. In this way, the outer layer of the HDL maintains a diffusion gradient for more cholesterol to be picked up. This system allows cholesterol to be removed from the tissues and taken to the liver. This completes the lipid transport cycle (Figures 11.3 and 11.4).

Because LDLs and HDLs are so intimately involved with cholesterol transport, they are believed to be closely associated with the development of atheroma and particularly of heart disease. Consequently, factors influencing the circulating levels of LDLs and HDLs have been extensively studied. It is believed that they are influenced by a number of factors, including genetics, hormone levels, age, gender, smoking, exercise and diet. One such gene, which appears to be particularly important, is that for apolipoprotein E. Several variants have been identified, which account for a proportion of the variation in LDL levels within a population. Variants may also determine the response of lipoprotein levels to changes in dietary factors and the rate of clearance from the circulation.

Storage: The Adipose Tissue

The body is able to store fat as an energy reserve, in specialized cells, called adipocytes, which are found in adipose tissue. The adipocytes extract triglycerides from passing lipoproteins by the action of the enzyme LPL. This enzyme is activated by insulin and is, therefore, most active in the postprandial phase (after meals). The triglycerides are broken down by LPL, taken into the adipose tissue cell and then reassembled into new triglycerides for storage. The storage and release of fat is a dynamic process, with a continuous flux of fats into and out of the cells. A great deal of fat storage occurs after meals, when there are increased numbers of chylomicrons and VLDLs in the circulation. In theory, fat may be synthesized from carbohydrate, but this happens only in exceptional circumstances of extremely high carbohydrate intakes and is very inefficient. Other sites in the body can also make fat, in particular, the liver and mammary gland during lactation. However, the liver does not normally store significant quantities of fat; a liver loaded with fat is generally diseased. The mammary gland is able to synthesize shorter chain fatty acids, with lauric and myristic acids predominating (C12 and C14).

Adipocytes make up only about half of the total cell numbers within adipose tissue; fibroblasts, macrophages and vascular tissue are other important components. Adipose tissue plays a major role in metabolism. Two types of adipose tissue have now been identified – the predominant form, white adipose tissue (WAT), and brown adipose tissue (BAT), which occurs in much smaller amounts. BAT differs from WAT in several respects, most noticeably, in having many more mitochondria, blood capillaries and nerve fibres than the white tissue. This type of fat is much more widespread in newborns and provides a means of heat generation at this critical stage of life, before shivering mechanisms develop. It used to be thought that brown fat then disappeared, but more recent research suggests that small amounts persist into adult life and may play a part in generating heat as a means of ridding the body of surplus energy.

The WAT cells store fat as a single droplet, which fills almost the entire cell contents, pushing the remaining organelles to the very edges of the cell. The fat stored in the body is a reflection of the type of dietary fat; thus, an individual eating a diet rich in polyunsaturated fats will have more of these in their adipose tissue. On the other hand, a person who has small fat stores and consumes little fat will have adipose tissue fats that are more typical of fat synthesized in the body containing mainly palmitic, stearic and oleic acids.

The number of fat cells has been estimated at about 5×10^{10} in the adult. There has been considerable debate about the means of expansion of fat stores. This can occur by hyperplasia, which is an increase in cell number, or by hypertrophy, which is an increase in size of existing cells. The size of adipocytes is related to their fat stores, so these will vary with the flux of fat into and out of stores. As fat stores increase, it is postulated that new cells are formed from pre-adipocytes already present in the body. Whether adipocytes can be lost on reduction of fat stores is still under debate, although there is evidence that apoptosis (programmed cell death) can occur, but the significance of this in individuals is unknown.

It has also become clear that adipose tissue depots to an extent may be self-regulatory and that depots in various parts of the body respond differently to physiological demands. In particular, there are differences between fat stored in the abdominal region and that in the thighs and buttocks. The fat adjacent to lymph nodes is proposed as having an important role in supporting the immune system and may become much larger in chronic inflammatory states at the expense of other fat depots, resulting in changes in body fat distribution. This has been noted in HIV infection and Crohn's disease.

The ability to store fat as an energy reserve offers an additional benefit, that of insulation and protection. Adipose tissue covers some of our more delicate organs, such as the kidneys, spleen, spinal cord and brain, to protect them from injury. This protective fat is used less readily as fuel in a fasting individual. Most of the fuel-storing adipose tissue is found under the skin, as subcutaneous fat. Here, it also provides insulation to facilitate the maintenance of body temperature. In hot climates, this can be a disadvantage, with overweight individuals sweating readily to lose heat. On the other hand, sufferers from anorexia nervosa, who have little subcutaneous fat, will feel cold even on a warm day and will dress in several layers of clothing both to provide extra warmth and perhaps to disguise their extreme thinness. The body also stores fat-soluble vitamins in its adipose tissue.

Adipose Tissue and Metabolic Regulation

Adipose tissue is now recognized as having a role as a source of many metabolic regulators, with more factors still being discovered. The most important of these has been leptin, discovered in 1994, which is produced predominantly by adipose tissue, but has also been shown to be secreted by other organs such as the stomach, mammary gland and placenta. Leptin receptors are also found in adipose tissue but are principally sited in the hypothalamus. Leptin has been shown to interact with neuropeptides in the brain to inhibit food intake. It also plays a role in energy expenditure, probably via BAT, and is a signal to the reproductive system in sexual maturation. Leptin release is under the control of the sympathetic nervous system.

There are many other factors released by adipose tissue with diverse actions and some as yet unidentified.

- Proteins involved in lipid and lipoprotein metabolism include LPL and cholesteryl ester transfer protein, important in accumulation of cholesteryl ester in WAT.
- Proteins that play a role in blood pressure regulation and blood clotting are also secreted and may be a link with disorders of these processes in obesity.
- Immune function is also influenced by secretory products from the adipose tissue, including cytokines (most notably tumour necrosis factor α (TNFα) and complement system products. The cytokines in turn appear to have a regulatory role in various aspects of adipose tissue function. The immune system uses up to 15% of the body's resting metabolic rate, and it may be that the close relationship between adipose tissue energy stores and the immune system is a means of ensuring that adequate energy can be provided when the immune system is under stress. TNFα inhibits fat storage and would, therefore, make fatty acids immediately available.
- Metallothionein is a stress response protein that acts as an antioxidant and may protect fatty acids in adipose tissue from damage by free radicals during high rates of oxygen utilization.

Fat Utilization

Substrate utilization for energy during exercise is covered in Chapter 22, pp. 423–426.

The body uses stored fat as its major energy supply, releasing non-esterified fatty acids (NEFA) into the circulation under the influence of noradrenaline released by the sympathetic nervous system. At most levels of activity, fat provides a significant proportion of the energy used. It is only when we exercise very intensively (e.g. running the 100 m sprint) that all the energy comes from carbohydrate, since fat cannot be metabolized sufficiently quickly. The lower the level of activity, the greater the proportion of energy that comes from fat. However, some glucose continues to be used for metabolism as the brain, nervous system and red blood cells require it. Under normal circumstances, glucose levels are maintained by hormones such as insulin, adrenaline and cortisol, which ensure that sufficient is present to fuel these essential tissues and organs. If there is no supply of glucose entering the body, organs such as the liver are capable of making glucose from protein residues and glycerol from fat breakdown (see Figure 11.5).

Fat breakdown to supply ATP occurs by the successive splitting of acetic acid molecules from the ends of long-chain fatty acids. These acetic acid molecules then enter the same common pathway that serves carbohydrate metabolism. For complete oxidation, some carbohydrate must be present.

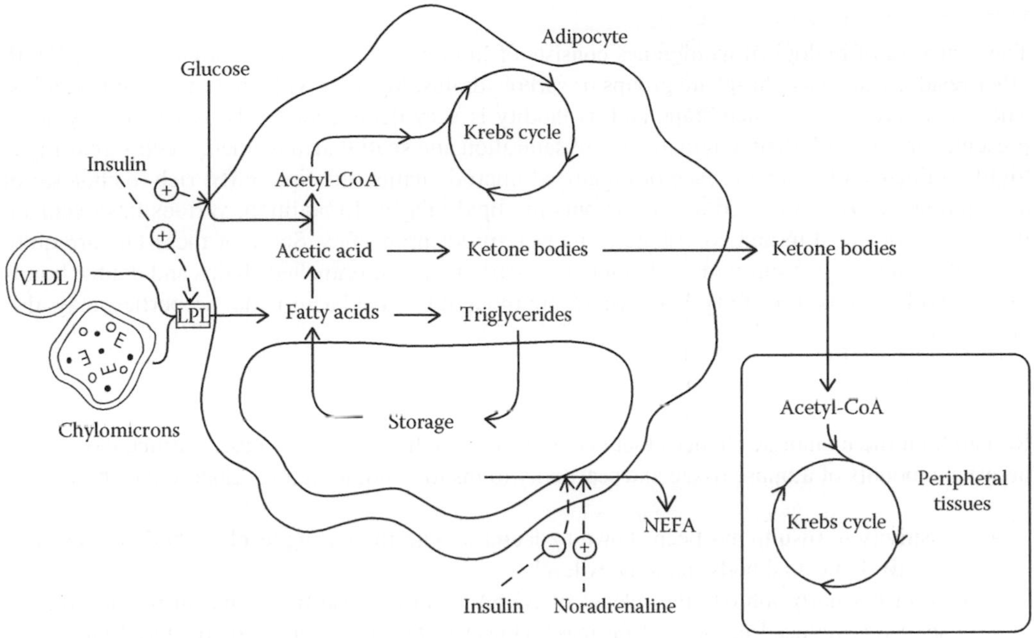

FIGURE 11.5 The role of adipose tissue in metabolism.

If there is no glucose or glycogen, then acetic acid molecules combine in pairs to form ketone bodies. Once formed, ketone bodies are sent to the peripheral tissues, where they can be converted back to acetyl coenzyme A and used in the normal Krebs (or citric acid) cycle. A mild rise in ketone body production (ketosis) will occur whenever fat mobilization occurs, for example, during moderate exercise, overnight fast and conditions associated with low food intake, such as acute gastroenteritis or the nausea and vomiting of early pregnancy. A more severe type of ketosis causing mental confusion or coma, as well as physiological changes (muscular weakness and overbreathing), may occur in severe states of these kinds and also in diabetes mellitus. In this case, insulin lack prevents normal glucose entry into cells and thus glucose oxidation. Symptoms associated with mild ketosis include lethargy, headache and loss of appetite. These are very general, however, and may be caused by many other factors.

If we fast, the body rapidly metabolizes body fat. Initially, there is also rapid breakdown of lean tissue as the body uses protein residues to maintain blood glucose supplies. After a number of days, however, the brain and nervous system adapt to the use of ketone bodies for energy, and survival using fat stores becomes possible. Inevitably, a fatter person will be able to survive longer than one with limited fat stores at the outset.

Functions of Fat in the Body

Fat occurs throughout the body, as part of the structure of every cell membrane, as well as being found in discrete areas as adipose tissue. Fat is essential in body composition and, as such, has many diverse functions in the body. These are the following:

- Structure
- Storage
- Metabolism

It should be remembered, however, that these categories are not separate and distinct from one another, and there is considerable overlap between them.

Structure of Membranes

The structure of biological membranes consists of lipid molecules that are often associated with other residues, such as phosphate groups or carbohydrates, together with cholesterol and proteins. The exact nature of the membrane and its fluidity is very dependent on the types of fatty acids present, varying with their length, degree of saturation and spatial arrangement – cell signalling is highly influenced by the presence of organized microdomains (the lipid rafts) rich in cholesterol and sphingomyelin compared to the surrounding lipid bilayer. In addition, various fats occur on the surface of the skin and contribute to its waterproof properties. Some of these fats are quite unusual, containing chains with odd numbers of carbon atoms, branched chains and double bonds in unusual locations. Free fatty acids, which are thought to have bactericidal properties, may also be present.

Link with Glucose Metabolism: Insulin Resistance

Research on the metabolic changes that occur in overweight and obesity has identified close links between amounts of adipose tissue and sensitivity to insulin and, therefore, glucose metabolism.

- Sensitivity to insulin has been shown to decrease with increasing levels of body fat, even at relatively normal body mass index levels.
- Insulin normally inhibits the release of NEFA from adipose tissue, but in obesity, this response is reduced per unit of fat mass. However, because there is more stored fat, the total amount of NEFA released is actually increased.
- The removal of triglycerides (as chylomicrons or VLDL) from the circulation by the action of LPL may also be depressed by reduced sensitivity of this enzyme to insulin.
- The overall consequence is a chronically raised level of circulating fats (lipaemia), which deposit in a number of tissues, including liver and skeletal muscle. This suppresses glucose utilization by muscle, stimulates the production of glucose in the liver and stimulates insulin release. High levels of NEFA may also damage the pancreatic β-cells that secrete insulin. Thus, there is interference with the normal insulin-mediated glucose disposal, owing to a failure of the buffer capacity of the adipose tissue (see Figure 11.6).

Steroid Metabolism

Cholesterol is essential in the body. It is the precursor for the synthesis of the steroid hormones, which include those produced in the adrenal gland, as well as the sex hormones. It is also a prerequisite for the formation of vitamin D in the skin. In addition, cholesterol is used in the manufacture of bile salts in the liver, which, as we saw earlier in this chapter, are vital in the normal digestion of dietary fats. The bile salts can be reabsorbed from the lower gut and reused by the liver. Some, however, can be trapped in the faeces and removed from the body. In this case, more bile salts have to be synthesized from cholesterol. Adipose tissue is a major site for storage of cholesterol.

Many of the steroid hormones are converted to their active form in the tissue. This includes formation of oestradiol from oestrone, testosterone from androstenedione and oestrogens from androgens. The last of these can form an important source of female hormones in overweight individuals, which may have positive benefits in terms of maintaining bone health after the menopause but also negative consequences in increasing the risk of hormone-dependent tumours.

Essential Fatty Acids

There are two major metabolic roles for the essential fatty acids. The presence of essential fatty acids in the membranes of cells and their organelles contributes to the stability and integrity of these membranes. Signs of deficiency include changes in the properties of membranes, particularly increases in permeability. These are accompanied by reduced efficiency of energy utilization and,

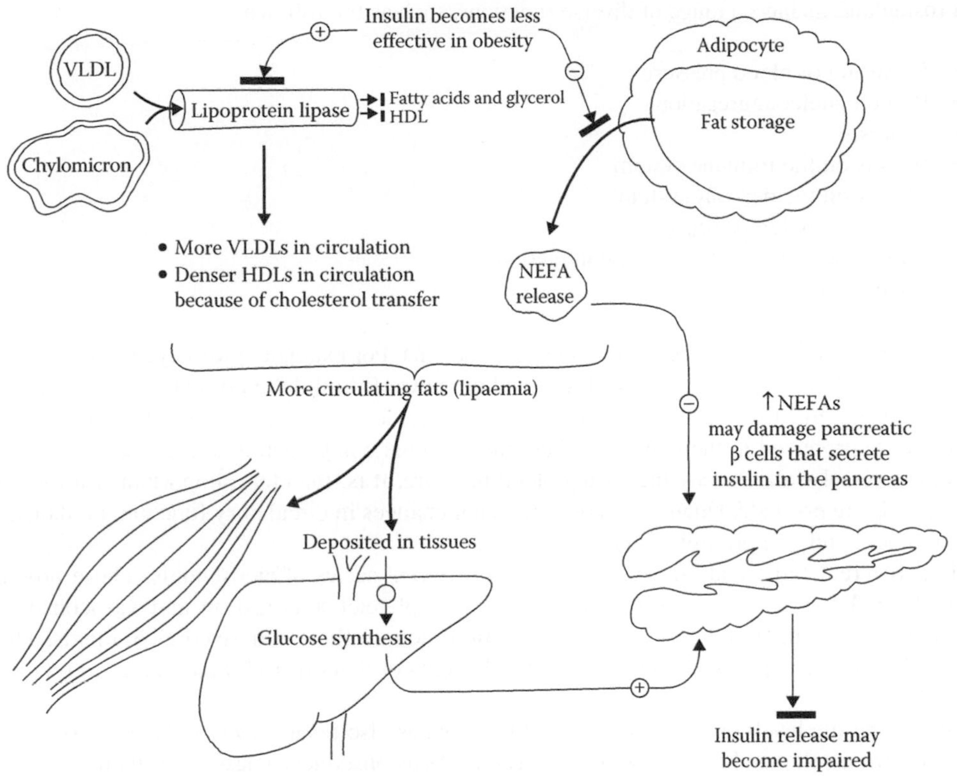

FIGURE 11.6 Aspects of insulin resistance.

therefore, poorer growth. The *n*-3 acids are of particular importance in the membranes of the nervous system and brain, as well as the retina. Docosahexaenoic acid (22:6) is particularly concentrated in the retina, and levels increase in the fetal brain and retina in the later stages of pregnancy. Development continues in early childhood, and a supply of these long-chain fatty acids is essential to optimize neurological development.

The role of fatty acids in coronary heart disease is covered further in Chapter 14, pp. 281–285.

In addition, essential fatty acids are the precursors of a family of bioactive compounds called eicosanoids, which act as metabolic regulators in a number of key functions. Two major pathways for eicosanoid production exist. Prostaglandins, prostacyclins and thromboxanes are made by the cyclooxygenase pathway, and leukotrienes are produced by the lipoxygenase pathway. Eicosanoids are derived from fatty acids with 20 carbon atoms. Thus, the majority originate from arachidonic acid (20:4), which is a member of the *n*-6 fatty acid family and is produced in the body from the essential fatty acid, linoleic acid. However, some are produced from eicosapentaenoic acid (20:5), which is a member of the *n*-3 family, made in the body from the essential fatty acid, alpha-linolenic acid. It is believed that a predominance of *n*-6 acids in the body may prevent the formation of eicosanoids of the *n*-3 series. Prostaglandins and other eicosanoids are very potent substances; therefore, they are produced at the site of action and very quickly inactivated. They are made from essential fatty acids contained in the phospholipids of cell membranes. Thus, although they may be described as 'hormone-like', they do not circulate in the blood in the same way. Their release is triggered by a variety of physiological stimuli, including hormones, such as adrenaline, antigen–antibody reactions and mechanical damage or injury.

Prostaglandins have a range of diverse functions, such as the following:

- Lowering of blood pressure
- Blood platelet aggregation
- Diuresis
- Effects on the immune system
- Effects on the nervous system
- Rise in body temperature
- Stimulation of smooth muscle contraction
- Gastric secretion

Some members of the eicosanoids have opposing actions. For example, prostacyclins are produced in the endothelial lining of the arterial wall and are powerful inhibitors of platelet aggregation, as well as causing the artery walls to relax. They, therefore, lower blood pressure. In contrast, thromboxanes are produced in the platelets, where they stimulate aggregation and cause contraction of the blood vessel wall, thereby increasing blood pressure. It is, therefore, important that these two eicosanoids are normally balanced, to prevent major changes in circulatory function. Leukotrienes, on the other hand, are pro-inflammatory.

The different fatty acid families give rise to different series of eicosanoids. Those produced from the *n*-3 family have less powerful effects on platelet aggregation and vasoconstriction (haemodynamic functioning) and on inflammation than do the *n*-6 derived eicosanoids. This is believed to be the explanation for the potential benefits of fish oils rich in *n*-3 acids in relation to heart disease.

Increasing the levels of *n*-3 fatty acids in the body has also been shown to displace some of the *n*-6 acids from cell membranes of white blood cells. As a consequence, less pro-inflammatory eicosanoids are produced as part of the immune response. In addition, *n*-3 acids may affect other parts of the immune response, such as cytokine activation. These effects are of potential benefit in chronic inflammatory conditions, and supplementation with fish oils has been shown to reduce symptoms in subjects with rheumatoid arthritis. There are potential benefits also in asthma, psoriasis and Crohn's disease, although more research is needed in these areas.

CARBOHYDRATES

Carbohydrates are an important source of energy for the body, providing glucose for immediate use and glycogen reserves. All the cells of the body require glucose and some, such as the brain, nervous system and developing red blood cells, are 'obligatory' users of glucose. We are able to make some glucose from proteins and fats in the process of gluconeogenesis. This enables the body to survive when the glycogen stores are depleted and no carbohydrate has been eaten. Almost all the body's amino acids (those known as glucogenic) and the glycerol part of triglycerides (about 5% of the weight of fat) but not the fatty acids can be converted to glucose. However, using protein to make glucose is potentially harmful, since tissue protein may be broken down. This happens in starvation both in the early stages before the body adapts to using more fats for essential energy and in the final stages when body fat stores have been depleted, and the body's structural protein is being used for energy.

A further problem arises when there is insufficient carbohydrate available to complete fat metabolism. In the absence of carbohydrate, acetyl coenzyme A accumulates and condenses to form ketone bodies. This state, known as ketosis, is associated with mild disturbances of cellular function and is an early indication of insufficient carbohydrate availability in the body. So, even though glucose can be produced from non-carbohydrate sources, the processes are inefficient and potentially harmful and indicate a specific need for carbohydrate in the diet to supply energy.

Carbohydrates Metabolism

Carbohydrate metabolism is an elegant yet complex set of biochemical events, which ultimately enable to store carbohydrates or mobilize them from storage.

Storage	Glycogenesis	Excess glucose is converted into glycogen as a cellular storage mechanism.
	Lipogenesis	Glucose is metabolized acetyl-CoA, which is converted to fatty acids as a storage mechanism.
Mobilization	Glycolysis	Glucose is oxidized to obtain ATP and pyruvate.
	Glycogenolysis	Glycogen is broken down into glucose.
	Gluconeogenesis	Specific amino acids are converted to glucose molecules (de novo synthesis).

Carbohydrate Storage

Glycogenesis

In discussing carbohydrate metabolism in the body, it is simpler to consider glucose, fructose and galactose. These travel in the bloodstream from the small intestine to the liver, where they are stored as long chains of glucose units in the form of glycogen. The liver stores one-third of the body's total glycogen (about 150 g). The remainder of the glucose may pass on to the muscles, where it is also stored as glycogen. Storage of glycogen is encouraged by insulin, the hormone produced by the β cells of the pancreas. Liver glycogen is readily transformed back into glucose whenever the blood sugar level falls below about 4 mmol/L. Thus, glucose can continue to supply energy to the brain, central nervous system and other organs whether the person has eaten or not. The glucose from the blood passes into these tissues where it is oxidized and energy is released by means of one of several pathways (glycolysis, tricarboxylic acid cycle, hexose monophosphate pathway), depending on circumstances. A number of vitamins are needed to achieve this oxidation, most notably thiamin, riboflavin and nicotinic acid. Insulin is also needed to facilitate the entry of the glucose into tissues (see Figure 11.7). Muscle glycogen is not used to maintain blood sugar levels; rather its role is to provide energy directly for muscle contraction.

Glycogen is stored in association with water and is a bulky way of storing energy. Thus, the body only contains enough glycogen to provide energy for relatively short periods of time, although new research suggests that glycogen stores are well controlled.

Lipogenesis

Longer-term energy stores are maintained in the form of fat and, as a last resort, as protein. If we take in more carbohydrate than we need, the body will use the glucose to fill its glycogen stores and then could convert the remaining glucose into the more permanent storage form – fat. Unlike the limited storage capacity for glycogen, the body can store unlimited amounts of fat. In practice, this does not occur in humans to any significant extent, and carbohydrate metabolism is stimulated to utilize the excess carbohydrate. As a consequence, energy from fat is not used and fat may be stored. Fat synthesis from carbohydrate only occurs when extremely large amounts of carbohydrate are consumed over a period of days.

Mobilization of Carbohydrates

Glycogenolysis/Glycolysis

Glycogenolysis takes place in liver and muscle tissue, to release glucose-6-phosphate. It is important for blood glucose homeostasis and mostly regulated by glucagon and insulin. Glycolysis is a different pathway, which converts glucose (and glucose-6-phosphate) into pyruvate; during this process, energy is released in the form of ATP and NADH. Glycolysis does not require oxygen.

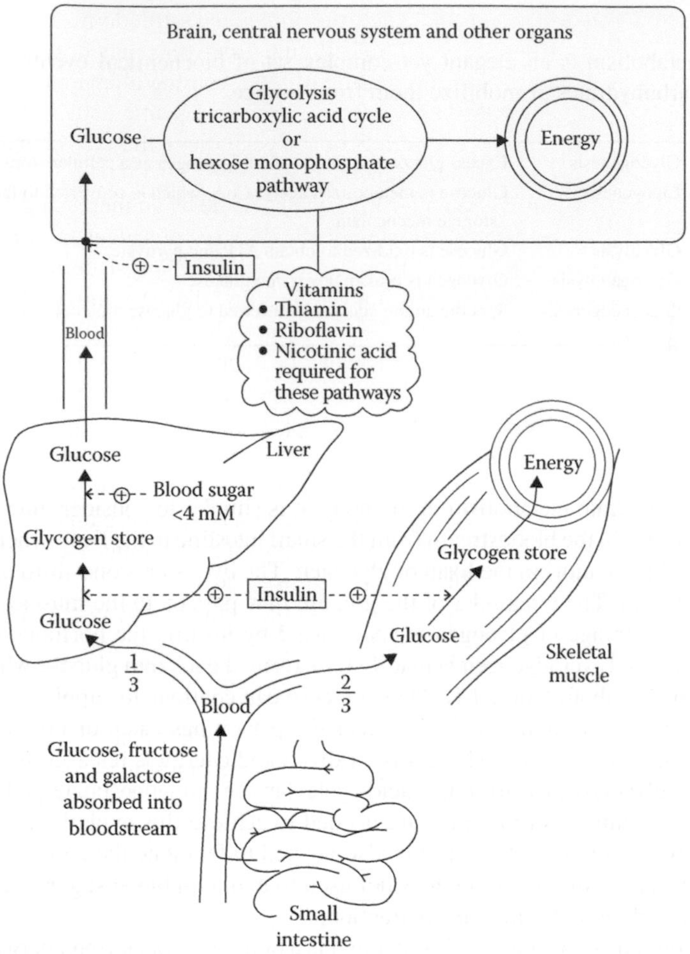

FIGURE 11.7 Metabolism of carbohydrates.

Gluconeogenesis

We are able to 'make' small amounts of glucose from proteins (glucogenic amino acids) and from the glycerol skeleton of triglycerides (but not the fatty acid chains) in the process of gluconeogenesis. This enables the body to survive when the glycogen stores are depleted and no carbohydrate has been eaten. However, using protein to make glucose is potentially harmful, since tissue protein has to be broken down. This happens in starvation both in the early stages before the body adapts to using more fats for essential energy, and in the final stages when body fat stores have been depleted, and the body's structural protein is being used for energy.

A further problem arises when there is insufficient carbohydrate available to complete fat metabolism. In the absence of carbohydrate, acetyl coenzyme A accumulates and condenses to form ketone bodies. This state, known as ketosis, is associated with mild disturbances of cellular function and is an early indication of insufficient carbohydrate availability in the body. So, even though glucose can be produced from non-carbohydrate sources and the brain can metabolize and obtain energy from ketone bodies, the processes are inefficient and potentially harmful, and indicate a specific need for carbohydrate in the diet to supply energy.

Metabolic Consequences of Sugar Intake

When sucrose is fed to subjects at levels of 18%–33% of total energy intake, a number of changes occur in the serum profile. It is believed that these results from a rapid influx of sugars into the circulation. The changes include the following:

- Increased fasting plasma triglycerides in men and postmenopausal women
- Decreased HDL cholesterol
- Increased fasting insulin levels

It is suggested that these effects are particularly noticeable in a subsection of the population, possibly about 15%, who are deemed 'carbohydrate sensitive'. These changes in serum lipids and insulin have all been associated with disease, although a direct casual link with sugars is not proven. Diseases that may be implicated include coronary heart disease, diabetes, gallstones, hypertension and kidney stones.

Other Physiological Roles of Carbohydrates

In addition to their primary role as a substrate for energy metabolism, carbohydrates have a variety of other physiological roles due to their diverse range of chemical and physical properties. They are used in the synthesis of various metabolically active complexes. Glycoproteins are important components of cellular membranes, in particular on the extracellular surface. They are also found as circulating proteins in blood or plasma. Glycolipids, such as sphingolipids and gangliosides, have roles at receptor sites on cells and in synaptic transmission.

Mucopolysaccharides have important water-holding or binding properties in many sites of the body; they occur in basement membranes and in intercellular cement and form an integral part of cartilage, tendon, skin and synovial fluid. Disorders of mucopolysaccharide metabolism have been associated with a number of disease states. Little is currently known about the influence of dietary sugars on these compounds or on specific quantitative requirements.

Gut Health

Carbohydrates that cannot be digested in the small intestine are delivered to the large intestine intact and play an important role in colon health. This includes non-starch polysaccharides (NSPs – cellulose and hemicelluloses such as pectins, xylans, gums and mucilages), oligosaccharides (fructo-/galacto-oligosaccharides [FOS/GOS], raftilose, maltodextrins, fructans, etc.) and resistant starch. These carbohydrates are either partially or completely fermented by colonic bacteria to form short-chain fatty acids acetate, butyrate and propionic acid. Those that are insoluble and therefore more resistant to fermentation, such as cellulose and some hemicelluloses, add faecal bulk and can therefore increase gut transit time and improve colon strength and muscle tone. Soluble NSPs, such as β-glucan, pectin, guar gum, increase the viscosity of the gut lumen contents and are more readily fermented by colonic bacteria. It has been shown that there is a positive relationship between their consumption and a decreased risk of cardiovascular disease, which is thought to be mediated by a reduction in LDL cholesterol (see Figure 11.8).

There are three possible mechanisms at play:

1. Increased viscosity in the small intestine reduces reabsorption of bile salts into the enterohepatic circulation, thus depleting bile salts in liver and necessitating the use of endogenous cholesterol to produce more.
2. Insulin activates HMG-CoAR which is required to synthesis cholesterol. Increased viscosity in the small intestine slows down glucose absorption and reduces insulin production which in turn reduces HMG-CoAR production.

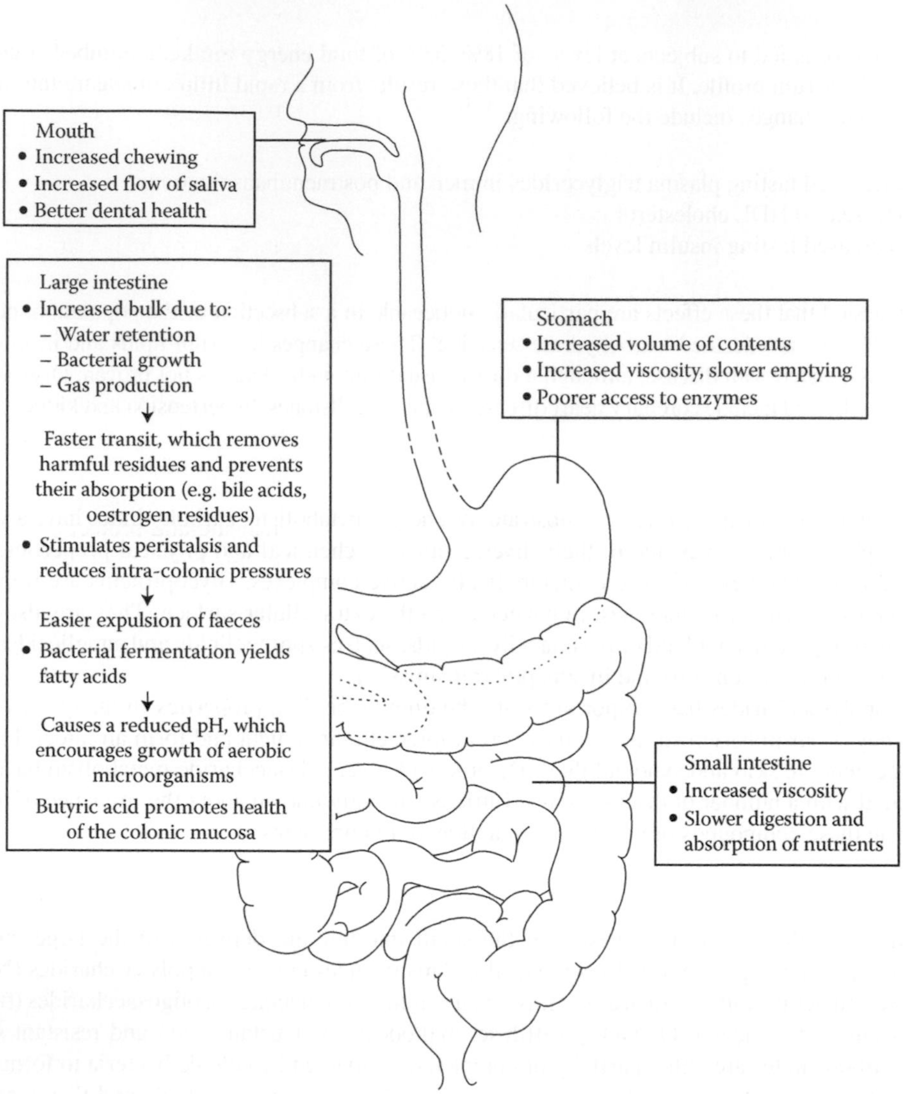
Mouth
• Increased chewing
• Increased flow of saliva
• Better dental health
Large intestine
• Increased bulk due to:
– Water retention
– Bacterial growth
– Gas production
Faster transit, which removes harmful residues and prevents their absorption (e.g. bile acids, oestrogen residues)
• Stimulates peristalsis and reduces intra-colonic pressures
Easier expulsion of faeces
• Bacterial fermentation yields fatty acids
Causes a reduced pH, which encourages growth of aerobic microorganisms
Butyric acid promotes health of the colonic mucosa
Stomach
• Increased volume of contents
• Increased viscosity, slower emptying
• Poorer access to enzymes
Small intestine
• Increased viscosity
• Slower digestion and absorption of nutrients

FIGURE 11.8 Summary of the effects of non-starch polysaccharides in the digestive tract.

3. Soluble NSPs are fermented to short chain fatty acids (SCFA) in the large intestine, which are also thought to inhibit HMG-CoAR and therefore reduce endogenous cholesterol synthesis, particularly propionate.

Oligosaccharides are found naturally in many plants and are particularly abundant in chicory root and Jerusalem artichokes. FOS and GOS consist of short chains of fructose and galactose molecules respectively and are a good substrate for colonic bacteria fermentation. As such, they are often added to functional foods as prebiotics. Different oligosaccharides are preferred by different colonic bacteria and therefore produce different SCFA profiles. Butyrate, in particular, is thought to be protective of colonic tissue, and an association has been suggested with a reduced risk of colon cancer and ulcerative colitis. Human breast milk is particularly rich in oligosaccharides (human milk oligosaccharides [HMOs]), and this is thought to confer a number of health benefits on the exclusively breastfed infant. A human baby is born with a sterile gut. Initial colonization occurs during the birth process, and HMOs have a prebiotic effect to promote the development of a healthy gut microflora, improve stool production, reduce constipation and protect against infection. A small percentage of HMO is believed to be absorbed intact in the small intestine and later excreted in the urine, which has prompted speculation on possible systemic effects, for example, in the immune system or in the context of neuronal development.

SUMMARY

1. Proteins fulfil many functions in the body, acting as hormones, enzymes, carriers and maintaining homeostasis.
2. As well as providing the primary substrate for energy metabolism, carbohydrates also have a key role in cell signalling (as glycoproteins) and at cell receptor sites and in synaptic transmission (as glycolipids).
3. Fat is transported in the circulation in the form of lipoproteins, which vary in their content of triglycerides and cholesterol.
4. Essential fatty acids are specifically needed in the diet in small amounts for membrane structure and synthesis of eicosanoids.
5. Stored fat is an important energy reserve and serves to insulate and protect the body. It also has important regulatory roles in metabolism and as a secretory organ for a number of bioactive factors.

STUDY QUESTIONS

1. Discuss the key aspects of carbohydrate metabolism of the body in the
   a. Fasted state
   b. Fed state
   c. Starved state
2. Discuss the metabolic fate of the NSP which escapes digestion and accumulates in the colon.
3. What are the main functions of dietary fatty acids in the body?

BIBLIOGRAPHY AND FURTHER READING

Asher, G., & Sassone-Corsi, P. (2015). Time for food: the intimate interplay between nutrition, metabolism, and the circadian clock. Cell, 161(1), 84–92.

Calder, P.C. 2012. Mechanisms of action of (*n*-3) fatty acids. *The Journal of Nutrition* 142(3), 592S–599S.

DoH (UK Department of Health). 1991. Dietary reference values for food energy and nutrients in the United Kingdom. Report on Health and Social Subjects No. 41. Report of the Panel on Dietary Reference Values of the Committee on Medical Aspects of Food Policy. London, UK: HMSO.

Gura, T. 2014. Nature's first functional food. *Science* 345(6198), 747–749.

Hardy, K., Brand-Miller, J., Brown, K.D., Thomas, M.G. and Copeland, L. 2015. The importance of dietary carbohydrate in human evolution. *The Quarterly Review of Biology* 90(3), 251–268.

Hu, T., Mills, K.T., Yao, L. et al. 2012. Effects of low-carbohydrate diets versus low-fat diets on metabolic risk factors: A meta-analysis of randomized controlled clinical trials. *American Journal of Epidemiology* 176(Suppl. 7), S44–S54.

Martens, E.A. and Westerterp-Plantenga, M.S. 2014. Protein diets, body weight loss and weight maintenance. *Current Opinion in Clinical Nutrition and Metabolic Care* 17(1), 75–79.

Pond, C.M. 2001. Long-term changes in adipose tissue in human disease. *Proceedings of the Nutrition Society* 60, 365–374.

Trayhurn, P. and Beattie, J.H. 2001. Physiological role of adipose tissue: White adipose tissue as an endocrine and secretory organ. *Proceedings of the Nutrition Society* 60, 329–339.

Tremaroli, V. and Bäckhed, F. 2012. Functional interactions between the gut microbiota and host metabolism. *Nature* 489(7415), 242–249.

Westerterp-Plantenga, M.S., Lemmens, S.G. and Westerterp, K.R. 2012. Dietary protein – Its role in satiety, energetics, weight loss and health. *British Journal of Nutrition* 108(S2), S105–S112.

12 Metabolism and Function of Micronutrients

AIMS

The aims of this chapter are to

- Describe the functions of vitamins and minerals in the body.
- Highlight the contribution of key vitamin and minerals to essential metabolic processed.
- Identify the deficiency diseases relevant to key micronutrients.

Overt micronutrient deficiency diseases are seldom due to dietary insufficiency in industrialized countries. Indeed, a main cause would be another clinical deficiency, such as vitamin B_{12} deficiency caused by failure to secrete intrinsic factor. Worldwide, the most common dietary deficiencies are vitamin A, iron and iodine, affecting women of child-bearing age and their offspring in particular.

The dietary sources of vitamins are covered in Chapter 4, pp. 61–74.

VITAMINS

The physiological functions of vitamins and the associated deficiency diseases are summarized in Table 12.1. The are broadly categorised as fat-soluble, with substantial storage thus resistant to periods of dietary insufficiency (vitamins A, D, E, K), and water-soluble, with little storage in the body so required daily (vitamins B and C).

Vitamin A

Most vitamin A is stored in the liver and the size of the stores can be used to assess vitamin status. It is transported to its target sites, attached to a specific retinol-binding protein (RBP), and a pre-albumin in the plasma. This double carrier molecule is too large to be excreted through the kidneys, which protects the body from loss of vitamin A, and is received on target tissues by specific receptors.

Retinol levels in the plasma do not reflect intake and are not a good indicator of vitamin status because of the size of liver stores. However, a normal status is indicated when levels are in the range of 20–50 mg/dL. Plasma retinol levels are generally tightly controlled, but may be altered during inflammatory disease states, when the synthesis of RBP is reduced.

Carotenoids, which have some antioxidant properties, also occur in the plasma and tend to reflect dietary intake; lutein comprises 10%–40% of plasma carotenoids and may be a useful marker of green vegetable intakes. Lycopene is the most potent antioxidant, found mainly in tomatoes and water melon. Beta-carotene, from many green vegetables as well as carrots, is responsible for the orange colouring of the palms of high-consumers.

The different forms of vitamin A appear to have differing functions in the body.

TABLE 12.1
Physiological Functions of Vitamins and Associated Deficiency Diseases

Vitamins	Physiological Functions	Known Deficiency Diseases
A – Retinol, beta-carotene	Visual pigments, gene expression, cell differentiation, antioxidant	Night blindness, xerophthalmia, keratinization of the skin
D – Calciferol	Calcium homeostasis, cell maturation in small intestine, insulin secretion	Rickets (poor mineralization of bone), osteomalacia (demineralization of bone)
E – Tocopherols	Antioxidant in cell membranes	Rare – serious neurological dysfunction
K – Phylloquinone, menaquinones	Coenzyme for enzymes of blood clotting and bone matrix	Impaired blood clotting, haemorrhagic disease
C – Ascorbic acid	Antioxidant, ↑ iron absorption, collagen synthesis, production of noradrenaline, ↓ production of nitrosamines in stomach	Scurvy (impaired wound healing, loss of dental cement, subcutaneous haemorrhage)
B_1 – Thiamine	Co-enzyme in pyruvate and 2-keto-glutarate dehydrogenase and transketolase, Poorly defined role in nerve conduction	Beri beri (peripheral nerve damage), Wernicke–Korsakoff syndrome (central nerve damage)
B_2 – Riboflavine	Co-enzyme in oxidation and reduction reactions, prosthetic group of flavoproteins	Lesions of corner of mouth, lips and tongue; seborrhoeic dermatitis
Niacin – Nicotinic acid, nicotinamide	Co-enzyme in oxidation and reduction reactions, functional part of NAD and NADP	Pellagra (photosensitive dermatitis, depressive psychosis)
B_6 – Pyridoxine, pyridoxal, pyridoxamine	Co-enzyme in transamination and decarboxylation of amino acids and glycogen phosphorylase, steroid hormone production	Disorders of amino acid metabolism, convulsions
B_9 – Folic acid	Co-enzyme in transfer of one carbon fragments	Megaloblastic anaemia, neural tube defects in babies
B_{12} – Cobalamin	Co-enzyme in transfer of one carbon fragments and metabolism of folic acid	Pernicious anaemia (megaloblastic anaemia with degeneration of the spinal cord)
Pantothenic acid	Functional part of coenzyme A and acyl carrier protein	Neuromotor disorders, mental depression, GI complaints and increased insulin sensitivity
Biotin	Co-enzyme in carboxylation reactions in gluconeogenesis and fatty acid synthesis	Impaired fat and carbohydrate metabolism, dermatitis

Source: Adapted from Combet, E. and Buckton, C., *Medicine*, 43(2), 66–72, 2015.

Vision

The retina is the light-sensitive cellular layer at the back of the eyes. It contains two types of cells: the rods (sensitive to dim light) and cones (sensitive to daylight and colour). In both types, the opsin proteins are associated with 11-*cis*-retinal, derived from retinol. Rhodopsin, found in rods, is much more sensitive to a lack of vitamin A than is the pigment in the cones.

When light strikes rhodopsin, the 11-*cis*-retinal changes to the all-*trans* configuration, triggering a series of complex changes resulting in the initiation and propagation of a nerve impulse, which is detected by the visual cortex. This occurs continuously in daylight so that rhodopsin is constantly being broken down. Most of our daylight vision is the result of changes occurring to the pigment in the cones.

Before it can be useful in dim light, rhodopsin needs to be resynthesized by conversion of the all-*trans* retinal back to the 11-*cis* isomer, for further visual signals to be detected. This can only occur in the dark, and when we blink in daylight. However, on entering a dark room, rhodopsin resynthesis occurs quickly, provided that there is a supply of retinol/retinal available, and we quickly become 'accustomed to the dark', and can see again. If there is insufficient supply of retinol to restore the rhodopsin, our dim light vision fails, and we suffer from 'night blindness' (see Figure 12.1).

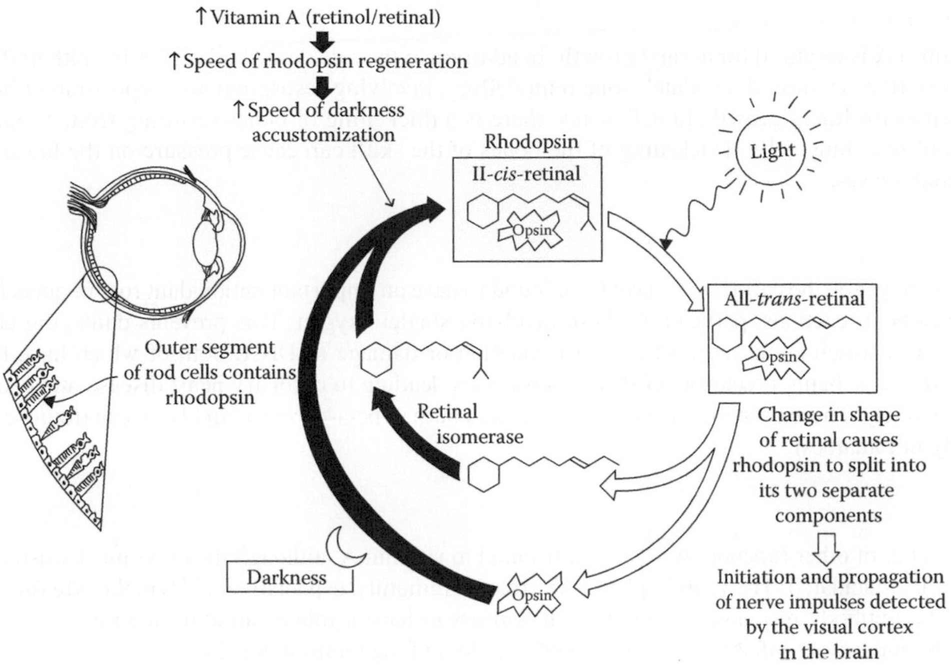

FIGURE 12.1 The role of vitamin A in vision.

The speed with which we can become accustomed to see in the dark is a measure of our vitamin A status. This is the basis of the dark adaptation test used to assess vitamin A status.

Cellular Differentiation

Retinoic acid appears to be the major form of the vitamin involved in gene expression and control of cellular differentiation. In particular, the differentiation of epithelial cells is under the control of vitamin A, which determines their mucus-secreting properties. There are specific binding sites on cellular nuclei, from which retinoic acid interacts with DNA and controls synthesis of proteins and gene expression.

Epithelia constitute most of the body's surfaces and linings, and the ability to secrete mucus and keep these surfaces lubricated and washed is essential to the body's defence. Thus, sites as varied as the conjunctiva of the eye, the trachea and lungs, the digestive tract linings, and the urethra and bladder are all dependent on adequate vitamin A to maintain their integrity and function.

A failure to maintain this epithelial integrity and mucus secretion results in one of the classic signs of vitamin A deficiency: xerophthalmia, or dry eye. In this condition, there is a failure of tear production and the eye lacks lysozyme to keep it clean. It becomes susceptible to bacterial infections, resulting in conjunctivitis and, ultimately, damaged patches develop, known as Bitot's spots. If left untreated, the xerophthalmia progresses to a full breakdown of the eyeball, known as keratomalacia and accompanying loss of sight.

Vitamin A has a key role as an anti-infective vitamin; this is now believed to be closely linked to its role in the maintenance of epithelial integrity. For example, impaired gastrointestinal epithelial integrity may allow the translocation of bacteria across the mucosa. Infection reduces the levels of circulating acute phase proteins that transport vitamin A, further exacerbating the problem of epithelial integrity. Children with vitamin A deficiency are also more susceptible to respiratory infections and measles. Supplementation of sick children with vitamin A has been shown to improve recovery rates.

Growth

Vitamin A is required for normal growth. In addition to the role described earlier in epithelial differentiation, vitamin A regulates bone remodelling, involving resorption and deposition of bone, required for linear growth. In deficiency, there is a thickening of bones resulting from a relative lack of resorbing cells. Thickening of the bones of the skull can cause pressure on the brain and cranial nerves.

Antioxidant Role

In recent years, the carotenoids have been found to have an important antioxidant role in quenching free radical reactions, particularly those involving singlet oxygen. This prevents damaging chain reactions, which could result in lipid peroxidation or damage to DNA, both of which have been postulated as being precursors of disease processes, leading to coronary heart disease and cancer, respectively. These properties have been attributed both to beta-carotene and lycopene (found especially in tomatoes).

Other Functions

A number of other functions have been attributed to vitamin A, although the exact mechanisms are not fully elucidated. The vitamin plays a key role in immunity, especially for T-lymphocyte function and the antibody response to infections. It appears to have a role as an anti-inflammatory agent. In addition, severe infections are associated with loss of the vitamin in urine.

There is a link between vitamin A and red blood cell formation, possibly involving the utilization or transport of iron; anaemia is a frequent finding in vitamin A deficiency, despite apparently adequate iron status.

Vitamin D

It is questionable whether 'vitamin D' is truly a vitamin. Under normal circumstances it is made in the skin during sun exposure. When people are removed from sunshine, or entirely clothed and covered, the only source is the diet. A great many health-related claims are made for vitamin D, most of which lack proper evidence. The principal physiological role of vitamin D is to maintain serum calcium and phosphorus concentrations at a level appropriate for the formation of bone, support of cellular processes, and functioning of nerves and muscles.

Calcitriol, the biologically active form, has a number of target tissues containing specific receptors for the vitamin, the most notable of which are the intestine, bone and kidney. In each case, the function of the vitamin is to cause an increase in the plasma level of calcium.

- In the intestines, this is achieved by the vitamin-stimulated synthesis of calcium-binding protein, required for absorption of calcium.
- In the bone, calcium can be mobilized by the action of the osteoclasts and is also made available for the osteoblasts to resynthesize bone. Thus, calcitriol enables appropriate amounts of calcium (and phosphorus) to be available in the bones for synthesis, while at the same time facilitating their release to maintain plasma levels.
- In the kidneys, calcium reabsorption is promoted by the action of vitamin D.

In summary, when plasma calcium levels fall, parathyroid hormone is released. This causes synthesis of calcitriol in the kidneys. In response, more calcium is absorbed by the gut, some calcium is mobilized by the bone and less calcium is lost at the kidneys. Overall, these changes raise plasma calcium levels, thus cancelling out the original stimulus.

If, however, the kidney is unable to respond to the original stimulus in this way (because there is insufficient 25-OH vitamin D being brought to the kidney, or the kidneys themselves are diseased), more parathyroid hormone will continue to be secreted. This can create a state of hyperparathyroidism, which may be a feature of vitamin D deficiency. Before the role of the kidneys in vitamin D and bone metabolism was fully understood, patients with kidney disease developed unexplained bone diseases. Treatment with active vitamin D can now prevent these problems arising.

Recent work has discovered calcitriol receptors in many other tissues, including placenta, gonads, skin and cells of the immune system, suggesting roles that are not directly linked to calcium homeostasis. Effects on cell proliferation and cell differentiation both in normal and malignant cells have been described. The vitamin may also be involved in down-regulating the immune response, and vitamin D defects may be involved in autoimmune reactions. However, these possible non-calcium-related actions are not well supported by experimental evidence, and most clinical trials have been negative. It is possible that vitamin D receptors in many tissues are redundant and not functional in life.

Vitamin E

The chemical structure of tocopherols and tocotrienols, with an –OH group on the ring structure, makes them very effective hydrogen donors. Therefore, vitamin E is a potent antioxidant and, as it is fat soluble, this activity is expressed particularly in lipid environments. In donating hydrogen, the vitamin E becomes oxidized itself, while preventing the oxidation of something more metabolically important, for example, polyunsaturated fatty acids in cell membranes. This is important when free radicals are present, as these highly reactive substances can attack double bonds, setting up chain reactions, with more free radicals being produced. In the case of damage to fatty acids, lipid peroxides are produced that alter the function of the cell membrane and cause possibly irreversible damage to metabolic pathways.

There is interaction between vitamin E and other nutrients, particularly selenium and vitamin C, in the antioxidant role. Vitamin C is involved in the regeneration of vitamin E.

Vitamin E is particularly important in those parts of the body where large amounts of oxygen are present, including the lungs and the red blood cells. In addition, the lungs are also exposed to environmental pollutants, which contain free radicals and, therefore, protection here is essential.

The antioxidant role of vitamin C & E and beta-carotene are covered further in Chapter 14, pp. 287–289, in relation to coronary heart disease, in Chapter 15, pp. 303–304, in relation to cancer, and in Chapter 22, p. 427, in relation to sport and exercise.

In summary, vitamin E is essential in maintaining cell membranes, contributing to their integrity, stability and function. Cell membrane function is closely related to their structure, and for this reason, vitamin E has been considered an important protective factor in the prevention of degenerative diseases, such as cardiovascular disease and cancer. There is some evidence that vitamin E plays a role in the prevention of cardiovascular disease, but the results of intervention trials have not been conclusive. It has also been proposed that vitamin E is essential for the maintenance of vascular integrity in the brain, where low levels may result in impairment of cognitive function and possibly contribute to dementia, platelet stickiness and improved immunity. In women taking vitamin E supplements, there is evidence of a lower incidence of strokes. Despite this, most nutritionists would recommend that vitamin E is obtained from a balanced diet, rich in grains, fruit and vegetables, rather than from vitamin supplements. At present, there is no evidence of harm from high doses of vitamin E secured via food intake – however, high dose vitamin E supplementation (10–5000 IU) in healthy people, singly or combined to other micronutrients, was associated with increased mortality.

Vitamin C

Free radical damage is covered further in Chapter 14, pp. 283–291.

Most of the roles of vitamin C in the body are related to its being a reducing agent, as the ascorbate is readily oxidized to dehydroascorbate. In this way, vitamin C can act as a hydrogen donor to reverse oxidation and, therefore, may be termed an antioxidant. As an anti-oxidant, vitamin C can react with free radicals and inactivate them before they cause damage to proteins or lipids. Once vitamin C has acted in this way, it must be regenerated. This is achieved by a number of reductase enzymes, which restore the ascorbate from dehydroascorbate, making it available for further reactions. Reductases that are used in this way include reduced glutathione and NADH and NADPH.

The other major role of vitamin C is as a cofactor for a number of hydroxylation reactions. This too may be an antioxidant role, whereby the vitamin is protecting metal ions, which act as prosthetic groups for these enzymes. Examples of hydroxylation reactions requiring vitamin C include the following:

- Formation of hydroxyproline and hydroxylysine, for collagen synthesis
- Synthesis of carnitine, needed for release of energy from fatty acids, especially in muscle
- Synthesis of noradrenaline
- Synthesis of brain peptides, including a number of hormone-releasing factors found in the brain

Vitamin C is closely linked to iron metabolism. It enhances iron absorption from food by reducing ferric iron to ferrous iron to facilitate absorption. It may also be involved in the incorporation of iron into ferritin. This may become a problem in individuals with excessive amounts of iron in the body. As always, caution should be exercised if large amounts of any single nutrient are taken.

Other roles have been proposed for vitamin C, including detoxification of foreign substances in the liver and the promotion of immune function. The latter has received a great deal of publicity and many people believe that consumption of large amounts (often several grams) of vitamin C will help prevent the occurrence of the common cold. Evidence has been reviewed and has failed to show a consistent effect on prevention of a cold. However, moderate doses (up to 250 mg/day) may reduce the severity of the symptoms of a cold. It should also be remembered that very high intakes of the vitamin are poorly absorbed (absorption may be 10% or less), may cause intestinal irritation and diarrhoea, and chronic ingestion may result in kidney stones.

Vitamin K

The major role of vitamin K is to take part in the gamma-carboxylation of glutamic acid residues. This is part of a cycle in which the vitamin changes from an oxidized form (quinone) to the reduced form (quinol). On completion of the carboxylation, the vitamin is converted back to the quinone form, and can be reused. The vitamin-K-dependent proteins (or gla-proteins) that are produced participate in many reactions in the body. The most important of these is the blood clotting cascade, in which four of the factors needed contain gamma-carboxyglutamate, namely prothrombin and factors VII, IX and X. It is thus clear why vitamin K deficiency has serious effects on blood clotting. Anticoagulants, such as warfarin, interfere with the regeneration of the reduced vitamin K, thus breaking the cycle.

Another gla-protein, found in bone, is osteocalcin, which is needed for the normal binding of calcium in bone matrix. It is now recognized that vitamin K supplementation may increase bone density in osteoporosis. Further evidence suggests that vitamin K may also inhibit bone resorption by causing osteoclasts to undergo apoptosis.

Vitamin K appears in the brain as menaquinone 4, where its role may be associated with the formation of a class of brain lipids. Other gla-proteins occur in many other organs in the body, although at present, their roles are unclear.

Thiamin (Vitamin B_1)

On absorption, thiamin is phosphorylated to thiamin pyrophosphate (TPP) (also called thiamine diphosphate), especially in the liver. The major tissues that contain thiamin are the skeletal muscle (about 50% of all thiamin), heart, liver, kidneys and brain.

The major role of TPP is as a cofactor in a number of metabolic reactions, especially involved with carbohydrate utilization. The most important of these is as a coenzyme for pyruvate dehydrogenase in the production of acetyl coenzyme A from pyruvate at the start of the Krebs cycle, through which 90% of the energy from glucose is released as ATP. Acetyl coenzyme A is also needed for the synthesis of lipids and acetylcholine (a neurotransmitter), and this demonstrates how thiamin is linked to nervous system function.

TPP is also required to complete the metabolism of branched-chain amino acids (large doses of thiamin may help in maple-syrup urine disease, which is caused by a genetic defect in this pathway). Interconversions between sugars of different carbon chain length also require TPP, acting as a cofactor for the enzyme transketolase.

Recently, thiamin triphosphate has been found to control a chloride ion channel in nerves and may be a further link to neurological functions of thiamin.

Thiamin status can be assessed by measuring the activity in the red blood cell of the enzyme transketolase, which is TPP dependent. There is also some evidence that magnesium is required for thiamin function, to activate RBC transketolase.

Riboflavin (Vitamin B_2)

In the tissues, riboflavin is converted into the coenzymes FMN and FAD, which constitute the active groups in a number of flavoproteins. Greatest concentrations are found in the liver, kidney and heart.

Both FMN and FAD act as electron and hydrogen donors and acceptors, which allows them to play a critical role in many oxidation–reduction reactions of metabolic pathways, passing electrons to the electron transport chain. Examples include the following:

- FAD is used in the Krebs cycle and in beta-oxidation of fatty acids, forming $FADH_2$.
- FAD also functions in conjunction with a number of oxidase and dehydrogenase enzymes, including xanthine oxidase (used in purine catabolism), aldehyde oxidase (needed in the metabolism of pyridoxine and vitamin A), glutathione reductase (selenium-requiring enzyme, used to quench free radicals), monoamine oxidase (for neurotransmitter metabolism) and mixed function oxidases (used in drug metabolism).
- $FADH_2$ is needed in folate metabolism.

The examples listed above show not only the crucial role that riboflavin has in macronutrient metabolism and energy release, but also the interrelationships that exist with other nutrients in the body.

Assessment of riboflavin status is most accurately performed using the activation of glutathione reductase (a riboflavin-dependent enzyme) in red blood cells.

Niacin (Vitamin B_3)

The main role of niacin in the body is in the formation of nicotinamide adenine dinucleotide (NAD) and NAD phosphate (NADP), which can be made in all cells. Once the niacin has been converted to NAD or NADP, it is trapped within cells and cannot diffuse out.

NAD and NADP act as hydrogen acceptors in oxidative reactions, forming NADH and NADPH. These, in turn, can act as hydrogen donors. On the whole, NAD is used in energy-yielding reactions, for example, glycolysis, the Krebs cycle and the oxidation of alcohol. The hydrogen they accept is eventually passed through the electron transfer chain, to yield water. NADPH is mostly used in energy-requiring, biosynthetic reactions, most importantly, for fatty acid synthesis. Overall, NAD and NADP play a part in the metabolism of carbohydrates, fats and proteins and are, therefore, central to cellular processes. In addition, they are involved in vitamin C and folate metabolism, and are required by glutathione reductase.

Pyridoxine (Vitamin B_6)

Pyridoxal phosphate is involved in many biological reactions, particularly those associated with amino acid metabolism. Some examples are as follows:

- Decarboxylation, for example production of histamine from histidine, production of dopamine and serotonin (important neurotransmitters)
- Transamination – for the synthesis of nonessential amino acids; synthesis of porphyrin (for haem), nicotinic acid from tryptophan and cysteine from methionine.

The formation of cysteine from methionine has homocysteine as an intermediate product, and there has been a great deal of interest in the possible role of vitamin B_6 as a factor for reducing homocysteine levels. At present, the evidence on its usefulness as a protective factor against hyperhomocysteinaemia is equivocal.

Vitamin B_6 also plays a role in the following:

- Fat metabolism, in the conversion of linoleic acid to arachidonic acid, and in synthesis of sphingolipids in the nervous system
- Glycogen metabolism, particularly in muscle

Some recent work has shown that vitamin B_6 may also have a role in modulating the action of steroid and other hormones at the cell nucleus.

Folate (Vitamin B_9)

Intracellular folate, as tetrahydrofolate (THF) is used to carry one-carbon units from one molecule to another. Thus, it can accept such single-carbon groups from donors in degradative reactions and then act as the donor of such a unit in a subsequent synthetic reaction. Such transfers are important in a number of steps during amino acid metabolism, for example:

- Synthesis of serine from glycine (and vice versa)
- Synthesis of homocysteine from methionine (and vice versa)
- Conversion of histidine to glutamic acid
- Synthesis of purine and pyrimidine bases, for DNA and RNA synthesis, which explains the crucial role of folate in cell division

The removal of the methyl group from 5-methyl THF is a particularly important step, which is catalysed by the vitamin B_{12}-dependent enzyme methionine synthase. Without the presence of vitamin B_{12}, the THF is 'trapped' in its methyl form and can no longer carry single-carbon units. This reaction is an essential link between the two vitamins and explains some of the common features of their deficiency states (see Figure 12.2).

Furthermore, the methyl group removed during this reaction is used to generate methionine from homocysteine. Evidence suggests that elevated homocysteine levels may be associated with an increased risk of some diseases, and thus, metabolic pathways that serve to reduce homocysteine levels have been extensively studied. The 5-methyl THF needed for methionine synthesis is formed from 5,10-methylene tetrahydrofolate, by the action of methylene tetrahydrofolate reductase

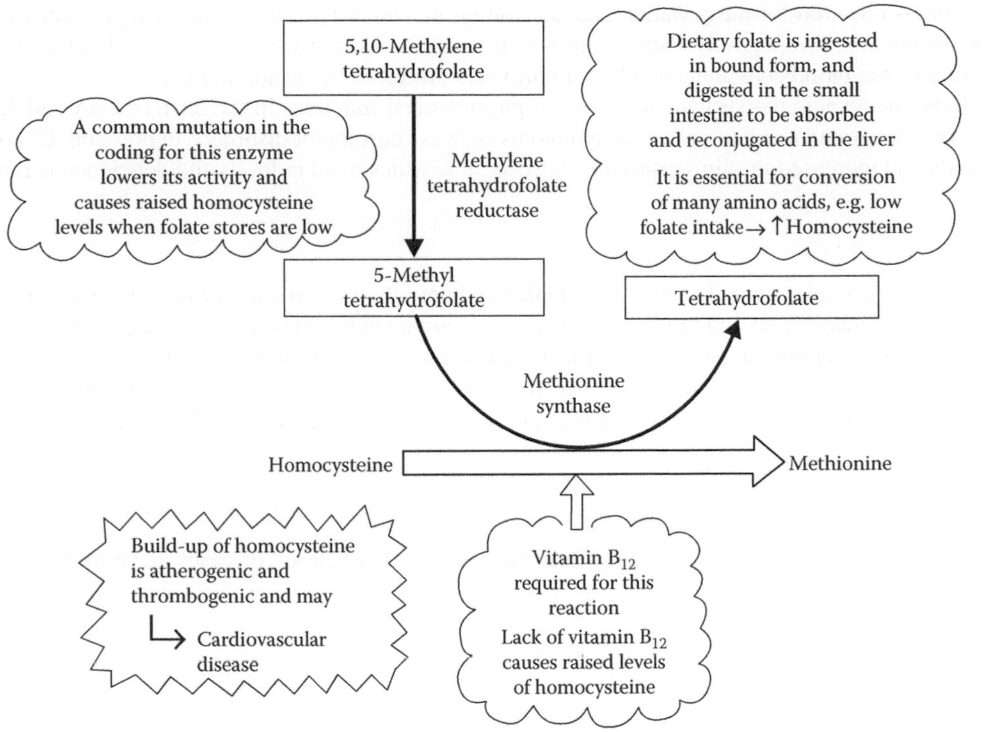

FIGURE 12.2 The metabolic role of folate in homocysteine metabolism.

(MTHFR). A recessive genetic mutation in the coding for this enzyme has been found, with 5%–18% of individuals estimated to be homozygous for this mutation. This results in a lower level of enzyme activity and, consequently, higher homocysteine levels when folate status is low. These findings may offer some explanation for the benefits of folate supplementation in certain circumstances, for example, the prevention of neural tube defects. Folate deficiency anaemia is very common, especially among elderly people and alcoholics. Folic acid supplementation is usual and the case for fortification of common foods is strong.

Cobalamin (Vitamin B_{12})

The metabolic role of vitamin B_{12} is associated with two enzyme systems, one involved in the availability of THF and the other in the metabolism of some fatty acids.

Vitamin B_{12} acts as a cofactor for methyltransferase, the enzyme needed to remove a methyl group from methyltetrahydrofolate, making THF available. Therefore, if vitamin B_{12} levels are low, folate deficiency is effectively caused. A further consequence is that an inadequate amount of methionine is produced. It is believed that this eventually results in damage to the myelin coating of nerve fibres.

Vitamin B_{12} is needed for the metabolism of fatty acids with an odd number of carbons in their chains.

Pantothenic Acid (Vitamin B_5)

Pantothenic acid is an integral part of the acylation carriers, coenzyme A (CoA) and acyl carrier protein (ACP). CoA is important in energy metabolism where it is needed to allow pyruvate to enter the tricarboxylic acid cycle (TCA cycle) as acetyl-CoA, and for α-ketoglutarate to be transformed to succinyl-CoA. CoA is also important in the biosynthesis of fatty acids, cholesterol and acetylcholine.

CoA is required for the acylation and acetylation in signal transduction and enzyme activation and deactivation, respectively. Pantothenic acid is needed to synthesize cholesterol and in the manufacture of red blood cells and a number of hormones produced in the adrenal glands.

Pantothenic acid has such a wide range of physiological functions in the form of CoA and ACP that deficiency can result in a range of symptoms such as neuromotor disorders, depression, GI complaints and increased insulin sensitivity. However, it is widespread in foods and deficiency is rare.

Biotin (Vitamin B_7)

Biotin is required for normal cellular functioning and growth. It is a coenzyme in carboxylation reactions in gluconeogenesis and fatty acid synthesis and amino acid catabolism. It is used to biotinylate histones and other nuclear proteins and affects gene expression at the non-transcriptional level. Biotin is also important for normal embryonic growth and is therefore a critical nutrient during pregnancy.

Biotin deficiency is rare as it is widely available in foods and can be synthesized by intestinal bacteria.

MINERALS

The physiological functions of minerals and the associated deficiency diseases are summarized in Table 12.2.

Calcium

In Bones

Calcium is principally located in bones, where it is found both in the dense cortical bone and in the less dense trabecular bone. The skeleton is an active reservoir of calcium. The mineral is continually being laid down (by osteoblasts) and resorbed (by osteoclasts) as bone growth (in childhood and adolescence), and maintenance (in adults) take place.

The dietary sources of minerals are covered in Chapter 5, pp. 83–97.

During growth in childhood and adolescence, there is a net gain of bone and, therefore, of calcium. In the early adult decades, the amount of bone remains relatively constant in health, although it is in a state of constant flux with a balance between the activities of osteoclasts and osteoblasts. However, if there is a period of immobility or changes in levels of some hormones, such as cortisol or oestrogens, then bone loss will occur. The amount of bone gradually declines with age. This happens earlier and more rapidly in women at the time of the menopause, particularly in the first 2–3 years. The gradual decline then continues as the rates of bone breakdown exceed bone repair. This may result in the bone becoming so fragile that it is easily broken; this condition is called osteoporosis.

The role of calcium in bone health, osteoporosis, and ageing is covered in Chapter 8, pp. 165–168.

In Blood and Body Fluids

The calcium present in body fluids is crucial to the normal homeostasis of the body and the levels are tightly regulated to remain within narrow limits of 2.2–2.6 mmol/L. This is achieved by the regulatory hormones, namely, parathyroid hormone, active vitamin D (1,25-dihydroxycholecalciferol) and calcitonin, acting on the gut, bones and kidneys in response to changes in circulating calcium levels (see Figure 12.3).

Overall, when plasma calcium levels are low (or phosphate levels are high), parathyroid hormone is secreted. This increases calcium levels by promoting synthesis of active vitamin D and, thus, increasing calcium absorption from the gut, reducing calcium excretion at the kidney and stimulating

TABLE 12.2

Physiological Functions of Minerals and Associated Deficiency Diseases

Minerals	Physiological Functions	Known Deficiency Diseases
Calcium	Skeletal growth and development, vascular and muscle contraction, nerve transmission, insulin release	Failure to attain peak bone mass, osteoporosis in later life
Chloride	Hydrochloric acid in the stomach, chloride shift in erythrocyte plasma membrane, regulation of osmotic and electrolyte balances	–
Chromium	Insulin action, carbohydrate, lipid and nucleic acid metabolism	Severe deficiency → insulin resistance
Copper	Immune, nervous and cardiovascular systems, bone health, iron metabolism, haemoglobin synthesis, regulation of mitochondria, other gene expression	Unlikely due to remarkable homeostatic mechanisms
Fluoride	Fluoroapatite in teeth and bones	↑ Risk of dental caries
Iodine	Thyroine hormones component, contributes to growth and brain development	Goitre, hypothyroidism, cretinism (collectively termed iodine deficiency disorders)
Iron	Oxygen transport and storage, catalytic centre for a broad spectrum of metabolic functions cell respiration and energy production, immune system, myelination and nerve development in fetus	Iron deficiency and iron deficiency anaemia, impairment of the immune response, adverse effect on psychomotor and mental development in children
Magnesium	Wide range of fundamental cellular reactions, >300 enzymatic steps in metabolism, skeletal development, gene regulation, nerve and muscle cell conduction	Secondary to GI losses with diarrhoea and vomiting, and poor intake/alcoholism. Promotes seizures.
Manganese	Catalytic co-factor for mitochondrial superoxide dismutase, arginase and pyruvate carboxylase	Rare – weight loss, dermatitis, growth retardation of hair and nails, decline of blood lipids
Molybdenum	Co-factor for the iron- and flavin-containing enzymes that catalyse hydroxylation	Rarely observed
Phosphorus	Hydroxyapatite in calcified tissues, phospholipids in biological membranes, nucleotides and nucleic acid, maintenance of normal pH, storage and transfer of energy, activation of catalytic enzymes by phosphorylation	Hypophosphataemia resulting in cellular dysfunction – may include anorexia, anaemia, muscle weakness, bone pain, rickets and osteomalacia, general debility, increased infections, paraesthesia, ataxia, confusion
Potassium	Major intracellular electrolyte – regulation of osmotic pressure and electrolyte balance, normal functioning of cardiovascular, respiratory, digestive, renal and endocrine systems, energy metabolism, cell growth and division	Low potassium intakes unlikely to lead to clinical potassium depletion and hypokalaemia except during starvation and anorexia nervosa
Selenium	Redox centre for the selenium-dependent glutathione peroxidases (antioxidant), thyroid hormone metabolism	Keshan's disease – a cardiomyopathy affecting children and women of child-bearing age Common secondary to poorly supervised diuretic drug use, causing postural hypotension
Sodium	Major extracellular electrolyte – regulation of osmotic and electrolyte balances, nerve conduction, muscle contraction, energy-dependent cell transport systems, formation of mineral apatite of bone	
Sulphur	Component of many proteins, energy metabolism as part of the electron transport chain	–
Zinc	Catalytic, structural and regulatory roles, >100 metalloenzymes involved in energy metabolism, DNA and RNA synthesis, protein synthesis, expression of multiple genes, protection of mucosal cells, functioning of immune and reproductive systems	Growth retardation, sexual and skeletal immaturity, neuropsychiatric disturbances, dermatitis, alopecia, diarrhoea, susceptibility to infection and loss of appetite

Source: Adapted from Combet, E. and Buckton, C., *Medicine*, 43(2), 66–72, 2015.

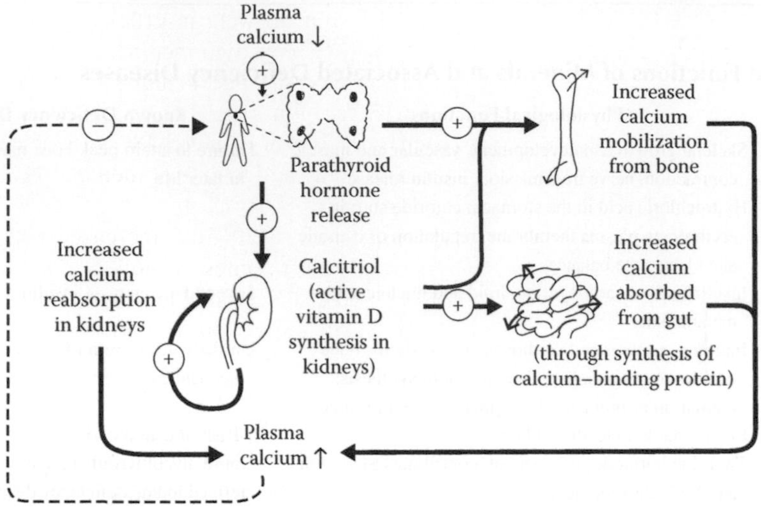

FIGURE 12.3 The regulation of plasma calcium.

calcium release from the bone. Conversely, high calcium levels cause the release of calcitonin from the thyroid gland. This inhibits bone mobilization and promotes calcium uptake into bone.

Why Does Plasma Calcium Need to Be Closely Regulated?

Calcium is essential for blood clotting; it is part of the clotting cascade by which insoluble prothrombin is converted into the thrombin of a blood clot by the action of fibrin and several other clotting factors. If calcium levels are insufficient, blood will not clot. Muscle contraction and nerve impulse transmission at nerve endings both involve the movement of calcium across the cell membrane, increasing intracellular levels and triggering contraction or depolarization.

Phosphorus

Phosphorus is a major mineral constituent of bone where it occurs as hydroxyapatite, and 85% of the body's phosphorus is found here. The remaining 15% is distributed within the soft tissues, as phospholipids in red blood cells and plasma lipoproteins, in DNA and RNA, and a small amount as inorganic phosphate. The inorganic phosphate compartment is, however, critical, as it receives phosphate from the diet and from bone resorption and loses phosphate to urine and bone mineralization. It is also the primary source for all of the biochemical reactions that require phosphates as the currency for energy transformations. It is, therefore, central to the functioning of the metabolic machinery. Phosphates are also critical as buffers to maintain normal pH in the body. Cells have limited storage capacity for phosphate and, therefore, draw on the inorganic phosphate pool for their needs.

Phosphorus levels in the body are regulated mainly by renal excretion under the influence of parathyroid hormone, which causes increased urinary loss (this allows plasma calcium levels to rise – a major function of the hormone). Abnormal levels of phosphate in the blood are generally the result of renal or parathyroid dysfunction, rather than dietary excess or deficiency, since there is extensive recycling of the mineral.

Magnesium

The magnesium found in bones is thought to act as a reservoir to sustain plasma levels. The remaining magnesium is largely found in muscle and other soft tissues. It occurs as part of cell membranes but is also an essential activator of over 300 enzyme systems. Most notably, it is involved in all enzyme systems utilizing ATP. In addition, magnesium is involved in protein synthesis, energy production, muscle contraction and nerve impulse transmission. Magnesium sometimes competes with or interferes with the action of calcium in the body. For example, magnesium inhibits the blood clotting process; it may also inhibit smooth muscle contraction by blocking the calcium binding sites. However, the actions of vitamin D and parathyroid hormones, which regulate calcium, both require the presence of magnesium. Magnesium is required for parathyroid action, to release calcium from bone. Magnesium deficiency presents as hypocalcaemia, and may cause seizures.

IRON

The main endogenous source of iron is the breakdown of red blood cells by the reticulo-endothelial system. This is added to the iron from the diet (exogenous iron) for use and storage.

Iron is carried in the body fluids attached to the protein transferrin, which takes it from sites of absorption or release to sites of iron utilization or storage. A substantial amount of iron is transported around the body each day; normal concentrations of transferrin are 2.2–3.5 g/L, which at any time are carrying 3 mg of iron. During the course of a day, 25–30 mg of iron is transported around the body in a very efficient 'recycling' mechanism.

Red blood cells have an average lifespan of 120 days, which means that, each day, 1/120th of the total red cell count is broken down and has to be replaced. The bone marrow requires 24 mg of iron per day to make red blood cells. This daily need for iron demonstrates how important it is that recycling of iron occurs in the body: it would be impossible to take in these quantities of iron on a daily basis. With an absorption rate of 10%, the diet would have to contain 240 mg of iron simply to meet the needs for red cell synthesis.

Iron is used

- Predominantly by the bone marrow, for red blood cell synthesis (between 70% and 90% is used here)
- By muscle cells for myoglobin synthesis
- In metabolically active cells for the production of cytochromes in mitochondria
- In synthesis of hormones and neurotransmitters
- In immune function

Losses of Iron

Small amounts of iron are lost daily from the digestive tract lining, skin cells, in bile, urine and any small blood losses. Overall, this 'obligatory' loss of iron amounts to approximately 0.9 mg/day in men. In women, there is a monthly loss of iron in menstrual flow, estimated to be equivalent to an additional 0.7 mg/day on average. However, up to 10% of women may have heavy menstrual losses, which may equate to an additional daily iron loss of up to 1.4 mg. Additional iron loss is generally associated with pathological changes in the digestive tract, such as ulcers or cancer causing bleeding. Some drugs such as aspirin, taken regularly, may also cause small blood loss into the gut, which, over time, can amount to a significant loss of iron.

Ideally, the obligatory losses are compensated by iron absorbed from the diet, which should be sufficient to restore iron balance. However, if insufficient iron is ingested, there will be a gradual depletion of iron stores, eventually resulting in iron deficiency.

Stored Iron

Iron in excess of immediate needs is taken to storage sites in the liver, bone marrow and spleen, where it is stored in association with a protein called ferritin. Ferritin can accommodate over 4000 atoms of iron in its interior and thus prevent any toxic effects. It has been suggested that even a moderate level of iron storage may be a risk factor for cardiovascular disease and cancer. Stored iron, acting as a pro-oxidant, has the potential to cause oxidative stress through the production of free radicals and thus dysregulate antioxidant–oxidant balance. Small amounts of ferritin are present in the circulation, and this can be measured to reflect the size of the iron stores. Plasma ferritin levels of 12 mg/L or less are suggestive of depleted iron stores. If the iron stores become very large, ferritin molecules can clump together to form haemosiderin, which allows safe storage of more iron. However, in excess, this too can be toxic and is associated with a serious condition called siderosis, in which liver function deteriorates.

Zinc

Zinc is essential, as a co-factor, for the activities of hundreds of enzymes and regulatory proteins, and plays a part in numerous, diverse functions of the body:

- The metabolism of all the macronutrients
- The production of energy
- Nucleic acid synthesis (and therefore cell division)
- Oxygen and carbon dioxide transport (in carbonic anhydrase)
- Antioxidant mechanisms (through superoxide dismutase)
- The immune system
- Protein synthesis especially important in wound healing and growth
- The storage and release of insulin, affecting glucose metabolism
- Nuclear transcription and activation of proteins that regulate gene expression – via zinc-finger proteins, present in transcription factors

With so many roles, it is not surprising that zinc is widely distributed throughout the body. Major sites are the muscle (60%), bone (30%), skin (4%–6%), with the remainder found in liver, kidney and plasma. There is no readily identified store of zinc, although in catabolic states, zinc is released from muscle and made available to the plasma. The liver provides 'fine-tuning' of plasma zinc levels, which are tightly controlled, by releasing zinc from metallothionein–zinc complexes in its cells. In infection, zinc is taken up by the liver metallothionein and plasma levels fall. Levels of zinc in other tissues, such as bone, brain, lung and heart, remain relatively stable in the event of low zinc intakes.

Excretion of zinc occurs mostly via the faeces through secretion into the digestive tract. Small amounts are lost in the urine and in skin cells. Large amounts can be lost with exudates from wounds such as burns, and in the urine of people with diabetes and with diuretic drug treatments.

Copper

Copper is found tightly bound to proteins, termed metalloproteins, some of which are cuproenzymes and take part in a variety of intracellular and extracellular reactions.

Of the total amount of copper in the body, 40% is found in muscles; the remainder is in the liver, brain and blood (in red cells and as caeruloplasmin in plasma). Essential for iron metabolism, caeruloplasmin converts ferrous iron into its ferric state. The ferric iron then binds to transferrin and enters cells. An absence of caeruloplasmin, therefore, results in accumulation of iron in liver and brain. Caeruloplasmin is also involved in the response to infection as one of the acute-phase proteins. Copper occurs as a component of several enzyme systems, including cytochrome oxidase, superoxide dismutase and various amine oxidases. Cytochrome oxidase is the essential final link of the electron transport chain for the production of energy as ATP. Copper is a component of the free-radical-quenching enzyme superoxide dismutase, which also has an important role in protecting the body from damage by products of the response to infection. Amine oxidase is used in cross-linkage formation in the connective tissue proteins collagen and elastin. Copper-containing enzymes are also involved in melanin production, in formation of myelin and for neurotransmitter synthesis (such as catecholamines, dopamine and encephalins). A summary of the roles of copper in the body is shown in Figure 12.4.

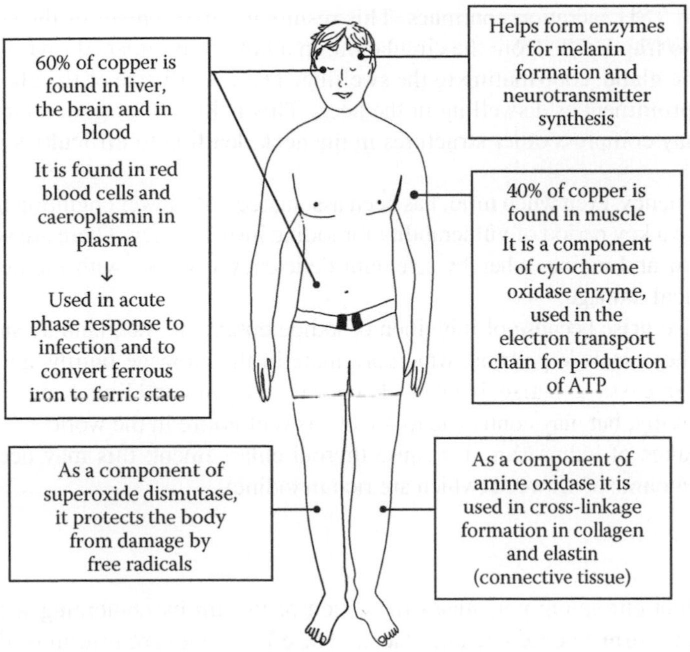
60% of copper is found in liver, the brain and in blood
It is found in red blood cells and caeroplasmin in plasma
↓
Used in acute phase response to infection and to convert ferrous iron to ferric state
Helps form enzymes for melanin formation and neurotransmitter synthesis
40% of copper is found in muscle
It is a component of cytochrome oxidase enzyme, used in the electron transport chain for production of ATP
As a component of superoxide dismutase, it protects the body from damage by free radicals
As a component of amine oxidase it is used in cross-linkage formation in collagen and elastin (connective tissue)

FIGURE 12.4 The role of copper in the body.

Selenium

Glutathione peroxidases are the major selenium-containing enzymes in the body. The enzymes occur in several variants, in different locations to provide protection against damage by reactive oxygen species. They occur both intracellularly and in plasma, within cell membranes, and have recently been found in sperm and in the gastrointestinal tract. Their role is to act as a catalyst for the reactions that remove hydrogen peroxide and other hydroperoxides to produce water or other harmless products. Glutathione peroxidase works in conjunction with other cellular enzymes, such as catalase and superoxide dismutase, as well as other dietary antioxidants such as vitamin E and C. Selenium is also involved in iodine metabolism in the conversion of thyroxine (T4) to its active form triiodothyronine (T3), in the thyroid gland.

Selenium plays a role in the normal functioning of the immune system. Defence against infection involves the production of reactive oxygen species, which must be removed by antioxidants to protect immune system cells from damage. It is suggested that selenium plays a key part in this, by protecting cells of the immune system in the lymph nodes, spleen and liver from damage.

The presence of a glutathione peroxidase in sperm has led to research on links between male subfertility and selenium status, with some positive results indicating improvements in sperm motility following supplementation with selenium in men with low status of this mineral.

Iodine

Most organ systems in the body are under the influence of thyroid hormones, which control metabolism. Iodine is important for neurodevelopment, and adequate intake is crucial during pregnancy, lactation and infancy. If the intake of iodine is insufficient, thyroid hormone levels fall and the pituitary responds by increasing secretion of thyroid-stimulating hormone (TSH, from the pituitary gland) to accelerate uptake of iodine by the gland. Normally, the resulting hormone shuts off the release of TSH. However, in the absence of iodine, insufficient hormone is produced to cause this and TSH secretion continues. This results in enlargement of the cells of the gland as they attempt to trap iodide from the circulation. In addition, unfinished thyroid hormones may accumulate in the gland, contributing to the swelling. The overall size of the gland increases and it may become prominent as a swelling in the neck. This is known as goitre. Gross enlargement of the thyroid may compress other structures in the neck, leading to difficulties in breathing and swallowing.

Iodine insufficiency, even when mild, has been associated with lower cognition in children; pregnancy is therefore a key period of vulnerability for iodine insufficiency. There are some interactions between selenium and iodine, whereby selenium deficiency together with iodine deficiency may reduce neurological damage.

Goitre may also arise because of inhibition of iodide uptake by the gland by substances known as goitrogens. These include goitrins, which originate in the cabbage family, and thioglycosides, which are found in cassava, maize, bamboo shoots, sweet potato and lima beans. They are largely destroyed by cooking, but may contribute to 4% of cases of goitre in the world.

Excessive intakes of iodine can also cause thyroid enlargement; this may occur when people consume large amounts of seaweed (which are rich in iodine).

Chromium

It is postulated that chromium potentiates the action of insulin by combining with nicotinic acid and amino acids to form glucose tolerance factor. The effectiveness of insulin is, therefore, greater with chromium than in its absence. In addition, chromium may have roles in lipid metabolism, specifically by affecting lipoprotein lipase activity and, in nucleic acid metabolism, by affecting the integrity of nuclear strands.

Sodium, Chloride and Potassium

Sodium is the major extracellular electrolyte. It is critical in the regulation of osmotic and electrolyte balances, nerve conduction, muscle contraction, energy-dependent cell transport systems and the formation of mineral apatite of bone. Sodium is critical in maintaining blood pressure and blood volume. Sodium is so widespread in the modern diet that deficiency is very unlikely and only occurs in clinical conditions such as major trauma, or with chronic over-treatment with diuretic (natriuretic) drugs.

Chloride is a key component of stomach acid (hydrochloric acid, HCL) and is important in the digestions of dietary fats. It is also necessary to maintain the body's acid balance and along with sodium helps to regulate osmotic and electrolyte balances. It is also important for the chloride shift in erythrocyte cell membranes.

As well as being the major intracellular electrolyte, potassium is essential for the correct functioning of all cells, tissues and organs in the body, including the cardiovascular, respiratory, digestive, renal and endocrine systems, energy metabolism and cell growth and division.

Potassium deficiency is also unlikely to occur for dietary reasons because of the widespread occurrence of the mineral in foods. However, low blood potassium may result from excessive losses of gastrointestinal fluids, for example, in vomiting, diarrhoea, purgative or laxative abuse. Certain diuretic drugs may also remove excessive amounts of potassium from the body. These result in mental confusion and muscular weakness. The muscular effects may affect the heart, causing sudden death, or the smooth muscle of the intestinal tract, resulting in paralytic ileus and abdominal distension. This may be a first sign of low plasma potassium in children.

High levels of blood potassium are generally associated with tissue breakdown, in catabolic states and starvation. More potassium is lost in the urine and the body gradually becomes depleted of potassium with shrinkage of the intracellular fluid volume. In uncontrolled diabetes mellitus, accelerated tissue breakdown will cause increased urinary loss of potassium.

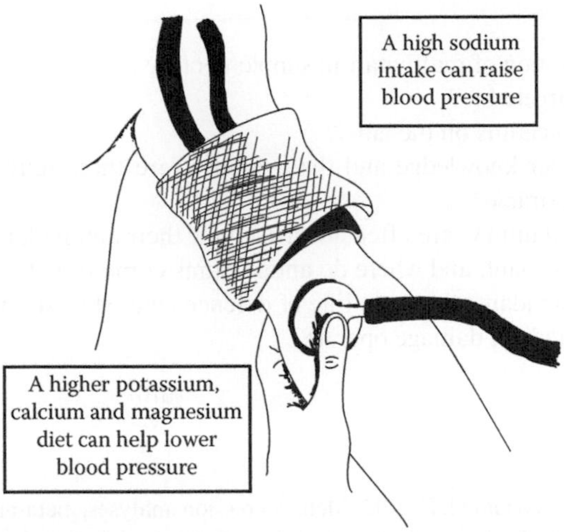

A high sodium intake can raise blood pressure
A higher potassium, calcium and magnesium diet can help lower blood pressure

FIGURE 12.5 Roles of electrolytes in blood pressure.

Treatment with insulin can cause plasma levels to fall dramatically, resulting in cardiac arrhythmias, and care must be taken to avoid this.

The major electrolytes have roles in regulating blood pressure; a summary is presented in Figure 12.5.

SUMMARY

1. Micronutrients play a central role in metabolism and in the maintenance of tissue function.
2. The physiological functions of micronutrients include acting as:
   i. co-enzymes in key metabolic reactions;
   ii. antioxidants in the control of damage caused by reactive oxygen species
   iii. modulators of gene transcription
   iv. components of and co-factors for enzymes
   v. structural components of tissues; and,
   vi. as regulators of osmotic pressure, electrolyte and fluid balance.
3. Micronutrients are also important in energy-dependent cell transport systems and in nerve conduction and muscle contraction, particularly the major electrolytes.

STUDY QUESTIONS

1. Construct tables to compare and contrast common features (food sources, function, signs of deficiency) of the following pairs of vitamins
   a. Riboflavin and niacin
   b. Vitamin B_{12} and folate
   c. Vitamins C and E
2. A number of minerals have a regulatory role in the body, including iodine, chromium and selenium.
   a. Explain these roles
   b. Discuss the likelihood of deficiency for an individual following a Western diet, and the consequences of a deficiency.

ACTIVITIES

12.1 Review the composition of multivitamin supplements available on the supermarket shelf.
- Who are they targeted to?
- Are there health claims on the label?
- According to your knowledge and the evidence, are these multivitamin preparations useful and/or desirable?

12.2 Vitamins such as vitamin C are often advertised for their antioxidant properties
- What is an antioxidant, and where do antioxidants come from?
- Are dietary antioxidants the main line of defence against oxidative stress?
- How does free-radical damage operate?

BIBLIOGRAPHY AND FURTHER READING

Bjelakovic, G., Nikolova, D. and Gluud, C. 2013. Meta-regression analyses, meta-analyses, and trial sequential analyses of the effects of supplementation with beta-carotene, vitamin A, and vitamin E singly or in different combinations on all-cause mortality: Do we have evidence for lack of harm? *PLoS One* 8(9), e74558.

Bjelakovic, G., Nikolova, D., Gluud, L.L., Simonetti, R.G. and Gluud, C. 2015. Antioxidant supplements for prevention of mortality in healthy participants and patients with various diseases. *Cochrane Database of Systematic Reviews* (2), CD007176.

Combet, E. and Buckton, C. 2015. Micronutrient deficiencies, vitamin pills and nutritional supplements. *Medicine* 43(2), 66–72.

Claessens, M., Contor, L., Dhonukshe-Rutten, R. et al. 2013. EURRECA – Principles and future for deriving micronutrient recommendations. *Critical Reviews in Food Science and Nutrition* 53(10), 1135–1146.

DoH (UK Department of Health). 1991. Dietary reference values for food energy and nutrients for the United Kingdom. Report on Health and Social Subjects No. 41. Report of the Panel on Dietary Reference Values of the Committee on Medical Aspects of Food Policy. London, UK: HMSO.

Fortmann, S.P., Burda, B.U., Senger, C.A., Lin, J.S. and Whitlock, E.P. 2013. Vitamin and mineral supplements in the primary prevention of cardiovascular disease and cancer: An updated systematic evidence review for the US Preventive Services Task Force. *Annals of Internal Medicine* 159(12), 824–834.

Jackson, M.J. 1999. Diagnosis and detection of deficiencies of micronutrients: Minerals. *British Medical Bulletin* 55(3), 634–642.

Shenkin, A. 2013. Micronutrient supplements: Who needs them? A personal view. *Nutrition Bulletin* 38(2), 191–200.

Vanderpump, M.P.J., Lazarus, J.H., Smyth, P.P. et al. 2011. Iodine status of UK schoolgirls: A cross-sectional survey. *Lancet* 377(9782), 2007–2012.

World Health Organization. 2014. Micronutrients. Available at: http://www.who.int/nutrition/topics/micronutrients/en/.

Section IV

Eating Behaviour and Nutritional Epidemiology

13 Habits and Influences on Eating Behaviours

AIMS

The aims of this chapter are to

- Discuss the reasons for eating and possible mechanisms that control eating.
- Describe food habits and discuss how food habits are determined.
- Explore the factors influencing food choice, the interactions between them and how they change.

Most people, if asked why they eat, would respond with 'to stay alive' or 'because I'm hungry'. Both of these are appropriate answers: the body has a physiological need for food and, when deprived, a sensation of hunger is soon experienced. This is a normal physiological response, which functions to balance the storage and utilization of nutrients with their input from food.

However, people eat for a number of other reasons. Eating becomes a matter of habit, and there are socially accepted 'mealtimes', when there is an expectation of eating, regardless of hunger, but food is usually widely available, often at all hours of day or night, and snacks between meals are heavily promoted. There are social norms associated with eating, which define what behaviour is and is not acceptable, but these can be changed by marketing.

Food provides us with sensory satisfaction, it is (usually) pleasant to eat, and this aspect of certain foods induces people to eat when they have no immediate physiological need to do so. Eating can be considered an addiction – one of a number of addictive behaviours which evolution has normalized for survival advantage.

We have very personal relationships with food. It is something that we deliberately take into our body and which becomes part of us. This can have very profound meanings for some people, but for everyone, there are psychological influences on eating.

Each of these influences on eating will be discussed in turn, to demonstrate that even something as basic as supplying the body with the energy for its survival involves more than an understanding of physiology.

REASONS FOR EATING

Habit as an Influence on Eating Behaviour

The physiological drivers for eating are covered in Chapter 9, pp. 186–190.

Conventionally, people eat at fairly clearly defined 'mealtimes', even when food is continually available. This behaviour has become a habit, and many Westerners believe that they should have three meals a day with the main meal either in the middle of the day or in the evening. This stereotype may itself have originated at a time of plenty. In other societies, especially among the poor, fewer meals are eaten, maybe only one or at most two within a day. Therefore, it appears that there is no physiological need to eat so frequently, but we have become accustomed to it. It is necessary to eat to satiation when mealtimes are infrequent, and it is easy to transfer this to the three-meal pattern. If eating is more continuous, the sensations of satiety or hunger may never be experienced. The brain, therefore, may fail to recognize these, which may result in poor regulation of eating behaviour at some point in life. A further complication is the relatively recent introduction of between-meal eating or snacking, which has become normalized within habit and behaviours, marketed with a vast range of new non-meal 'snacks'.

Psychological Drivers for Eating

Eating is a pleasurable activity and can satisfy some of our internal needs. Boredom provides a major incentive to eating and may fill many empty hours for people. Depression or anxiety can also make people turn to food for comfort. This is believed to stem from the reassurance given by food provided by parents to children, linking positive feelings about parental care and love with the food. It is important that the 'food as comfort' response is not made too frequently, as it is likely to result in overweight, often with associated emotional problems.

We may also offer food to people to distract or comfort them; for example, a child who has fallen and been hurt may be cuddled and then offered something to eat (often a sweet or biscuit). After a funeral, people may come together to share food. This acts as a comforting gesture for both those providing the food and those eating it. Children with learning disabilities are often given excess food and become habituated to overeating. If we remember that provision of food is linked with loving and caring, it is easy to see how rejection of the food by the intended recipient can be hurtful and painful. This happens with young children who are learning about food but can become manipulative and cause their carers considerable hurt. They may use food rejection to express feelings of anger, jealousy or insecurity or to gain attention. Children who have to follow a special diet for health reasons may be particularly at risk of this type of behaviour. Using food as a weapon can become a habit maintained into adult life.

The sensory stimuli which trigger food seeking and eating may become confused. A bored, lonely person sitting watching TV commonly perceives a signal to get up, go to the fridge and eat. The physiological need may actually be to get up and exercise.

Sensory Appeal

The way in which a food stimulates our senses by its appearance and smell, taste and texture may also increase our desire to eat it. Most people claim that the taste of the food is the prime consideration, although for adolescents, the appearance also rates highly.

The visual appeal of the food, although important to attract the eye, can be quite deceptive, however, and gives no indication of nutritional value. Most sighted people would be very wary of accepting and eating a food they could not see. Our expectations of the taste of a food are prepared by its appearance – we expect an orange-coloured drink to have a sweet, citric taste; anything else might lead to rejection. The food industry is well aware of the importance of the 'correct' visual stimulus and uses a range of colorants to produce an acceptable finished appearance. However, the numbers of these are less than they were 10–20 years ago as consumers become more concerned about safety aspects and are increasingly prepared to buy foods with a more 'natural' colour.

The smell of the food must also meet our expectations. We use this to detect if food has 'gone off', and we are enticed to eat by pleasant aromas. We can recognize many foods purely from their smell. Smell and taste interact to produce the flavour of the food; if the sense of smell is lost, for example, when suffering from a cold, food may seem tasteless. The number of taste buds is highest in children, who have them on the insides of the cheeks and throat, as well as over the surface of the tongue. These begin to decrease from adolescence and are considerably reduced by the age of 70.

Children's food preferences and choices are driven primarily by taste. Relative to adults, young children have a preference for very sweet taste and avoid bitter tastes. The liking for intense sweetness declines into adolescence, more so in girls than boys. There is also a link between energy density and sweetness, and this is believed to be a means by which intake of high-energy foods is assured to support growth and development in children. Once adulthood is reached, the need for such energy-dense foods is reduced, and the liking for intense sweetness tends to disappear. The aversion to bitter tastes also declines, and adults accept and enjoy bitter tastes. With increasing age, there is also a move to less energy-dense foods, which are often those associated with a healthier diet. Taste perception can change in certain circumstances: pregnant women, surgical patients and people with cancer or liver disease all report an altered ability to taste certain foods. It has been suggested that zinc status plays a role in this. Unusual appetites for particular foods may also develop. People can become accustomed to a particular taste if this is perceived to be an advantage. The bitter tastes found in beer, quinine (in tonic water) and coffee appear to be an acquired taste for many people. Taste and small sensations can be lost after a stroke and with dementia, and appetite can be declined.

The texture and taste of the food in the mouth provide us with the pleasurable aspects of eating. The feel of the food in the mouth can include its texture, temperature and even any pain it produces. We expect particular foods to be presented at a certain temperature (e.g. ice cream or hot tea). Extremes of temperature can cause pain to the mouth and teeth. Chilli contains a chemical substance (capsaicin), which irritates the nerve endings, triggering pain. Some substances can cause a local anaesthetic effect in the mouth – chewing coca leaves (widespread practice in parts of South America) has this effect; its purpose is to dull the hunger sensation among people who have little food.

Food technologists can measure optimal levels of various sensory characteristics (such as sugar content, aroma, water content, temperature), which are associated with the highest level of pleasure. These are aptly named 'bliss points'. These are not fixed forever and can become modified if the diet changes, although the initial alteration to the diet will be associated with a reduction in pleasure. For example, an individual who normally takes two spoonfuls of sugar in their tea probably will have that concentration of sugar as their 'bliss point'. Cutting out sugar will result in a reduction in 'bliss'. In time, the subject is likely to adapt to the newer taste, the level of 'bliss' is restored at a lower sweetness, and drinking tea with the original level of sugar will no longer be acceptable. This sequence will apply to other changes made to the diet that have sensory implications, including cutting down fat or salt intakes. Removing all added salt from food makes food taste bland for about 10 days, but a normal perception of food then returns.

Variety encourages us to eat. Studies on both animals and humans have shown clearly that, when offered a variety of food, total intake is greater than when just a single food is offered. Thus, it is possible to make rats overweight by offering them a 'cafeteria diet', containing chips, burgers, crisps, chocolate, etc., rather than ordinary rat pellets; they eat more of the mixed diet. Humans will also overeat when offered something new; for example, having apparently eaten their fill of a main course, many people will still manage to have a dessert afterwards. It has also been noted that more food is eaten when meals are accompanied by wine and taken in a social setting. These factors occurring together can promote an unconscious overconsumption. Overweight is much less common in communities around the world where only a few foods appear regularly in the diet – it seems that monotony imposes its own limits on eating. On the other hand, organizing food into different courses, with different flavours, seems to enhance the food intake. In a sense, this is counter-physiological. With greater variety, there is a better spread of nutrients, so less food is required, not more.

Social Influence

Food is used in a social context to please or displease others. Offering food or drink is recognized as a gesture of hospitality, and refusal may be interpreted as rejection. This may extend to the obligation to eat food that is not wanted or even disliked, to avoid offending the giver. This may be a particular problem for visitors to other countries, who may be presented with unknown or even unacceptable food yet feel obliged to consume it.

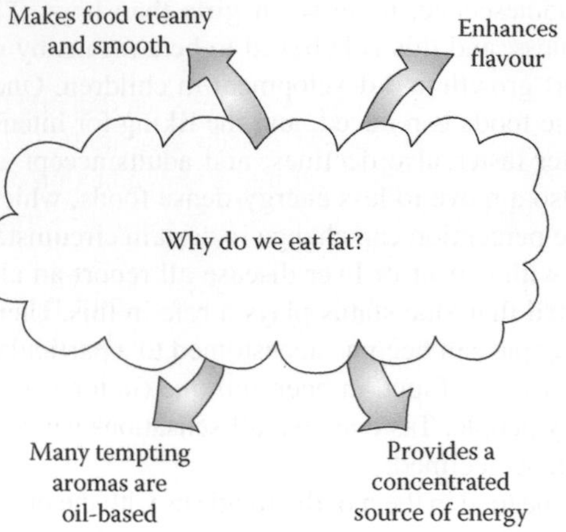

FIGURE 13.1 Why do we eat?

In situations where food is scarce or budgets are very restricted, wasting food may be socially unacceptable, and individuals may feel it necessary to eat everything provided. The opposite may also apply – waste may be quite acceptable where food supplies are plentiful or where leftover food can be put to other uses, such as feeding pigs or poultry.

All of these influences and some of their interrelationships are summarized in Figure 13.1.

FOOD HABITS

So far, we have learned that the primary reason for eating is to satisfy our hunger and that what and when we eat can also reflect who we are, the society we live in, our upbringing and how we perceive ourselves. We can identify typical food habits of a particular group of people in relation to food, which provide important signals of the identity of the group. They determine food choice, as well as eating times and numbers of meals, size of portions, methods of food preparation and who takes part in the meal. Food habits are a product of the environmental influences on a culture, and they are resistant to change, but if change is improved, perception, taste and habits change quite rapidly.

Some of the components of an individual's food habits are shown in Figure 13.2.

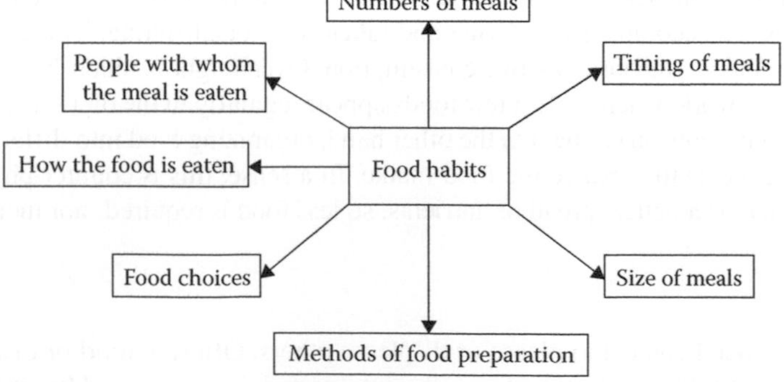

FIGURE 13.2 Some of the main components of a person's food habits.

Acquisition of Food Habits

The acquisition of food habits is largely unconscious, since they are acquired at a young age from parents, which incidentally ensures transmission between generations. The strongest influence on a child in its acquisition of food habits has generally its mother, who is likely to be the most closely involved with the provision of food. Children learn what is acceptable as food and what is not. Foods that are associated with good times are often preferred to those that do not have these connotations. We may remember particularly foods that we ate on holiday and seek these out to relive happy memories. Children are dependent on the food practices and beliefs of the adult caregivers; this may restrict a child's opportunities to try many foods, if they are not part of the adult's food choice. In addition, some foods may be seen as inappropriate for children and, therefore, not offered.

After the initial socialization within the home environment, children learn more food practices from other people or institutions outside the home. A major force may be school, where behaviour is learned from other children, as well as through the food provided in school meals and tuck shops, and more formal teaching about food in lessons. All of these will broaden the child's view of food and will affect the food practices.

Later still, other people may influence food habits as different views are encountered with a widening social circle. Foreign travel also provides experience of different food habits.

Changing Food Habits

Although food habits are resistant to change, they are not static. Change may come from within the culture. For example, the increase in female employment in the West has resulted in a dramatic increase in the availability of convenience food. Fewer households now eat meals prepared from basic ingredients on a regular basis. Weekday meals in particular are composed to a great extent of convenience items, with perhaps the addition of a home-prepared vegetable or starchy staple (such as rice or potato). The prevalence of microwave ovens, together with widespread ownership of freezers, has meant that meals can be ready in minutes and that even quite young children can prepare themselves something hot to eat with little risk of accident. The consequence of this has been that, in many families, mealtimes are no longer taken together. Instead, individual members of the family may eat at times convenient to themselves, often heating up different meals in the microwave. In addition, around 30% of meals eaten are likely to be consumed away from home, in work or school canteens, in cafes, in fast-food outlets, in restaurants or in the car. The National Food Survey rolling survey (UK, 2008–2012) showed that a quarter of adults ate out once a week or more, while a fifth brought takeaway meals for consumption at home; this represents 26% of the expenditure on food.

Another source of change is the increase in the availability of information about world cookery. Examples of the cuisine of different cultures are found in restaurants, supermarkets and as cookery programmes on the television, and the wide availability of many exotic ingredients makes it possible for these 'foreign' dishes to be included into traditional food habits. Many books describe how to prepare these dishes.

The media are also responsible for changing food habits. This may occur through the following:

- Advertising and promotion of new food products (although the information given here may be biased).
- Programmes or articles that aim to increase people's knowledge about food, perhaps in the context of nutrition and health.

- Providing role models in the form of characters in programmes and advertising. These contribute a subtle force towards change in food habits by the food they eat and the attitudes they express. Some of the messages put forwards are not necessarily conducive to health; for example, there is believed to be a prevailing message that only thin women are healthy and attractive, which causes often disastrous changes to food habits among the female population.

One prominent media activity which appears not to alter cooking on eating habits is celebrity cooking programmes, whose educational value is close to zero.

Food habits may have to change when an individual suffers from an illness requiring dietary alteration for its management. The difficulty of changing food habits is best seen in such subjects, who often struggle to maintain dietary changes, even when there are very good health reasons for doing so.

Nutrition educators and health promoters aim to change food habits towards a healthier balance. This is a very complex process because of the multifaceted influences on food habits. Different influences may be at work in determining what is eaten from day to day or even from meal to meal. A further factor is the strength of the attitude of the subject towards food and healthy eating. If they are ambivalent about either of these, change may be difficult to bring about. Finally, the subjective recognition that change is needed to the diet is a powerful influence in determining whether it is undertaken.

Therefore, an educator may need to consider the strength of the subject's belief:

- That food and healthy eating are important
- That these can influence their individual health in a beneficial way
- That making changes to food and eating has a high priority among factors that influence food choice

Studies have identified many barriers to making changes towards healthy eating that are more prevalent among those subjects who make fewer changes. In a study by Margetts et al. (1998), these included the following:

- A perception that there is a lack of clear messages about healthy foods
- A belief that the tastiest foods are the ones that are 'bad'
- Confusion about what to eat
- Difficulty of eating healthy food away from home
- Costs of healthy eating
- Lack of concern about what is eaten

In addition, changes towards healthier eating are less likely to be found among younger, lower-income groups and those who smoke. This emphasizes that dietary change is closely linked to other lifestyle indicators in complex ways.

Food Choices

Within the context of a culture's food habits, each individual makes their own, personal food choices, which are likely to be different from those of anyone else. There are many ways to study individual food choices, and much has been written about them. There are still areas of uncertainty, however, and research into determinants of food choice, especially within family groups, is ongoing. Viewpoints may be anthropological, economic, physiological or administrative, political, psychological or sociological, as well as nutritional. The following is a nutritional perspective on food choice.

In very broad terms, people can only choose from the range of food available and accessible to them; thus, factors that determine food supply and distribution are important. Given a range of foods, an individual will not necessarily choose to eat all of them. The choice will depend on what is acceptable to them, personally, and here affordability is a key component. Hence, the four main

TABLE 13.1

Factors Influencing the Availability of Foods

Physical/Environmental	Legislative	Economic	Food Handling
Locality (soil/climate)	National/international laws	Money	Access to shops
Transport/marketing		Budget priorities	Cooking skills
Distribution costs	Health recommendations	Cost of foods	Knowledge
Perishability		Significance of foods	Cooking facilities
		Variety	Time available
Factors affecting accessibility of foods			
Family status			
Mobility/car ownership			
Disability			

determinants of food choice all begin with 'a': availability, accessibility, acceptability and affordability (Tables 13.1 and 13.2).

Availability

Physical/Environmental Factors

In the West, these factors are less important now than they were 20 or more years ago. Food preservation, storage and distribution around world markets are so efficient that it rarely matters whether the local area produces a food or not. It can generally be imported from elsewhere. This creates a uniformity of foods available, and there is concern that many interesting varieties of locally produced foods are being lost or remain available only in a speciality market. Differences exist, however, in what food is available to buy in a locality. This will be dependent on factors such as population density and, therefore, the number of shops in the vicinity and ease of access, which will determine the cost of transporting food into the area. The perishability of a food will also determine the range over which it can be transported. For these reasons, rural areas in most countries generally have a smaller range of food available than urban areas.

However, in places not reached by the world market, where locally grown produce is eaten, physical factors, such as type of soil, rainfall or transportation, are important determinants of what food is actually available. The perishability of food and the means of preservation available will also determine how long food can be kept. Thus, for a subsistence family in a developing country, physical factors are extremely important determinants. The range of foods available for local trading will have a major impact on the food they eat.

TABLE 13.2

Factors Influencing the Acceptability of Foods

Cultural	Physiological	Social/Psychological
National identity	Physiological need	Status (of self/of foods)
Culture group	Hunger/satiety	Group identity
Meal patterns	Appetite/aversion	Communication
Religious ideology	Sensory appeal	Ritual
Taboos/prohibitions	Personal preference/choice	Emotional support
	Therapeutic diets	Reward/punishment

Legislative Factors

Government legislation aims to ensure that food available for purchase is of a suitable quality and has not been adulterated. There is also agricultural policy, which regulates the prices received by the producers of crops. Trade agreements and sanctions may operate at particular times between different countries. In addition, the United Kingdom, as a member state of the European Union, is subject to Europe-wide laws relating to food and agricultural production. All these factors will influence the type of food available for sale in shops and its exact composition, especially in terms of additives and minimum standards of composition.

In recent years, the labelling of foods has become more explicit, with more information about the nutritional composition appearing on the label. The quality of this information is ensured by public agencies, the European Food Safety Authority (EFSA) in Europe, the Food and Drug Administration (FDA) in the US. This is to be applauded as an important means of educating people about nutrition, as well as providing useful information for anyone who wishes to understand more about the food they eat.

Legislation has also been needed to control the introduction of some of the new foods resulting from developments in food technology. Recent introductions in Britain have included irradiated foods, items produced from research in genetic engineering and foods containing synthetic substitutes (e.g. for fat). In addition, there is a growing market in 'functional foods'. All have been the subject of safety testing and have needed to obtain government approval before being marketed. There are regulated processes for making health claims about foods, through agencies like EFSA in Europe, FDA in US, but the sheer numbers of foods, and the complex nuances of claims which can increase sales, has made health claims difficult to police.

Affordability, Cost and Taxation

The cost of food is a major determinant of what people perceive as available to them; it ranks only after taste in general surveys of influences on choice. Within the range of foods available to them, people can only eat what they can afford or choose to afford. The second point is important, since it brings into consideration the priorities that exist in spending money. The annual DEFRA statistics (2014) point out that, on average, people in Britain spent 11.4% of their budget on food, although this is less among the better off and can be much more (up to 30% or more) among lower-income groups. Food prices have risen since 2007, 18% in real term to 2012, with a slight decrease since. People see their food budget as one of the more flexible items in their expenditure; other expenses such as fuel, rent, cigarettes and alcohol may take priority. When income is small and food budget cuts are made, food distribution within the family may change, food treats may still be bought, and the children's likes and dislikes may be attended to. The variety of foods eaten becomes smaller and the diet becomes more monotonous. Since 2007, lowest-income households purchased less beef, bacon, butter, fish, fruit, tea and biscuits/cakes and bought more pork, poultry and eggs. Interestingly, the steepest price increases affected sugar/confectionaries, fish and alcohol, while the price of potatoes, vegetables, coffee, tea, coca and fruit fell. Recent attempts have been made to limit the consumptions of certain foods high in saturated fats, and high in sugars, using selective taxation. This is clearly effective, at least in the short term, sales falling with increasing tax, provided the purchaser can see the added cost.

Accessibility

If food is available and there is money with which to buy it, getting to the shops, bringing it home and preparing it for eating remain as possible areas of difficulty. Particular difficulties face large families, mainly if there is no car. Many supermarkets in Britain have moved to peripheral locations outside towns, which makes shopping easier for the car-owning customers who spend a lot of money, but very difficult for those families living further away, without transport. The sheer weight of fruits and vegetables required by a large family, if it is to meet nutritional guidelines, presents difficulty for access and transport, as well as storage. These foods need to be purchased most days as they will deteriorate. They are commonly not accessible without a car. These then rely on the local shops, which inevitably keep less stock, thereby restricting choice. Special problems of accessibility face the elderly and disabled.

Once the food is in the kitchen, most of it has to be prepared in some way for eating. This will depend largely on the knowledge and skill of the cook, facilities and time available. Cooking skills are variable; it has been suggested that fewer people now know how to cook which restricts access to available food in an edible state. This has been attributed to the escalating reliance on pre-prepared convenience foods, which eliminate the need for cooking skills. Often the only skill required is the ability to open a packet or can and heat the contents. Some foods can even be eaten cold out of the packaging in which they were bought. In families where cooking does take place, the complexity of the preparation of the food will reflect the cook's personal experience of food and cooking, education, interest and time available.

Acceptability

Cultural Factors

Each cultural group possesses its own typical food selection patterns. These may be similar to those of related cultural groups, but are unlikely to be the same. Even within a relatively small country such as the United Kingdom, there are different regional foods, such as haggis in Scotland, laver bread in Wales and jellied eels in London. However, all these groups also share similar 'British' food choices, such as fish and chips or roast beef. It is not just the choice of food that may vary between the cultures, but also the way in which it is cooked, the seasonings and flavourings used and the way it is served.

Traditional foods confer a sense of identity and belonging. This is very deeply held, since for most people, it derives from the socialization process in childhood, discussed earlier. The strength and persistence of this cultural identity may be illustrated by two examples. First, when people holiday in another country, many will seek out foods with which they are familiar. Although they may be prepared to try the local dishes, it is often with a sense of curiosity and a preconceived idea that they will be strange. More importantly, when people emigrate to another country for long-term settlement, they often suffer a sense of alienation or difference from the adopted environment. They may adopt the host country's style of dress and speak the language, but the food that is eaten in the privacy of their home may remain very traditional. This provides a link with the homeland and support in an alien environment.

If in addition to providing a cultural identity, the food is also associated with religious beliefs, and traditional food habits may persist longer still. Studies on migrants to Britain show that first-generation members adhere strongly to traditional food practices. With the second generation, these practices are less widespread, unless they are associated with religious prescription. Conflict may arise between the generations as a result. Short-term migration does not, however, bring about changes to the diet, with evidence pointing to a reluctance to include host-country foods and an adherence to traditional foods, even if they are hard to find.

The types of foods that may be served to form a meal are culturally determined. People may classify foods in different ways: for example, 'sweet' and 'savoury', 'healthy' and 'less healthy', 'snack food' (or 'junk food') and 'proper meal'. Nutritionists categorize foods more systematically in terms of their main nutritional role in the diet. Currently, most Western countries use five food groups: cereal/grain (or starchy) foods, fruit and vegetables, meat and meat substitutes, milk and dairy products and fatty and sugary foods. An appropriate amount of each group should be eaten to provide a nutritionally balanced diet.

As well as providing the accepted norms for what can be eaten, cultural identity will also determine what should not be eaten. Each culture has clearly defined ideas about what is 'food' and 'non-food'. In many instances, these distinctions have arisen for sound reasons, including scarcity of a particular plant or animal or its potential harmfulness. In addition, there may be prohibitions on particular foods at certain times of life, particularly in infancy and during pregnancy. Many cultures have prohibitions associated with pregnancy, based on beliefs about possible effects on the fetus. Although generally harmless, some may restrict intakes of foods, such as meat or other useful sources of iron, for which needs are increased in pregnancy. It is also believed by some that eating a particular mixture of foods around the time of conception can influence the gender of the embryo.

A taboo that occurs in most world cultures is that against cannibalism, but even this deep-rooted taboo is not universal. There are records throughout history of people reverting to cannibalism in times of severe hardship, such as wartime siege or following an air crash in an inaccessible region, as well as some cases of murder followed by cannibalism.

Many world religions also forbid the eating of particular foods completely or at special times. These include a prohibition on pork among Muslims and Jews, and on all animals among the Hindus and Jains.

Physiological Factors

Since the 1980s, research into the obesity epidemic has revealed a complicated physiological neuroendocrine regulation of appetite and eating. Over 20 peptides secreted from the gut and adipose tissue affect appetite (Lean and Malkova, 2016).

Appetite is associated with memories of particular foods and is the desire for a specific food or foods. In animals, there is some evidence that such desires for particular foods are linked to a specific nutritional need. This is very difficult to demonstrate in humans and has, therefore, not been proven. The opposite is an aversion to a specific food; this is often linked to an unpleasant memory of that food or an experience associated with it.

Personal preferences for foods are usually linked to a liking for the sensory attributes of the food, which contribute to the pleasure of eating it. Liking a food is frequently given as the main reason for choosing it; however, people will eat foods they feel neutral about or even dislike in certain circumstances, for example, to please others. Most people select their food from a relatively small number of items that appear frequently in their diet. New foods may be tried on occasions, often as a result of advertising or promotion of the product in the media. The wealthier members of society include more variety in their choices than those on a low income. Compared with traditional hunter–gatherer societies, who would eat a wide range of wild products from the land at different seasons, our Western diet is quite limited.

Children are considered to be the age group most reluctant to diversify their diet, with some individuals eating so few foods that they threaten their nutritional status.

Because of the importance of personal preference in making food choice, it is important that individuals are allowed to exercise some control over what is eaten. Loss of control can lead to loss of appetite. This can be a reason for poor intakes in hospitalized patients or residents in other institutions, where menus are centrally determined, perhaps repetitive, and little choice is offered.

The need to follow a special diet for therapeutic reasons will affect personal food selection and is a further area where loss of control and self-determination may cause problems with compliance. This is a particular problem in adolescents, who may refuse to comply with dietary restrictions, as part of the maturing process. Food selection may be deliberately restricted in those wishing to control their weight: eating behaviour becomes inhibited, and less food than is required to alleviate hunger may be eaten. Also, specific food groups (the 'fattening foods') may be avoided, while others are eaten in their place (the 'slimming foods'). If the inhibition of intake is broken, for a number of reasons, food intake may become excessive, resulting in binge eating, until the inhibitory influence is restored. This pattern of restrained eating appears to exist, to a greater or lesser extent, in up to 80–90% of women in Western society. In some, it results in clinically recognized conditions of anorexia or bulimia nervosa.

Special diets may be adopted for moral or ideological perspectives, and these will impose constraints on individual food choice. Of these, vegetarian diets have become the most prevalent in Britain in recent years. The extent to which people stop eating all animal produce varies and some of those claiming to be vegetarian may still actually consume some animal foods, even white meat as well as fish, eggs, cheese and milk. The reasons for choosing this diet may stem from abhorrence of the killing of animals (and the methods used) and concern about the exploitation of animals reared in cramped conditions for food. More recent publicity about aspects of food safety related to foods of animal origin, such as beef, chicken, eggs and milk, has convinced others that avoiding these foods may be healthier.

Whatever the rationale for the special diet, the individual's freedom of choice is restricted. It makes the person different from the rest of their culture group (this may be one of the objectives!). Consequently, it may create barriers to the sharing of food, causing alienation and possibly avoidance of social eating situations or lack of compliance with therapeutic diets. Giving as much freedom of choice as possible within the constraints of a special diet will help the individual to regain their self-determination and enhance compliance.

Choosing to follow a 'healthy' diet is a positive choice made by an increasing number of people. This has arisen from the recognition that many of the diseases prevalent in Western society may have a dietary origin. The understanding of these links may not be very accurate and even confused, as may also the understanding of what constitutes a 'healthy' diet. A common belief is that eating too much fat causes heart disease in men or that too much chocolate will make women fat. Thus, one or two aspects of current dietary guidelines may be adopted, while others are ignored. Only a tiny percentage of the population manage to achieve all of the dietary guidelines, most focus on one or two isolated foods, and the idea of a 'whole-diet' approach to healthy eating has not been widely recognized. The concept of 'healthiness' becomes blurred by food safety issues, including concerns about additives in foods, genetically modified products, food that is not fresh, ready-made foods containing unknown ingredients and possible contamination by microorganisms, such as *Listeria* or *Salmonella*. Most commonly, a 'healthy' diet is equated with a 'slimming' diet, and men frequently hold the view that 'healthy eating' is something for girls to do.

To attempt to clarify this, nutritionists tend to avoid the term 'healthy' as applied to food or diets. 'Healthful' is better, but still open to misinterpretation.

Social/Psychological Influences

Although our own physiological needs and wants are important determinants of what we find acceptable to eat, we are nevertheless also influenced in our actions by the prevailing social conditions, as well as our own psychological makeup.

Food and the way it is presented can be used to express status in society. The most obvious distinction is that between having and not having food. Every fisherman understands this distinction. The wealthy generally have access to more and varied food, while the poor have less choice and are more likely to go hungry. In some societies, it is a sign of wealth and status to be obese.

Individual foods may also have differing status: those that are more expensive or difficult to get, such as grouse, venison or caviar, will be perceived as being high status. On the other hand, foods such as tripe or pig's trotters may be equally unusual, but because of their association with low-income diets, usually have a low status. Everyday staple foods, such as potatoes, rice and pasta, will also have relatively low status. The status of foods may change with time, depending on how they are valued. For example, in the nineteenth century, brown bread was considered coarse and fit only for the lower classes; now it is seen as healthy and desirable in the diet, and its status has increased considerably. Sausages in Italy or France are high-status foods, renowned for their place of origin and unique blends of constituents, texture and flavours. In United Kingdom, sausages are mass produced, homogenous in texture and flavour and made largely from high-fat waste products. They have low status.

What is eaten in particular circumstances is likely to reflect the assumed status of the food. When eating alone, it does not matter what we eat, and people may 'treat' themselves to combinations of foods that they would not eat in company. As soon as food is eaten in company, value judgements are made on the basis of the foods. The status of the foods served reflects the implied status in which the diners are held. Thus, the type of food shared in a meal implies more than satisfying a physiological need. Sharing food with others is very symbolic: it confirms previously established links and a sense of mutual identity. There is also powerful peer pressure to conform with social norms in food selection.

Relationships within groups of people are confirmed in the sharing of food: usually the most powerful or most important members of the group are served first. This confirms their superiority and allows them to choose the prime parts of the meal.

The food preferences of men and women often differ; in most cultures, men consume more meat and women consume more fruit and vegetables. Women are expected to be thinner, to eat less and tend to eat more of the foods that are regarded as 'healthy'. It is suggested that these differences are associated with the traditional gender roles, which still exist in society. Women remain in charge of the food-related activity; therefore, they tend to know more about food. Information about healthy diets tends to be seen more by women, as it features in women's magazines or in leaflets available from supermarkets or in doctors' surgeries. However, despite this greater knowledge or level of information, decisions about what is eaten are shown to be dictated in many families by the men and children rather than the women. Studies of changes in food intake on marriage show that both partners make some adjustments, with husbands adopting more of the wives' habits initially but reverting to their original habits in time. Married men tend to have healthier diets and better health prospects than single men.

Differences have also been reported in the way food is eaten, with men taking gulps and mouthfuls, whereas women nibble and pick. As a consequence of this, it is suggested that some foods are more appropriate for women (such as fish or fruit) and other foods for men (red meat, bread).

Food can be a powerful means of communication. A box of chocolates given as a present is perhaps the most widely used example of food acting as a token of affection. Some may find it easier to give the chocolates than to put into words what they are feeling. A cup of tea is a typical British answer to a difficult social situation, when words are hard to find. A family eating a meal together is sharing not only food but also the affection they feel for each other. Rejecting the meal in this situation can, therefore, be a very potent dismissal of the love being offered. Reciprocal invitations to meals or parties by both adults and children strengthen the social bonds. Children may exchange small items of food, such as sweets, to communicate their friendship. In Scotland, they are called play-pieces.

A special form of communication by means of food exists in the ritual use of food. Many religions use foods as offerings to their deities as sacrifices or in shared eating. Christians use bread and wine. The end of the growing season and the harvest are marked in many communities by a festival, with a sample of the crops being offered in thanksgiving, often to the poorest members of the community.

Certain life events are marked by specific ritual meals – baptismal feasts, wedding breakfast and funeral wake. Group membership may also be marked by rituals involving food or drink, for example, the pre-wedding ritual of stag night and hen party, where men and women separately undergo a 'rite of passage', usually involving large amounts of alcohol. Danakil tribesmen would go to battle without a bellyful of camel milk.

Food represents security from the earliest age, so that in times of stress, it can form an important support. Anxiety can provoke eating as a means of coping with tension, although in some individuals stress can result in a loss of appetite and an inability to eat. Anxiety may also lead to feeding others, for example, anxious mothers may overfeed their children to relieve their own anxiety about them. Abnormal eating patterns have also been linked with uncertainty about a person's role or position in society. It has been suggested that both overweight and anorexia nervosa may originate from a dissociation between the socially desirable body image and that with which the individual feels psychologically at ease.

In the case of obesity, it is argued that overeating occurs as a deliberate attempt to add substance to the body (generally female) in an effort to cope with the demands of the world. In anorexia nervosa, the body size is deliberately reduced to escape from the pressures of society on the adult female and return to the child shape.

SUMMARY

1. Apart from the physiological need and neuroendocrine drivers to eat, human food intake is also heavily influenced by psychological needs, social influences and the sensory satisfaction obtained from eating and habit.
2. What is eaten is also influenced by many factors that determine the availability of food, its accessibility, acceptability and affordability to the individual.
3. Despite many differences between cultures in actual foods eaten, influences on eating and food choice are similar.
4. The interaction of influencing factors may be a key determinant in achieving dietary change.

STUDY QUESTIONS

1. The sensory appeal of food is very important. Give examples of some situations where
   a. Sensory properties may not be detected by the eater
   b. Additional care needs to be taken to enhance sensory appeal
2. Consider the food habits of members of your family or your immediate friends.
   a. Have they changed in the last 10 years? 30 years?
   b. If so, can you account for any changes?
   c. If they have remained the same, what have been the major factors maintaining this consistency?
3. Suggest ways in which government action could influence food habits. What barriers to change might this encounter?
4. In what ways can the following influence food habits:
   a. Travel
   b. Education
   c. Multi-ethnic societies
   d. Owning a microwave oven

ACTIVITIES

13.1 Before studying this chapter, spend a little time thinking about
a. Why you eat
b. What you eat
c. What are some of the reasons for choosing the particular foods

You may find that this is a surprisingly difficult task. We are generally quite unconscious of our reasons for eating and choosing particular foods. Only when we have a basic framework with which to study these influences can we begin to gain insight into our own behaviour related to food.

13.2 Using your experience, try to identify which of the factors given in Figure 13.2 are likely to be most important for the following people:

a. Yourself
b. A preschool-age child
c. A mother with young children
d. A teenage girl/boy
e. An elderly woman, living on her own

Account for your answers.

BIBLIOGRAPHY AND FURTHER READING

Adams, J., Goffe, L., Brown, T. et al. 2015. Frequency and socio-demographic correlates of eating meals out and take-away meals at home: Cross-sectional analysis of the UK national diet and nutrition survey, waves 1–4 (2008–12). *International Journal of Behavioral Nutrition and Physical Activity* 12(1), 51.

Blundell, J.E. and Halford, J.C.G. 1994. Regulation of nutrient supply: The brain and appetite control. *Proceedings of the Nutrition Society* 53, 407–418.

Burnett, C. 1994. The use of sweets as rewards in schools. *Journal of Human Nutrition and Dietetics* 7, 441–446.

Charles, N. and Kerr, M. 1988. *Women, Food and Families*. Manchester, UK: Manchester University Press.

Cotton, J.R., Burley, V.J., Weststrate, J.A. et al. 1994. Dietary fat and appetite: Similarities and differences in the satiating effect of meals supplemented with either fat or carbohydrate. *Journal of Human Nutrition and Dietetics* 7, 11–24.

Craig, P.L. and Truswell, A.S. 1994. Dynamics of food habits of newly married couples: Who makes changes in the foods consumed? *Journal of Human Nutrition and Dietetics* 7(5), 347–362.

DEFRA. 2001. National Food Survey 2000: Annual report on food expenditure, consumption and nutrient intakes. London, UK: The Stationery Office.

DEFRA. 2014. *Food Statistics Pocketbook 2014*. London, UK: The Stationery Office.

Lean, M.E.J. and Malkova, D. 2016. Altered gut and adipose tissue hormones in overweight and obese individuals: cause or consequence? *International Journal of Obesity* 40, 622–632.

Lee, S., Kim, Y., Seo, S. and Cho, M.S. 2014. A study on dietary habits and food intakes in adults aged 50 or older according to depression status. *Journal of Nutrition and Health* 47(1), 67–76.

Margetts, B.M., Thompson, R.L., Speller, V. et al. 1998. Factors which influence 'healthy' eating patterns: Results from the 1993 Health Education Authority health and lifestyle survey in England. *Public Health Nutrition* 1(3), 193–198.

Mennell, S., Murcott, A. and van Otterloo, A.H. 1992. *The Sociology of Food: Eating, Diet and Culture*. London, UK: SAGE Publications.

Stubbs, R.J., Harbron, C.G., Murgatroyd, P.R. et al. 1995. Covert manipulation of dietary fat and energy density: Effect on substrate flux and food intake in men eating ad libitum. *American Journal of Clinical Nutrition* 62(2), 316–329.

Weststrate, J.A. 1996. Fat and obesity. *British Nutrition Foundation Nutrition Bulletin* 21, 18–25.

Wilding, J.P. 2002. Neuropeptides and appetite control. *Diabetic Medicine* 19, 519–527.

Wood, R.C. 1995. *The Sociology of the Meal*. Edinburgh, UK: University Press.

14 Diet and Coronary Heart Disease

AIMS

The aims of this chapter are to

- Define what is meant by coronary heart disease and describe its development.
- Describe the lipid hypothesis for heart disease aetiology.
- Study some of the ways in which evidence about heart disease causation has been collected.
- Identify some of the suggested risk factors.
- Describe the suggested role of dietary factors in the development and prevention of heart disease.

Coronary heart disease, together with other cardiovascular diseases are responsible for more than 17.3 million deaths per year and are the leading causes of death in the world. Throughout Europe, cardiovascular disease accounts for about 40% of overall mortality; the majority of these deaths are attributable to coronary heart disease, most of the remainder to stroke. Across Europe, there is an East–West gradient, with higher mortality rates in central and Eastern Europe than in Western Europe. The differential between the highest and lowest mortality approaches a factor of 5. There are also higher rates of coronary heart disease, but not stroke, in Northern Europe than in the South, and the variation between North and South is approximately 2.5.

Death rates from coronary heart disease vary between the countries of the United Kingdom. The rates are highest in Scotland and the North of England, lowest in the South of England and intermediate in Wales and Northern Ireland. The premature death rate for men living in Scotland is 63% higher than in South West of England and 100% higher for women. These rates have been consistently highest in Scotland for more than 25 years. Almost half (46%) of all deaths from cardiovascular disease are from coronary heart disease. Heart disease rates among women in the United Kingdom are some of the highest in the world. In Scotland, the rate among women aged 35–74 is 10 times greater than that in Japanese women.

People born in the Indian subcontinent living in the United Kingdom have heart disease rates 36% higher than those in the population as a whole. Those in people originating from the Caribbean countries are lower than in the population as a whole, by 55% in males and 24% in females.

In the United Kingdom, the age-standardized death rate of people under 65 from circulatory diseases was 35 per 100,000 of the population in 2008 (half of the age-standardized death rate in 1995). In France, which has the lowest rate in Europe, the death rate was 36 per 100,000 in 1995 and 15 in 2008. In comparison, in Belarus, the age-standardized death rate of people under 65 from circulatory diseases was 207 per 100,000 of the population in 2008 (216 per 1,000,000 in 1995). In 2012, coronary heart disease caused about 1 in 7 male deaths and 1 in 10 female deaths in the United Kingdom – a total of around 74,000 deaths. In addition, angina and other circulatory disorders, some resulting in stroke, are leading causes of ill health and disability.

CHANGES IN RATES OF CARDIOVASCULAR DISEASE

Most Western European countries, including the United Kingdom, have experienced a downward trend in heart disease rates since the 1980s and early 1990s. There has been a dramatic decline in coronary heart disease mortality in the United Kingdom from 1981 to 2000. Coronary heart disease death rates have been falling fastest in the 55 and over age group and more slowly in the younger age groups. Rates have fallen by 44% in the 75 age group in the last 10 years. However, in the countries of Eastern Europe, such as Hungary, Poland and Romania, rates increased. Cardiovascular mortality rates have declined substantially in high-income countries over the past two decades. Evidence shows that population-wide primary prevention and individual healthcare intervention strategies have both contributed to these declining mortality trends. For example, during the 10-year period covered by the World Health Organization (WHO) Multinational Monitoring of Trends and Determinants in Cardiovascular Disease initiative (WHO MONICA Project), coronary heart disease and stroke mortality rates have declined dramatically in many of the 38 MONICA populations.

In the United States, Australia, New Zealand and Japan, rates have shown dramatic reductions in the last 15–20 years, but the causes are unclear. Perhaps the most remarkable decline in incidence of coronary heart disease has been seen in Finland, where a comprehensive coronary prevention programme was instituted, reducing production an consumption dietary sodium and saturated fats, and encouraging physical activity.

Traditionally, coronary heart disease has been viewed as a disease of men because, in middle age, mortality is higher in men. However, after the menopause, women become increasingly susceptible to the disease and death rates of the two sexes are similar. Since women generally live longer than men, many more suffer from heart disease in old age. As a result of this perception, much of the early research has been focused on the disease in men, and both research and treatment in women has lagged behind. More recent studies have included women among the subjects.

There are many changes that occur in diet and environmental influences that make it very difficult to pinpoint those having the major effects. Positive factors may include health education that affects, for example, the intake of fats, fruit and vegetables and increases physical activity. On the other hand, negative factors may include the societal shift in dietary intake to more 'fast food', as well as political changes (such as in Eastern Europe during the 1990s), which cause stress, and increase alcohol intake and smoking rates.

Projections for the future indicate that prevalence of cardiovascular disease will remain high, and possibly increase among women because of relatively high smoking rates in women, now that smoking has declined among men. There is now better treatment and survival after heart attack, albeit with increased morbidity. By 2030, it is projected that almost 23.6 million people will die from cardiovascular disease mainly from heart disease and stroke. A further reason is the age profile of most populations, with an increase in the proportion of older people, who are at increased risk of these diseases.

This chapter will focus on coronary heart disease, as this is the major manifestation of cardiovascular disease in Western Europe. In addition, more of the research in this area has been on the dietary determinants of coronary heart disease rather than stroke.

WHAT IS CORONARY HEART DISEASE?

A heart attack 'acute coronary syndrome' occurs when the blood and hence oxygen supply to a part of the heart fails because of a blockage in the vessels supplying the muscular walls of the heart. This makes the heart unable to continue working normally to supply blood to the heart muscle itself, causing cardiac chest pain, and to all the parts of the body and, most crucially, to the brain. If a large part of the muscle is deprived of oxygen, the heart attack may be fatal. Failure of a smaller part of the heart muscle may allow the rest of the heart to continue working and maintain the circulation.

If part of the heart muscle dies during an acute coronary syndrome (i.e. 'myocardial infarction'), then there may be permanent functional loss, with chronic heart failure, breathlessness and oedema.

These events are, however, usually the culmination of a process that may have been developing gradually over a long period of time, involving a series of changes to the walls of the coronary arteries. The process may be described in terms of atherogenesis and thrombogenesis (see Figure 14.1).

Injury to the Coronary Arteries

The blood vessel walls are continually exposed to wear and tear by the flow of blood. The wall is not completely smooth, especially where there are divisions of the vessels into smaller channels and associated branching. Blood flow becomes turbulent here, rather like the flow of a river where streams are joining or there is some obstruction to the flow.

Prolonged raised blood pressure will also increase stress on the walls. As a result, the wall of the vessel is continually repairing itself in response to the damage, using the blood platelets and forming minute blood clots. New collagen and smooth muscle cells may be laid down to strengthen the wall. Over a long period of time, these areas may become thicker and, since they are no longer perfect, become more permeable to substances and particles in the blood. Many factors contribute to the normal functioning of the endothelial surface of the blood vessel, including relaxing factors and growth factors, and these are considered to be important in maintaining functional integrity.

Fibrous Plaque Formation

The progression from the previous stage is not completely clear. It is normal for blood vessel walls to be permeable to substances required by the tissues, such as lipid-soluble material needed for metabolic processes. It is now believed that partly oxidized lipids present in low-density lipoprotein (LDL) entering the blood vessel wall are recognized as 'foreign' and are not allowed to pass through the endothelium of the blood vessel. Their presence attracts monocytes (a type of white blood cell), which adhere to and then enter the blood vessel wall. Various factors are now known to influence the adhesion of the monocytes, including nitric oxide (endothelial relaxing factor) and antioxidants (particularly vitamin E).

Having penetrated the blood vessel wall, the monocytes are converted to macrophages, which are scavenger cells whose purpose is to destroy the damaged lipids. However, the macrophage itself then cannot leave the wall and so these scavenger cells accumulate, laden with fat, and gradually coalesce to produce 'foam cells'. When these die, the fat they contain remains in the wall and becomes the origin of the fatty streaks that are believed to be a contributing factor in the atherogenesis of the heart disease process.

The fatty streaks also attract blood platelets and fibrin, which attempt to 'seal off' the damaged area. In the process, these clot-forming entities actually contribute to thickening, producing a fibrous plaque and ultimately hardening the blood vessel wall. Smooth muscle cells are laid down under the influence of growth factors, derived from platelets and other blood components. The plaque area grows, protruding progressively into the lumen of the vessel and further interfering with the blood flow.

Thrombosis and Heart Attack

Eventually, the fibrous plaque becomes unstable and ruptures, releasing fatty contents into the circulation. These attract components of the clotting mechanism, and a thrombus (or clot) is likely to form. If the blood vessel is already narrow at this point, the clot may block the flow of blood. The fibrous plaque components themselves may also become lodged in the vessel. Both of these processes will cause a myocardial infarction, if the blockage is in a coronary blood vessel. When the narrowing and thrombosis occur in a blood vessel supplying the brain, a stroke (or cerebrovascular accident) will be the result.

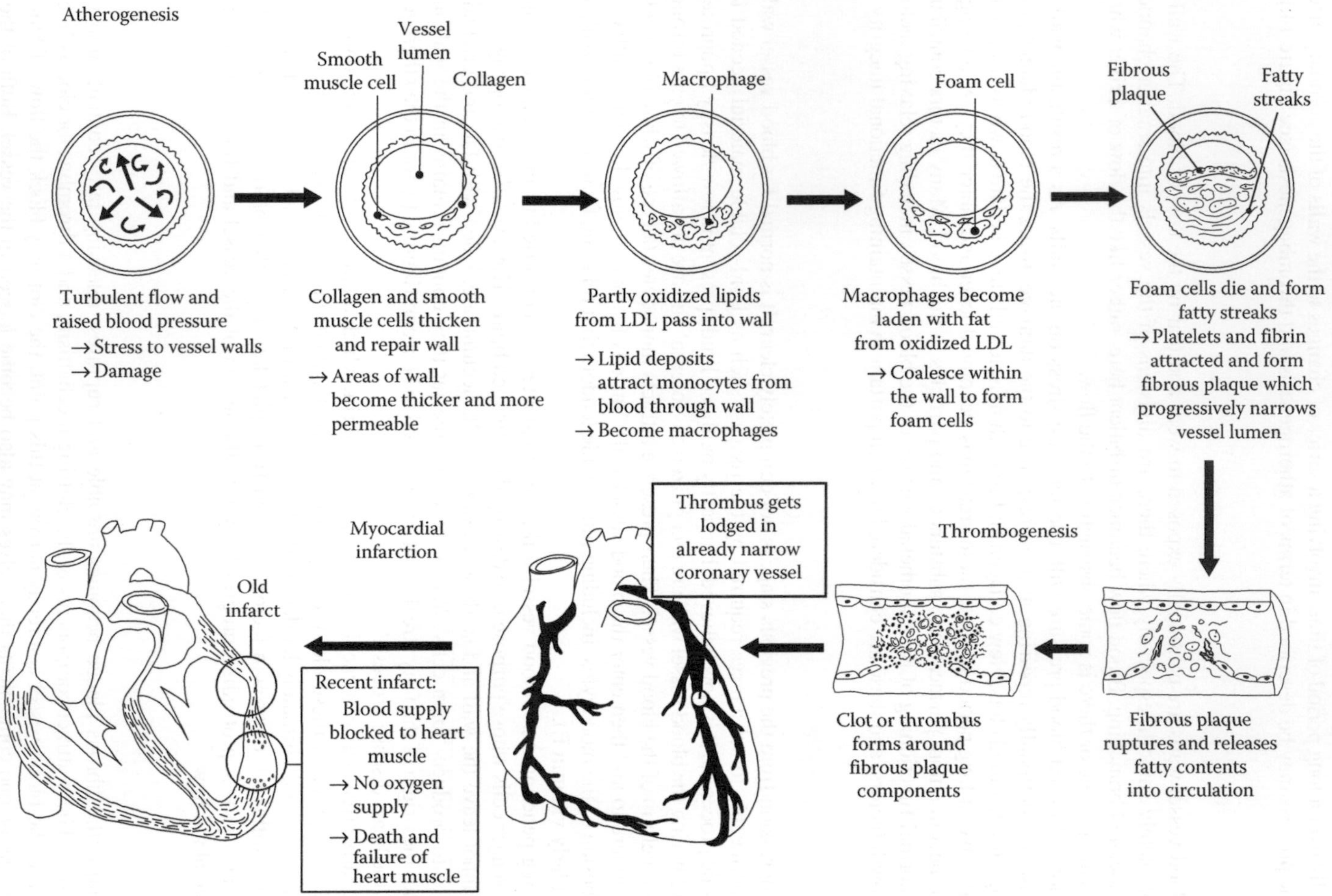

FIGURE 14.1 The development of coronary heart disease. Low-density lipoprotein.

Various physiological and dietary factors are involved in the processes described earlier. An understanding of these is emerging from the many studies of coronary heart disease and its associated risk factors. The developments in molecular biology have added a new dimension to these studies, so that mechanisms that were originally only suggested as a possibility are now being described in detail at the molecular level. As more information becomes available, it clarifies some aspects, but it also demonstrates that the picture is highly complex.

STUDYING CORONARY HEART DISEASE

The study of coronary heart disease is hampered by the absence of a close animal model for myocardial infarction, although aspects of the disease process can be mimicked in various animals. However, to obtain the most relevant data, studies are performed on human populations and, for ethical reasons, are limited in the scope of experimental work that can be done. Much of the research is, therefore, based on epidemiological data obtained from populations with high and low rates of heart disease and attempts to associate these with diet and lifestyle characteristics. A number of approaches have been used. Dietary lipids have been the main focus of attention because of the lipid nature of the fibrous plaque contributing to the narrowing of the blood vessels.

ORIGINS OF THE LIPID HYPOTHESIS

Cross-Community Comparisons

The most widely known of the early studies is Keys' Seven Country Study, which compared fat intakes and serum cholesterol levels with subsequent 10-year coronary heart disease incidence in men aged 40–59 from seven countries (Keys, 1970). The strongest correlation was found between the percentage of energy derived from saturated fat in the diet and increased risk of heart disease. These results were compared more recently in a 25-year follow-up of the subjects. In communities with a high incidence of heart disease, the intake of saturated fatty acids (SFAs) typically ranges between 15% and 25% of the energy intake. At the extremes, saturated fat intakes in East Finland were 22% and in Crete 8% of energy. The corresponding rates of coronary heart disease were 1,074 and 26 per 10,000 (age-standardized rate), respectively. There was also a weaker, negative correlation between intake of polyunsaturated fats and heart disease.

Although these relationships could be seen across different population groups, with varying diets and cultures, they are more difficult to find in comparisons of individuals within one country. Nevertheless, it has been possible to produce an equation that predicts the change in serum cholesterol, given changes in the dietary intake of saturated and polyunsaturated fats. Two such equations have been produced by Keys and Hegsted. The Keys formula shows that SFAs (excluding stearic acid, C18) raise plasma cholesterol levels by twice as much as polyunsaturated fatty acids (PUFAs) can lower it. This may not always be exactly so predictable for any one individual because of other behavioural or genetic factors. However, the ratio of polyunsaturated (P) fatty acids to saturated (S) fatty acids is a useful means of expressing the desirable proportion in the diet. Where the ratio is low (P/S = 0.2), the population generally has a high blood cholesterol level and a high risk of coronary heart disease. Increasing the P/S ratio to 0.5–0.8 has been considered a desirable goal, as heart disease rates are lower in populations where the normal diet approaches these proportions.

This basic premise is the first principle of the lipid hypothesis and is widely accepted. However, the biochemistry is complex, and as a result of attempts to simplify the story, views have become polarized and a lack of consensus has been widely publicized in the media, with resulting confusion for both health professionals and the general population. Much of that confusion has arisen because of the blanket term 'saturated fat', assumed to be universally hazardous. The evidence in fact only really incriminates the aturated fatty acids with 12, 14 and 16 carbon atoms. Shorter-chain saturated fatty acids, found particularly in milk, appear not to be harmful. Moreover, it matters what replaces saturated fat: *n*-6 fatty acids can also be harmful in large amounts, so a mix of complex carbohydrates and *n*-3 fatty acids appears better.

Prospective Studies

These involve studying a cohort of individuals over a number of years and measuring those parameters that are believed to be related to heart disease. Over time, some individuals will develop the disease; it is assumed that they share particular characteristics, not seen in the unaffected members of the population. One of the best known of these studies is that in Framingham, Massachusetts, where a cohort of more than 5000 individuals was first recruited in 1948. Data regarding their cardiovascular health and many possible causal factors have been systematically collected, using standardized methods of measurement. Data from the Framingham study have shown that raised serum cholesterol, high blood pressure and cigarette smoking are three major contributory risk factors in heart disease. The study also showed the comparative level of risk with increasing serum cholesterol levels. As newer risk factors are discovered, the data from Framingham can be reviewed to investigate other relationships. A newer data set is information from a sample of more than 100,000 female nurses in the United States, from whom medical and dietary information has been collected and who are being followed up prospectively. A review of 10 within-population studies (Caggiula and Mustad, 1997) showed a positive significant relationship between intakes of saturated fat and coronary heart disease. The WHO (2011) reported that prospective epidemiological studies have shown a relationship between overweight or obesity and cardiovascular morbidity, cardiovascular mortality and total mortality. Obesity is strongly related to major cardiovascular risk factors such as raised blood pressure, glucose intolerance, type 2 diabetes and dyslipidaemia.

Intervention Studies

The second principle of the lipid hypothesis suggests that if a raised serum cholesterol level is associated with an increased risk of heart disease, then lowering it should reduce the risk. Many trials have attempted to demonstrate this by using advice, dietary manipulation, lifestyle changes or drug intervention either separately or in varying combinations.

In some studies, those with no pre-existing evidence of heart disease have been targeted (primary prevention). The main drawbacks of this approach are the size of the subject group needed to demonstrate any benefits and the difficulty of evaluation.

Some community projects have been successful, most notably the North Karelia project in Finland, where a programme of health education was targeted at the whole community, aimed at reducing the very high incidence of heart disease. Evaluation has found measurable improvements in the average values for key parameters, most notably a 13% decrease in serum cholesterol. This was attributed to changes from butter to vegetable oil margarines, from whole fat to low-fat milk and from boiled to filtered coffee. In addition, blood pressure fell as a result of reduced salt intakes and an increase in fruit and vegetable intake. Overall, coronary heart disease mortality declined by 55% in men and 69% in women. These results imply that some individuals have achieved substantial changes. However, such large projects can also have very disappointing results. For example, the WHO collaborative study, targeting factory workers in several European countries, achieved some reduction in heart disease mortality in Belgium and Italy but not in the United Kingdom.

More specifically, focused trials recruiting those at high risk of heart disease have had mixed results. The Multiple Risk Factor Intervention Trial found that both the study and control groups showed an improvement in mortality rates. This demonstrated the difficulty of human studies, where diet is not a constant variable. Figure 14.2 shows the relationship between plasma cholesterol and heart disease from this study.

A review by Truswell (1994) of 14 studies from the 1960s and 1970s, in which SFAs were exchanged with PUFAs, found that the average cholesterol level was lowered by 10%. This was associated with a 13% reduction in coronary events and a 6% reduction in mortality. Where cholesterol reduction was more than average, there was an even greater decrease in coronary events and mortality.

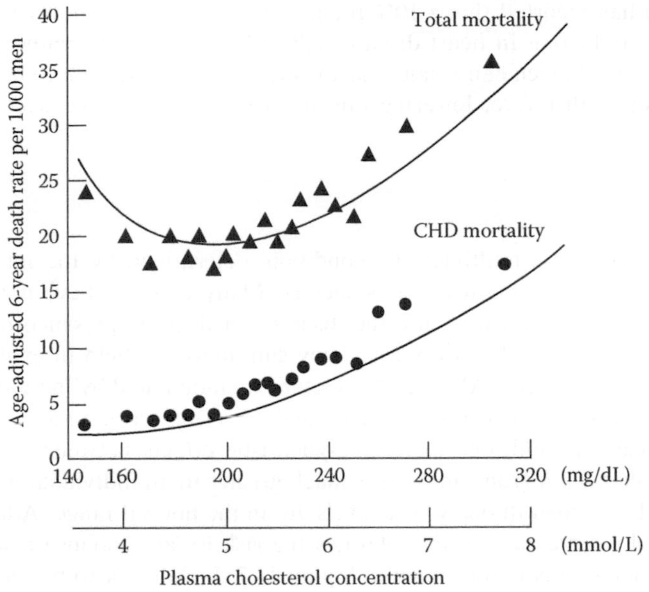

FIGURE 14.2 The increase in risk with increases in serum cholesterol levels. Coronary heart disease. (Reprinted from Martin, M.J. et al., *Lancet*, ii, 933, 1986. With permission.

Trials using cholesterol-lowering drugs (e.g. Helsinki Heart Study, Lipid Research Clinic Trial) have also demonstrated that it is possible to reduce heart disease mortality. However, both of the trials mentioned also found an increase in non-cardiovascular mortality in the study group. The findings of this nature led to concern about the safety of cholesterol lowering in subjects who have not experienced heart disease. The Scandinavian Simvastatin Survival Study (1994) achieved a 25% reduction in plasma cholesterol and 42% fewer coronary deaths and no excess mortality in the treated group.

Secondary prevention targets those who already possess signs or symptoms of heart disease or who have suffered a heart attack. In recent years, interventions have introduced other dietary manipulations as the lipid hypothesis has become more sophisticated. Some of these studies have achieved excellent results. Diet and Reinfarction Trial (The DART) study (Burr et al., 1989) showed that advice to eat fatty fish resulted in a reduction of 29% in mortality within 2 years; this was not seen in a group advised about fat intakes or about cereal fibre intake. The Lyon Diet Heart Study (De Lorgeril et al., 1994) increased the levels of alpha-linolenic acid as part of the dietary intervention and achieved a 70% reduction in mortality and 73% fewer non-fatal coronary events. Addition of long-chain *n*-3 fatty acids to the diet resulted in a 20% reduction in coronary heart disease mortality (GISSI Prevenzione Investigators, 1999).

It is clear that the lipid hypothesis does not fully explain all the causes of coronary heart disease. In particular, the following applies:

- The saturated/polyunsaturated fat relationship is an oversimplification of the link between diet and heart disease.
- Some of the SFAs have more potent effects than others.
- The role of different PUFAs in the atherosclerosis process is determined by the position of the first double bond in the chain and hence the fatty acid family.
- Further evidence suggests that monounsaturated fatty acids (MUFAs) are important in determining development of coronary heart disease.
- The *trans* fatty acids that are found in the diet may also have a role.

The WHO (2010) has reported that a 10% reduction in serum cholesterol in 40-year-old men resulted in a 50% reduction in heart disease within 5 years and the same serum cholesterol reduction for 70-year-old men can result in an average of 20% reduction in heart disease occurrence within 5 years; therefore, lowering raised serum cholesterol reduces the risk of heart disease.

RISK FACTORS

Coronary heart disease is a multifactorial condition, determined by the interaction of different combinations of factors, known as risk factors. Many of these have now been identified. A risk factor does not necessarily cause the disease nor does its presence mean that an individual will definitely develop heart disease. They can, however, help to explain cross-cultural and inter-individual differences. Although the factors are modulated by individual susceptibility, the presence of several factors in any one individual does suggest that there is a greater chance of developing disease. In addition, there are synergistic effects between the risk factors. For example, the calculated risk from smoking is much greater in an individual who also has raised blood cholesterol levels than in one whose levels are in the normal range. Adding the extra risk factor for raised blood pressure further elevates the risk by an amount greater than that seen for hypertension alone. This is illustrated in Figure 14.3. It should also be remembered that the development of heart disease is a process and that risk factors may be involved at different stages. Therefore, some may contribute to the laying down of fatty deposits in the blood vessels, and others influence the formation of a thrombosis or determine the response of the heart muscle to a lack of oxygen supply.

The main risk factors associated with heart disease are shown in Figure 14.4. Some of the factors are believed to increase risk and others to reduce risk. Therefore, any high risk factors can be ameliorated by enhancing those that reduce the risk. A large percentage of cardiovascular diseases are preventable through the reduction of several behavioural risk factors such as unhealthy diet, physical inactivity, tobacco use and harmful use of alcohol. In terms of attributable deaths, the leading cardiovascular risk factor is raised blood pressure (to which 13% of global deaths is attributed), followed by tobacco use (9%), raised blood glucose (6%), physical inactivity (6%) and weight gain and obesity (5%).

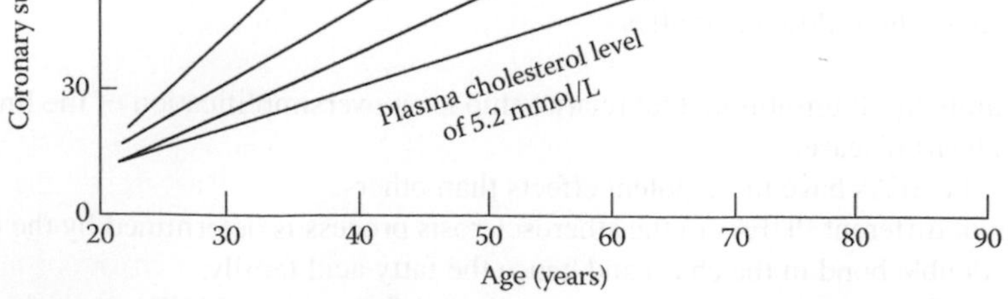

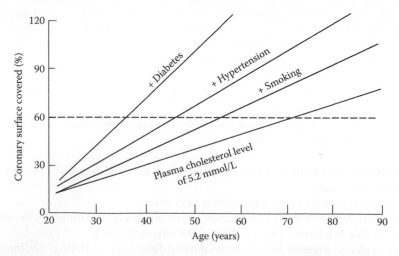

FIGURE 14.3 Additive effects of risk factors on damage to coronary arteries. (From Grundy, 1988. Copyright 1988, American Medical Association.)

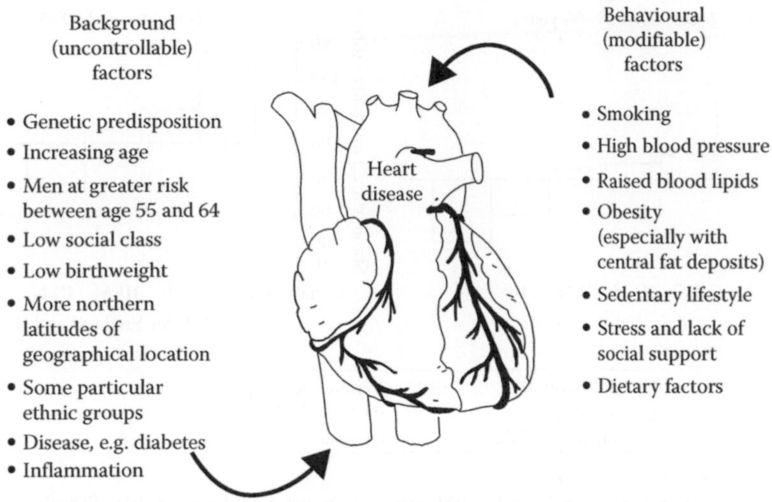

FIGURE 14.4 Main risk factors in the development of coronary heart disease.

Genetic Predisposition

This may be associated with increased risk. Often those who develop heart disease have a strong family history of the disease. It has even been suggested that any advice to reduce heart disease risk should only be targeted at those with a family history, as this will account for most of the new cases. Equally, it should be remembered that there may be a genetic predisposition to not develop heart disease.

Age

It was stated earlier in this chapter that the risk of heart disease increases with age in both men and women. Morbidity statistics show the peak age in men to be 55–64 and in women 75–84. This implies that the disease develops over a period of time, which is in line with the proposed mechanisms described earlier. In women, there is a relative protection against the disease during the reproductive years and an increase in incidence after the menopause. This also accounts for the gender differences in risk in middle age, with a higher risk seen in men than women before the ages of 50–55. In 2008, deaths caused by coronary heart disease in the United Kingdom increased with increasing age and they were overall higher in men than in women.

Social Conditions and Social Inequality

Contrary to some common perceptions, it is not the 'stressed businessman' who is most likely to develop heart disease. The highest incidence of the disease is among the more socially deprived. Standardized mortality ratios for England and Wales show this quite clearly for both genders. Furthermore, improvements in heart disease rates have been largest in the professional classes, so that the health inequality between these and the unskilled groups is widening (Figure 14.5). There are many mechanisms which contribute to different rates of heart disease according to life-choices and life-circumstances. Smoking, habitual diet composition, physical activity all interact. Behind all of these are the issues around chronic stress associated with limited opportunities for self-determination through social position. There is also a difference in height between social classes in the United Kingdom, those in the higher social classes being taller. This results in an inverse relationship between heart disease and height.

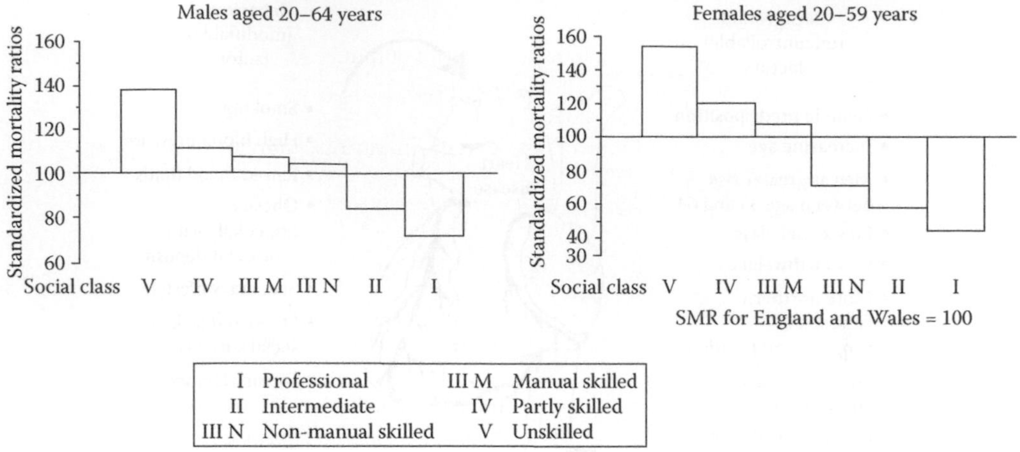

FIGURE 14.5 Socioeconomic and gender differences in heart disease mortality. Standardized mortality ratio (SMR) compares the true mortality of population with the experience that would have been expected if it had a standard mortality rate. An SMR above 100 indicates mortality rates higher than expected in a standard population. (Reproduced from DoH [UK Department of Health], Nutritional aspects of cardiovascular disease, Report on Health and Social Subjects No. 46, Report of the Cardiovascular Review Group of the Committee on Medical Aspects of Food Policy, HMSO, London, UK, 1994. With permission.)

Birthweight

Individuals who were born small for gestational age have been shown in a number of studies to have a higher risk of coronary heart disease. In addition, there is an increased risk of many of the risk factors, such as hypertension, raised cholesterol levels and higher levels of the blood clotting factors. Those individuals who were thin at birth, with less well-developed skeletal muscle are also at risk of glucose intolerance, which may result in type 2 diabetes in adult life. This in its turn may also result in a higher risk of coronary heart disease, as it is associated with some of the other factors mentioned earlier. The risk seems to be greatest in those people who become overweight as adults, after having been small infants. Maintenance of a normal body weight helps to minimize the risk. The WHO (2011) reported that low birthweight is associated with an increased risk of adult diabetes and cardiovascular disease (CVD). There is an increasing evidence that exposure to undernutrition in early life increases an individual's vulnerability to these disorders by 'programming' permanent metabolic changes.

The fetal origin of diseases is covered further in Chapter 7, pp. 110–113.

Geographical Location and Sunlight

Crude heart disease prevalence trends indicate that the disease occurs more commonly in northern latitudes and is less common nearer the equator. It has been suggested that low levels of ultraviolet light during winter months may, in some way, be responsible perhaps via a mechanism involving vitamin D levels. Recent evidence suggests that the mechanism may indeed be a lack of sunlight, but the link is not vitamin D. Instead, it may be the normal action of ultraviolet light on skin to synthesise the vasodilator, nitric oxide, from nitrate stored in skin. This would also link with the increased incidence of heart attacks in winter. Immigrants from more southerly origins tend to experience the heart disease risk of their host country after a relatively short period of time. However, as has already been mentioned, it has been found that some of the immigrant groups in the United Kingdom have much higher heart disease rates than the indigenous population. Thus, although environmental factors play an important part, other mechanisms are also involved.

Disease

Of the many diseases affecting humans, diabetes is one of the most prevalent, and people with type 2 diabetes have an increased risk of heart disease, often associated with obesity, high blood pressure, and raised lipid levels. The insulin resistance syndrome that occurs in these cases is associated with central fat distribution and a number of metabolic abnormalities, affecting carbohydrate and fat metabolism and resulting in raised lipid levels and poor oxidative capacity in skeletal muscle and liver. Cardiovascular disease accounts for about 60% of all mortality in people with diabetes. The risk of cardiovascular events is from two to three times higher in people with type 1 or type 2 diabetes, and the risk is higher in women. The current guidelines on dietary management of diabetes stress reduced fat intakes to minimize the risk. Previously, recommended diets controlled carbohydrate intakes strictly and allowed much higher fat intakes, which exacerbated the problem of heart disease.

There is some reported evidence that a chronic inflammatory state associated with the presence of infective organisms (e.g. *Helicobacter pylori*, found in the stomach, *Chlamydia pneumoniae*, which can cause respiratory infection or even oral bacteria that cause gum disease) may elevate cytokine levels, which affect the endothelial function of the blood vessel, and may facilitate immune responses and trigger clotting mechanisms. Patients with periodontal disease have been shown to have higher levels of plasma clotting factors. Conversely, bacteria responsible for periodontitis have been found in atherosclerotic plaques. C-reactive protein, a marker of inflammation, has now been shown to correlate with incidence of heart disease.

Smoking

Smoking is the major external cause of all ischaemic cardiovascular diseases, especially coronary heart disease. The rates of smoking are now, with better awareness and education, falling in Western countries. In UK the rate has fallen from over 40% to about 20% over the last 50 years. Part of that fall has been from increased taxation of tobacco, but the most recent drop has resulted from bans on smoking in public places and at work, to protect others from passive smoke exposure. It is no longer fashionable for young people to smoke. Persuading at-risk subjects to stop smoking can result in a significant reduction of their heart disease risk. It is thought that the free radicals that enter the body from cigarette smoke contribute to the disease process by causing peroxidation of lipids. The altered lipids are then taken up by macrophages in the blood vessel walls and contribute to the fatty streaks. A further potential effect of smoking is the reduction in oxygen-carrying capacity of the red blood cells owing to higher levels of carbon monoxide, which can exacerbate ischaemia in tissues fed by narrowed blood vessels. Dietary intake studies also show that smokers tend to have poorer diets and consume lower levels of antioxidants from fruit, which compounds the risks from free radicals. There appears to be a clear linear relationship between the numbers of cigarettes smoked per day and heart disease risk. There is a large body of evidence from prospective cohort studies regarding the beneficial effect of smoking cessation on coronary heart disease mortality. A 50-year follow-up of British doctors demonstrated that, among ex-smokers, the age of quitting has a major impact on survival prospects: those who quit between 35 and 44 years of age had the same survival rates as those who had never smoked (WHO, 2011).

High Blood Pressure

The INTERHEART study has estimated that 22% of heart attacks in Western Europe and 25% of heart attacks in Central and Eastern Europe were due to a history of high blood pressure. The British Heart Foundation (2010) reported that in 2008, 32% of men and 29% of women in England and 34% of men and 31% of women in Scotland were hypertensive. The prevalence of high blood pressure increases with age and, for women but not men, it is more prevalent in the lowest income quintile.

Raised blood pressure is one of the main contributors to heart disease, possibly because it potentiates the damage to blood vessel walls and increases the transfer of substances across the blood vessel wall. Both of these may play a part in the development of the fibrous plaque. Blood pressure levels have been shown to be positively and progressively related to the risk of stroke and coronary heart disease. In some age groups, for each incremental increase of 20/10 mmHg of blood pressure, starting as low as 115/75 mmHg, the risk of cardiovascular disease doubles. Reduction of blood pressure by drug treatment, weight loss or dietary modification is likely to be of benefit. Better control of hypertension may account for some of the reduction in heart disease seen in Western countries in recent years.

Raised Blood Lipids

Above normal levels of cholesterol, especially in the LDL fraction, are strongly linked with increased risk of heart disease, as evidenced by many studies. Those individuals with familial hyperlipidaemias have a well-recognized high risk of developing heart disease, often at a very young age. Recent interest has focused on the possible role of lipoprotein (a), closely related to LDL, but carrying an additional apoprotein molecule. Raised levels of this molecule appear to be more strongly linked to myocardial infarction than even LDL. These may explain the high incidence of heart disease in South Asians in the United Kingdom. Chylomicrons and very-low-density lipoprotein (VLDL), both of which are rich in triglycerides, are elevated in some individuals, resulting in prolonged lipaemia (presence of fats in the blood) after meals. These raised levels seem to be caused by a defective rate of clearance from the circulation by the enzyme lipoprotein lipase. Both chylomicrons and VLDL are likely to be atherogenic and constitute risk factors. More attention is now being focused on dietary factors that contribute to raised levels of the VLDL fraction. Measures to reduce blood lipid levels in individuals as well as population groups could result in reduced incidence of heart disease. The INTERHEART study estimated that abnormal blood lipids causes 45% of heart attacks in Western Europe and 35% of heart attacks in Central and Eastern Europe and that people with abnormal blood lipids are over three times more likely to have a heart attack compared to people with normal blood lipids.

Weight

Early studies, such as the Seven Countries Study by Keys, failed to find a causative effect of overweight on heart disease risk because many of the other risk factors are also aggravated by a higher body fat content. Using more sophisticated analyses, it is now clear that excess body fat is a direct contributor to coronary heart disease, as well as acting indirectly through many of the risk factors, such as diabetes, hypertension and raised blood lipids. In particular, when body fat distribution is taken into account and people are divided into 'apples' (those with predominantly abdominal fat deposits) and 'pears' (peripheral fat deposits, mostly around the buttocks and hips), a strong relationship with heart disease is seen for 'apples'. In general, the relative risk of cardiovascular disease for individuals with a body mass index (BMI) > 30 is about two to three times that of people with a BMI < 25. In 2008, 34% of adults over the age of 20 were overweight (33.6% of men and 35% of women) and 9.8% of men and 13.8% of women were obese compared to 4.8% for men and 7.9% for women in 1980. The use of waist circumference as a guide to the need for weight loss is a useful quick measure to indicate increased risk. Action levels for weight loss based on waist measurements are discussed in Chapter 13. Weight loss by dietary restriction and with physical activity can improve all the modifiable risk factors and thus reduce the risk of coronary heart disease.

Physical Activity

A proportion of people have been shown to have minimal levels of physical activity. In 2008, 31.3% of adults aged 15 or older (28.2% men and 34.4% women) were insufficiently physically active. The prevalence of insufficient physical activity is higher in high-income countries compared to low-income countries partly due to the use of vehicles for transport in high-income countries. High-income countries have more than double the prevalence of insufficient physical activity compared to low-income countries for both men and women, with 41% of men and 48% of women being insufficiently physically active in high-income countries compared to 18% of men and 21% of women in low-income countries.

People who are insufficiently physically active have a 20–30% increased risk of all-cause mortality compared to those who engage in at least 30 minutes of moderate intensity physical activity most days of the week. Many long-term studies have found lower mortality in those who have a more active lifestyle, compared with more sedentary controls, and therefore, exercise has been promoted as desirable in the reduction of heart disease risk. Changes to activity levels are followed by changes in risk of death, with an improvement of risk seen in previously sedentary subjects who begin an activity programme. Even moderate levels of activity appear to confer benefit, although the evidence is stronger for men than women. The mechanisms involved are unclear but, at a basic level, activity helps in the maintenance of energy balance and prevents development of overweight. Exercise has been shown to increase the beneficial high-density lipoprotein. Abdominal fat deposits appear to be particularly sensitive to mobilization by exercise, and in individuals with central obesity, even moderate exercise can produce improvements in the metabolic profile. Other possible beneficial effects include changes in clotting factors (linked to endurance-type exercise) or in the density of capillaries in the tissues, which provides protection against ischaemic damage, if blood vessels become narrowed. Inactivity may be as important a risk factor as hypertension, smoking or hypercholesterolaemia. Many studies that have examined the association between physical activity and cardiovascular disease have reported reduced risk of death from coronary heart disease and reduced risk of overall cardiovascular disease, coronary heart disease and stroke.

Psychosocial Factors

These are less well defined than other factors. Data from the Whitehall studies show higher rates of heart disease in lower employment grades, with the gradients being steeper for women than men (see DoH, 1994; Ashwell, 1996). It is suggested that stress and lack of social support may be linked to coronary heart disease.

Dietary Factors

There are several constituents of the diet for which there is evidence of a link with heart disease. Most notably, this applies to the fats that have been linked with lipid levels in the blood. In addition, other components, such as total energy intake, dietary fibre (non-starch polysaccharides), sugar, salt, alcohol and antioxidant nutrients, have all been studied in relation to stages in the development of heart disease. The dietary risk factors are summarized in Figure 14.6.

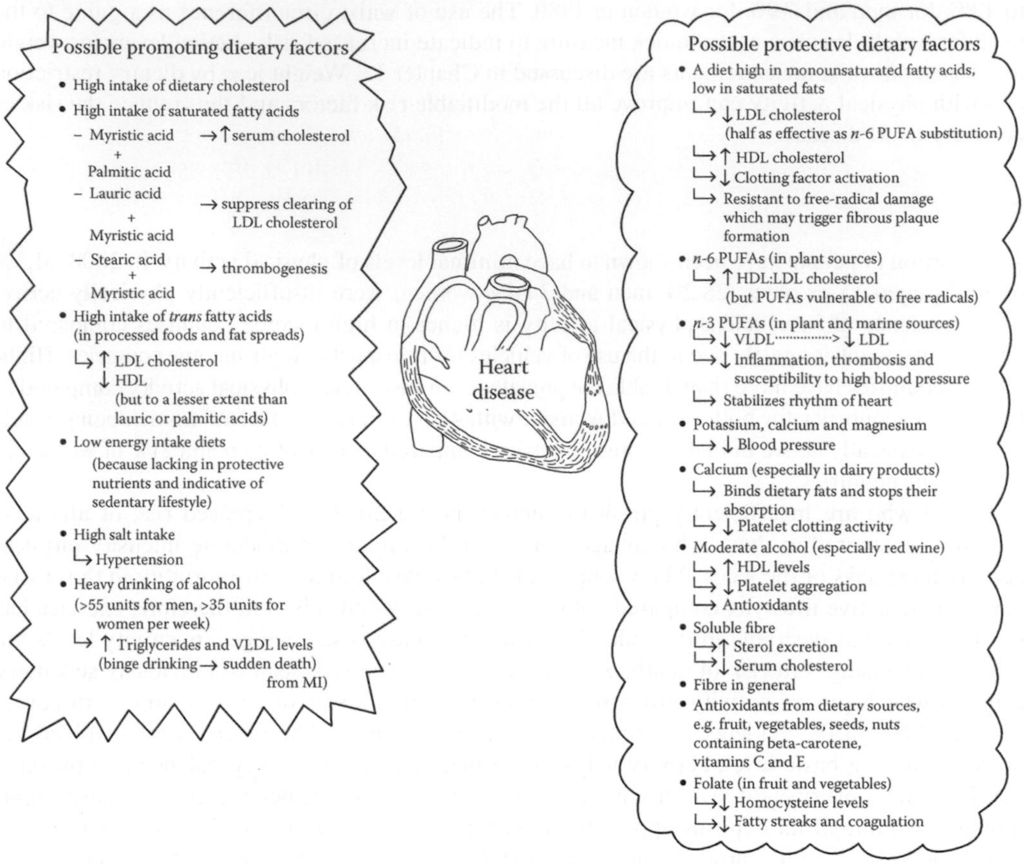

Possible promoting dietary factors
• High intake of dietary cholesterol
• High intake of saturated fatty acids
– Myristic acid + Palmitic acid → ↑ serum cholesterol
– Lauric acid + Myristic acid → suppress clearing of LDL cholesterol
– Stearic acid + Myristic acid → thrombogenesis
• High intake of trans fatty acids (in processed foods and fat spreads)
↳ ↑ LDL cholesterol
↓ HDL (but to a lesser extent than lauric or palmitic acids)
• Low energy intake diets (because lacking in protective nutrients and indicative of sedentary lifestyle)
• High salt intake
↳ Hypertension
• Heavy drinking of alcohol (>55 units for men, >35 units for women per week)
↳ ↑ Triglycerides and VLDL levels (binge drinking → sudden death) from MI)
Heart disease
Possible protective dietary factors
• A diet high in monounsaturated fatty acids, low in saturated fats
↳ ↓ LDL cholesterol (half as effective as n-6 PUFA substitution)
↳ ↑ HDL cholesterol
↳ ↓ Clotting factor activation
↳ Resistant to free-radical damage which may trigger fibrous plaque formation
• n-6 PUFAs (in plant sources)
↳ ↑ HDL:LDL cholesterol (but PUFAs vulnerable to free radicals)
• n-3 PUFAs (in plant and marine sources)
↳ ↓ VLDL ·········> ↓ LDL
↳ ↓ Inflammation, thrombosis and susceptibility to high blood pressure
↳ Stabilizes rhythm of heart
• Potassium, calcium and magnesium
↳ ↓ Blood pressure
• Calcium (especially in dairy products)
↳ Binds dietary fats and stops their absorption
↳ ↓ Platelet clotting activity
• Moderate alcohol (especially red wine)
↳ ↑ HDL levels
↳ ↓ Platelet aggregation
↳ Antioxidants
• Soluble fibre
↳ ↑ Sterol excretion
↳ ↓ Serum cholesterol
• Fibre in general
• Antioxidants from dietary sources, e.g. fruit, vegetables, seeds, nuts containing beta-carotene, vitamins C and E
• Folate (in fruit and vegetables)
↳ ↓ Homocysteine levels
↳ ↓ Fatty streaks and coagulation

FIGURE 14.6 A summary of dietary risk factors for coronary heart disease. High-density lipoprotein, low-density lipoprotein, myocardial infarction and polyunsaturated fatty acid.

Fats

Dietary Cholesterol

Meat, egg yolks and dairy products contain fairly large amounts of cholesterol, and many people concerned about their blood lipids have in the past attempted to reduce their intake of these foods. However, changing the amount of cholesterol in the diet has only limited effects on blood cholesterol concentrations in most people. This is because several compensation mechanisms exist. Only about half of the cholesterol ingested is absorbed from the gut; a typical dietary intake of 400 mg/day will, therefore, only result in the absorption of 200 mg of cholesterol. The essential nature of cholesterol in the body means that the body synthesizes the remainder of its needs, about 1 g of cholesterol per day. If dietary intake increases, the amount synthesized is reduced to compensate; this is achieved by regulating one of the enzymes – hydroxymethylglutaryl-coenzyme-A reductase – in the cholesterol synthesis pathway in the liver through a negative feedback mechanism. In addition, HDL activity can also increase to scavenge excess cholesterol from the tissues for removal in bile.

However, control is not exact and an increase in cholesterol intake in the diet can raise blood cholesterol levels. It has also been shown that there are individual, genetically determined differences in response to dietary cholesterol, with hyporesponders and hyperresponders. This makes it difficult to generalize about the effect of dietary cholesterol.

Saturated Fatty Acids

Originally, it was postulated that all SFAs in the diet were equally harmful, causing an elevation of blood cholesterol/LDL levels. It is now recognized that myristic acid (C14) is the main fatty acid responsible for raising the serum cholesterol level. This contributes to the formation of fibrous plaques and is described as atherogenic. Both lauric acid (C12) and myristic acid also suppress the clearing mechanism at LDL receptors, which removes LDL cholesterol from the circulation, thus contributing to raised circulating levels. Palmitic acid (C16) has probably less effect on cholesterol levels in the blood than originally suggested by Keys. However, palmitic acid is the main SFA in most diets and, therefore, has an important effect because of its prevalence. In addition, the different fatty acids appear to have varying effects on the formation of thrombi in the blood. Myristic acid and stearic acid (C18) are considered to be the most thrombogenic, together with *trans* fatty acids. A reduction in thrombogenic effects is associated with MUFAs, seed oils and fish oils.

Monounsaturated Fatty Acids

MUFAs, particularly oleic acid (18:1), were originally believed to be neutral in their effect on blood cholesterol levels and were not included in the original equations of Keys and Hegsted. Studies of heart disease prevalence among people in Mediterranean countries showed a lower rate than expected. The diet in these countries (particularly Greece and southern Italy) contains more MUFAs, especially oleic acid from olive oil, than is found in northern European diets. This led to the suggestion that this type of fatty acid may be protective against heart disease. It should, however, be remembered that there are many other features of a Mediterranean diet and lifestyle, such as large intakes of fruit, vegetables and wine, which may better explain the lower prevalence of heart disease. However, a number of studies have now confirmed that substitution of some of the saturated fats in the diet by MUFAs results in a reduction of LDL cholesterol, equal to about half of that achieved by *n*-6 PUFA substitution. In addition, however, there is an elevation of HDL cholesterol, an effect not obtained with *n*-6 PUFAs.

The proposed mechanism is an increase in LDL clearance by the liver as a result of increased receptor activity. In addition, as MUFAs contain only one double bond, they are more resistant to the harmful effects of free radicals, which attack PUFAs and can lead to the early stages of fibrous plaque formation. Observed effects on thrombogenesis have also been reported, with reduced levels of clotting factor activation. Overall, MUFAs are considered to be a beneficial component of the diet, with no harmful effects on the known risk factors for coronary heart disease. New equations predicting the change in total serum cholesterol consequent on modifications to the dietary intake of MUFAs, in addition to SFAs and PUFAs, have now been developed based on metabolic ward studies (e.g. Mensink and Katan, 1992). It should, however, be remembered that, in terms of weight control, the intake of MUFAs, as of other fats in the diet may need to be regulated.

Polyunsaturated Fatty Acids

PUFAs in the diet originate from two main sources: *n*-6 acids from plant foods and *n*-3 acids mainly from marine foods, and it is now recognized that the two families have different effects on coronary heart disease risk factors.

Fatty acids metabolism and functions are covered further in Chapter 11, pp. 220–226.

n-6 PUFAs. Fatty acids from this family have a LDL cholesterol-lowering effect, independent of any change in saturated fat intake. It is believed that the effect is achieved, by increasing the removal of LDL from the circulation by enhancing the activity of the LDL receptor sites, which thus opposes the effect of the SFAs on these receptors. Although *n*-6 PUFAs are also reported to reduce HDL levels in the blood, this is to a smaller extent than the effect on LDL and, consequently, the HDL/LDL ratio increases.

The *n*-6 PUFAs in membrane lipids are, however, vulnerable to free radical attack, resulting in peroxidation. Once established, this produces a chain reaction with further peroxide formation and potential for further damage. At present, there is little evidence that high intake of *n*-6 PUFAs in any way contributes to enhanced peroxidation in the body, but the vulnerability of the double bonds in these molecules suggests that this could be a possibility. Accordingly, it is advisable to be cautious about excessively high intakes of PUFAs and intakes should be below 10% of total energy. European recommendations (EURODIET, 2001) are that intakes of *n*-6 PUFAs should not exceed 5% (range 4%–8%) of total energy.

n-3 PUFAs. The *n*-3 fatty acids reduce VLDL levels and hence may eventually cause a reduction in LDL. The effect is linked to a more rapid clearance of VLDL rich in *n*-3 PUFAs than those containing SFAs, resulting in less post-prandial lipaemia on a *n*-3 PUFA-rich diet. However, the main interest in these fatty acids is associated with their action on blood clotting, which arose from studies on Greenland Eskimos who, despite a diet high in fat, have very low rates of heart disease. In addition, these subjects have prolonged bleeding times. Their diet contains a large amount of marine foods providing high levels of long-chain *n*-3 PUFAs. The *n*-3 series of prostaglandins and eicosanoids has less aggregating potency than those made from the *n*-6 family. In addition, the vasoconstricting effects on blood vessel walls are less. The overall effect is that the *n*-3 series is less likely to produce inflammation, thrombosis or increases in blood pressure. All of these responses are likely to reduce the risk of heart attack. Ingestion of significant amounts of *n*-3 PUFAs is believed to displace the *n*-6 series from enzyme sites, so that *n*-3 series eicosanoids are produced. Research has attempted to ascertain the ratio of *n*-6:*n*-3 PUFAs in the diet that could ensure optimal outcomes in respect of coronary heart disease. Current advice for populations based on EURODIET (2001) is that *n*-3 PUFAs should constitute 1% of total energy, providing a *n*-6:*n*-3 ratio of 5:1.

Data from the DART study (Burr et al., 1989) also suggested that the higher intake of *n*-3 acids stabilizes the rhythm of the heart and allows it to continue beating normally during a heart attack, ensuring a higher chance of survival. The Lyon Heart Study (De Lorgeril et al., 1998) demonstrated a significant protective effect of additional alpha-linolenic acid together with a Mediterranean diet. Supplementation with long-chain *n*-3 PUFAs in the GISSI trial (GISSI Prevenzione Investigators, 1999) caused a reduction in total mortality. It is on the basis of studies such as these that an increase in *n*-3 PUFA intake is recommended, either by increasing fish consumption or inclusion of more sources of alpha-linolenic acid in the diet.

Trans *Fatty Acids*

The naturally occurring unsaturated fatty acids have a *cis* orientation; *trans* fatty acids are produced by chemical alteration of the molecule. This occurs in the stomachs of ruminants and results in a dietary intake of naturally formed *trans* fatty acids in foods such as milk, dairy products, beef and lamb. In addition, the diet contains artificial *trans* fatty acids produced during food processing or manufacture of fat spreads by hydrogenation (approximately 65% of the total intake). These fats are used in the manufacture of biscuits, pies, cakes and potato crisps. Most *trans* fatty acids have so far been monounsaturated, predominantly *trans*-oleic acid. The manufacture of high PUFA margarines, using emulsifier technology and the deodorizing of vegetable oils has resulted in increased levels of *trans* PUFAs, including both *n*-6 and *n*-3, and there could be an increased intake of *trans*-alpha-linolenic acid in the future.

Studies suggest that large amounts of *trans* fatty acids (greater than currently consumed in the United Kingdom) raise LDL cholesterol and depress HDL, albeit to a smaller extent than seen with lauric and palmitic acids. Other evidence points to an elevation of lipoprotein (a) by up to 30%. Current intakes in the United Kingdom are in the range of 4–6 g/person, but the top 2.5% of consumers may take in more than 12 g/day. Intakes are higher in the United States, with an average of 8.1 g/person/day.

Overall, *trans* fatty acids have an adverse effect on both LDL and HDL, and this appears to be greater than that following an equal amount of SFAs. Nevertheless, since saturated fat represents a greater proportion of fat intake, reducing these is of greater importance. Consideration should perhaps be given to including information about *trans* fatty acids in nutritional labelling. It is recommended that *trans* fatty acids should comprise no more than 1% of total energy intake.

Conjugated linoleic acid is a *trans* fatty acid formed during the conversion of linoleic acid to oleic acid by rumen bacteria. It is found in milk and dairy produce and in beef and lamb. Animal studies have shown an anticancer and antiatherogenic activity by this acid, and current research is investigating potential health benefits.

Total Fat

When total fat intake was studied by Keys (1970) in the Seven Countries Study, it was found that there was an association with serum cholesterol levels and heart disease mortality. However, this effect was dependent on the saturated fat intake. More recent data have suggested that the total fat intake may be closely linked with the activity of factor VII, one of the clotting factors, and may thus have a role to play in the thrombosis phase of the aetiology of heart disease. The current view is that total fat intake needs to be controlled in individuals who are not within the ideal body weight range. In these cases, a reduction in fat, together with increased physical activity, is a useful contribution to reducing the risk of coronary heart disease. In people who are at or near their ideal body weight, the balance of fats should be the main focus rather than aiming to change total fat intakes.

Total Energy

A low energy intake has been associated with a high incidence of heart disease. Low levels of food intake not only contain small amounts of energy but also low nutrient levels, including many of the other protective factors that are necessary to sustain normal physiological functioning in the body. It is thought possible that this level of intake is a consequence of a low energy output and a sign of a sedentary lifestyle. In addition, low levels of physical activity are associated with increased body weight, which in itself is considered to be a risk factor. The incorporation of physical activity into everyday life is probably the best way to escape from this cycle.

Salt

Since hypertension is a recognized risk factor in coronary heart disease, it can be argued that reducing salt intake in those who are susceptible might reduce their risk of heart disease. However, it is now clear that a broader dietary approach can be more effective in reducing blood pressure. Data from the Dietary Approaches to Stop Hypertension (DASH) trial showed a dietary change that included low-fat dairy products, nuts, fruit and vegetables resulted in greater reductions in blood pressure than salt restriction alone (Appel et al., 1997). The DASH diet included increased intakes of potassium, calcium and magnesium, as well as lower sodium intakes, and it is now recognized that all of these factors are effective in changing blood pressure. These findings add further support to the importance of potassium intakes in the control of blood pressure. There is increasing emphasis on prevention of hypertension throughout life, as a measure to reduce coronary heart disease. There is clear evidence, leaving no doubt that even small reductions in sodium consumption at a population level will result in significant lowering of blood pressures and reduction in heart disease and stroke. The problem is the very large amount of salt added to foods during manufacture, with the consequence that people's palates have become accustomed to most foods tasting salty. Thus if the salt is removed suddenly, foods temporarily taste unpleasant. It takes about 10–14 days for the palate to readjust to a low salt diet. It is estimated that decreasing dietary salt intake from the current global levels of 9–12 g/day to the recommended level of 5 g/day would have a major impact on blood pressure and cardiovascular disease. Recent campaigns to reduce salt in manufactured foods have gained traction in many countries, with falls in consumption and indications that blood pressures are indeed also falling. However the greatest need is to protect infants and children from excessive salt from weaning onwards, because early chronic high-sodium exposure appears to elevate the renal and adrenal regulation of blood pressure for life.

Calcium

For many years, it has been noted that the incidence of coronary heart disease is lower in those geographical areas that have hard water. Several mechanisms have been put forward, with supporting evidence. Dietary calcium combines with fats, especially SFAs producing soaps, which remain unabsorbed and are excreted from the body. In a study of British and French farmers, calcium intake was inversely related to blood levels of triglycerides. In addition, there was an inverse relationship with platelet clotting activity. Finally, as discussed earlier, calcium intakes are inversely related to blood pressure, as has been demonstrated in a number of large cohort studies. In general, calcium intakes, especially from dairy produce, appear to be associated with a lower risk of coronary heart disease, and low-fat cheese may be considered a constituent of healthy diets.

Alcohol

Heavy drinking in excess of 55 units for men and 35 units for women per week is associated with raised triglyceride and VLDL levels and thus increases heart disease risk. In addition, binge drinking has been associated with sudden death due to myocardial infarction or stroke. However, a moderate alcohol intake (within 'safe' limits) has been shown to have a protective effect against heart disease. The mechanisms appear to involve both the atherogenesis and thrombogenesis aspects of coronary heart disease. A number of studies have found an increase in HDL levels on alcohol consumption, which falls within 24 hours when alcohol intake stops. The elevation of HDL is approximately similar to that achieved by physical activity. In addition, moderate alcohol intake has been shown to reduce platelet aggregation. In large amounts, alcohol can cause platelet aggregation. In this case, alcoholic beverages that contain antioxidants, such as red wine, may be protective.

The relationship between alcohol consumption and heart disease is usually found to follow a J-shaped curve, with increased risk in non-drinkers and heavy drinkers. The lowest risk occurs in the middle range of alcohol intakes, taking 2–4 drinks per day on 3–4 days per week. Ideally, consumption should be with meals, as is seen in Mediterranean countries. There has been debate about the type of alcoholic drink that may be most beneficial, and many studies suggest that red wine has the greatest protective effects. However, in general, it appears that the consistent effects are attributable to the alcohol per se rather than additional constituents particular to a specific beverage. However, antioxidants in red wine, most notably resveratrol, may contribute an additional protective benefit.

Some concern has been expressed by health educationists about the desirability of promoting alcohol consumption as a means of preventing heart disease because of the implications for health of alcohol in amounts greater than 'moderate'.

Fibre (Non-Starch Polysaccharides)

Sources of soluble fibre, especially from oats, have been shown to reduce serum cholesterol levels, although the effects are not large. Insoluble fibre does not appear to have a similar effect on cholesterol. Nevertheless, a significant inverse relationship between fibre intake and myocardial infarction and coronary mortality has been demonstrated in two prospective studies, in Finland and the United States, in large cohorts of men. The relationship was strongest for cereal fibre and persisted when confounding variables were taken into account. It has been suggested that the effects occur due to the satiating effect of fibre-rich foods that results in a lowered fat intake and possibly a reduced total energy intake.

However, soluble fibre may increase sterol excretion from the body, thereby lowering cholesterol levels. High fibre intake has been associated with a decrease in the level of insulin and increased insulin sensitivity, thus improving metabolic function. Additionally, a high-fibre diet also affects the clotting factors and may be associated with a lower blood pressure. Overall, it is likely that the effects of fibre on heart disease are not mediated through a single mechanism and no adverse harmful effects have been reported from increased sources of fibre in the diet.

Antioxidants

The inability of the lipid hypothesis to explain the link between diet and heart disease fully and the completion of studies that show inconsistent or contrary results have led over the years to a search for other influencing factors. Several studies demonstrated that levels of antioxidants in both diet and serum exhibit good correlations with heart disease incidence – often higher levels of correlation than are seen in the same studies for fat indices. In particular, the MONICA study (Gey et al., 1991) has shown inverse relationships between heart disease mortality and intakes of beta-carotene, vitamin C and vitamin E. The strongest correlations ($p < 0.001$) were seen with alpha-tocopherol, vitamin C and beta-carotene in food supplies and the rate of coronary heart disease. Correlations also existed with the dietary sources of these nutrients, most notably vegetables, vegetable oils, sunflower seed oil, seeds, nuts and fruit. In the United States, two large prospective studies (of male health professionals and female nurses) found a lower incidence of coronary heart disease in the subjects who consumed vitamin E supplements.

However, these results were not replicated in a series of intervention studies in various countries, in which supplements of the major antioxidants, mainly vitamin E and beta-carotene, were assigned to subjects. In general, these studies showed either no beneficial effect of supplementation with these antioxidants or an adverse effect of supplementation, with a higher rate of coronary heart disease or cancer than the control groups. It is suggested that antioxidant nutrients can act as pro-oxidants in certain conditions, which may include the administration of large amounts of a single antioxidant.

Thus, it is likely that antioxidants work together to produce the effects seen in whole diet studies and that advice should be targeted towards fruit and vegetable consumption. It is possible that fruit and vegetables contain other substances that have not yet been taken into account and that have even more effect on heart disease development. There is interest in other factors found in fruit and vegetables, such as polyphenols or flavonoids. The recommendation of the WHO is to eat five servings of fruit and vegetables per day. Approximately, 1.7 million (2.8%) of deaths worldwide are attributable to low fruit and vegetable consumption.

There are good grounds for believing that the antioxidant nutrients do play a preventive role in the formation of fibrous plaques. It is appropriate at this point to summarize all of the functions of antioxidants in protection against free radicals.

Mechanisms of Action of Antioxidants

Free radicals are produced by most of the oxidative reactions in the body. The most important of these radicals are the following:

- The hydroxyl radical – OH
- Superoxide radical – O_2
- Singlet oxygen – $^1O_2$
- Nitric oxide – NO

Also included are the peroxyl radical, hydrogen peroxide and hydroperoxyl. All share the common property of having an exceedingly short lifespan and, therefore, are very unstable. They can attack vital cell components, inactivate enzymes and damage genetic material. It is, therefore, reasonable to assume they play a part in degenerative diseases.

The body has a complex antioxidant defence system to counteract these radicals. This is made up of endogenous and exogenous components.

- Endogenous antioxidants are mainly enzymes that catalyze radical quenching reactions (many of these are dependent on dietary minerals for activation) or bind pro-oxidants, which might catalyze free-radical reactions.
- Exogenous antioxidants are mainly vitamins that quench free radicals.

Endogenous Antioxidants

The antioxidant enzymes include the following:

- Superoxide dismutase, which neutralizes the superoxide radical and which requires zinc and copper or manganese for activation
- Catalase, which is specific for hydrogen peroxide and requires iron for its activity
- Glutathione peroxidase, which removes peroxides and is a selenium-requiring enzyme

Many minerals are clearly involved in activating these enzymes. However, copper and iron can also act as pro-oxidants when freely present. This explains why there are binding proteins present to prevent this happening, most notably caeruloplasmin and albumin to bind copper and transferrin and ferritin to bind iron.

Exogenous Antioxidants

The most important of these are vitamins C and E and the carotenoids. Plant flavonoids and other phenolic compounds are possible members of this group.

Vitamins C and E quench free radicals by providing H atoms to pair up with unpaired electrons on free radicals. This inactivates the vitamins, which then need to be regenerated. Glutathione is believed to regenerate vitamin C, and vitamin C can regenerate vitamin E (Figure 14.7). In its turn, vitamin E may promote the antioxidant activity of beta-carotene against lipid peroxidation. It is suggested that vitamin C is the primary antioxidant in the plasma and is consumed first in destroying free radicals. Vitamin E is the major antioxidant in the lipid parts of membranes. Lipid peroxidation does not begin

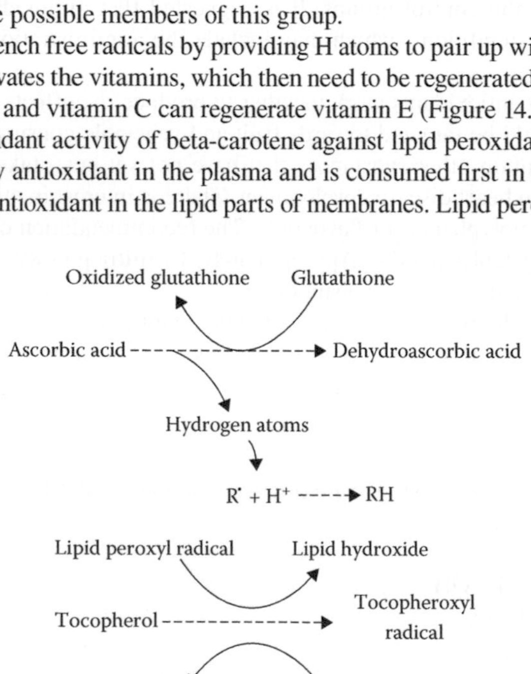

FIGURE 14.7 Interactions between glutathione, vitamin C and vitamin E during antioxidant activity. R, free radical.

until after the vitamin C has been used. It is important that regeneration can take place, however, so that a continued supply of the vitamins is available. These interactions highlight the importance of maintaining a balance between the different exogenous antioxidants supplied to the body.

In conclusion, the theories about antioxidants allow some of the other factors discussed earlier to be linked together. It has been suggested that the desire for weight loss, which preoccupies so many women and which encourages them to eat low-calorie fruits and vegetables, helps to protect them from heart disease by adding more antioxidants to their diet. Smokers, who have a greatly increased risk of heart disease, are recorded as having very low intakes of fruit and vegetables and consequently poor vitamin C status. When linked to the increased burden of free radicals, this may explain their greater risk. Finally, alcoholic beverages, most notably wines, contain phenolic substances that also act as antioxidants. This may explain why there are lower rates of coronary heart disease among populations in wine-drinking countries.

Homocysteine and Folate

It has been known since the late 1960s that raised levels of homocysteine in the blood are associated with severe arteriosclerosis. Initially, this was considered to be a problem in individuals with inborn errors in the metabolism of homocysteine. However, in recent years, it has been found that raised homocysteine levels are an independent risk factor for vascular disease, and the effect is graded. The evidence for this comes from a range of different studies, including retrospective case-control, cross-sectional and prospective studies. The metabolism of homocysteine is linked to that of methionine and cysteine and utilizes a number of B vitamins as cofactors. These include folate, pyridoxine, riboflavin and vitamin B_{12}. Deficiencies in the metabolism of homocysteine, with resultant elevated plasma levels, are associated with mutations in one of the enzymes (methylene tetrahydrofolate reductase) involved in the metabolic pathway. Lower activity levels of the enzyme have been identified in approximately 30% of the population, with a smaller percentage being homozygous for the mutation. The reference range of homocysteine in the plasma is still debated, but the following are generally accepted:

5–15 μmol/L normal range
15–30 μmol/L moderate elevation
30–100 μmol/L intermediate elevation
>100 μmol/L severe elevation

It has been proposed that homocysteine may be directly toxic to endothelial cells, through a mechanism involving nitric oxide that normally causes endothelial relaxation. This would facilitate monocyte adhesion and promote the process of fatty streak formation. A further possible mechanism is through an increased coagulation tendency, by an inhibition of the normal fibrinolytic mechanisms that disperse blood clots. However, neither of these mechanisms has yet been conclusively proven and much remains to be discovered about the relationship of homocysteine to the processes of vascular disease.

Dietary interventions can lower homocysteine levels. Most importantly, folate status is inversely associated with homocysteine levels, with as little as 200 μg/day of folate causing a reduction in plasma homocysteine levels. Evidence is less conclusive for supplementation with riboflavin, pyridoxine or vitamin B_{12}, although a combination of these may be beneficial. It should also be remembered that folate is provided by fruit and vegetables in the diet, so that an increase in these foods in line with other aspects of dietary intervention will also help to increase folate status. Fortification of grain products with folic acid, at a rate of 1.4 μg/g of product, has been introduced in the United States since 1999. Early indications are that, in the first year after this was introduced, there was a 3.4% reduction in mortality from stroke and heart attack. Mean homocysteine levels have fallen, and mean plasma concentrations of folate have increased.

Sources of folate are covered in Chapter 4, pp. 71–72. Folate metabolism and function is covered in Chapter 12, p. 242.

More controlled studies in this field are still required.

FUTURE DIRECTIONS

There is still a huge amount to learn about coronary heart disease. Developments in molecular biology and the human genome project may in the future allow research to identify the interaction between risk factors and particular genes. Animal models with specific genetic modifications are already being used to study mechanisms to understand existing knowledge. Improved targeting of dietary intervention and drug therapy may be a consequence.

SUMMARY

1. The role of diet in the aetiology of coronary heart disease is complex.
2. Early hypotheses about links with fat have been discovered to explain only part of the relationship.
3. New findings about the roles of other fats, such as MUFAs, *n*-3 fats and *trans* fatty acids, have modified the original lipid hypothesis.
4. The importance of other dietary factors, in particular the antioxidants, provides opportunities to link some of the earlier findings together.
5. Dietary guidelines promoting lower fat and increased fruit and vegetables intakes address many of the postulated mechanisms relating to coronary heart disease. Weight control and promotion of physical activity remain important preventive factors.

STUDY QUESTIONS

1. Distinguish between atherogenesis and thrombogenesis, and describe the mechanisms that are currently offered as explanations of these processes.
2. Which dietary factors are thought to be involved in following?
   a. Atherogenesis
   b. Thrombogenesis
3. What are the main tenets of the lipid hypothesis and what changes to it have been suggested in recent years?
4. a. Explain what you understand by the antioxidant nutrients.
   b. Produce a diagram to show how they might play a part in protecting against heart disease.
5. Discuss with a colleague how you believe the theories about the dietary links with heart disease are reflected in current dietary guidelines. Can you explain all of the guidelines on a scientific basis?
6. Produce a poster or leaflet to summarize the main aspects of dietary advice for the prevention of coronary heart disease. Make the information as practical as possible.

BIBLIOGRAPHY AND FURTHER READING

Appel, L.J., Moore, T.G., Obarzanek, R. et al. 1997. A clinical trial of effects of dietary patterns on blood pressure. *New England Journal of Medicine* 336, 1117–1124.

Bellizzi, M.C. 1995. Wine and vegetable oils: The French paradox revisited. *British Nutrition Foundation Nutrition Bulletin* 20, 256–265.

Berger, S., Raman, G., Vishwanathan, R., Jacques, P.F. and Johnson, E.J. 2015. Dietary cholesterol and cardiovascular disease: A systematic review and meta-analysis. *The American Journal of Clinical Nutrition* 102, 276–294.

Brown, A.A. and Hu, F.B. 2001. Dietary modulation of endothelial function: Implications for cardiovascular disease. *The American Journal of Clinical Nutrition* 73, 673–686.

Burr, M.L. 1993. Fish and ischaemic heart disease. *World Review of Nutrition and Dietetics* 72, 49–60.

Caggiula, A.W. and Mustad, V.A. 1997. Effects of dietary fat and fatty acids on coronary artery disease risk and total and lipoprotein cholesterol concentrations: Epidemiologic studies. *The American Journal of Clinical Nutrition* 65(Suppl.), 159S–610S.

Chen, A.F., Chen, D.D., Daiber, A., Faraci, F.M., Li, H., Rembold, C.M. and Laher, I. 2012. Free radical biology of the cardiovascular system. *Clinical Science* 123(2), 73–91.

De Lorgeril, M., Renaud, S., Mamelle, N. et al. 1994. Mediterranean alpha-linolenic acid-rich diet in secondary prevention of coronary heart disease. *Lancet* 343, 1454–1459.

DoH (UK Department of Health). 1994. Nutritional aspects of cardiovascular disease. Report on Health and Social Subjects No. 46. Report of the Cardiovascular Review Group of the Committee on Medical Aspects of Food Policy. London, UK: HMSO.

DoH (UK Department of Health). 1999. Saving lives – Our healthier nation. London, UK: The Stationery Office.

Erens, B. and Primatesta, P. (eds.). 1999. *Health Survey for England: Cardiovascular Disease'98*. Vol. 1: *Findings*. London, UK: The Stationery Office.

Estruch, R., Ros, E., Salas-Salvadó, J. et al. 2013. Primary prevention of cardiovascular disease with a Mediterranean diet. *New England Journal of Medicine* 368(14), 1279–1290.

EURODIET. 2001. Report and proceedings. *Public Health Nutrition* 4(2A).

Gey, K.F., Puska, P., Jordan, P. et al. 1991. Inverse correlation between plasma vitamin E and mortality from ischaemic heart disease in cross-cultural epidemiology. *The American Journal of Clinical Nutrition* 53, 3265–3345.

GISSI Prevenzione Investigators. 1999. Dietary supplementation with *n*-3 polyunsaturated fatty acids and vitamin E after myocardial infarction, results of the GISSI Prevenzione trial. *Lancet* 354, 447–453.

Halliwell, B. 1994. Free radicals, antioxidants and human disease: Curiosity, cause or consequence? *Lancet* 344, 721–724.

Hegsted, D.M., Ansman, L.M., Johnson, J.A. et al. 1993. Dietary fat and serum lipids: An evaluation of the experimental data. *The American Journal of Clinical Nutrition* 57, 875–883.

Hu, H., Stampfer, M.J., Manson, J.E. et al. 1997. Dietary fat intake and the risk of coronary heart disease in women. *New England Journal of Medicine* 337, 1491–1499.

Hulshof, K.F.A.M., van Erp-Baart, M.A., Anttolainen, M. et al. 1999. Intake of fatty acids in Western Europe with emphasis on trans fatty acids. The TRANSFAIR study. *European Journal of Clinical Nutrition* 53, 143–157.

Keys, A. (ed.). 1970. Coronary heart disease in seven countries. *Circulation* 41(Suppl.), I186–I195.

Kinane, D.F. and Lowe, G.D.O. 2000. How periodontal disease may contribute to cardiovascular disease. *Periodontology* 23, 121–126.

Kromhout, D. 2001. Epidemiology of cardiovascular disease in Europe. *Public Health Nutrition* 4(2B), 441–457.

Law, M.R., Wald, N.J. and Thompson, S.G. 1994. By how much and how quickly does reduction in serum cholesterol concentration lower risk of ischaemic heart disease? *British Medical Journal* 308, 367–372.

Li, J. and Siegrist, J. 2012. Physical activity and risk of cardiovascular disease – A meta-analysis of prospective cohort studies. *International Journal of Environmental Research and Public Health* 9(2), 391–407.

Martin, M.J., Halley, S.B., Browner, W.S. et al. 1986. Serum cholesterol, blood pressure and mortality: Implications from a cohort of 361622 men. *Lancet* ii, 933–936.

McKinley, M.C. 2000. Nutritional aspects and possible pathological mechanisms of hyperhomocysteinaemia: An independent risk factor for vascular disease. *Proceedings of the Nutrition Society* 59, 221–237.

Mensink, R.P. and Katan, M.B. 1992. Effect of dietary fatty acids on serum lipids and lipoproteins – A meta-analysis of 27 trials. *Atherosclerosis and Thrombosis* 12, 911–919.

Mozaffarian, D., Micha, R. and Wallace, S. 2010. Effects on coronary heart disease of increasing polyunsaturated fat in place of saturated fat: A systematic review and meta-analysis of randomized controlled trials. *PLoS Medicine* 7(3), e1000252.

Nichols, M., Townsend, N., Luengo-Fernandez, R., Leal, J., Gray, A., Scarborough, P. and Rayner, M. 2012. *European Cardiovascular Disease Statistics 2012*. Brussels, Belgium: European Heart Network.

Renaud, S. and Lanzmann-Petithory, D. 2001. Coronary heart disease: Dietary links and pathogenesis. *Public Health Nutrition* 4(2B), 459–474.

Rimm, E.B., Klatsky, A., Grobbee, D. et al. 1996. Review of moderate alcohol consumption and reduced risk of coronary heart disease: Is the effect due to beer, wine or spirits? *British Medical Journal* 312, 731–736.

Sattelmair, J., Pertman, J., Ding, E.L., Kohl, H.W. and Haskell, W. 2011. Dose response between physical activity and risk of coronary heart disease. A meta-analysis. *Circulation* 124, 789–795.

Scandinavian Simvastatin Study Group. 1994. Randomised trial of cholesterol lowering in 4444 patients with coronary heart disease: The Scandinavian Simvastatin Survival Study (4S). *Lancet* 344, 1383–1389.

Schaefer, E.J. 2002. Lipoproteins, nutrition and heart disease. *The American Journal of Clinical Nutrition* 75, 191–212.

Shaper, A.G. and Wannamethee, G. 1991. Physical activity and ischaemic heart disease in middle-aged British men. *British Heart Journal* 66, 384–394.

Slavin, J., Martin, M.C., Jacobs, D.R. et al. 1999. Plausible mechanisms for the protectiveness of whole grains. *The American Journal of Clinical Nutrition* 70, 459S–463S.

Townsend, N., Williams, J., Bhatnagar, P., Wickramasinghe, K. and Rayner, M. 2014. *Cardiovascular Disease Statistics, 2014*. London, UK: British Heart Foundation.

Troisi, R., Willett, W.C. and Weiss, S.T. 1992. Trans fatty acid intake in relation to serum lipid concentrations in adult men. *The American Journal of Clinical Nutrition* 56, 1019–1024.

Truswell, A.S. 1994. Review of dietary intervention studies: Effects on coronary events and on total mortality. *Australia and New Zealand Journal of Medicine* 24, 98–106.

Various authors. 2000. Symposium on reducing cardiovascular disease risk: Today's achievements, tomorrow's opportunities. *Proceedings of the Nutrition Society* 59, 415–440.

15 Diet and Cancer

AIMS

The aims of this chapter are to

- Describe what is meant by cancer.
- Discuss the ways in which the relationship between diet and cancer is studied.
- Identify the main relationships that have been indicated.
- Describe the guidelines on healthy eating for the reduction of cancer risk.

Cancer affects one in three people in the United Kingdom and United States at some time in their life, and is responsible for approximately one-quarter of all deaths. Worldwide, lung cancer is the most common cancer contributing 13% of the total number of new UK cases diagnosed in 2012. In men the top three cancers; lung, prostate and colorectal, contributed nearly 42% of all cancers. In women breast cancer was the second most common cancer and colorectal the third with nearly 1.7 and 1.4 million new UK cases, respectively, in 2012.

More people now die from cancer than was the case 100 years ago. However, this is a reflection of a longer life expectancy and larger numbers of elderly people in the population, and at the same time, with better treatments more people than ever are living with or after cancer. Because risk increases with age, the majority of cancer deaths occur in people aged over 65 years. Different cancers show different trends, however. Deaths from lung cancer are clearly linked to smoking and these have followed trends in smoking throughout the century. Melanoma, a cancer of the skin, has increased in recent years, probably as a result of increased sudden exposure to powerful sunlight with sunburn, as more people have indoor jobs and take holidays abroad. On the other hand, stomach cancer rates have declined dramatically since the 1950s. Several explanations may be offered for this, including dietary changes. However, a major factor recently discovered is the role of *Helicobacter pylori* in the development of the disease. Antibodies to this bacterium are much more common among people brought up in overcrowded housing conditions, who then have a higher risk of stomach cancer. Improvements in housing provision may have had the added benefit of reducing exposure to this bacterium and, consequently, contributed to reduced rates of stomach cancer. This example illustrates the often multifactorial nature of the aetiology of cancer, and the consequent difficulties of study.

Other factors that need to be taken into account in studying statistics on cancer are the improvements in detection and diagnosis, and advances in treatment, both of which may increase figures for the apparent incidence of the disease. Thus, we are not working with a static baseline from which to explore trends. It is also important to note that changes in the environment and lifestyle factors may impact on cancer statistics, and these must be continuously studied to give more clues about the aetiology of cancer at various sites.

According to the statistics, there have been no marked changes in cancer incidence rates that could be attributed to toxic hazards, such as pesticides and pollution at average levels of exposure. However, when groups of individuals are exposed to abnormal levels, for example of radiation, as happened after the nuclear accident in Chernobyl in 1986, then higher rates of particular cancers are found. Unusual occurrences of cancer in a community are always suspicious, since they may be coincidental or linked to a particular environmental event. Finding an answer can help to further our understanding of the development of the disease.

Around the world there are also differences in the occurrence of particular cancers. In Africa, Asia and Latin America, there tends to be a higher rate of cancers of the upper respiratory and digestive systems (aerodigestive system) (mouth, pharynx, larynx and oesophagus), the stomach, liver and cervix. Conversely, cancers of the breast, endometrium, prostate, colon and rectum are more common in Europe, North America and Australia. Cancers of this latter group are now increasing in the urbanized areas of the developing countries. Lung cancer is the commonest cancer worldwide. Migration from one type of community to another is often associated with a change in the pattern of cancers seen in the migrants.

WHAT IS CANCER?

Cancer is now accepted as an acquired genetic disorder of somatic cells, in which an accumulation of genetic changes causes a normal cell to give rise to one which is abnormal in form or function. There may be an underlying genetic predisposition to certain cancers, such that some people, and some families, are prone particularly to endometrial, breast, and colon cancers. There are now genetic tests to identify individuals at risk, for closer surveillance and even preventive surgery. Generally, several changes have to occur for cancer to develop, varying between different types of cancer. The fundamental change occurs within the genetic material of the organ in which a cancer arises, and may be inherited or, in the great majority of cases, occurs sporadically. Environmental factors, including diet, can contribute to initiating cancerous change, to the rate of growth and metastasis, and to responses to treatment.

The resulting abnormal cells fail to respond to some or all of the regulatory signals and immune system mechanisms that normally control division, growth, differentiation and programmed cell death (apoptosis). In addition, the affected genes may malfunction in their role, for example, as tumour suppressors, 'proof readers' of encoded material or repairer of genes. There are many types of cancers. They have different characteristics, which probably originate in varying ways, occur in different parts of the body, have different courses of development and require various treatments.

The developing tumour causes damage to its host by interfering with the normal functioning of the tissue or organ where it grows. It also draws on the host for nutrients to support its growth. Some cancers produce factors, which cause increased catabolism of the body's own tissues, resulting in a state of rapid weight loss and deterioration.

Although the process of development of cancer (or carcinogenesis) is not fully understood, it is clear that there are several stages that take place over a period of time (Table 15.1). The boundaries between the stages may not be as clear as implied here, but they provide a useful framework. The exact duration of each stage is unknown, but opportunities may arise for the process to be stopped, and possibly reversed, before it reaches the later stages.

STUDYING THE RELATIONSHIP BETWEEN DIET AND CANCER

In 2007, the World Cancer Research Fund (WCRF) and the American Institute for Cancer Research (AICR) published their second expert report, a systematic review of the scientific evidence on food, nutrition, physical activity and cancer entitled 'Food, nutrition, physical activity, and the prevention of cancer: A global perspective'. This review is the largest of its kind involving a panel of 21 expert scientists who systematically assessed the available scientific evidence in order to make recommendations for public health goals and personal actions in order to reduce cancer risks. Many approaches to the study of cancer exist and new evidence is continually emerging. It is, therefore, essential that such a review is kept up to date. The WCRF/AICR Continuous Update Project (CUP) is an ongoing review of cancer prevention research that provides up-to-date evidence on how people can reduce their cancer risk through diet and physical activity. The CUP database is thought to be the biggest database of evidence in the world on how food, nutrition, physical activity and body fatness affect cancer risk.

TABLE 15.1
Summary of Stages in Cancer Development

Stage of Development	Associated Change
Initiation	Exposure to harmful agent (e.g. chemical carcinogen, virus, free radical, radiation) or error in transcription may permanently alter the DNA material.
	The cell may remain in this state for a long period.
	It is also possible for the DNA damage to be repaired or the damaged cell to be destroyed by the body's normal regulatory systems.
	Molecular biology research suggests that there are genes that can both promote and suppress these changes. This may explain the increased risk of certain cancers in families.
Promotion	Substances that increase the rate of cell division may cause the damaged DNA to replicate before it has been repaired or destroyed.
	This may not happen for 10–30 years after the first step.
	Promoters are believed to include oestrogens, dietary fat and alcohol.
	There may also be inhibitory agents, including antioxidants, dietary fibre, calcium, other constituents in plant foods and additives.
Progression	The cells undergo further development and begin to grow in an uncontrolled manner, producing a tumour.

Worldwide, the occurrence of cancer is greater in industrialized than in developing countries, with up to 30-fold differences in rates of particular cancers. This suggests that there may be important environmental factors involved in the aetiology. Many of these have been investigated in observational studies comparing different communities, groups within communities and migrant groups moving from one community to another. However, such studies do not provide evidence of causality or information about biological mechanisms and must be supported by experimental findings. Developments in identification and measurement of biological markers and rapid gains in information about human genetics will provide opportunities to link observational data with molecular mechanisms.

Much of the current evidence is based on many epidemiological studies, whose results allow researchers to calculate the relative risk, or odds ratio of disease, resulting from exposure to a particular factor. It is on the basis of such data that risk factors for the development of various cancers can be proposed.

Ecological or Correlational Studies

These aim to show an association between the incidences of specific cancers in populations with a high or low occurrence of a particular environmental factor. This type of evidence can only point to the need for further, more detailed studies as the existence of a correlation does not imply causality. Changes over time in either the diet or the incidence of the cancer, and evidence from migration studies, may provide further clues.

Case–Control Studies

These studies attempt to identify individuals with cancer and closely match each one with a control individual without disease. Comparison of environmental factors, including diet, can then be made, with the objective of identifying differences that may have contributed to the development of the cancer. In addition to the difficulties of obtaining accurate measurements of dietary intake, there are a number of other drawbacks to this approach.

- Studies that rely on information about dietary intake several years ago are imprecise. This is particularly true for a person who has recently been given a diagnosis of cancer, which tends to be a devastating event. In addition, the development of symptoms associated with the disease may have already resulted in dietary changes.

- Cancer is believed to develop over a long period of time; differences in diet a short time before the diagnosis may not reflect differences when the cancer was initiated or promoted.
- Control cases may in fact have undiagnosed or pre-clinical cancer, or develop the cancer later.

Prospective Cohort Studies

These offer the most promising approach. They involve the recruitment of a large cross-section of the population and follow up the sample over a number of years, thus monitoring development of disease. Data about diet and lifestyle factors, together with biochemical measurements are taken initially and at intervals. The use of biomarkers, for example, biological function tests, blood or urine levels of substances, carries less risk of measurement error. Thus, if and when disease does occur, data will be available that cover the period when the disease was developing. A study of this type – the European Prospective Investigation into Cancer and Nutrition (EPIC) – is currently taking place in 10 countries in Europe. Recruitment started in 1992, has recruited more than 520,000 subjects and first results were reported in 2001. The major disadvantage of this type of study is the need for very large numbers of subjects. Research on 'fetal programming' and evidence from studies on growth that point to relationships with later disease, may indicate that even a prospective study over 10 or 15 years may be of insufficient duration to identify factors that may trigger the cancer process. The UK Biobank aims to provide a resource for researchers seeking to improve the prevention, diagnosis and treatment of a wide range of chronic non-communicable diseases including cancer, long into the future. From 2006 to 2010 the UK Biobank recruited 500,000 people aged between 40–69 years from across the country to take part in this project. They have undergone health and lifestyle measures, provided blood, urine and saliva samples for future analysis, provided detailed information about themselves and agreed to have their health followed. Over many years this will build into a powerful resource to help scientists discover why some people develop particular diseases and others do not, although there may be limitations because the UK Biobank had a response rate of only about 5%, so the individuals included may be unusual.

Meta-Analysis

Data from separate studies can be reanalysed by 'meta-analysis'. By cooperating with the investigators, it is possible to record all the outcomes of a number of studies in a similar way and thus increase the power of the analysis. In this way, it may become possible to quantify the relationship between exposure to a hazard and the risk of a particular disease obtained by epidemiological study, even when that risk is only moderate. It is important that only those studies that have similar methodologies are used, and that all relevant studies are included, irrespective of their results, for the analysis to be unbiased and worthwhile. More such analyses will no doubt be carried out in the future.

ENVIRONMENTAL CAUSES OF CANCER

Various attempts have been made over the last 20 years to evaluate the environmental contribution to the development of cancer; some estimates suggest that this may be up to 80%. It has been estimated that about one-third of cancers in developed high-income societies are attributable to factors relating to food, nutrition and physical activity.

Of these, the most important factors are:

- Diet, which may account for an average of one-third of cancer deaths (although the suggested range for different cancers is between 10% and 70%). Alcohol is increasingly recognised as an important cause of some cancers.

- Smoking, which is causal in 30% of cancer deaths (range between 25% and 40%)
- Physical activity, which contributes to maintenance of a normal body weight, prevention of excessive adiposity and is an important protective factor

In comparison other factors believed to be important causes of cancer, such as food additives, pollutants, industrial products and geophysical factors, taken together probably account for 6% of all known cancer deaths (range 0%–13%). It should be noted that some food additives, like antioxidants and preservatives, may actually be protective against cancer.

In looking at the above data, it is not surprising that there is a growing interest and urgency in modifying diets and lifestyles in an attempt to reduce cancer risk. The World Cancer Research Fund estimated that attention to diet, smoking and physical activity could reduce cancer incidence by 30%–40%, preventing 3–4 million cases of cancer worldwide annually.

Role of Diet

Food or nutrients may contribute to the development of cancer in a number of ways, broadly classified as follows:

- Foods may be a source of pre-formed (or precursors of) carcinogens.
- Nutrients may affect the formation, transport, deactivation or excretion of carcinogens.
- Nutrients may affect the body's resistance to carcinogens and, therefore, be important protective factors.

Diets are extremely complex and their measurement is subject to error. This is particularly a problem in a population whose diets are relatively similar. If the error is not consistent and is greater than the variation in intakes, it can result in misclassification of individuals and a miscalculation of risk. Random errors can also reduce the power of studies to detect relationships between intake and disease, but these errors can be minimized by repeated measurements or the use of large cohorts. Other difficulties arise because of the co-variation in particular nutrients. For example, fat intakes and energy intakes may change simultaneously, meat intakes may reflect the protein content of the diet, fruit and vegetables in the diet affect the overall intake of non-starch polysaccharide (NSP). RCT studies attempting to isolate the effects of specific nutrients often use supplements as the intervention and the results of such studies do not reflect the effect of dietary sources of the nutrients, or the impact of the food matrix. Finally, there is good evidence from many studies that subjects tend to underreport their dietary intake, and this does not happen in a systematic manner with some nutrients more likely to be underreported, in particular protein, sugars and fat missed from a diet record. Again, this can be taken into account in large prospective studies, if they are well designed. Despite these difficulties, epidemiological evidence from the last 15 years has identified a number of consistent trends in the relationship between diet and some cancers. Detailed mechanisms underlying these associations remain to be elucidated.

The WCRF (2007) report classifies the evidence associated with diet and physical activity factors on cancer risks at 18 possible cancer sites. Evidence is categorised under eight headings:

1. Convincing evidence of a decreased risk
2. Probable evidence of a decreased risk
3. Limited suggestive evidence of a decreased risk
4. Limited suggestive evidence of an increased risk
5. Probably evidence of an increased risk
6. Convincing evidence of an increased risk
7. Evidence that a substantial effect on risk is unlikely
8. Limited evidence – no conclusion possible.

Possible Promoting Factors

According to the WCRF, there is currently convincing evidence of the following lifestyle factors increase the risk of specific cancers:

Lifestyle Factor	Convincing Evidence of Increased Risk of
Consumption of red and processed meats	Colorectal
Body fatness	Oesophageal, pancreatic, colorectal, breast postmenopause, endometrial and kidney
Abdominal fatness	Colorectal
Alcohol consumption	Mouth, oesophageal, colorectal (men), breast pre- and postmenopause
Adult attained height	Colorectal and breast postmenopause
Aflatoxins	Liver
Arsenic in drinking water	Lung
Beta-carotene supplements	Lung

Total Energy Intake

Restricting the food intake of mice without modifying the proportion of the individual nutrients has long been known to halve the incidence of spontaneous tumours of the mammary gland and lung and to reduce susceptibility to known carcinogens. This effect of restricted energy intake appears to be independent of any reduction in fat content of the diet. In mice, increased activity was as effective at reducing tumour development as restricted energy intake. Increased exercise may promote activity of the immune system, thereby increasing resistance. The evidence that obesity, weight gain and also overweight short of obesity increase the risk of a number of cancers is more impressive than was the case in the mid-1990s.

In humans, rapid growth in childhood, and especially growth in height, may also, in ways as yet unknown, contribute to a higher risk of cancer. Data from the National Health and Nutrition Examination Survey (NHANES) 1 study found a positive correlation with height and a number of cancers, including colorectal cancer. Follow-up of children under 16 years, first studied by Boyd Orr in 1937–1939, has also shown a significant positive association, with a 20% increased risk of all cancers not associated with smoking, for every 1 MJ greater daily energy intake (Frankel et al., 1998). Potential confounding variables, such as social class and household size, were taken into consideration in the analysis.

High energy intakes also contribute to risk by leading to greater adiposity and, therefore, overweight, if not accompanied by increased energy expenditure. Therefore, restriction of energy intake and avoidance of overweight are probably important at key stages of life. In women, being overweight at puberty and after the menopause appear to be linked to increased breast cancer risks, but premenopausal overweight may be protective. These findings are linked to presensitization of breast tissue to oestrogens in the young adolescent and unopposed production of oestrogens by adipose tissue after the menopause. Both may promote the development of oestrogen-dependent tumours. Levels of ovarian hormones appear to be influenced by nutritional status; thus, a high caloric intake may increase production and thereby risk of breast cancer. A correlation between breast cancer risks, sex hormone levels and energy intakes has been found in countries across the world. Sex hormones produced or modified by adipose tissue may also play a part in cancer of the endometrium in women and possibly the prostate in men.

A review of data on energy intake and cancers also indicates a positive relationship with large bowel cancer. This may reflect greater exposure to carcinogens with the greater food intake but more evidence is needed in this area.

Fat Intakes

Fat has been described as a promoter of carcinogenesis, although the effect of dietary fat is often difficult to distinguish from that of energy intake, as fat obviously contributes to the total energy content of the diet. Associations with fat intake have been reported for cancers of the breast, colon and prostate, as well as weak relationships for cancer of the ovary, kidneys and pancreas.

In the case of breast cancer, there is still considerable controversy. Estimated fat consumption in different countries of the world shows a strong positive correlation with age-adjusted death rates from breast cancer. In the United States, the Nurses' Health Study (Willett et al., 1992) found no association between total fat intake or intake of fibre and the incidence of breast cancer in both pre- and postmenopausal women. It is possible that the prevailing higher fat intakes lead to earlier menarche in girls, thereby prolonging the exposure of breast tissue to circulating oestrogens and increasing risk. This has not, however, been fully investigated. Although in animals there is evidence of a promoting effect of *n*-6 fatty acids and an inhibitory effect of *n*-3 fatty acids on mammary tumour growth, this effect has not been demonstrated in humans. It has been suggested that *n*-6 fatty acid intakes may already be above the threshold of this promoting effect, after which no further increase is seen. This may explain the absence of evidence in women. Nevertheless, it is probably prudent to limit fat intakes, even if this simply reduces total energy intake and thereby provides some protection.

Dietary changes in Japan in the last 40 years have included a dramatic increase in fat intake, paralleled by a reduction in complex carbohydrates. Associated with these dietary changes has been an increase in colon cancer, suggesting a link. Evidence for the involvement of fat intake is stronger in the case of colon cancer, particularly in relation to fat of animal origin, cholesterol and red meat consumption. Further evidence from the U.S. Nurses' Health Study has shown a 2.5-fold increase in risk of colon cancer in women consuming beef, pork and lamb daily, compared with those eating these meats less than monthly. Association with chicken and fish was negative, and there was no association with cholesterol intakes. It has been proposed that dietary fat causes a greater secretion of bile acids; these may be fermented by anaerobic bacteria in the colon to produce mutagenic compounds, leading to abnormal cell proliferation in the colon. However, other dietary factors may modify this process, most notably NSPs and protective factors in fruit and vegetables. The lowered pH of the bowel as a result of soluble NSP fermentation may be protective.

Prostate cancer has also been weakly associated with a high fat intake, but more evidence is needed to support this. Overall, it remains problematic to separate the effects of higher fat intakes from those of a high energy intake and overweight.

Alcohol

There is an association between consumption of alcohol and cancers of the aerodigestive tract (mouth, throat and oesophagus), as well as the liver, colorectum and breast both pre- and postmenopause. The EPIC study has confirmed that the risk of these cancers is nine times greater in those drinking 60 g ethanol or more (7–8 units) a day compared with those drinking 30 g or less. The effects of alcohol as a causative agent are potentiated by smoking, with those smoking more than 20 cigarettes a day having a 50-fold greater risk than nonsmoking, moderate alcohol drinkers. The risks of oral and pharyngeal cancers can be offset to some extent with a high intake of fruit and vegetables.

Oesophageal cancer has been increasing since the early 1970s in the United Kingdom, which parallels the increase in alcohol consumption, with a latency of 15–20 years. It is not clear if the relationship is simply with the amount of alcohol consumed; some evidence suggests that spirits are more harmful than beer and wine. Oesophageal cancer also occurs in parts of the world, where alcohol consumption is low. In these cases, it is thought to be related to micronutrient deficiencies in the diet.

Alcohol consumption, above a moderate level, has also been shown in the EPIC study to be associated with a rise in breast cancer, although there was no evidence of a dose–response relationship with wine consumption.

Salt

Salt and salt-preserved foods have been suggested as probable causative factors in stomach cancer (WCRF, 2007). This was found to be true between countries, between different regions of the same country and different subgroups of the population. Salt has high osmotic activity and has been reported to cause gastritis in animals, resulting in early damage to the mucosa. Other factors are also important, most notably the presence of *H. pylori*, which is now known to be a major cause of chronic atrophic gastritis and which must be taken into account in future studies on the exact role of salt as a factor in causation of stomach cancer.

In addition to sodium chloride, other forms of preservation using nitrates and nitrites as well as pickling have been associated with stomach cancers. Nitrates occur in the diet as preservatives in foods, such as ham, bacon and sausages, and in beer and are naturally present in vegetables as well as in the drinking water, particularly in agricultural areas owing to contamination from fertilizers. Dietary nitrates may not cause cancer per se, but it has been proposed that the conversion to nitrites and subsequently to carcinogenic nitrosamines is more likely in the presence of low gastric acidity. Both *H. pylori* infection and a high salt intake are thought to cause low gastric acidity and this may complete the link with nitrites.

The decline in both stroke mortality and gastric cancer over the last 20–30 years may be explained by decreases in salt intake with advances in food preservation. Refrigeration and deep freezing have reduced the use of salt as a preservative for meat, fish and vegetables. In addition, there has been much greater all year round availability of fruit and vegetables. The vitamin C content of these inhibits the formation of nitrosamines in the stomach and may be an important protective factor. Conversely, nitrosamine formation is promoted by thiocyanates from cigarette smoke, and smokers have been shown to have higher rates of gastric cancer. The decline in smoking may also have had an effect on the incidence of this disease.

Meat and Fish

The evidence that heavily cooked (eg barbecued) red meats and processed meats are a cause of colorectal cancer is convincing. A substantial amount of data from cohort and case control studies shows a dose–response relationship. A recent meta-analysis of 15 prospective cohort studies reported a summary effect estimate of 1.28 (95% CI 1.18–1.39) per 120 g of red meat consumed per day. In addition Cantonese-style salted fish is a probable cause of nasopharyngeal cancer (this latter finding does not apply to other types of fish).

Nitrogenous residues from meat digestion, as well as other proteins, may be metabolized in the large bowel to produce ammonia, and the amount produced increases with meat consumption. Ammonia has been shown to induce cell proliferation in human colonic cells and to produce adenocarcinomas in rats. Other products from meat ingestion that may contribute to the promotion of colon cancer are *N*-nitroso compounds, which increase with red meat (but not white meat or fish) intake, and heterocyclic amines. The latter are formed during the cooking of meat and are dependent on temperature, duration and amount and type of fat in the meat. High-temperature cooking, for example, grilling, barbecuing and frying, also produces polycyclic hydrocarbons and has been associated with higher cancer risk. Molecular biology has identified 'fast' and 'slow' acetylators amongst human subjects. The conversion of heterocyclic amines to carcinogenic products in 'fast acetylators' appears to increase their risk of developing adenomatous polyps, which are considered to be precancerous. Subjects who are slow acetylators appear to be much less at risk.

Processed meats, including ham, sausages and bacon, have also been linked to moderately increased risk of colon cancer, which has been shown in the EPIC study to be 50% greater in those subjects consuming 60 g/day of processed meat than in those consuming none. Early results from the EPIC study have not, however, shown a significant increase in colon cancer with red meat intake, but some protective effect was indicated from white meat and fish intakes, and further results are awaited. Based on its reports from 2007 and 2011, the WCRF advises

TABLE 15.2
Some Proposed Links between Dietary Components and Cancers

Dietary Component	Suggested Link with Cancer Site	Mechanism/Interpretation
Moulds: aflatoxin	Liver	Grows on peanuts; important cause of cancer in some countries in Africa
Iron	Colon and rectum	Relates to tissue levels of iron, not dietary intakes; may represent a breakdown of iron regulatory mechanisms
High maternal adiposity	Testicular cancer	Endocrine environment of developing fetus affected, predisposes both to undescended testes and cancer
Calcium	Colon and rectum	Weak relationship; possible action through binding of intestinal fats and thus reduces bile acid secretion
Vitamin D	Colon and rectum	May control cell growth and differentiation; weak association
Folate	Colon and rectum	Inverse relationship between plasma levels and colorectal polyps; aggravated by high alcohol intake
Smoked, grilled or barbequed foods	Stomach	Limited suggestive evidence; effect of charring food

eating no more than 500 g of red meat each week, and little (if any) processed meat. Meanwhile, a recent press release (2015) classified processed meat as carcinogenic to humans (Group 1), based on the evidence gathered so far in humans that the consumption of processed meat causes colorectal cancer.

A number of other cancers have been linked in some studies with meat consumption. These include cancer of the breast, lung, prostate and pancreas, but in all cases, the evidence for an association is weak. There is some evidence that stomach cancer may be linked with consumption of processed meat (see the 'Salt' section). The great variety of ways in which people preserve and cook meat across the world makes this a particularly challenging area for study.

Other Promoters of Cancer

A number of other dietary factors have been linked with the promotion of cancers (Table 15.2), although in most cases the supporting evidence is limited suggestive evidence and no firm connections have been proved. In most cases, it is difficult to separate the effect of the proposed factor from that of associated dietary components. Because only a small part of the environmental causes of cancers, research is very actively hunting for other factors. For example, recent evidence that some emulsifiers in processed foods may damage the mucus layer of the gut and promote colitis has stimulated a new line of enquiry. The unexpected discovery of acrylamide in some heat-stressed cereal products led to immediate changes in manufacture, as acrylamide is a well-known carcinogen.

Possible Protective Factors

According to the WRCF, there is currently convincing evidence for only two lifestyle factors as possibly protective factors against specific cancers:

Lifestyle Factor	Convincing Evidence of Decreased Risk of
Physical activity	Colorectal cancer
Lactation	Breast cancer pre- and postmenopause

Other possibly protective factors such as dietary fibre, nonstarchy vegetables, fruits, pulses, milk, foods containing folate, carotenoids, selenium, vitamin E and selenium as a supplement have been classified as probably reducing the risk of certain cancers at sites such as the mouth, pharynx, larynx, oesophagus, stomach, colorectum, pancreas, lung and prostate.

Nonstarch Polysaccharides (Dietary Fibre)

Early observations, such as those of Burkitt et al. (1972), found a low incidence of diseases of the bowel in communities that had a large consumption of plant foods. This was developed into a theory about the protective effects of dietary fibre in a number of diseases. Knowledge about this fraction, now called NSPs in the United Kingdom, is currently much more extensive. It is believed that NSPs may protect against colon cancer by three possible mechanisms:

1. High levels of NSP in the diet lead to increased bulk, mainly due to an increase in colonic bacteria, and, therefore, faster transit time through the colon. As a result, potentially harmful carcinogenic substances are present in a more dilute form and are in contact with the colonic mucosa for a shorter time.
2. Fermentation of soluble NSP (as well as resistant starch) in the colon yields a number of short-chain fatty acids, which influence epithelial cell function. Most notable is butyric acid, which has been shown to be an anti-proliferative and differentiating agent, able to induce apoptosis (programmed cell death) in the large bowel epithelium.
3. As a result of the formation of the short-chain fatty acids, NSP in the diet reduces the pH of the bowel. This allows primary bile acids to bind to calcium, preventing them from being converted to mutagenic secondary bile acids. The lower pH also increases the number of aerobic bacteria, which do not produce carcinogenic products from bile acids. More of the bile acids are excreted, bound to components such as lignin. Studies in which subjects were supplemented with wheat bran showed a reduced mutagenicity in stool samples.

In their 2007 report, the WCRF panel judged that there was evidence of a probable decreased risk of colorectal cancer and a limited suggestive decreased risk of oesophageal cancer, associated with increased consumption of dietary fibre. The assessment of the evidence for colorectal cancer was upgraded to convincing as part of the continuous update project in 2011 (WCRF, 2011). Meta-analysis was possible on eight studies, giving a summary effect estimate of 0.90 (95% confidence interval [CI] 0.84–0.97) per 10 g/day increment.

However, problems with interpreting studies on intakes of 'fibre' and the incidence of cancer arise because of confusion over the definition of the fractions of fibre in the diet and the lack of detailed food composition data on this. Controversy over which fractions of fibre intake are more important in prevention of colon cancer continues, with some studies supporting a role for fruit and vegetables, and others for cereal fibre. Further difficulties arise from the effects of a change of NSP content in the diet on its other constituents, which may also be involved in cancer development.

It is also possible that a high intake of vegetables and fruit, and perhaps cereals, indicates an increased intake of other substances, such as antioxidants or flavonoids, which may be protective, rather than just the NSP they contain. The EPIC study has reported a 40% lower incidence of colon cancer in subjects eating a high-fibre diet (32.5 g), compared with those eating only 12 g of fibre.

In the case of breast cancer, women consuming 'high-fibre' diets have been found to excrete more inactivated conjugated oestrogen in the faeces, with resultant lower plasma levels. However, evidence that high-fibre diets are protective against breast cancer is weak. Recent evidence suggests that soya products may offer some protection against breast and prostate cancer because of the presence of phyto-oestrogens. These are believed to increase the synthesis of oestrogen-binding proteins and thereby reduce the levels of these hormones in both men and women. Related compounds called lignans may be found in whole cereals, seeds and fruit, and may in part account for some of the findings attributed to 'dietary fibre' in protection against breast cancer.

Fruit and Vegetables

One of the most consistent findings in all of the literature on diet and cancer is that incidence is lower where fruit and vegetable intakes are high. Non-starchy vegetables probably protect against cancers of the mouth, pharynx, and larynx, and those of the oesophagus and stomach. There is limited evidence suggesting that they also protect against cancers of the nasopharynx, lung, colorectum, ovary, and endometrium. Allium vegetables probably protect against stomach cancer. Garlic (an allium vegetable, commonly classed as a herb) probably protects against colorectal cancer. There is limited evidence suggesting that carrots protect against cervical cancer; and that pulses (legumes), including soya and soya products, protect against stomach and prostate cancers. Fruits in general probably protect against cancer of the mouth, pharynx, and larynx, and those of the oesophagus, lung, and stomach. There is limited evidence suggesting that fruits also protect against cancers of the nasopharynx, pancreas, liver, and colorectum. Conversely, there is little recorded increased risk of any cancer associated with fruit and vegetable consumption, the only exception being some limited evidence that consumption of chilli could be a cause of stomach cancer.

The initial understanding of the mechanisms involved was that the antioxidant nutrients present in fruit and vegetables were responsible for the protective effect. The suggested mechanism links the antioxidant nutrients to the prevention of oxidative damage to the DNA by free radicals, and hence the initiation of damage. These nutrients also protect lipids in cellular membranes. Fruit and vegetables are also a source of NSPs and many other nutrients, which may play a role through different mechanisms. In addition, fruit and vegetables contain a wide variety of other chemically active substances that may play an important role in the overall effect, and research in this area is still relatively new. A problem associated with studies of fruit and vegetables is the inconsistency of definition of terms used. For example, potatoes or pulses may or may not be included in the vegetables group. Tomatoes may be included as either fruit or vegetables and in some studies, fruit and vegetables are subdivided into smaller groups by colour. In reviews of evidence, therefore, the whole group of fruit and/or vegetables may be considered in general.

The antioxidant mechanism of action of dietary compounds is covered in Chapter 14, pp. 287–289.

Antioxidant Nutrients

Fruit and vegetables provide the three most studied antioxidants, namely, vitamin A (and carotenoids), C and E. Proposed mechanisms of action for a protective effect have been explored, but no firm conclusions have been possible.

Retinoids (vitamin A family) regulate epithelial cell differentiation and could, therefore, influence tumour growth in tissues. Carotenoids are powerful quenchers of singlet oxygen and, therefore, act as antioxidants to minimize damage. It has also been postulated that the role of carotenoids may be mediated through potentiation of immune system activity.

Initial epidemiological studies had suggested that vitamin A (as retinol) was protective against lung cancer. More recent data have shown a consistent inverse relationship between the incidence of lung cancer and intakes of various carotenoids (precursors of vitamin A) as well as high plasma levels of beta-carotene. Nevertheless, results of supplementation trials have not been encouraging. Supplementation of 30,000 Finnish male smokers with either beta-carotene and/or vitamin E or placebo resulted in an increased mortality from lung cancer and coronary disease in the carotene group (Alpha-Tocopherol, Beta-Carotene Cancer Prevention Study Group, 1994). Similar results have occurred in at least two other trials. Studies on lung cancer are often difficult to interpret because of the strong confounding effect of smoking. However, excessive amounts of any single antioxidant are undesirable, since an imbalance can promote some prooxidant activity. Supplementation with beta-carotene has also been associated with an increased risk of colon cancer in two studies.

The Nurses' Health Study in the United States found a 20% rise in breast cancer rates between the highest and lowest intakes of vitamin A and carotenoids. Amongst women with the lowest dietary intake of vitamin A, the use of a supplement reduced the risk of breast cancer. Results for stomach and prostate cancers, however, do not show a consistent trend.

Vitamin C may also be an important protective factor against cancers of the oesophagus, stomach and pancreas. This role may be linked to its antioxidant properties, especially in association with vitamin E. It also has a protective role for the mixed function oxidase systems in the liver, which are important for destroying foreign and harmful substances. The most researched function of vitamin C is its role in inhibiting nitrosamine formation in the stomach, thereby reducing the risks of stomach cancer. Levels of vitamin C in the stomach are reduced by *H. pylori* infection, which results in a loss of gastric acid secretion and consequent increase in stomach pH. This situation favours bacterial colonization and increased formation of nitrites and nitroso compounds.

Results of studies into the relationship between vitamin E and cancers at various sites are inconclusive, with better results obtained in smokers than nonsmokers. Results are complicated by the interaction of vitamin E with selenium status and plasma cholesterol levels. A supplementation study with various combinations of nutrients in a poorly nourished population in Linxian, China, achieved a significant reduction in mortality from stomach cancer in those subjects receiving vitamin E, beta-carotene and selenium (Blot et al., 1993). It is likely that initial intakes were low, thus contributing to the positive finding.

Most of the findings described earlier relate to fruit and vegetable intakes as part of the whole diet. It is perhaps unsurprising, therefore, that attempts to replicate the results with single constituents of these foods have been unsuccessful. What is more concerning is that unexpected adverse effects have occurred. This emphasizes once again the need for a balance of nutrients in the diet, to provide appropriate amounts for their metabolic role at cellular level.

Other Chemically Active Constituents

A number of phenolic compounds are found in fruit and vegetables. These include flavonoids, such as quercetin and catechins, which act as antioxidants and may have roles in gene blocking or suppression. However, no convincing evidence exists at present of a protective role in cancer. Phytooestrogens are also a class of phenolic compounds; the most important examples are isoflavones, found in soya, and lignans, which occur in linseed, lentils, asparagus, broccoli and leeks. These compounds can act as oestrogen agonists (promote or mimic the action) and antagonists (oppose the action), depending on the receptors to which they bind. It is this potential to prevent a normal oestrogen response that may offer protection against hormone-dependent tumours, such as breast and prostate. However, the evidence base to support this proposal is weak at present.

Members of the brassica vegetable family (cabbage, broccoli, cauliflower, Brussels sprouts) are particularly rich in glucosinolates, which have been shown to have blocking and suppressing properties in the development of cancers. However, large amounts may also be potentially toxic, so a cautious approach and more research are needed. Garlic, onions and leeks, all of which belong to the Allium family, also have potential blocking and suppressing properties, which have been demonstrated in rats to suppress the formation of gastric cancer. Epidemiological studies suggest a possible protective role in humans.

Further research is needed, however, to demonstrate if the positive effects of fruit and vegetables in the prevention of cancer may be attributed to any of these constituents.

Calcium

In recent years, a number of studies have indicated an inverse relationship between the intake of calcium, particularly in the form of dairy products, and colon cancer. It is suggested that calcium binds fatty acids and bile acids in the colon, preventing them from causing damage to the mucosa. It is possible that calcium itself has an antiproliferative action on the colonic cells, thus preventing tumour formation. In addition, a role for vitamin D in prevention of colon cancer has also been proposed, linked to its function in control of cell proliferation. Milk may produce benefits in other ways. Whey proteins are rich in cysteine, which is a precursor of the antioxidant glutathione.

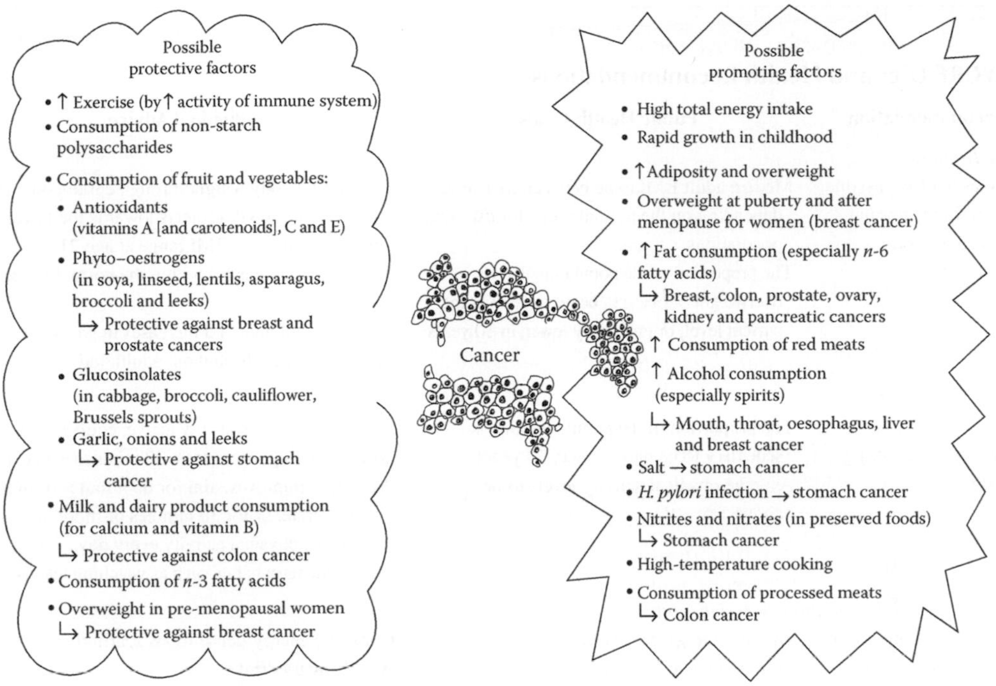

Possible protective factors
• ↑ Exercise (by ↑ activity of immune system)
• Consumption of non-starch polysaccharides
• Consumption of fruit and vegetables:
• Antioxidants (vitamins A [and carotenoids], C and E)
• Phyto–oestrogens (in soya, linseed, lentils, asparagus, broccoli and leeks)
↳ Protective against breast and prostate cancers
• Glucosinolates (in cabbage, broccoli, cauliflower, Brussels sprouts)
• Garlic, onions and leeks
↳ Protective against stomach cancer
• Milk and dairy product consumption (for calcium and vitamin B)
↳ Protective against colon cancer
• Consumption of n-3 fatty acids
• Overweight in pre-menopausal women
↳ Protective against breast cancer
Cancer
Possible promoting factors
• High total energy intake
• Rapid growth in childhood
• ↑ Adiposity and overweight
• Overweight at puberty and after menopause for women (breast cancer)
• ↑ Fat consumption (especially n-6 fatty acids)
↳ Breast, colon, prostate, ovary, kidney and pancreatic cancers
↑ Consumption of red meats
↑ Alcohol consumption (especially spirits)
↳ Mouth, throat, oesophagus, liver and breast cancer
• Salt → stomach cancer
• H. pylori infection → stomach cancer
• Nitrites and nitrates (in preserved foods)
↳ Stomach cancer
• High-temperature cooking
• Consumption of processed meats
↳ Colon cancer

FIGURE 15.1 Possible promoting and protective factors in the diet in relation to cancer development.

In addition, milk contains lactoferrin, which can bind iron in the digestive tract, making it less available to act as a prooxidant.

Supplementation studies have again produced equivocal results, once more indicating that attention to foods rather than individual nutrients may be the key to prevention. Figure 15.1 summarizes possible promoting and preventive effects of nutrients.

PREVENTION OF CANCER

In the United Kingdom, healthy eating policy is embodied in the 'Eight Guidelines for a Healthy Diet', the Department of Health Dietary Reference Values (DoH, 1991) and the eatwell guide. All of these give advice about a diet that aims to reduce the intake of foods containing fats and sugars and to increase the intakes of starchy carbohydrates, fruit and vegetables. Ensuring a moderate intake of sources of protein, from meat, fish, dairy products and their alternatives for vegetarians, will also provide other minerals and vitamins. Maintaining a normal body weight through adequate but not excessive energy intakes and exercise is also important.

In 1998, the Department of Health report on Nutritional Aspects of the Development of Cancer published a number of specific recommendations in this area. In essence, they do not differ from the broader guidelines on healthy eating.

They are as follows:

- To maintain a healthy body weight within the body mass index (BMI) range 20–25 and not to increase it during adult life.
- To increase intakes of a wide variety of fruit and vegetables
- To increase intakes of non-starch polysaccharides (dietary fibre) from a variety of food sources
- For adults, individuals' consumption of red and processed meat should not rise; higher consumers should consider a reduction and, as a consequence of this the population average will fall

TABLE 15.3

WCRF Diet and Health Recommendations

Recommendation	Public Health Goals	Individual Advice
Body fatness		
Be as lean as possible within the normal range of body weight	Median adult BMI to be between 21 and 23, depending on the normal range for different populations The proportion of the population that is overweight or obese to be no more than the current level, or preferably lower, in 10 years	Ensure that body weight through childhood and adolescent growth projects towards the lower end of the normal BMI range at age 21. Maintain body weight within the normal range from age 21. Avoid weight gain and increases in waist circumference throughout adulthood.
Physical activity		
Be physically active as part of everyday life	The proportion of the population that is sedentary to be halved every 10 years Average physical activity levels to be above 1.6	Be moderately physically active, equivalent to brisk walking, for at least 30 minutes every day. As fitness improves, aim for 60 minutes or more of moderate, or for 30 minutes or more of vigorous, physical activity every day. Limit sedentary habits such as watching television.
Foods and drinks that promote weight gain		
Limit consumption of energy-dense foods and avoid sugary drinks	Average energy density of diets to be lowered towards 125 kcal per 100 g Population average consumption of sugary drinks to be halved every 10 years	Consume energy-dense foods sparingly. Avoid sugary drinks. Consume 'fast foods' sparingly, if at all.
Plant foods		
Eat mostly foods of plant origin	Population average consumption of nonstarchy vegetables and of fruits to be at least 600 g (21 oz) daily Relatively unprocessed cereals (grains) and/or pulses (legumes), and other foods that are a natural source of dietary fibre, to contribute to a population average of at least 25 g NSP daily	Eat at least five portions/servings (at least 400 g or 14 oz) of a variety of nonstarchy vegetables and of fruits every day. Eat relatively unprocessed cereals (grains) and/or pulses (legumes) with every meal. Limit refined starchy foods. People who consume starchy roots or tubers as staples also to ensure intake of sufficient nonstarchy vegetables, fruits and pulses (legumes).
Animal foods		
Limit intake of red meat and avoid processed meat	Population average consumption of red meat to be no more than 300 g (11 oz) a week, very little if any of which to be processed	People who eat red meat to consume less than 500 g (18 oz) a week, very little if any to be processed.
Alcoholic drinks		
Limit alcoholic drinks	Proportion of the population drinking more than the recommended limits to be reduced by one-third every 10 years	If alcoholic drinks are consumed, limit consumption to no more than two drinks a day for men and one drink a day for women.
Preservation, processing, preparation		
Limit consumption of salt and avoid mouldy cereals (grains) and pulses (legumes)	Population average consumption of salt from all sources to be less than 5 g (2 g of sodium) a day Proportion of the population consuming more than 6 g of salt (2.4 g of sodium) a day to be halved every 10 years Minimize exposure to aflatoxins from mouldy cereals (grains) or pulses (legumes)	Avoid salt-preserved, salted or salty foods; preserve foods without using salt. Limit consumption of processed foods with added salt to ensure an intake of less than 6 g (2.4 g sodium) a day. Do not eat mouldy cereals (grains) or pulses (legumes).

(*Continued*)

TABLE 15.3 (*Continued*)

WCRF Diet and Health Recommendations

Recommendation	Public Health Goals	Individual Advice
Dietary supplements		
Aim to meet nutritional needs through diet alone	Maximize the proportion of the population achieving nutritional adequacy without dietary supplements	Dietary supplements are not recommended for cancer prevention.
Breastfeeding		
Mothers to breast feed, babies to be breast fed	The majority of mothers to breastfeed exclusively, for 6 months	Aim to breastfeed infants exclusively up to 6 months and continue with complementary feeding thereafter.
Cancer survivors		
Follow the recommendations for cancer prevention	All cancer survivors to receive nutritional care from an appropriately trained professional	If able to do so, and unless otherwise advised, aim to follow the recommendations for diet, healthy weight and physical activity.

Source: World Cancer Research Fund/American Institute for Cancer Research, Food, nutrition, physical activity, and the prevention of cancer: A global perspective, AICR, Washington, DC, 2007.

BMI, body mass index; PAL, physical activity level.

These recommendations should be followed in the context of the Committee on Medical Aspects of Food Policy (COMA)'s wider recommendations for a balanced diet rich in cereals, fruits and vegetables. In addition, it was recommended that:

- Beta-carotene supplements, as a means of avoiding cancer, should not be used
- Caution should be exercised in the use of high doses of purified supplements of other micronutrients, as they cannot be assumed to be without risk

The World Cancer Research Fund has identified the 'five-star' foods for cancer prevention:

1. Foods rich in beta-carotene – spinach, carrots, broccoli and tomatoes
2. Foods rich in vitamin C – citrus fruits, berries, melons, green vegetables, tomatoes, cauliflowers and green peppers
3. Foods rich in selenium – bran, wheat germ, tuna fish, onion, garlic and mushrooms
4. Foods rich in vitamin E – wholegrain cereals, wheat germ, soya beans and leafy greens
5. Foods rich in complex carbohydrates – bread, cereals, beans and peas

These foods should be eaten in place of fattier items and can help to reduce overweight. They may also contain other important substances that may help the body's resistance to cancer.

The World Cancer Research Fund Report, published in 2007, took a global perspective on the prevention of cancer and made recommendations that were also consistent with the prevention of other diseases. They contain policy goals and advice for individuals. It was, however, intended by the report that the relative importance of the different recommendations would vary in different parts of the world, for their populations. They are summarized in Table 15.3.

In addition to the recommendations detailed earlier, the WCRF also identified safe storage, preservation and preparation of foods as well as the presence of additives and residues as important areas for public health policy. Recommendations were also made against the use of dietary supplements and tobacco use. Overall, the recommendations shown in Table 15.3 go further than those of the United Kingdom in recommending a move to a more traditional, evolutonary, more plant-based diet. It is not necessary to adopt a radical stone-age or 'paleo' diet, and selecting a diet from the eatwell guide in the proportions recommended will provide a good balance of the nutrients needed. What is also needed is the motivation and the desire to be healthy, and willingness to make permanent health-oriented changes to cusomary diet and lifestyle. That rarely happens overnight, except after a cancer is diagnosed, when it is not entirely too late but failing to make an earlier change is regretted bitterly. Taking vitamin supplements cannot provide what a balanced diet does, and may accelerate cancers. Although much research is still required to further elucidate the role of dietary factors in certain cancers, we already have sufficient information to make recommendations that can significantly reduce the risk.

SUMMARY

1. Diet may play a major role in the development of cancer.
2. Particular aspects of the diet that may be involved as promoters and protective factors have been identified.
3. Dietary guidelines for the prevention of cancer have been proposed. These include a high intake of fruit and vegetables and avoidance of excess intakes of fat and energy and maintenance of a healthy weight. Protein intake, especially from meat sources, should also be moderated. Lifestyle changes, including regular physical activity, are needed to support the dietary adjustments.

STUDY QUESTIONS

1. Why is it difficult to study the relationship between nutrition and cancer?
2. a. In what ways have dietary fats been linked with the development of cancers?
   b. Why is it difficult to distinguish the effects of fats from those of total energy intake in cancer causation?
3. List the reasons why an increase in NSPs (dietary fibre) intake might protect against some cancers.
4. How does the advice on diet for cancer prevention compare with general healthy eating guidelines?
5. a. In what ways might the antioxidant nutrients be useful in the prevention of cancers?
   b. Does the scientific evidence currently support this theory?

ACTIVITIES

15.1 Looking at the findings in the WCRF (2007) report 'Food, nutrition, physical activity, and the prevention of cancer: A global perspective', how would you use this information to develop public health messages designed to change dietary and lifestyle patterns in the United Kingdom and reduce the risk cancer?

- How would you segment your audience?
- What would your key messages be?
- What communication channels would you use?
- What else might you do to try to influence healthy eating and lifestyle behaviours?

15.2 How might you convince government agencies, such as the Food Standards Agency, to invest in your campaign to reduce the risks of cancer in the United Kingdom? What arguments would you use – financial or others?

BIBLIOGRAPHY AND FURTHER READING

Alpha-Tocopherol, Beta-Carotene Cancer Prevention Study Group. 1994. The effect of vitamin E and beta-carotene on the incidence of lung cancer and other cancers in male smokers. *New England Journal of Medicine* 330(15), 1029–1035.

Bingham, S.A. 1999. High meat diets and cancer risk. *Proceedings of the Nutrition Society* 58, 243–248.

Blot, W.J., Li, J.-Y., Taylor, P.R. et al. 1993. Nutrition intervention trials in Linxian, China: Supplementation with specific vitamin/mineral combinations, cancer incidence and disease specific mortality in general population. *Journal of the National Cancer Institute* 85, 1483–1492.

Burkitt, D.P., Walker, A.R.P. and Painter, N.S. 1972. Effect of dietary fibre on stools and transit times and its role in the causation of disease. *Lancet* ii, 1408–1412.

Burr, M.L. 1994. Antioxidants and cancer. *Journal of Human Nutrition and Dietetics* 7, 409–416.

Cancer Research UK. 2012. *Cancer Stats: Key Facts.* London, UK: Cancer Research UK.

DoH (UK Department of Health). 1991. Dietary reference values for food energy and nutrients for the United Kingdom. Report on Health and Social Subjects No. 41. Report of the Panel on Dietary Reference Values of the Committee on Medical Aspects of Food Policy. London, UK: HMSO.

DoH (UK Department of Health). 1998. Nutritional aspects of the development of cancer. Report on Health and Social Subjects 48. London, UK: The Stationery Office.

Frankel, S., Gunnell, D.J., Peters, T.J. et al. 1998. Childhood energy intake and adult mortality from cancer: The Boyd Orr cohort study. *British Medical Journal* 316, 499–504.

Key, T. 1994. Micronutrients and cancer aetiology: The epidemiological evidence. *Proceedings of the Nutrition Society* 53, 605–614.

Milner, J. A. (2006). Diet and cancer: facts and controversies. *Nutrition and Cancer*, 56(2), 216–224.

National Dairy Council (NDC). 1995. *Nutrition and Cancer.* Fact File 12. London, UK: NDC.

Riboli, E. 1991. Nutrition and cancer: Background and rationale of the European prospective investigation into cancer and nutrition (EPIC). *Annals of Oncology* 3, 783–791.

Riboli, E. and Norat, T. 2001. Cancer prevention and diet: Opportunities in Europe. *Public Health Nutrition* 4(2B), 475–484.

Willett, W.C., Hunter, D.J., Stampfer, M.J. et al. 1992. Dietary fat and fibre in relation to role in breast cancer. *Journal of the American Medical Association* 268, 2037–2044.

World Cancer Research Fund/American Institute for Cancer Research. 2007. Food, nutrition, physical activity, and the prevention of cancer: A global perspective. Washington, DC: AICR.

World Cancer Research Fund/American Institute for Cancer Research. 2011. Keeping the science current—Colorectal cancer 2011 report. Washington, DC: AICR.

Section V

Dietary and Nutritional Assessment

16 Energy: Intake and Expenditure

AIMS

The aims of this chapter are to

- Present the concepts of energy intake and energy output.
- Study energy intake and how it can be measured.
- Study energy output and its component parts.
- Consider the different requirements for energy in various individuals in different activities.

The term 'energy' is confused or poorly understood because in lay language it is often used to refer to a subjective feeling of alertness. In nutritional science, 'energy' refers to the metabolic fuel needed for all bodily functions. We need a continuous supply of energy for the basic physiological functioning of the body, particularly at cellular level in active transport pumps, but also more apparent functions, such as breathing, digestion and excretion. The most energy-demanding organ is the brain. In addition, our muscles require energy to function, the heart to keep blood circulating to the tissues and our skeletal muscles to maintain posture, balance and mobility. For any activity, whether it has to do with our occupation, movement, domestic activity or leisure, more energy must be supplied. Even when we are asleep, we are using energy. In the early years of life and during pregnancy and lactation, additional energy is required for growth.

This energy has to be provided from the macronutrients in our food, which are broken down into their constituent parts by digestion and metabolized in the tissues. Some of the energy will be used immediately and some will be stored. If more is eaten than is needed, there is a net increase in the body's energy content and the size of the stores increase. Conversely, if the current energy needs are greater than the intake of energy, then some will have to be provided from stored energy. These are the fundamentals of energy balance.

UNITS OF MEASUREMENT OF ENERGY

Two units of measurement are traditionally used in nutrition to quantify energy, reflecting two different products of energy. The calorie is widely used by the public, appears on food labels, underpins most weight control diets and is often preferred by scientists. One calorie raises the temperature of 1 mL of water through 1°C. Measurements of energy in nutrition are in units of 1000 cal or kilocalories (kcal). One kilocalorie is commonly called a Calorie (capital C) in diets and magazines.

The kilojoule (or megajoule for larger amounts of energy) is the SI unit for energy. The joule was originally defined as the amount of energy exerted when a force of 1 N was moved through a distance of 1 m. Like the calorie, it is a small unit (1 cal = 4.18 J) and so normally appears as the kilojoule (1 kJ = 1000 J) or the megajoule (1 MJ = 1000 kJ) in nutrition.

The rate of energy supply or energy utilization (or metabolic rate) is measured as energy per unit time. A typical man might have a 24 hour energy expenditure or 24 hour metabolic rate of 11 MJ (or 2600 kcal) per day, which is about 100 J/s or 100 W.

ENERGY INTAKE

Energy intake is the study of both the quantity of food eaten by an individual, as well as its energy content.

See Chapter 9 for more on the physiological regulation of food intake, pp. 186–190.

Energy Content of Foods

Different foods provide different amounts of energy for a given weight or serving size. This is determined by their content of the 'macronutrients', carbohydrate, fat, protein and alcohol which contribute to its energy content. After eating, digestion and absorption, it is the products of these macronutrients which release energy when they are finally metabolized to CO_2 and water. Some of this energy is wasted as heat, but most is trapped chemically, for use in the cells of the body. The micronutrients, vitamins, minerals and water do not contribute directly to energy supply, but some are necessary for its release and use.

In order to study energy intake, nutritionists need to know the energy content of foods that may be eaten, digested, absorbed and then oxidized in the body. Various methods have been developed to obtain these values.

Bomb Calorimeter

In a laboratory, the amount of energy contained in a food is determined with a bomb calorimeter (Figure 16.1). This is a steel vessel with a tight-fitting stopper. It is filled with oxygen under pressure, and a weighed amount of the food is placed into the crucible within. The whole apparatus is sunk in a water bath of known volume and temperature. The food is ignited electrically and burns explosively as the energy held in the chemical bonds is released in the form of heat. The heat of combustion is measured from the rise in water temperature.

An alternative measurement is to determine the amount of oxygen used during the combustion of a food to carbon dioxide and water.

For pure macronutrients, a bomb calorimeter will typically reveal the following figures:

	kJ/g	cal/g
Starch	17.2	4.1
Glucose	15.5	3.6
Fat	39.2	9.37
Protein (egg)	23.4	5.58

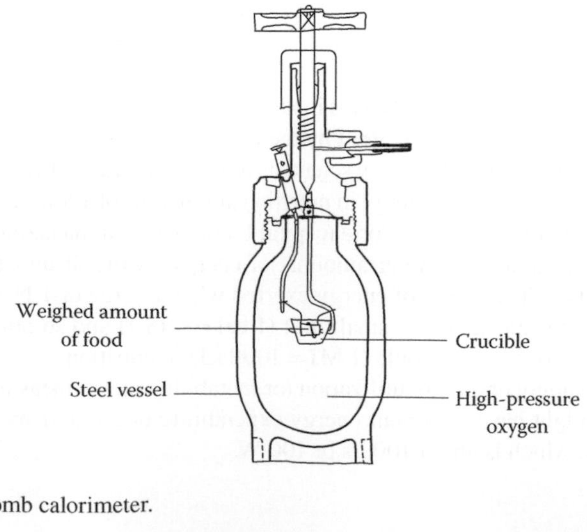

FIGURE 16.1 The bomb calorimeter.

These figures represent the gross energy of the isolated macronutrient, which is greater than the true quantity of energy obtained by the cells of the body for a number of reasons. Small amounts of the potential energy are lost during the processes of digestion and absorption, which are not 100% efficient, even in health. In illness, the losses may be substantially greater owing to vomiting, diarrhoea and inefficient digestion and absorption.

Bomb calorimetry of foods may reveal slightly different (lower) energy content than is predicted from a chemical analysis of the macronutrient content, as oxidation may not be complete. However, there is a larger, obligatory, loss of energy available to the body during metabolism and storage. In general, fat (triglyceride) in food is digested, absorbed, reassembled, transported and either directly oxidized or stored, very efficiently, so the theoretical 9.49 kcal/g in dietary fat is reduced to 9 kcal/g of available energy. For carbohydrates and protein, the energy costs of metabolism are greater, so available energy is reduced to about 3.75 kcal/g for carbohydrates and 4.0 kcal/g for protein. Dietary fibre or non-starch polysaccharide only releases energy (as fatty acids) after fermentation by caloric bacteria, at about 2–3 kcal/g.

Estimates suggest that digestion rates in healthy people are as follows:

Carbohydrates	99%
Fats	95%
Protein	93%

Proximate Principles

The amount of energy that the body receives from a food, called the metabolizable energy, can be calculated from values known as 'proximate principles'. These are based on extensive, meticulous experimental work, some of which dates back to the early years of the twentieth century. Such was the accuracy of this work that few changes have had to be made to the values obtained with the more sophisticated techniques now available. The proximate principles provide a value for the amount of energy that is available for metabolism from each macronutrient contained in a food. Thus, after analyzing a food to determine its content of fat, protein, 'available' carbohydrate (starch and sugars) and alcohol, it becomes possible to calculate the amount of energy provided for each 100 g of the food. These are the figures that appear in the food composition tables used in the United Kingdom (Food Standards Agency, 2002b) shown in Table 16.1.

There may be substantial losses of metabolizable energy in illness. For example, in poorly controlled diabetes, energy in the form of glucose is lost in the urine; in nephrotic syndrome, large amounts of protein, another potential source of energy, are excreted. Many gastrointestinal diseases involve a degree of major, clinically obvious malabsorption, with pale, floating stools and undigested food present. This usually indicates more than about 10 g of fat malabsorption per meal. Lesser degrees of malabsorption, below 10 g of fat per meal, can be completely asymptomatic.

TABLE 16.1
Energy Conversion Factors Used in Food Composition Tables

	kJ/g	kcal/g
Protein	17	4
Fat	37	9
Carbohydrate (available monosaccharide)	16	3.75
Alcohol	29	7

TABLE 16.2
Percentage of Energy from Carbohydrate, Protein and Fat in Selected Foods

Food	Total Energy Content of 100 g Serving (kJ)	Energy (%) from Protein	Fat	Carbohydrate
Wholemeal bread	922	17	10	73
Cornflakes	1601	8	2	90
Boiled rice	587	8	8	84
Milk, semi-skimmed	195	30	32	38
Cheese, cheddar type	1725	25	75	0
Butter/margarine	3042	1	99	0
Low-fat spread	1519	7	91	2
Egg, boiled	612	35	65	0
Beef stew	570	45	42	13
Chicken, roast	742	63	37	0
Baked beans	355	25	6	69
Peanuts	2491	17	79	5
Peas	291	35	11	54
Potatoes, boiled	306	10	1	89
Chocolate	2177	6	52	42

Sources: Data calculated from Food Standards Agency, *Food Portion Sizes*, 3rd edn., The Stationery Office, London, UK, 2002a; Food Standards Agency, *McCance and Widdowson's The Composition of Foods*, 6th summary edn., Royal Society of Chemistry, Cambridge, UK, 2002b.

This may be difficult to identify as a cause of weight loss. After an acute attack of gastroenteritis, there is often a transient loss of the normal digestive enzymes from the gut, which results in a transient intolerance to certain foods. There is often a loss of lactase, resulting in transient post-infective lactose intolerance. To some degree, the absorption capacity of the gastrointestinal tract reflects current diet. A sudden increase, for example, in milk or vegetables, may lead to transient malabsorption until the digestive capacity has had time to adapt.

Knowledge of the macronutrient content of foods in the diet allows us to calculate the amount of energy the body will derive assuring normal digestion, absorption and metabolism. Most such analyses ignore the contribution of dietary fibre so can underestimate total energy consumption. Using this approach, it is also possible to find out what proportion of the total energy intake has been provided by the individual macronutrients. Dietary guidelines are generally formulated in these terms. Data for selected foods are shown in Table 16.2.

Most foods do not contain the ideal proportions of the macronutrients as given in dietary guidelines. It is the combination of different foods within a complete diet that determines whether the balance of the diet is right. For this reason, it is misleading to speak of 'bad' foods and 'good' foods in terms of the proportions of energy they supply from the macronutrients. All foods can be useful, when combined with others in a mixed diet. However, if a diet contains too many foods that all have a similar pattern of energy provision, perhaps containing high percentages of energy from fat, then the total diet risks being too high in fat. It is, therefore, only an overdependence on particular types of food, resulting in a diet which is a long way from that suggested by dietary guidelines that might be termed 'a bad diet'. It should be remembered, however, that even such a diet can be redeemed by including foods that redress the balance of macronutrients.

Dietary Assessment

The research methodology associated with dietary assessment is described in detail in Chapter 18, pp. 343–358.

Information about the energy content of foods can be applied in a practical way to assess energy intakes of groups of the population. Usually, this is performed using survey techniques. Many such studies have been undertaken, using the methodologies described in Chapter 18. However, it is very difficult to obtain accurate information about what people actually eat. In recent years, it has become clear that, in most surveys of food intake, the subjects have under-reported their consumption levels. The UK National Diet and Nutrition Survey (NDNS) report in 2014 provided combined results for years 2008/2009–2011/2012 and revealed that the average daily energy intake per person was 8.8 MJ (2111 kcal) for men and 6.78 MJ (1613 kcal) for women (including household food, food eaten out and alcohol). This is clearly still well below the true average, around 80% and 76% of the estimated average requirement (EAR) for men and women, respectively. However, these figures are still used to estimate proportional macronutrient intakes. The percentages of the reported total energy supplied by the different macronutrients (excluding alcohol) were as follows:

Carbohydrates	48.0%
Protein	17.4%
Fats	34.6%
Saturated fats	12.6%

This clearly provides insufficient energy for any significant amount of activity as part of daily life and is unlikely to be the true picture. In the light of evidence on the prevalence of overweight and obesity in the population, it was concluded that these values must be an underestimate of the true intakes. Large dietary surveys usually reveal huge ranges in reported energy intakes. To some extent, these may reflect day-to-day variation in true intake, but there is also substantial intentional misreporting, so about one-third of normal people intentionally under-report and one-third intentionally over-report what they actually eat.

This pattern of reported macronutrient intake is remarkably consistent, but we do not know which foods or nutrients are under-reported. The proportion of protein has risen over the years, and fat has fallen slightly.

Contribution from Food Groups

It is also possible to obtain information from the NDNS on how the major food groups contribute to our overall energy intake. The latest survey data reveal that the average total energy intakes for adults from the main food groups are as follows:

Cereals and cereal products (including bread and breakfast cereals)	31%
Meat and meat products	17%
Fruit and vegetables (including potatoes)	14%
Milk, dairy and cheese (including eggs)	11%
Soft drinks, sugar and confectionary	9%
Alcoholic drinks	6%
Fish and fish dishes	3%
Fat spreads	3%

TABLE 16.3
Revised Population Estimated Average Requirements Values for Energy

	Men			Women		
		EAR			EAR	
Age Range (Years)	Height (cm)	MJ/Day	(kcal/Day)	Height (cm)	MJ/Day	(kcal/Day)
19–24	178	11.6	(2772)	163	9.1	(2175)
25–34	178	11.5	(2749)	163	9.1	(2175)
35–44	176	11.0	(2629)	163	8.8	(2103)
45–54	175	10.8	(2581)	162	8.8	(2103)
55–64	174	10.8	(2581)	161	8.7	(2079)
65–74	173	9.8	(2342)	159	8.0	(1912)
75+	170	9.6	(2294)	155	7.7	(1840)
All adults (as an average for a group)	175	10.9	(2605)	162	8.7	(2079)

Source: Reproduced from Scientific Advisory Committee on Nutrition (SACN), *Dietary Reference Values for Energy*, HMSO, London, UK, 2011. With permission.

Careful inspection of these average figures shows that the majority (almost 80%) of the energy in the UK diet is actually obtained from staple foods such as bread, cereals, pasta, potatoes, meat, fish, dairy products, fruit and vegetables. Nearly 10% of energy is provided by foods that contain only simple carbohydrate (sugars), such as sugar, soft drinks and confectionery. Often referred to as 'empty energy', these energy sources provide no other nutritional value. Thus, most energy in the diet is accompanied by micronutrients; however, the ranges are wide, so many people and possibly particular population subgroups have poor macronutrient balances. In 2011, the population average requirements for energy were revised, as presented in Table 16.3.

ENERGY OUTPUT

The components of energy output or expenditure have been studied extensively and will be considered in turn (see Figure 16.2). They are the following:

- BMR
- Thermogenesis (related to food intake)
- Physical activity

Basal Metabolic Rate

The single largest component of a person's daily energy output is the BMR. In a sedentary individual, it represents 65%–70% of total 24 hour energy expenditure. BMR is the total of the minimal activity of all the cells of the body under steady state resting conditions. BMR is measured when no digestion or absorption of food is taking place (at least 12 hours after eating) and in a subject who is in a state of physical and mental relaxation. At other times, a resting metabolic rate (RMR) will be somewhat higher than the BMR.

Most of the BMR is expended in driving the osmotic pumps that maintain the differences between extracellular and intracellular fluids and for the synthesis of proteins and other macromolecules. Only about 10% of BMR is used in internal mechanical work, for the functioning of the heart, respiratory system and digestive tract.

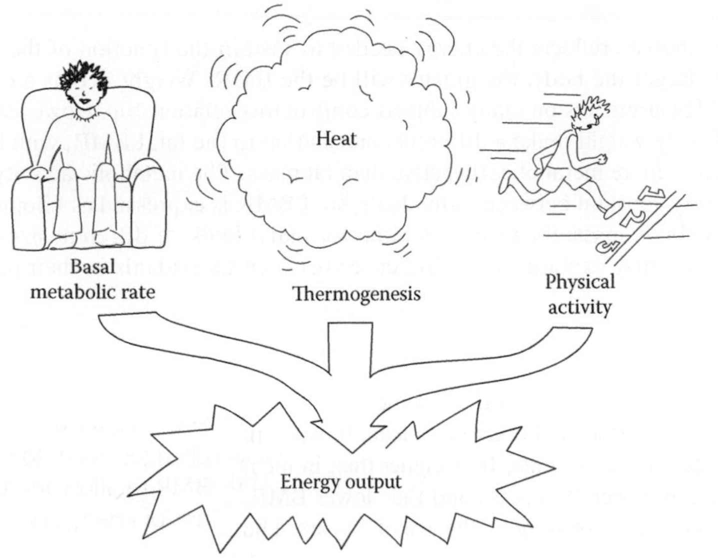

FIGURE 16.2 The components of energy output.

BMR values are quoted as kcal or kilojoules per hour. As a general rule, the BMR for men averages 4.2 kJ (1.0 kcal) per minute and for women 3.75 kJ (0.9 kcal) per minute. Metabolism in subjects during deep sleep (called minimal metabolic rate) may be 5–10% lower than BMR. Metabolic rate may be expressed per kg body weight.

Various factors, both external and internal, can affect the BMR of an individual, and these are now considered (Figure 16.3).

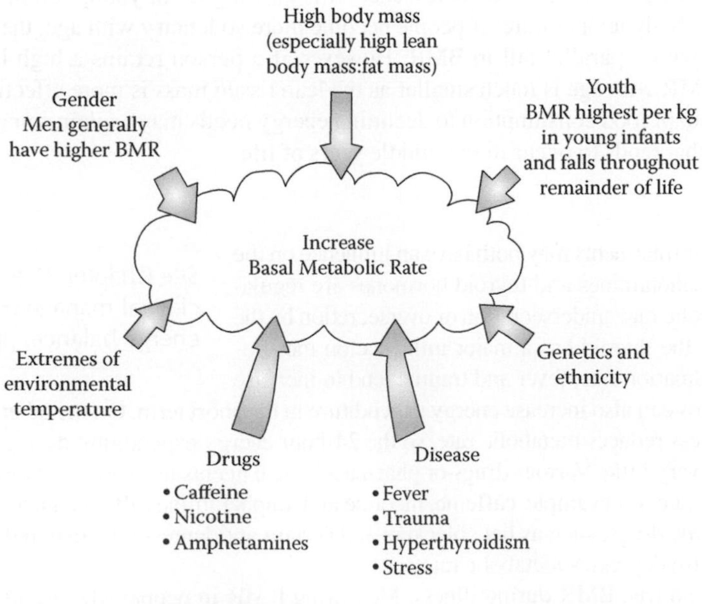

FIGURE 16.3 Factors affecting basal metabolic rate.

Influence of Body Weight

Since basal metabolism reflects the energy needed to sustain the function of the body tissues, it is clear that the larger the body, the greater will be the BMR. Weight is thus a critical determinant of BMR. Measurements on many subjects confirm this relationship. However, the two major components of body weight make a different contribution to the total BMR, with lean body mass being considerably more metabolically active than fat mass. The metabolic activity of lean tissue, at rest, is relatively constant between individuals, so if BMR is expressed as kilojoules or kcal per kilogram of lean body mass, the result is similar for individuals, of different sizes. Subtle differences in this figure may explain some differences between individuals in their predisposition to weight gain.

Influence of Gender

The BMR for women is lower than that for men because of differences in the proportions of body fat to lean. In women, the body fat content is, on average, 10% higher than in men, with a consequently lower lean mass and thus lower BMR. This gender difference is apparent by the age of 2 years. The BMR per kg lean mass is similar for men and women. A further aspect is the energy demand made on the mother's body during pregnancy and lactation to support the growth of the fetus.

See Chapter 6 for more on changes occur to the maternal BMR to allow for a more efficient use of energy, pp. 104–106.

Influence of Age

Children have relatively less body fat than adults, and their lean tissues are more metabolically active. The BMR is lower, in absolute terms, in young children than in adults, but when expressed per kg, it is highest in young infants and falls throughout the remainder of the life cycle. The decline is relatively slow in children and adolescents; in particular, once adulthood has been reached, there is a gradual progressive decline of approximately 2% per decade after the age of 30 years. This is related to the amounts of metabolically active tissue present at different ages, as well as the rapid rates of growth in early infancy and adolescence. It is also higher in young infants because of the need to maintain body temperature. If people become more sedentary with age, the amount of lean tissue declines, with a parallel fall in BMR. However, if a person retains a high level of activity, the decline in BMR with age is much smaller as the lean tissue mass is more effectively preserved.

A failure to adapt food consumption to declining energy needs may explain some of the increase in body weight that tends to occur in the middle years of life.

Influence of Disease Status

Diseases and their treatments may both have an influence on the BMR. Since catecholamines and thyroid hormones are regulators of the metabolic rate, undersecretion or oversecretion by the adrenal gland or the thyroid has a major influence on metabolism. Any inflammation sate, fever and trauma tend to increase metabolism. Stress can also increase energy expenditure in the short term. On the other hand, inactivity during acute illness reduces metabolic rate, so the 24-hour energy expenditure during illness may end up being altered very little. Various drugs or pharmacological agents have an effect on metabolism and may increase the rate, for example, caffeine, nicotine and amphetamines all potentiate the action of catecholamines. Some drugs, such as beta blockers and certain antidepressants, may reduce metabolism. Undernutrition also depresses metabolic rate.

See Chapter 21 for more on the clinical management of negative energy balance, pp. 400–402.

There can be no true BMR during illness. Measuring RMR in people who are ill may help guide energy needs at different stages of the disease. Anxiety, blood transfusions, effect of pre-test treatments or feeding regimes all influence the RMR. In translating the RMR result into a total energy expenditure, it should also be remembered that a bedridden patient will have a much lower level of physical activity, so that energy requirements overall may be less than in health, even if RMR is elevated.

Thermogenesis

As mammals, humans are warm-blooded; our bodies need to generate heat to maintain the constant body temperature at which our tissues function optimally. This is known as thermoregulatory thermogenesis, and the energy expenditure required is a variable component of our energy balance. Mostly, we exist well fed and in environments at a comfortable or thermoneutral temperature, and we adjust our clothing so that little extra energy is used to keep warm. Eating affects energy expenditure because the body uses energy in eating, digesting and absorbing the food, transporting the nutrients and incorporating them into the cells. It represents the inefficiency of the body's processing of its food intake. This is usually called the 'thermic effect' of food or 'diet-induced thermogenesis'. In the past, this was known as 'specific dynamic action' and thought to derive specifically from proteins. All the macronutrients of the diet contribute to this heat production, although fats contribute very little and proteins and carbohydrates the most. Total diet-induced thermogenesis accounts for about 10% of the total energy eaten in a meal. Thus, if a meal containing 3 MJ (750 cal) is eaten, the amount of energy available to the body for metabolic use will be 10% less than this. Diet-induced thermogenesis contributes usefully to thermoregulation of thin people and in cold conditions, but may cause a problem with heat dissipation for obese people or in hot conditions, when sweating after a meal is a frequent consequence.

Thermogenesis also occurs as a result of cold exposure, hormonal states or drug intake.

Physical Activity

This is the aspect of our total energy expenditure over which we have most control. We can choose to undertake a range of different activities during the course of a typical day, walking to work or school, taking part in sports and having hobbies that involve movement. On the other hand, we can drive or take the bus to work, we can sit during our break and lunch hours, and, on returning home, we can spend the evening in front of the television. Clearly, such contrasting lifestyles are associated with different levels of energy expenditure.

It has been shown by careful measurements that the amount of energy expended in activity is related to the size of the body being moved and, consequently, to the BMR. Therefore, two individuals, both weighing 60 kg, will expend a similar amount of energy performing the same task. In contrast, a person weighing 100 kg will use twice as much energy in a given task as a 50 kg person. This is an important finding, as previous calculations of energy expended in activities made no reference to the size of the person performing them. Many figures have been derived that quantify the average amount of energy used, as a function of the BMR, for specific activities, known as physical activity ratios (PARs) or metabolic equivalents (METs). By expressing the energy cost of an activity in terms of the BMR, a single PAR or MET value for each activity can then be applied to all individuals, regardless of age, size or gender, since these will already have been taken into account in the calculation of the BMR itself.

See Chapter 22 for an introduction to sport nutrition and energy needs in sport, pp. 421–430.

In deriving PARs, some assumptions have to be made. A certain amount of activity is common to most people; this includes the general 'personal maintenance' activity associated with washing, dressing, preparing and eating food and generally moving about from room to room in the home environment. It is assumed that this makes similar demands on the body for all individuals, and a factor of 1.4 is attributed to it. Sleeping has a PAR of 1.0 as there is no increment above BMR. Various occupational activities may also be grouped together, based on the usual and average

TABLE 16.4

Physical Activity Ratios for Calculation of Energy Expenditure

Activity	PAR
Lying at rest/sleeping	1.0
Quiet sitting activities (e.g. reading, TV)	1.2 (range 1.0–1.4)
Active sitting activities (e.g. driving, playing piano)	1.6 (range 1.5–1.8)
Stationary standing activities (e.g. ironing, laboratory work, washing-up)	1.6 (range 1.5–1.8)
General mixed standing/sitting (e.g. personal activities, washing, dressing, eating)	1.4
Activities involving moving about (e.g. cleaning, tidying, cooking, bowling)	2.1 (range 1.9–2.4)
Walking, average speed, making beds	2.8 (range 2.5–3.3)
Gardening, playing table tennis	3.7 (range 3.4–4.4)
Walking quickly, dancing, swimming	4.8 (range 4.5–5.9)
Jogging, football, tennis	6.0

Source: Reproduced from DoH (UK Department of Health), Dietary reference values for food energy and nutrients for the United Kingdom, Report on Health and Social Subjects No. 41, Report of the Panel on Dietary Reference Values of the Committee on Medical Aspects of Food Policy, HMSO, London, UK, 1991. With permission.

amount of physical activity involved. It must be recognized that average figures can never exactly indicate the energy expenditure of an individual; PAR/MET values make no judgement about the intensity with which the work is carried out and, if it continues for a period of time, whether intensity varies. Some examples are shown in Table 16.4.

Measurement of Energy Output

The body converts the energy of food into ATP with an efficiency of approximately 50%, with the remaining energy being employed or lost (depending on ambient temperature, clothing activity, etc.) as heat. When the ATP itself is used by the body to do work, a further loss of heat occurs, equal to approximately 50% of the energy in the ATP. Finally, the work itself generates heat. Thus, a body's total heat production gives a measure of the amount of energy that has been used.

Because of this, it is possible to use calorimetry or the measurement of heat production, to quantify the amount of energy expenditure. If heat is measured directly, the technique is known as direct calorimetry. However, an indirect approach is usually used, based on the utilization of oxygen in respiration. The rate of oxygen consumption is proportional to the amount of ATP synthesis, and each mole of ATP synthesized is accompanied by production of a given amount of heat.

It is possible to see from the chemical equations for the oxidation of carbohydrates and fats how much oxygen is used and how much carbon dioxide is produced:

Glucose oxidation

$$C_6H_{12}O_6 + 6O_2 \rightarrow 6H_2O + 6CO_2 + 15.5 \text{ kJ/g of energy}$$

Starch oxidation

$$(C_6H_{10}O_5)_n + 6nO_2 \rightarrow 5nH_2O + 6nCO_2 + 17 \text{ kJ/g of energy}$$

Fat oxidation

For example, glyceryl butyro-oleostearate (the main fat in butter)

$$C_3H_5O_3 \cdot C_4H_7O \cdot C_{18}H_{33}O \cdot C_{18}H_{35}O + 60O_2 \rightarrow 43CO_2 + 40H_2O + 39 \text{ kJ/g of energy}$$

TABLE 16.5
Energy Yields Obtained from the Oxidation of Different Substrates

Nutrient	Oxygen Consumed (L/g)	Carbon Dioxide Produced (L/g)	Respiratory Quotient	Energy Equivalent (kJ/kcal/L of Oxygen)
Starch	0.829	0.829	1.0	21.2/5.06
Glucose	0.746	0.746	1.0	21.0/5.01
Fat	2.019	1.427	0.71	19.6/4.69
Protein	0.962	0.775	0.81	19.25/4.66

It can be seen that, for carbohydrate oxidation, the volume of carbon dioxide produced equals the volume of oxygen used. When fat is oxidized, however, the volume of carbon dioxide produced is about 70% of the volume of oxygen consumed. These values are usually expressed as a fraction: CO_2 produced/O_2 consumed, known as the respiratory quotient (RQ). The RQ for carbohydrates is 1.0 and for fats averages 0.71 (different fats have slightly different values). Most amino acids in proteins are oxidized like carbohydrates, but some like fats, so an average RQ figure is usually assumed for protein, intermediate between fats and carbohydrates at 0.83.

The RQ value can in principle be used to discover the amount of energy production for each litre of oxygen consumed, since this is also predictable from the equation. The body always uses a mixture of substrates for its metabolism, and the metabolic mixture being used which varies through the day, with feeding and with exercise, can be determined from a measurement of RQ. Thus, a value close to 0.7 suggests that mainly fats are being metabolized; conversely, a value close to 1.0 would indicate carbohydrate-fuelled metabolism. In practice, the usual metabolic mixture provides an RQ of around 0.8. These figures only apply during a state of 'energy balance'. If there is excess energy supply at the time of measurement, there will be some fat synthesis from carbohydrate, and the measured RQ can then exceed 1.0.

In summary, if one can determine oxygen usage and/or carbon dioxide production, it is possible to calculate the amount of energy released during metabolism. With information about both oxygen and carbon dioxide, it is possible to derive the actual RQ that applies. However, if only one of the gases has been measured, an RQ of 0.8 is usually assumed (as this represents the average metabolic mixture). It is estimated that not adjusting for the actual RQ across the range of commonly consumed diets probably introduces an error of 3%–4%, which is generally acceptable for most purposes.

Tables 16.5 and 16.6 provide the RQ and oxygen utilization values used in these measurements.

TABLE 16.6
Effect on Energy Yield of Different Metabolic Mixtures and Respiratory Quotient

		Energy (%) Derived from	
RQ	kJ/L of Oxygen	Carbohydrate	Fat
0.71	19.6	1	99
0.75	19.8	16	84
0.80	20.1	33	67
0.85	20.3	51	49
0.90	20.6	68	32
0.95	20.8	84	16
1.00	21.1	100	0

Direct Calorimetry

The original human calorimeter was designed by Atwater and Rosa in 1905. This was the size of a small room that contained a bed and stationary exercise bicycle. The walls were well insulated to prevent any heat loss, and all heat dissipated by the subject was transferred to circulating water in the walls of the chamber. Increases in water temperature could be measured, and these represented the subject's heat loss.

In addition, the gases flowing into and out of the chamber could be analyzed, giving additional information about the subject's metabolism. Such calorimeters are still in use today. The major difference lies in the methods by which the heat output is measured in the walls of the chamber; modern calorimeters use microchips and computers for this. There is also a reduction in size, with some modern calorimeters being the size of a phone booth or even smaller.

The major drawback of the human calorimeter (apart from its cost) is that it only allows a limited amount of activity and is thus not usable for 'real-life' measurements.

If the calorimeter is large, the length of time taken for any changes in heat to be measurable is longer. At a minimum, a calorimeter of 1.6 m^3 provides a response in 3 minutes; one with a size of 20 m^3 takes 2 hours to show a response. The accuracy of measurements with a direct calorimeter is of the order of 1–2%. It is not more accurate than indirect calorimetry.

Indirect Methods

Respiratory Gas Analysis

The principle of indirect calorimetry is based on the relationship between oxygen use and carbon dioxide production, described earlier. To apply this, the method used must be able to measure either or possibly both of the gases over a period of time. Equipment used for this purpose ranges from the large and stationary to more portable versions. Obviously, stationary equipment can only be used when subjects are resting; more mobile activities require portable equipment.

Originally, the respiration chamber itself was used, with the gases inspired and expired by the subject sampled and analyzed. More recently, a hood or small plastic tent is placed over the recumbent subject to collect the gases, which these days pass straight into automated analyzers linked to computers, providing instant data. This type of measurement is useful in hospital patients who may be confined to bed. The equipment must be mobile and moved to the bedside.

Mobile equipment has largely been of the backpack variety, worn by the subject during physical activity. The necessary link between the equipment and the subject's respiratory system is by way of a corrugated tube, mouthpiece and nose clip. This is not especially comfortable and can both limit the duration of the measurement and affect the normal pattern of breathing.

Isotope Methods

The doubly labelled water technique, enriched with a known amount of stable (non-radioactive) isotopes of hydrogen and oxygen (^2H and ^{18}O), has been referred to as 'doubly indirect calorimetry'. The subject drinks a small volume of labelled water. The hydrogen equilibrates in the body water pool (producing hydrogen-labelled water), the oxygen in both the water (as oxygen-labelled water) and in the carbon dioxide pools. Thus, the ^{18}O is contained in both the carbon dioxide and water, and the ^2H is contained only in the water; as both CO_2 and H_2O are lost from the body, the labelled oxygen is lost from the body faster than the labelled hydrogen.

The rates of loss of the isotopes are generally measured in a series of samples of body fluid, such as urine, over a period of up to 21 days. The difference between the rates of loss of the two isotopes represents the loss of carbon dioxide and can be used to calculate carbon dioxide and, hence, heat production. In turn, this can be used to derive energy expenditure.

Several assumptions are made with this technique, most notably about isotope fractionation in the body and the rate of water loss. In addition, as oxygen usage is not measured, the RQ has to be estimated. However, if a concurrent food intake record is kept, then the RQ value from the intake can be calculated, assuming there is energy equilibrium. Body weight must be checked at the beginning and end of the measurement period.

This technique provides a useful, safe and non-intrusive way of measuring carbon dioxide turnover and, hence, metabolism over periods of time. As a result, a large amount of information has been derived in recent years about energy expenditure in groups of subjects that previously have been difficult or unethical to study, such as the elderly, pregnant and lactating women, and young infants and children.

Measurements of 24 hour energy expenditure can be made by a relatively novel isotope technique, the bicarbonate–urea method. This technique uses the isotope dilution principle. Labelled CO_2, given subcutaneously as bicarbonate, is diluted by endogenous CO_2; the extent of this dilution is measured by the isotope activity in urinary urea produced over a 24 hour period. This allows the CO_2 produced in the body to be calculated, and energy expenditure found using values for the energy equivalent of CO_2.

Other Methods

A number of other techniques have been used to estimate energy expenditure, including

- Activity diaries
- Heart rate monitoring
- Skeletal muscle recording (electromyography)
- Pedometers (to record movement) or accelerometers
- Radar measurement of fidgeting or minor 'non-exercise activity thermogenesis'

All of these give less reliable results than calorimetry but may be of value when groups of subjects are being studied, to provide data on specific components of energy expenditure.

Some of the methods listed earlier can provide estimates of the intensity of exercise or patterns of activity during a period of exercise that may provide useful additional information. Activity diaries are prone to some omissions, especially of small habitual movements, but more importantly systematically over-report structured or intense activity and over-report total physical activity when compared to measurements with accelerometers.

CALCULATION OF ENERGY EXPENDITURE

In order to calculate total energy expenditure, it is necessary to obtain a figure for the BMR. Various equations, such as the du Bois and Harris–Benedict equations, have been derived and are based on experimental measurements of BMR in subjects. Most widely used at present are those derived by Schofield, based on measurements made on more than 10,000 subjects, and derived as regression equations from the plots of results. These, together with some more recent data on elderly subjects, are used in the dietary reference values report (DoH, 1991) and were the basis of the FAO/WHO/UNU (1985) recommendations on energy intake, which have not been superseded. It is important to recognize that these published equations have variability when applied to individuals, commonly ±10% of the true (measured) figure. They were not derived for sick malnourished people or for obese. There were very limited data for the elderly or for racial and ethnic variations and should therefore be used with great caution when applied to these groups.

The equations for adults are given in the following (DoH, 1991):

	BMR	
	MJ/Day	cal/Day
Males		
18–29	0.063 W + 2.896	15.1 W + 692
30–59	0.048 W + 3.653	11.5 W + 873
60–74	0.0499 W + 2.930	11.9 W + 700
Females		
18–29	0.062 W + 2.036	14.8 W + 487
30–59	0.034 W + 3.538	8.3 W + 846
60–74	0.0386 W + 2.875	9.2 W + 687

W, body weight (kg).

Calculation of 24-Hour Energy Expenditure: An Example

Bill is a 40-year-old advertising executive. He is a keen 5-a-side football player and weighs 70 kg. His BMR is calculated as follows: (0.048 × 70) + 3.653 = 7.01 MJ/day. Therefore, his hourly BMR 7.01/24 = 292 kJ/hour.

He recorded his daily activity pattern as shown in the following. Energy expenditure is, therefore, calculated as follows, with the appropriate PAR values and using his hourly BMR:

	Duration (Hours)	×	PAR/MET	×	BMR/Hour	=	Energy Used (kJ)
Sleeping	7		1.0		292		2044
Driving	2		1.6		292		934
Personal activities	3		1.4		292		1226
Watching TV	3		1.2		292		1050
Playing football	1		6.0		292		1752
Sitting at work	8		1.2		292		2803
Total							**9809 = 9.8 MJ**

Thus, Bill expended 9.8 MJ in the course of this day.

In comparison with his BMR, which is 7.01 MJ, it is possible to calculate his physical activity level (PAL) throughout the day. This represents the amount of extra energy that he expended, above his BMR, and is calculated as energy expenditure/BMR, that is, 9.8/7.01 = 1.4. This means that, over the day, he used 40% more energy than that simply needed for his BMR – PAR = 1.4.

Because Bill played football, he might consider himself physically active – or even fit; this is in fact a very average figure for a relatively sedentary population, typical of the United Kingdom. Moreover, it is likely that Bill did not play football every day. PAR 1.4 forms the basis for the EARs for energy, summarized in Table 16.4.

SUMMARY

1. Energy intake is the metabolizable energy of foods, generally calculated from the proximate principles. Dietary surveys tend to underestimate energy intakes.
2. Energy output comprises BMR, thermogenesis and physical activity.
3. BMR is influenced by a number of factors, including age, gender and body weight.
4. Energy expenditure in activity is related to the BMR and can be calculated by the use of factors known as PARs. The overall daily energy expenditure can be compared with the BMR in the form of the PAL.

STUDY QUESTIONS

1. Distinguish between and account for any differences in the yield of energy from a food when
   a. It is combusted (burned) in a bomb calorimeter
   b. Its constituents become available for use at cellular level in the body
2. Would a diet with a low fat content (e.g. 15% of energy from fat) be appropriate for
   a. Healthy child with an average (not large) appetite
   b. An elderly, housebound person

   Explain your viewpoint.
3. Including the energy from alcohol in calculating the contribution from each macronutrient to the total energy intake can make important differences to the results. Comment on the following cases:
   a. *Harry*: total energy intake = 12.8 MJ
      Fat 33%, protein 15%, carbohydrate 40%, alcohol 12%
   b. *Alex*: total energy intake = 10.6 MJ
      Fat 40%, protein 12%, carbohydrate 48%
   c. *Sam*: total energy intake = 15 MJ
      Fat 28%, protein 13%, carbohydrate 34%, alcohol 25%
4. In the example calculation of energy expenditure (Bill) earlier, answer the following:
   a. What is Bill's BMR per kg lean mass (approximately)?
   b. If Bill got a dog and walked it for 1 hour instead of watching TV, how would this affect his energy expenditure?
5. Critically discuss the principles of indirect calorimetry, including the use of different assumptions and its application for measurement of RMR and total energy expenditure.

ACTIVITIES

16.1 Susan has a diet that provides her with a total of 8.8 MJ (2100 cal) per day but wishes to know if it contains the appropriate proportions of the macronutrients in line with dietary guidelines. On analysis, the nutritionist finds that the diet contains the following:

Carbohydrate	200 g
Protein	95 g
Fat	100 g
Alcohol	10 g

The energy obtained from these macronutrients can, therefore, be calculated and expressed as a percentage of the total amount of energy in the diet.

Carbohydrate: 200 × 16 = 3.2 MJ. Therefore, % of total is 3.2/8.8 × 100 = 36%.
Protein: 95 × 17 = 1.6 MJ. The % of total is 1.6/8.8 × 100 = 18%.
Fat: 100 × 37 = 3.7 MJ. The % of total is 3.7/8.8 × 100 = 42%.
Alcohol: 10 × 29 = 0.29 MJ. The % of total is 0.29 /8.8 × 100 = 3%.
Check these figures against the dietary guidelines (Chapter 3), and draw some conclusions about Susan's intake.

16.2 Using your own diet record, calculate the percentage of the energy in your diet coming from the different macronutrients.

- How do your figures compare with the dietary guidelines?
- Can you identify particular foods in your diet that are contributing to an especially high/low intake of one of the macronutrient groups?

Compare your results with those of other students; if possible, produce a table of results for a whole group.

- How similar are the results?
- Which macronutrient is the most variable?
- What difference does including alcohol in the total energy intake make to the individual macronutrient percentages? (Check in the dietary reference values report (DoH, 1991) to see how the guidelines vary when alcohol is included or excluded.)

16.3 Keep a record of your own activities for two periods of 24 hours. They need not be consecutive but should represent differing levels of your own activity. Find your body weight and use this to calculate your BMR. Then construct a chart similar to the worked example earlier, to allow you to calculate your total energy expenditure over the 2 days. Work out the ratio of your total energy expenditure with respect to your BMR: this is your physical activity level.

- Is there anything that surprises you about the results for the 2 days you have chosen – for example, is the difference between them more or less than you expected?
- Which component of your daily activity has made the largest contribution to the total – is it your BMR or a particular activity?
- If you had a period of strenuous exercise, what proportion of the total did this constitute? Is this more or less than you expected? For what period of time would you need to continue this level of exercise for it to equal half of your BMR expenditure?
- Did you have different periods of sleep during the two recorded days? Did this make a difference to your output?
- Compare your results with those of others. What differences can you find? Can you account for them?

16.4 Three friends have undertaken a study of their activity. They are all male, aged 25 years, with body weights of 60 kg (Tom), 70 kg (Sam) and 80 kg (Harry). The results of their activity diaries are given in the following:

Tom		**Sam**		**Harry**	
Activity	**Duration (Hours)**	**Activity**	**Duration (Hours)**	**Activity**	**Duration (Hours)**
Work: sedentary	8	*Work*: mixed standing/sitting	8	*Work*: mainly moving about	8
Other		*Other*		*Other*	
Personal activities	3	Personal activities	2	Personal activities	2
Watching TV	4	Watching TV	1	Watching TV	2
Drive to work	1	Walk to work	1	Drive to work	1
		Walking dog (brisk)	1	Football	1
		Gardening	2	Swimming	1
		Tidying house	1	Playing computer games	1
Sleeping	8	Sleeping	8	Sleeping	8
Total hours	24		24		24

Calculate each man's daily energy expenditure, and express the answer as the physical activity level, to allow comparisons to be made between them.

- What similarities and differences are there?
- What impact do their various leisure activities have on the total expenditure?
- How important is the level of work activity?
- What conclusions can you draw about the optimal way of increasing daily energy output?

BIBLIOGRAPHY AND FURTHER READING

Bates, B., Lennox, A. and Prentice, A. 2012. *National Diet and Nutrition Survey. Headline Results from Year 1, Year 2 and Year 3 (Combined) of the Rolling Programme (2008/2009–2010/2011).* London, UK: Food Standards Agency/Department of Health.

DEFRA. 2001. National food survey, 2000. Annual report on food expenditure, consumption and nutrient intakes. London, UK: The Stationery Office.

DoH (Public Health England). 2014. *National Diet and Nutrition Survey: Results from Years 1–4 (Combined) of the Rolling Programme (2008/09–2011/12).* London, UK: PHE.

DoH (UK Department of Health). 1991. Dietary reference values for food energy and nutrients for the United Kingdom. Report on Health and Social Subjects No. 41. Report of the Panel on Dietary Reference Values of the Committee on Medical Aspects of Food Policy. London, UK: HMSO.

Dugas, L.R., Harders, R., Merrill, S., Ebersole, K., Shoham, D.A., Rush, E.C., Assah, F.K., Forrester, T., Durazo-Arvizu, R.A. and Luke, A. 2010. Energy expenditure in adults living in developing compared with industrialized countries: A meta-analysis of doubly labeled water studies. *The American Journal of Clinical Nutrition* 93(2), 427–441.

FAO/WHO/UNU. 1985. Energy and protein requirements. Report of a joint FAO/WHO/UNU Expert Consultation. WHO technical report no. 724. Geneva, Switzerland: WHO.

Food Standards Agency. 2002a. *Food Portion Sizes*, 3rd edn. London, UK: The Stationery Office.

Food Standards Agency. 2002b. *McCance and Widdowson's The Composition of Foods*, 6th summary edn. Cambridge, UK: Royal Society of Chemistry.

Halsey, L.G., Shepard, E.L.C. and Wilson, R.P. 2011. Assessing the development and application of the accelerometry technique for estimating energy expenditure. *Comparative Biochemistry and Physiology Part A: Molecular & Integrative Physiology* 158(3), 305–314.

Institute of European Food Studies. 1999. A Pan-EU survey on consumer attitudes to physical activity, body weight and health. Dublin, UK: IEFS.

Millward, D.J. 2013. The use of protein: Energy ratios for defining protein requirements, allowances and dietary protein contents. *Public Health Nutrition* 16(5), 763–768.

Murgatroyd, P.R., Shetty, P.S. and Prentice, A.M. 1993. Techniques for the measurement of human energy expenditure. *International Journal of Obesity* 17(10), 549–568.

Schofield, W.M., Schofield, C. and James, W.P.T. 1985. Human nutrition. *Clinical Nutrition* 39C(Suppl.), 1–96.

Scientific Advisory Committee on Nutrition (SACN). 2011. *Dietary Reference Values for Energy.* London, UK: HMSO.

Square, T. and Lane, B. 2013. *Health Survey for England – 2013.* Office of Population Censuses and Surveys. London, UK: HMSO.

Tetens, I. 2013. *EFSA Panel on Dietetic Products, Nutrition and Allergies (NDA); Scientific Opinion on Dietary Reference Values for Energy.* Parma, Italy: European Food Safety Authority.

Watson, L.P.E., Raymond-Barker, P., Moran, C., Schoenmakers, N., Mitchell, C., Bluck, L., Chatterjee, V.K., Savage, D. B. and P.R. Murgatroyd. 2014. An approach to quantifying abnormalities in energy expenditure and lean mass in metabolic disease. *European Journal of Clinical Nutrition* 68(2), 234–240.

17 Energy Balance

AIMS

The aims of this chapter are to

- Present the components of energy balance: energy intake and energy output.
- Consider the factors influencing energy intake and output.
- Review the adaptation and control mechanisms relevant to energy balance.
- Consider the consequence of energy imbalance.

ENERGY BALANCE

Many people maintain their bodies in a state of energy balance within quite narrow limits, as evidenced by a constant body weight over a prolonged period of time. However, everyone has days, even weeks, of substantial energy imbalance. Over time, short periods of energy excess are balanced by energy deficit. This compensation is difficult to detect and occurs subconsciously. When there is energy imbalance sufficient to cause weight gain or loss, this is usually a very small imbalance, of the order of 1%–2% over a long period of time. Again this usually goes unnoticed, and the mismatch is too small to be measured.

Energy intake derives from the food we eat and is regulated by a number of different factors, including physiological (such as hunger), psychological (appetite or mood), social and environmental factors, all of which interact in complex ways, and are thus difficult to study and to control. Energy output represents the energy used to maintain physiological and biochemical activities (as BMR), to digest and process the food we eat and to fuel all physical activities. When these two aspects are in equilibrium, energy intake is sufficient to meet the energy output (see Figure 17.1).

$$\text{Energy intake} = \text{energy output (BMR + thermogenesis + physical activity)}$$

Evidence suggests that overall, there is a stability of body weight, and data from a long-term study of the population in Framingham, Massachusetts, shows that, over a period of 18 years, most people were at a body weight within 5 kg of their original weight. This energy imbalance represented less than 0.5% of the total turnover in energy, implying that reasonably efficient regulation was occurring. Subjects whose weight changed the most (up or down) were also the most likely to suffer from disease.

Nevertheless, weight changes do occur. In most countries, statistics shows that overweight and obesity among the adult population are increasing rapidly. Parallel trends of increased weight are also seen in children, often from a very young age. In all of these cases, there is an increase in fat stores. Thus, the energy balance equation has to be rewritten as

$$\text{Energy intake} = \text{energy output} \pm \text{energy stores}$$

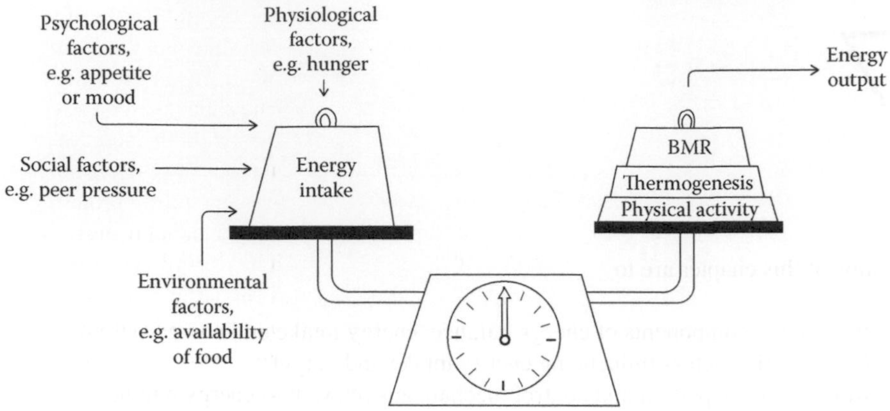

FIGURE 17.1 Components of energy balance.

Influences on Energy Intake

Regulation of food intake will control the input side of the energy balance equation. Food intake may change or be adjusted intentionally in a number of ways such that energy intake levels fluctuate. As well as altering total energy intake, a change in food consumption will affect the nutritional composition of the diet.

See Chapter 9 for more on the physiological regulation of food intake, pp. 186–190.

In some diseases, there may be interference with the process of digestion or absorption as well as changes in food choice. Disease of the digestive tract may prevent normal digestion, so that food is either lost by vomiting or passes undigested through the gut. Malabsorption may also affect the transfer of the digestion products ('nutrients') into the blood. Altered bowel anatomy with fistulae (short-circuits between upper and lower bowel), altered bacterial activity (e.g. small bowel overgrowth) or a reduced absorptive area following partial removal of the bowel will have similar consequences.

Some psychiatric eating disorders result in the deliberate interference with digestion and absorption, either by inducing vomiting after eating, or by using purgatives to prevent the food being absorbed.

Finally, orlistat, a drug used in the management of obesity, inhibits the enzyme responsible for the normal digestion of fat, so that malabsorption occurs and undigested fat is lost in the faeces. This has the effect of reducing the energy available from the food eaten. Another drug, acarbose, used in diabetes treatment blocks the digestion of some starch, which is malabsorbed in the small bowel and enters the colon. There, it is avidly hydrolyzed and metabolized by bacteria, and the side effects of flatulence and diarrhoea limit its acceptability.

Influences on Energy Output

Adaptations to Basal Metabolic Rate

Changes in basal metabolic rate (BMR) are most likely to occur as a result of changes in body weight or body composition. BMR is influenced particularly by lean body mass, so any alteration in this will affect the rate of metabolism. Ageing is accompanied by a reduction in lean body mass, and therefore, there is a gradual fall in BMR. Immobility as a result of illness or ageing will cause a loss of lean tissue and a consequent reduction in metabolic rate.

See Chapter 16 for more on components of energy expenditure, pp. 318–321.

Conversely, training which involves exercising the whole body or specific blocks of muscles will gradually increase the lean muscle mass and can result in an elevation of the metabolic rate. However, this may be compensated for by a loss of adipose tissue resulting in no net weight change and specific measurements of body composition are needed to identify the changes in these components.

An increase in overall body weight is most commonly associated with an increase in body fat. In this case, there is an increase in BMR, because the larger tissue mass requires more energy to sustain it and the associated increase in supporting cellular structures, including protein-containing cell wall material and water. There are also increases in the heart and skeletal muscles, digestive tract and liver to cope with the increased demands put on them. The overall effect on the BMR is smaller as a result of an increase in fat rather than lean tissue, as the latter is more metabolically active. Nevertheless, it is important to remember that a heavier person or obese will always have higher BMR and a greater metabolic cost of physical activity than a smaller, thinner individual. This fact is sometimes overlooked by people that are overweight, who claim that their problem is the result of 'slow metabolism'. Obese people actually have higher BMR and 24EE, so a 'faster' metabolism. They need to increase their energy intake to avoid weight loss.

When weight is lost, there is a reduction in BMR, arising from a fall in the mass of metabolically active tissue. This is one of the problems encountered by dieters. As they lose weight, the smaller body requires less energy to sustain it. The energy deficit becomes smaller as the metabolic rate falls by about 25%, and the rate of weight loss will slow down.

BMR can be drastically reduced after major amputations, if large amounts of muscle are lost. However, the impact on 24-hour energy expenditure may be counterbalanced by a greater energy cost of physical activity using prosthetic limbs. Loss of kidneys, liver (e.g. in cirrhosis) and other organs also reduce BMR. The most metabolically active tissue of all is the brain, and BMR can be significantly reduced by the loss of brain tissue, for example, after a stroke.

Adaptations to Thermogenesis

This comprises the thermic effect of food as well as possible 'adaptive thermogenesis'. Obese people may have a smaller thermic response to food than the non-obese, but both exhibit an increase in thermic effect on overfeeding. Adaptive thermogenesis is energy expended as heat in response to a number of stimuli, such as cold, infection, injury or cancer cachexia as well as overfeeding. It is particularly important during hibernation in animals, in the very young mammal as a means of controlling body temperature, before the capacity to shiver has developed, or in adults to avoid the functional impediment from shivering. In both cases, it is a particular type of fat cell, known as brown adipose tissue (BAT), which is responsible for the production of heat. The cells of BAT have a rich blood supply and extensive sympathetic innervation, a high concentration of mitochondria in each cell and the presence of myoglobin for oxygen transport.

The role for BAT in the control of energy balance in humans was demonstrated initially in rats overfed on 'cafeteria foods' typical of some human diets. Some of the rats remained at a normal weight, whereas others gained weight and became obese. These rats that were able to control their weight were shown to have more active BAT, which dissipated the excess energy as heat rather than storing it as fat. This response of BAT is under the control of the sympathetic nervous system and several key receptors have been identified, of which the most important is the BAT-specific, unique, β_3-adrenergic receptor. A specific uncoupling protein (UCP) that allowed production of heat in BAT was identified in the inner mitochondrial membrane. Contrary to the earlier view that BAT was only present in human infants, there is a small amount of BAT in adults which can function to generate heat on uncoupled respiration. A mutation associated with reduced β_3-receptor activity has been identified and linked with increased abdominal fat deposition, reduced metabolism and a greater capacity for weight gain. Genes for UCP have also been identified and variants discovered. The physiological importance of BAT in normal subjects is probably small; it may possibly account for up to 10% of energy balance, but usually only 1%–2% and it is difficult to detect. Physiologists have believed for many years that there might be a mechanism that allows subjects to 'adapt their energy expenditure to match the intake'. It is possible that BAT is one component of this mechanism, and it certainly contributes to massive weight loss when chronically stimulated by catecholamines, with pheochromocytoma.

Adaptations to Physical Activity

This is the aspect of our daily energy output that is most variable, both between and within individuals and, therefore, provides the greatest potential to modify energy balance.

There has been a major change in the level of activity of people in most Western countries in the last 30–40 years, and particularly in the last decade. The advances in technology have reduced the need for physical effort in all four of its major categories: domestic, work, transport and leisure activities. Few people now have very physically demanding jobs, compared with 30 years ago. Many tasks related to everyday life are now less physically demanding, for example, shopping with a supermarket trolley and car, compared to carrying shopping from the local high street, and making a bed with sheets and blankets, compared with straightening a duvet. Leisure activities themselves have become more sedentary, with television, video and computer games constituting a substantial proportion of many people's entertainment. Children play outside much less and are generally transported to school more, with the result that the pattern of low activity levels is established at a young age. School sport has also decreased, as pressure on the curriculum for academic subjects, as well as the loss of school playing fields to building and development have their effects.

There is considerable concern about the steady decline in activity levels and various initiatives exist to raise awareness about the importance of activity. Current advice in the United Kingdom is that adults should aim to be active daily. Over a week, activity should be up to at least 150 minutes (2½ hours) of moderate intensity activity in bouts of 10 minutes or more – one way to approach this is to do 30 minutes on at least 5 days per week. Alternatively, it is suggested that comparable benefits can be achieved by undertaking 75 minutes of vigorous intensity activity spread across the week, or in combinations of moderate and vigorous intensity activities. Associated with this is an increasing emphasis on incorporating more 'routine' activity into the lifestyle. This may include using the car less or walking up stairs; the intention is to include activity as part of the normal day, rather than separating it into 'exercise', which tends to become a chore and often stops when the initial enthusiasm wears off. Many schemes exist to encourage physical activity, including 'the walking bus' to take a number of children to school, 'exercise on prescription' to prevent or treat disease and many 'get fit' campaigns promoted in the media and local leisure centres. There are indications that a small increase in moderate to vigorous activity has taken place both in Europe and the United States. However, this is seen among the better-educated and better-off groups, rather than in the more deprived sectors, for whom physical labour is strongly associated with low social status. In addition, this small increase is insufficient to compensate for the downturn in 'lifestyle' activity that has been occurring.

Most people in Western countries are classed as having light occupational activity levels and sedentary leisure activity; an overall physical activity level (PAL) of 1.4 or less is therefore assumed. Studies of free-living populations confirm these assumptions, with some studies finding average PAL as low as 1.27. This means that the amount of energy expended during 24 hours is only an additional 27% of the BMR, representing minimal physical effort.

Spontaneous low-level activity, or fidgeting, is also of interest. It has been noted that subjects in overfeeding studies varied substantially in their levels of fat storage, some of which was attributed to differences in 'non-exercise activity thermogenesis', or fidgeting. This is also related to sympathetic nervous system activity, but the exact involvement of this aspect of activity in total energy output is as yet unclear.

Current interest has focussed on physical activity as well as activity. Developed societies have certainly reduced physical activity, but the most radical change in the past 30 years has been a massive increase in the time spent completely inactive. The time spent sitting in front of a screen (e.g. work computer, television, computer games) commonly adds up to 6–8 hours a day – often longer. Research has shown that the high risks of obesity, type 2 diabetes and heart disease which are associated with inactivity cannot completely be overcome even by periods of intense exercise.

HOW WELL IS ENERGY BALANCE CONTROLLED?

Humans consume different amounts of food each day, with differing proportions of macronutrients, and expend different amounts of energy in varying activities. The preceding sections have discussed the components of energy balance and shown how changes can occur in each component, consciously or unconsciously, which might bring about a restoration of energy balance. The body functions best in a stable state of homeostasis, and a number of mechanisms appear to operate in order to balance energy intake to energy expenditure and thus needs. The regulation of energy balance is neither perfect nor rapid and, as a consequence, changes in weight occur, reflecting these fluctuations in energy balance.

By adjusting food intakes in experimental subjects and concurrently measuring energy expenditure, it can be shown that changes in weight and energy expenditure are not matched precisely. Both experimental and long-term observational studies show that the body resists an energy deficit, whether this is induced by diet or exercise, and there is a powerful drive to compensate for this either by increasing energy intake in subsequent days, or reducing energy expenditure. Over 30 different neural and endocrine mechanisms exist which modify appetite, mostly to increase it. These results confirm that maintaining a weight loss can be difficult. Strong cognitive control, or will power, may be needed to resist the physiological neuroendocrine drive to restore energy appetite and balance. Exercise has been shown to help in the maintenance of weight over the long term, but it has complex, and to an extent, conflicting effects on appetite and eating. It can lead to muscle and joint damage with an acute inflammatory response mediated by cytokines such as IL-1, IL-6 and TNF. Appetite is reduced, but at a cost, and this is not a sustainable way to avoid weight gain. Moderate exercise, if sustained on a long-term basis, will ultimately increase appetite and energy consumption to match the demand, but this appears to happen only when body composition is near-ideal. When obese people take regular, moderate, physical activity, their appetites actually fall to allow a loss of body fat (and thus more efficient function during exercise). Restoration of energy balance during or following overfeeding is less effective, especially if high-fat diets are consumed. Exercise appears to be an important adjunct to maintaining energy balance on high-fat diets. However, there are varied responses to these disturbances of energy balance between individuals and between genders.

The relative ease of weight gain and difficulty of maintaining weight loss associated with physiological mechanisms for homeostasis means that some individuals demonstrate a fluctuation in weight over a period of time, as weight lost is regained. This has been termed 'yo-yo dieting'. Long-term studies of population cohorts have shown that there is an increased morbidity and mortality in people whose weight fluctuates (unintentionally) compared with those who have a stable weight. It is not, however, possible to state that weight fluctuation is the cause of the increase health risks: it may be that poorer health is the cause of weight fluctuation. It is possible that weight loss followed by weight regain, repeated on many occasions, is detrimental to the psychological well-being of the individual. However, intentional, maintained, weight loss brings consistent health benefits to overweight and obese people.

CONTROL MECHANISMS

For almost 50 years, it had been suspected that body weight is controlled by signals that monitor the quantity of adipose tissue. The nature of that signal was identified in 1994, when the protein 'leptin' produced by adipose tissue was identified. The amounts of leptin in the circulation are correlated with measures of adiposity, such as BMI and percentage body fat. Leptin is present in the circulation in both bound and free forms. Receptors for leptin were found originally in the hypothalamus, but many other tissues are now known to contain leptin receptors. These include organs involved in energy storage, metabolism and digestion. Other sites that contain leptin receptors include tissues or organs involved with immunity, blood pressure regulation and reproductive organs; the role of leptin in these functions is still being investigated, but its primary role may be signal, with a rising concentration that there is sufficient body fat for a woman to become pregnant and thus to ovulate. The very high levels seen in human obesity may be beyond the range which has a regulatory function.

Most of our understanding of leptin comes from laboratory animals, some of which are genetically deficient in leptin or its receptors. Leptin levels provide information to the brain about the abundance of body fat. Energy balance is regulated by the actions of leptin in the hypothalamus resulting in inhibition of food intake and increase in energy expenditure. Food intake is regulated through the release of neuropeptides, most notably neuropeptide Y, which is associated with increases in food intake. An increase in leptin levels will inhibit neuropeptide Y and, therefore, reduce food intake. The central action of leptin also stimulates the sympathetic nervous system, which in animals has been linked to thermogenesis in BAT, allowing dissipation of energy as heat. In subjects with a high fat mass, evidence suggests that a failure of the leptin receptors to respond, that is, leptin resistance, results in a breakdown of energy balance, allowing fat deposition to occur (see Figure 17.2).

There are close links between leptin and insulin. Insulin has similar effects in the hypothalamus, to reduce food intake and increases energy expenditure. It is now clear that insulin is involved in the secretion of leptin from adipose tissue, and also that leptin can inhibit insulin secretion. Therefore, when food is eaten, polypeptides (such as glucose-dependent insulinotropic polypeptide [GIP]) released from the intestine, together with absorbed metabolites (glucose, amino acids), stimulate insulin release. Glucose metabolism in adipocytes eventually causes leptin release, which acts on the brain to cause a reduction in food intake. This pathway will be most effective

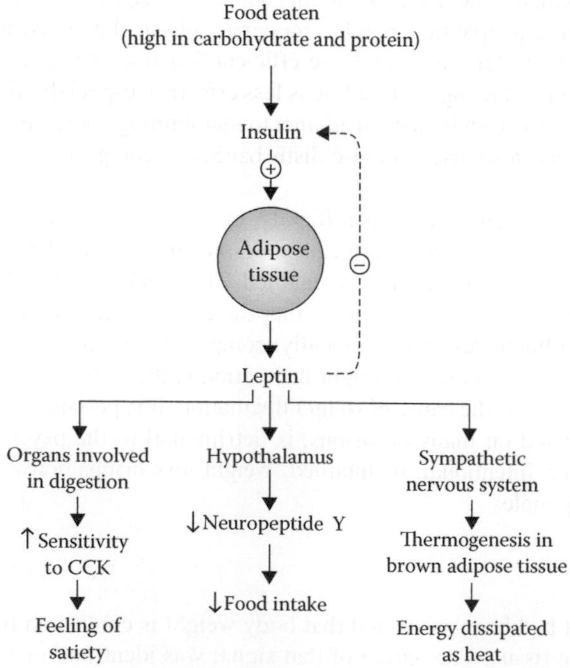

FIGURE 17.2 Actions of leptin. CCK, cholecystokinin.

with foods that trigger insulin release, such as carbohydrate- and protein-containing foods, and ineffective with high-fat foods. It, therefore, seems probable that the balance of macronutrients in the diet may influence leptin secretion.

The feedback loop described earlier identifies the role of leptin in a medium- to long-term control of energy balance. Leptin is also involved in short-term control of food intake, by increasing the sensitivity of the response to cholecystokinin (CCK). This is one of the gut hormones associated with satiation, released when food enters the duodenum. Leptin levels are not constant in an individual, as they exhibit a peak around midnight, which for many people is approximately 4–6 hours after an evening meal. The timing of the peak changes if meal times are altered. Levels are reduced during fasting and cause increases in hunger even before any change has occurred in body fat levels. This is not helpful for weight reduction, but is a normal physiological response to an energy deficit. A great deal of research effort has been focused on the potential use of leptin, its analogues or triggers, in order to manipulate energy balance, but results have been disappointing. Obese people already have high circulatory leptin concentrations, and fail to respond to it, possibly because it fails to enter the 'brain'. The transport process requires catecholamines. Investigations into the genetic codes for various leptin receptors and intermediaries in the pathways are ongoing, seeking factors in the aetiology of obesity, but research to date has found very few individuals in whom mutations in genes for leptin production or leptin receptors are the cause of overweight. It has recently been noted that pre-term babies, who were assigned to receive an enriched formula rather than human milk, had higher leptin levels relative to fat mass, at adolescence. This suggests that the leptin feedback mechanism may already be less sensitive at this age, and early feeding may programme the later development of overweight.

See Chapter 9 for more on the physiological regulation of food intake, pp. 186–190.

ENERGY BALANCE AND IMBALANCE

Humans are well adapted, through our evolution, to cope physiologically with both positive and negative energy imbalances. Our food supply is intermittent, as meals an historically we faced seasonal famines and we probably did not often have ample food every day at any time during evolution. The energy we consume during a meal usually exceeds the immediate need, so some is held in store to be used as required later. Thus, between each meal, there is commonly a period of positive energy balance, followed by a period of negative energy balance. These periods vary from an hour or two up to a whole day for individuals who eat only once daily. Excess food energy is stored as glycogen, with a limited capacity of about 400 g (i.e. 1600 kcal) in liver and muscle, and as fat in adipose tissue, whose capacity is almost unlimited in healthy people.

NEGATIVE ENERGY BALANCE

Negative energy balance occurs when the energy intake does not match the expenditure. Although the homeostatic response of the body is to try to minimize the energy deficit, weight may ultimately be lost by mobilization of fat stores and lean tissue in an attempt to maintain the energy supplies to the tissues. Eventually, when stores become depleted, the organs themselves may be broken down, resulting in death. The length of time that a person can withstand such negative energy balance depends on the initial size of the stores, and the magnitude of the negative energy balance. Individuals on hunger strike who continue to take liquids may survive for periods up to 100 days. If food is eaten, even in small amounts, then survival can be for much longer. After the first few days, when weight loss can be quite rapid, fasting results in a loss of about 0.5 kg/day in the obese subject and 0.35 kg/day in a non-obese subject. A smaller energy deficit results in slower weight loss; for example, diets providing 5.9–7.9 MJ (1400–1900 cal) may result in a weight loss up to 0.20 kg/day in obese males and up to 0.12 kg/day in obese females.

The Fasted State

When the immediate nutrient supply from meal digestion has finished, usually in about 2–3 hours, the body must provide the necessary constant energy in supply from the stores. Initially, this is mainly as glucose, released from glycogen stores, but there is always some supply of fatty acids released and transported from adipose tissue. As time goes by, the proportion of energy supplied from fat increases. Glycogen stores dwindle, but some is retained even into quite prolonged starvation. There is a need to continue some supply of glucose to the brain, the kidneys and as a reserve for any sudden muscular activity. After 2–3 days without food, however, glycogen stores are empty, and all the energy required by body tissues has to come from triglyceride in fat stores. The glycerol component of triglyceride does provide a small amount of glucose, but not enough for the brain, which then has to obtain its energy from the end-products of beta-oxidation of fatty acids, known as 'ketone bodies'. The best-known ketone body is acetone (nail polish remover), which gives a characterization fruity smell to the breath. This also occurs, more markedly, in untreated insulin-deficient diabetic patients, who cannot utilize glucose. The need to release glucose and ketone bodies as energy sources for vital organs during starvation, together with a loss of enzymatic functional capacity with starvation and infection, leads to an accumulation of re-assembled fatty acids which cannot be transported as lipoproteins. The result is a paradoxical fat-filled liver in advanced starvation.

Starvation

The hierarchy of functional, energy-saving adaptations during negative energy balance – or starvation – has been described from observations during famines, and from careful studies of volunteers and prisoners in the 1940s – metabolic rate is maintained, or even increased by a stress response over 24 hours of food deprivation. It then starts to fall, to a point 15%–20% below normal, as non-essential organ functions reduce. The signals for these compensatory changes are unknown and include a fall in thyroid hormone, insulin, growth hormone and testosterone.

See Chapter 21 for more on the clinical management of negative energy balance, pp. 400–402.

Their evolutionary value is obvious for a species faced with intermittent and seasonal famines. Voluntary physical activity drops, with a sense of fatigue. Sleeping time increases, and thermogenesis falls so people feel cold and tend to curl up to conserve heat. Blood pressure and pulse rates both fall, reducing cardiac output and work. Cellular metabolism for protein synthesis and maintenance of ionic gradients fall, which contributes to the appearance of oedema, if there is superadded infection. The immune system becomes underactive, risking infections. While brain function is maintained, there are often profound psychological effects of starvation. A particularly serious consequence of food deprivation is a rapid loss of bowel mucosa, through atrophy. This means that re-introducing normal amounts of food will cause diarrhoea, with fast bowel transit and failure to absorb nutrients. Food re-introduction must therefore be cautious and gradual, starting with about half of the actual requirements for energy balance.

With prolonged negative energy balance, changes in body composition become apparent. Initially, most of the energy deficit is made up from body fat. Adipose tissue provides about 7000 kcal/kg, so weight loss is relatively slow. The first fat to be used comes mainly from the most metabolically active internal, intra-abdominal sites (omentum, etc.), so there may be little to see externally, other than subtle changes in the shape of the face. As starvation (or dieting) progresses, more subcutaneous fat is lost, and particularly with physical inactivity, muscle is lost too. Muscle contains only 1000 kcal/kg, so weight loss is much more rapid when muscle is lost – a very bad sign, indicating that there is also infection with an inflammatory process, or that the remaining fat stores are critically depleted. A normal, non-obese individual can survive 6–8 weeks with no food at all.

Obese people can survive longer. Women are smaller than men, but have a greater proportion of fat stores, so their survival time during starvation is very similar.

Humans survived the competitive pressures of evolution, by developing the capacity to function remarkably well during periods of under-nutrition and an appetite sufficient to seek and to store relatively large amounts of energy during periods of excess. Few other species can reliably survive 40 days of starvation (or biblical fasting).

See Chapter 20 for more on the complex issues around energy balance and obesity, pp. 383–397.

Positive Energy Balance

The condition of unrelenting positive energy balance, and progressive accumulation of body fat, would have been exceedingly rare during our evolution, so we have developed few mechanisms to regulate appetite, or behaviour, or metabolism, under prolonged positive energy balance. It is evident that some people can store colossal amounts of body fat, increasing their BMI as high as 100 kg/m^2 – five times an optimal, healthy, body weight. There are major physical metabolic, psychological and social consequences of severe obesity, but they vary greatly between individuals, with degree and duration of positive energy balances. For many people, fat accumulation with a rise in BMI above 25 kg/m^2, or waist circumference above 80 cm in women or 94 cm in me, is sufficient to overload the fat-storage capacity of vital organs (liver, pancreas, heart) and to cause serious metabolic consequences. The primary, underlying, cause of type 2 diabetes, and much heart disease, is fat accumulation in pancreas and liver. This occurs with a BMI below 30 kg/m^2 for half of all people with type 2 diabetes. The conclusion from this is that quite modest chronic accumulation of body fat can be very dangerous. However, it needs to be recognised that, for presumed genetic reasons, many people can become seriously obese without developing diabetes or related metabolic consequences. Suffice to say here that there are adverse effects on health and well-being for all obese people, but with varying patterns between individuals and at different ages. The factors contributing to positive energy balance are summarized in Figure 17.3.

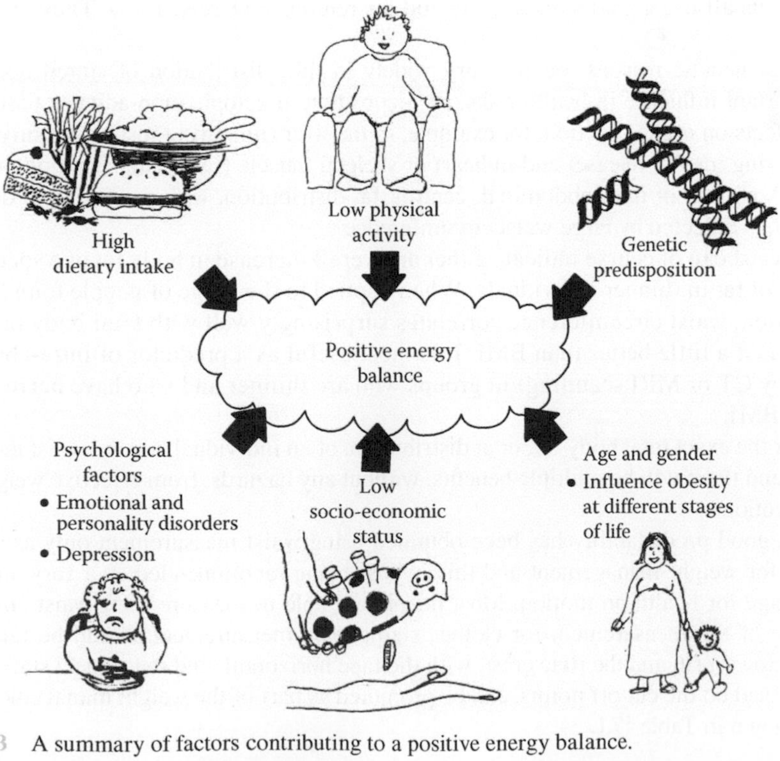

FIGURE 17.3 A summary of factors contributing to a positive energy balance.

Energy Balance and Body Composition

See Chapter 18 for a detailed account of body composition assessment, pp. 348–358.

When an individual is in energy balance over a period of time, the body weight and composition stay constant. A growing child, or an athlete in training aiming to increase muscle bulk, will need to be in positive energy balance to accrue body mass. On the other hand, an individual who is aiming to lose weight will need to be in negative energy balance. Measuring the body mass and its composition is, therefore, important. Most people assume that, in adults, a gain in weight is associated only with an increase in body fat, but some increase in supporting tissues also occurs. Subjects who are physically active and engaging in training schedules may gain weight as a result of an increase in muscle (lean) mass. Similarly, when weight is lost, there is always some loss of lean tissue, particularly if rapid weight loss occurs. This might be the result of a badly planned slimming diet, or perhaps due to illness. The functional consequences are very different, and the requirements to restore normal body composition will also be very different. It would be more accurate to describe people as overfat rather than overweight, to differentiate between the heavy, but lean individual and the person with a high percentage of fat in the body. Similarly, a light person may still have a relatively high percentage of fat in their body, but this may be not apparent if their lean mass has shrunk, that is, sarcopenia. This may be true of an older adult who has become very sedentary. A rise in waist circumference, with little or no increase in BMI, is now common in older adults and probably indicates replacement of lean tissue with fat mass.

Height is an important indicator of growth, and achieved growth (which may be less than the height potential, or growth capacity, conferred by genes). Weight is a measure of body size, important for many reasons, but it varies for different reasons: more may be good if it is muscle, but bad if it is fat. A variety of methods are used to quantify the two compartments: fat mass/total body fat and lean mass/fat free mass (of which muscle is a major variable component). These methods all use a gold standard method for reference (UNW, D_2O). They are covered in Chapter 18.

Mainly for genetic reasons, people vary widely in thin distribution of stored body fat. This has an important influence in health risks. Fat deposition in ectopic (non-adipose tissue) sites has profound effects on organ function, for example, in the liver (impairing insulin sensitivity), in pancreas (impairing insulin release) and in heart or skeletal muscle (impairing function and substrate oxidation). A pattern of intra-abdominal, central, fat distribution, with ectopic lipid deposition in these organs, is reflected by large waist circumference.

A large waist can of course indicate either an overall increase in body fat or a specific central distribution of fat in thinner individuals. When applied to the range of people found in the general population, waist circumference correlates surprisingly well with total body fat ($R^2 = 0.8$), which is in fact a little better than BMI. It is most useful as a predictor of intra-abdominal fat (measured by CT or MRI scanning) in groups who are thinner and who have narrow ranges of body fat or BMI.

Whatever the exact total body fat, or at distribution, of an individual, a large waist indicates high health risk, and there will be multiple benefits, without any hazards, from effective weight management intervention.

Recently, good predictability has been obtained using waist measurement only as an indicator of the need for weight management and this is now being recommended as a very simple public health message for health promotion. Most people are able to measure their waist circumference or are aware of the measurement for clothes sizing. The measurement should be taken midway between the lowest rib and the iliac crest, with the tape horizontal, and the subject standing. Levels for action, based on the cut-off points, can be promoted as part of the weight management message. These are shown in Table 17.1.

TABLE 17.1

Action Levels for Weight Management Based on Waist Circumference

Level of Health Risk	Waist Circumference – Men (cm)	Waist Circumference – Women (cm)
Healthy/normal	<94	<80
Action level 1		
Increasing risk – no further weight should be gained	94–102	80–88
Action level 2		
High risk – medical advice should be sought for weight management	>102	>88

Source: Adapted from Scottish Intercollegiate Guidelines Network (1996).

SUMMARY

1. Energy balance represents the relationship between energy intake and energy output.
2. Energy balance can be affected by changes in energy intake, energy output, or both of these.
3. Changes in energy intake may be the result of deliberate manipulation or secondary to changes in appetite perhaps related to disease.
4. Changes in body composition occur as a result of alterations in energy balance as the body tries to re-establish homeostasis.
5. There is an increased prevalence of overweight in the United Kingdom, which may be linked to a high-fat diet. Low levels of activity may also play a part. Weight loss can only be achieved by measures that cause a negative energy balance.

STUDY QUESTIONS

1. Discuss the potential impact of intermittent fasting on physiological systems related to energy balance.
2. Use your knowledge of the components of energy balance to analyse this case fully. Ann is a reasonably fit 40-year-old woman, weighing 58 kg. She takes regular exercise. This includes swimming for 1 hour three times each week, walking her dog for 1 hour each day and spending about 1 hour each day gardening. Recently, Ann broke her leg in a skiing accident and has been immobile for 6 weeks. She finds that her body weight is now 64 kg, although she has not increased her food intake.
   a. Explain what has happened, in terms of the energy balance process.
   b. Once her leg has healed and she starts to walk again, what could she do to return to her previous weight as quickly as possible?

BIBLIOGRAPHY AND FURTHER READING

Conway, J.M. (ed.). 1995. Advances in human energy metabolism: Review of current knowledge (symposium). *American Journal of Clinical Nutrition* 52(5), 1033–1075.

Durnin, J.V. and Womersley, J. 1974. Body fat assessed from total body density and its estimation from skinfold thickness: Measurements on 481 men and women aged from 16 to 72 years. *British Journal of Nutrition* 32(1), 77–97.

Ferro-Luzzi, A., Sette, S., Franklin, M. et al. 1992. A simplified approach of assessing adult chronic energy deficiency. *European Journal of Clinical Nutrition* 46, 173–186.

Fruhbeck, G. 2001. A heliocentric view of leptin. *Proceedings of the Nutrition Society* 60, 301–318.

Gibney, G.R. 2000. Energy expenditure in disease: Time to revisit? *Proceedings of the Nutrition Society* 59, 199–207.

Hardie, D.G., Ross, F.A. and Hawley, S.A. 2012. AMPK: A nutrient and energy sensor that maintains energy homeostasis. *Nature Reviews Molecular Cell Biology* 13(4), 251–262.

Han, T.S., van Lee, E.M., Seidell, J.C., Lean, M.E.J. 1995. Waist circumference action levels in the identification of cardiovascular risk factors: prevalence study in a random sample. *BMJ* 311, 1401–1405.

Lean, M.E.J., Han, T.S. and Deurenberg, P. 1996. Predicting body composition by densitometry from simple anthropometric measurements. *The American Journal of Clinical Nutrition* 63, 4–14.

Manning, S. and Batterham, R.L. 2014. The role of gut hormone peptide YY in energy and glucose homeostasis: Twelve years on. *Annual Review of Physiology* 76, 585–608.

Rosenbaum, M. and Leibel, R.L. 2014. 20 Years of leptin: Role of leptin in energy homeostasis in humans. *Journal of Endocrinology* 223(1), T83–T96.

Scottish Intercollegiate Guidelines Network (SIGN). 1996. Obesity in Scotland - integrating prevention with weight measurement. Edinburgh: Royal College of Physicians.

Westerterp, K.R. 1999. Body composition, water turnover and energy turnover assessment with labelled water. *Proceedings of the Nutrition Society* 58, 945–951.

White, A., Nicolaas, G., Foster, K. et al. 1993. *Health Survey for England 1991.* Office of Population Censuses and Surveys. London, UK: HMSO.

Wycherley, T.P., Moran, L.J., Clifton, P.M., Noakes, M. and Brinkworth, G.D. 2012. Effects of energy-restricted high-protein, low-fat compared with standard-protein, low-fat diets: A meta-analysis of randomized controlled trials. *The American Journal of Clinical Nutrition*, 96(6) pp 1281–1298.

18 Dietary and Nutritional Assessment

AIMS

The aims of this chapter are to

- Describe the main forms of dietary assessment.
- Evaluate ways in which dietary information is collected.
- Conceptualize the nutritional status of individuals and assessment of its components.
- Outline the applications of dietary and nutritional assessment.

NUTRITIONAL STATUS

Central to any study, or action, in nutrition is the concept of nutritional status. This has been defined as the capacity to perform the range of functions required in health and the metabolic competence to respond to stresses ('the biological condition of an individual in respect of parameters dependent to a greater or lesser extent on diet, whether or not other factors are involved'). Measurement of nutritional status includes the measurement of anthropometric, biochemical and clinical indicators and the nutritional status of an individual therefore incorporates an understanding of

- *The past*: Genetic endowment defining potential and needs
  - Dietary exposure
  - Other past influences in food/nutrient utilization, for example illness
- *The present*: Current form and behaviour, including habitual diet
- *The future*: Capacity for growth, activity recovery and resistance to infection reproduction

There are three interacting but distinct components of nutritional status: what we eat, what we are and what we can do. To be able to assess nutritional status, all three must be evaluated, using different methods and dietary intake assessment is just one method of gleaning information about an individual's nutritional status.

What We Eat: Diet Composition

These rely on the dietary assessment techniques presented earlier in this chapter.

- Self-reported intake
- Objectively observed food consumption
- Estimated or measured nutrient consumption

What We Are: Body Composition

- Water content
- Two-compartment (fat/lean tissue)
- Bone mass/tissue composition

What We (Can) Do: Function

- Metabolic, cellular
- Organ/whole-body function
- Physical, mental and social activities

What We Pass On

An important legacy of our nutritional status forms a fourth component – what we pass on. Recent evidence is accumulating that, amongst other factors, the three components of nutritional status affect the growth and development of offspring by epigenetic mechanisms which modify gene expression. Although we cannot measure this at present, an epigenetic legacy is clearly a fourth element within nutritional status.

WHAT WE EAT: DIETARY ASSESSMENT

Information on the dietary intake of individuals is usually obtained by asking subjects to keep a record of everything they have eaten over a period of time. The level of precision with which this is carried out, and the duration of the study have been subject to debate. In general, the more exact the method of measurement tries to be, the less it is likely to reflect the normal, freely chosen diet of the subject.

The exact method used will be determined by the aims of the study. Decisions have to be taken by the researcher to determine the reliability and validity of the methods used. In other words, if the method chosen provides results that can be reproduced on a subsequent occasion, it has a reasonable degree of reliability. A second more difficult question to answer relates to the validity of the information, that is how well it measures the subject's intake. Since food and, therefore, nutrient intakes are not constant from day to day for the majority of people, an average intake over a period of time would reflect 'habitual' intakes. The duration over which food intake has to be recorded to obtain a valid measure of habitual intake has been studied and shown to vary for different nutrients. Ultimately, the decision on how long a recording period should be depends on the nutrients to be analysed. For example, for energy and macronutrient intake, Black (2001) reports that a 7-day intake record will provide a result within 15%–20% of the true level of intake. For micronutrients, the variability is up to 30%–40% for those that are widely distributed in foods, and very large for vitamins, such as A and C, which occur in large amounts in fewer foods. Fish is still commonly eaten only 1 day per week, so average intakes of individuals cannot be assessed in this way. Some of the methods used are discussed in the following text. Some are retrospective and rely on recollection of events (such as the food frequency questionnaires [FFQs] and the dietary recall), and others are prospective and rely on active involvement of the participant in real-time-recording of information relevant to food consumption (e.g. weighed dietary records).

The Weighed Inventory (or Weighed Dietary Record)

This is considered to be the 'gold standard' of dietary intake studies. In this method, all the food eaten by the subject during a period, usually 1 week, is weighed and recorded, together with any plate waste. It is a prospective method. Actual nutrient intakes are then calculated, using data from food composition tables applicable to the particular country (in the United Kingdom, McCance and Widdowson's tables, published by the Royal Society of Chemistry, are the most widely used – see Food Standards Agency, 2002b). The major drawback of the method is that it requires a considerable degree of motivation and cooperation on the part of the subject. It is quite an intrusive method, which takes time at meals and may thus deter a busy person. The numbers willing or able to complete a 7-day weighed food inventory are low, so it is common to use 3 or 4 days, including weekend days. If Fridays are not included, it may appear that nobody eats fish.

Most subjects tend to under-record their habitual food intake, possibly because they actually eat less during the study period, or forget/omit to record some of the foods eaten. This seems to be a particular problem in those who are trying to restrain their food intake in some way. Snack foods are often omitted, perhaps because of inconvenience or forgetfulness. Recent work has shown that the fat and carbohydrate intakes are underreported to a greater extent than protein intakes. Food choice may also be altered to facilitate weighing.

Food Diaries (or Estimated Dietary Records)

In this (prospective) technique, the food eaten is simply recorded in a notebook, without being weighed, usually for 7 days. Comprehensive instructions are provided to the subject to explain the procedure. Cooking methods, brand names and recipes are requested. The respondent is asked to provide an estimate of the portion size using household measures, for example spoons, cups, units, slices or recording packet weights. The researcher then has the task of quantifying portions eaten. Food models or pictures may help in the quantification of portion sizes. A number of photographic atlases of food portions have been developed and validated in recent years. Other visual images, including those generated by computer or digital camera may be used, but will also need to be validated. Average portion sizes have been described in the United Kingdom, based on measurements of typical portions. Database information is available for a large number of typical servings of foods, although they remain only an estimate for each particular subject. A large database, known as DINER (Data Into Nutrients for Epidemiological Research), has been developed as part of the EPIC study, which contains information on over 7000 foods and portion sizes. The food diary method requires that the subject is literate and physically able to write. Alternative ways of recording the size of portion eaten include photographing the meal and the use of computerized scales with an associated tape recorder, for example, the PETRA (Portable Electronic Tape Recording Automated) scales system, which can both weigh and store a description of the meal. In both cases, however, the data still require interpretation and collation by the researcher.

The diary method remains subject to possible changes in the diet by the respondent and failure to record all foods eaten. However, if respondents are adequately instructed, reasonably comprehensive records can be obtained. Generally, women produce more reliable records by this method than men.

A record of foods eaten with no attempt to assess the quantity (a menu record) is a further modification of this approach. Average servings can be used by the researcher and, although the accuracy of individual intake calculation is reduced, this method can provide an overview of dietary patterns.

A simpler and more straightforward approach used increasingly is to compile a food intake record based on food groups, such as those in the 'Eatwell Guide'. This allows an overall profile of the diet to be obtained and the balance to be assessed against a standard desirable pattern.

Food Frequency Questionnaires (FFQs)

These provide an inexpensive means of studying intake retrospectively. It can be self-administered by large numbers of people and requires only a short period of time. This tool is often used in epidemiological research. It has the advantage that current diets are not altered by the recording method used. Analysis of the data can be done rapidly using a computerized scoring system. Disadvantages are that the results are culture-specific and a different group may require a new questionnaire. Additionally, individuals with unusual diets within the study group may not fit the predetermined criteria for coding. Even for people with a relatively consistent dietary pattern, it can be quite a complicated task to convert information about a habitual food intake into a frequency over a week, for specific foods. This is complicated further by trying to assess portion sizes of these foods. This type of questionnaire often looks at a subset of foods providing specific nutrients, rather than at the whole diet, and is generally tailored to the aims of a particular study.

A large number of nutrient-specific, or disease- specific, FFQs have been used, and some properly validated, for specific purposes, for example, to assess consumption of calcium or iodine. The Scottish Dietary Targets Monitor was developed (and validated) to assess the intakes of foods which contribute to seven dietary targets but does not attempt to quantify energy intake, etc. In general, questionnaires can give useful information, sufficient to rank individuals within groups into subsets according to intake, rather than to provide precise data on actual individual intakes.

The Diet Interview

This technique is widely used by dieticians to obtain a general picture of a person's food intake. It requires a skilled interviewer to elicit an accurate picture of a person's diet history. The time frame is usually 7 days. This can be sufficient to pinpoint potential excesses or deficiencies. The interview may be more or less detailed, depending on the type of information required and its purpose. It usually consists of questions about the daily eating pattern, along the lines of 'What do you usually have for breakfast, mid-morning, lunch, etc.?' It then aims to draw a more precise picture by focusing on the current (or previous) day's intake, by asking 'What did you have for breakfast, mid-morning, lunch, etc. today, or yesterday?' Many people have little awareness of what they eat, so that it may be quite difficult for them to remember even the previous day's food intake. An estimation of portion sizes may also be made, often with the help of food models. A checklist of foods may be used to remind subjects about foods that they do eat, but forgot to mention.

Some of the limitations of a diet history are that it requires both a skilled interviewer and a subject with a reasonable memory. For the latter reason, it is unlikely to be suitable for children and for anyone with a failing memory. It also depends on the subject having a recognized dietary pattern, and a 'usual intake'. In addition, it is time-consuming both to complete the interview and to carry out any subsequent analysis of the data collected. Hand-held computers with dietary analysis packages can simplify the process, allowing information from the subject to be entered directly.

A dietary recall interview can be simplified to focus just on the previous 24 hours and obtain a 'snapshot' of a typical intake. This can be done by telephone and need not take more than 15–20 minutes. However, bias is introduced as the day chosen may be atypical. It is also likely that food portion sizes are inaccurate, and the completeness of the record is memory dependent.

Practical Issues in Dietary Assessment Methods

The way in which food is perceived by the subject may affect what is recorded. This might include perceptions of what their culture group believes they *should* be eating as well as what the interviewer might expect.

Obtaining dietary intake information from children and adolescents poses particular challenges. With young children, below the age of 8 years, the limiting factors include suspicion, knowledge of the names of foods, limited attention span and memory. The use of a parent as surrogate reporter may introduce bias. As children become older, the ability to record the food intake increases, but at the same time, there may be a greater desire to *please* the interviewer and accuracy of records may be low. There are no easy solutions to collect dietary intake data in these age groups, and new or refined survey methods are needed. Some of the problems found in this group include underreporting and non-response, which are also discussed in the following text.

Misreporting

There is now recognition among nutritionists that much of the dietary intake data that are collected contain an element of misreporting, and increasingly among the overweight and obese, underreporting. Misreporting can occur through errors, or memory lapses, but intentional misreporting is surprisingly common. People resist telling the whole truth about many behaviours, and that includes food access and eating. As many as 50% of all women said they would intentionally report either more (mostly thin people) or less (mostly obese people) than they actually eat. This is confirmed by comparison of energy intake with calculated or measured energy expenditure in many different groups. Measurements of energy expenditure using the doubly labelled water technique are available in some research settings. Biomarkers such as urinary nitrogen levels can also be used to confirm the accuracy of food intake records, although these increase the intrusion of the method, and could reduce compliance.

General findings, for example, based on studies of 77 groups (reported by Black, 2001) show a ratio of reported-energy intake to energy expenditure of 0.83 (when a ratio of at least 1.0 is required to avoid weight loss). In addition, there is variability between subjects in the extent of misreporting. For 29% of the groups studied, results for energy were within 10% of those for expenditure. In 69% of the groups, energy intake figures were more than 10% below energy expenditure. Only in 2% of the groups were the intake results more than 10% greater than the expenditure results.

In summary, food intakes are usually underreported. This has implications for the calculation of energy intakes, but also nutrient intakes. If nutrient intakes are expressed in relation to the total energy intake, a measure of the nutrient density of the diet can be obtained, expressed as the weight of nutrient/MJ or 1000 cal. This can then be used for comparison between individuals, even if underreporting has occurred. These findings raise concerns about the accuracy of dietary intake studies, and underline the need for new methods to be developed that can more accurately capture information about individual intakes. Alternatively, more precise techniques for validating the intake records are needed.

Measurement Errors, Bias and Precision

There are two types of error occurring during dietary assessment: random errors and systematic errors. Random errors occur by chance or by mistake, and contribute to decreasing the precision of an assessment tool. However, random errors do not affect the accuracy of the assessment tool. The difference between precision and accuracy is illustrated in Figure 18.1. It is possible to overcome the lack of precision introduced by random errors by taking more measurements.

Systematic errors, on the other hand, are the result of a flaw in study design and execution, which is consistent, and leads to the introduction of a bias. Systematic errors make the assessment tool less accurate, and it is not possible to remedy bias in dietary assessment.

Examples of sources of random and systematic errors are illustrated in Table 18.1

Validity

It is important to validate assessment tool to evaluate how well they perform at measuring a specific dietary parameter. As such, validation studies rely on several (different) methods to measure the same dietary parameter, in order to compare a *new* method to an established reference (sometime gold-standard) method. This is the study of relative validity. It is useful to include a biomarker as one of the reference methods in validation studies. Biomarkers are present in biological fluids

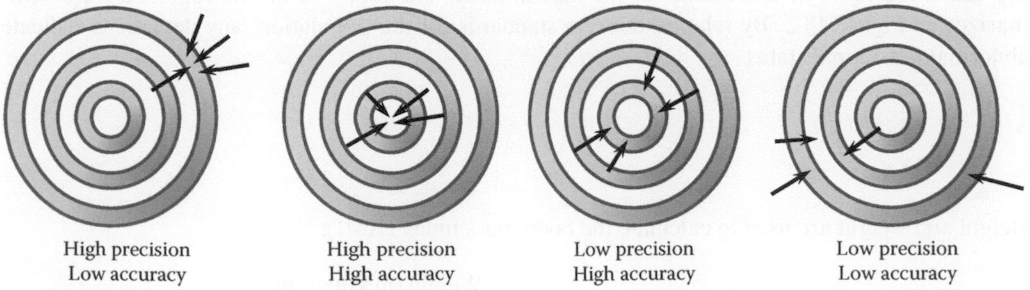

FIGURE 18.1 Accuracy and precision.

TABLE 18.1
Examples of Random and Systematic Errors in Dietary Assessment

Source	Random Errors	Systematic Errors
Measurement of quantity of food by the subject	Occasional error in recording portion sizes: forgetting to tare the kitchen scale, or by writing down incorrect weights.	The instrument (such as kitchen scales) is not properly calibrated and consistently show the wrong amount.
Reporting of intake by the subject	A food is forgotten, by mistake, on a specific occasion.	A group of food is never (or most often) reported.
Burden associated with the study	A high burden triggers occasional mistakes.	A high burden means that subjects adapt their diet to make the assessment exercise more bearable.
The researcher	The researcher changes his or her interview style on a given occasion, and elicits a different answer compared to the standard interviewing technique.	The researcher asks questions in a way that primes the subject to favour a certain type of answers.
The technique used	Instructions to the subject are confusing or not clear, leading to potential misinterpretation of what needs to be done.	The method used is not adequate to measure a specific nutrient or food group and, as a result, does not provide a true picture of intake.
Data analysis	Typing errors are made when entering food quantities or food codes in a spreadsheet.	The database has significant gaps which leads to the under-/over-estimation of specific nutrients in the diet.

(often blood or urine) and provide an objective way to assess nutrient intake, independently of food intake. Examples of biomarkers include urinary nitrogen (a 'recovery' biomarker, useful to validate tools measuring protein intake), plasma carotenoids (a 'concentration' biomarker, useful to validate tools measuring carotenoid intake, or more generally, fruit and vegetable intake) or metabolites of polyphenolics in urine (a proxy biomarker for intake of plant foods rich in polyphenols).

Statistical analysis of the dietary data measured by each of the method used in the validation exercise, and the difference between each method, enables the determination of bias, precision and agreement between methods. Agreement alone is not sufficient to validate a new method: indeed, good agreement may only reflect the fact that both methods tested have a similar level of errors.

WHAT WE ARE: BODY COMPOSITION

Assessing body composition involves firstly quantifying overall size, then sizes of major organ or tissue compartments, and finally assessing the structure and nutrient or chemical contents of tissues. All are influenced by diet, and all affect functions. Anthropometric (literally 'measuring of man') indicators are basic measurements of the human body. The methods of anthropometry are summarized in Figure 18.2. By relating these to standards for the population, any deviations indicate abnormal nutritional status.

MEASURING BODY COMPOSITION

Body Mass Index

Height and weight are used to calculate the body mass index (BMI):

$$\text{BMI (or Quetelet's index)} = \frac{\text{Weight (in kilograms)}}{[\text{Height (in metres)}]^2}$$

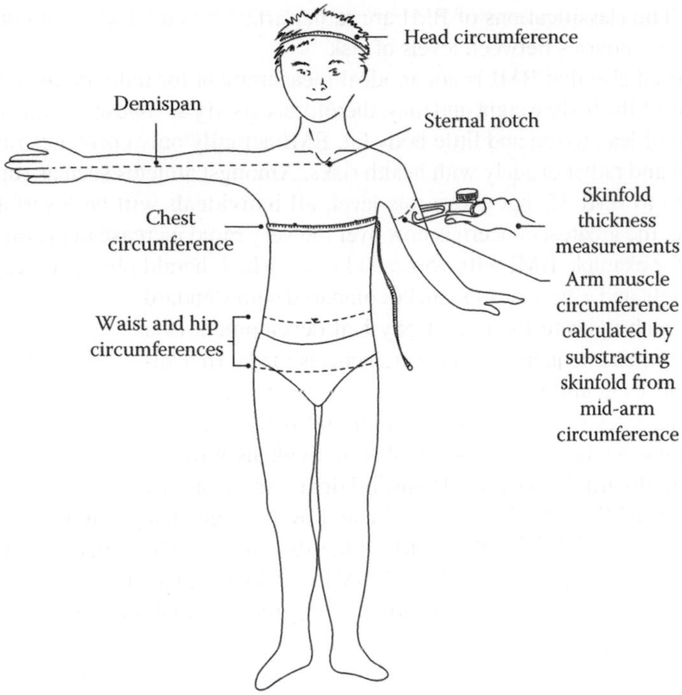

FIGURE 18.2 Summary of the main methods of anthropometry.

Standard procedures are available for accurate measurement of weight (using scales, either digital or mechanic) and weight (using stadiometers, with the head in the Frankfurt plane position).

BMI correlates modestly with total body fat, $r = 0.75$, and is used to categorize overweight in epidemiology. The World Health Organization (WHO) has recommended that the following categories be used for adults in epidemiology:

BMI (kg/m²)	Grade
<18.5	Underweight
18.5–24.99	Normal weight
25.0–29.99	Overweight
30.0–34.99	Obese (grade 1 obesity)
35–39.99	Obese (grade 2 obesity)
≥40.0	Obese (grade 3 obesity)

The relationship between energy balance and body composition is covered in Chapter 17, p. 340.

These data are based on the greater health risks associated with increasing weight, as shown by actuarial life expectancy tables, as well as information about morbidity. In general, risks increase with rising BMI, even within the band categorized as 'normal'. For example, for women, the risk of coronary heart disease in an American study was shown to be twice as great at a BMI between 25 and 29 as at a BMI of less than 21. Above a BMI of 29, the risk was almost 3.5 times greater. For diabetes, the prevalence is about three times greater for people with a BMI above 28.5 than for those whose BMI is below 24.4 and that is already increased three times above the lowest risk, with BMI below 22 kg/m^2. The classifications of BMI are rather arbitrary and useful for convenience, rather than being major boundaries between levels of risk.

It should be noted also that BMI is not an ideal measurement for individuals. It takes no account of the components of the body weight and may, therefore, classify as 'obese' a trained athlete who has a high percentage of lean tissue and little body fat. BMI actually only correlates rather weakly with body fat ($r^2 = 0.5$) and rather crudely with health risks. Amongst athletes such as rugby players, body fat may be low up to BMI 35, but above this level, all individuals will be 'overfat'. From a public health perspective, the greatest concern is now over the very rapid increase in prevalence of very high BMI categories, for example BMI >40, >50, >60 kg/m^2, which herald physical incapacity.

In children, height and weight results can be compared with standard growth curves, which indicate the rate of physical development of a child, particularly when a sequence of measurements is made. In addition, head and chest circumference measures can also be useful in children to indicate rates of growth of the brain and body. The patterns of growth vary, but healthy, well-nourished individuals follow a predictable path: malnutrition causes a downward drift away from the predicted path. The BMI of children is complicated by its huge change, and the effects of puberty. Age-standardized BMI is plotted on the centile of the 1991 survey. The 98th centile is used to indicate obesity in children. It corresponds broadly with BMI > 25 kg/m^2 in adulthood.

Growth during childhood is covered in Chapter 7, pp. 136–138.

BMI is also useful for crude classification of degrees of malnutrition in adults, as follows (Ferro-Luzzi et al., 1992):

BMI	Grade of Malnutrition
<16	3
16–16.9	2
17–18.4	1

Because BMI is conceptually complicated, a chart may be used to check the degree of overweight (see Figure 18.3).

Skinfold and Skeletal Measurements

Skinfold (or fatfold) measurements are a useful and inexpensive way of obtaining a measurement of body fat content. Skinfold thickness measurements at mid-triceps, mid-biceps, subscapular and supra-iliac sites using Harpenden or similar callipers give a surprisingly accurate value for body fat, when used by a skilled person. In the hands of an experienced operator, the specially designed callipers can yield results within 3%–5% of those obtained by more complicated and accurate methods, such as hydrostatic weighting (see the following text). Figure 18.4 illustrates the technique. The results from skinfold measurements can be used simply to quantify the subcutaneous fat at specific sites and monitor this in a particular individual over a period of time.

A drawback of this technique is that it may not be suitable in individuals who are very fat, elderly (fat is more compressible in older age groups) or highly trained (muscular development makes it difficult to pinch a fatfold). In addition, it should be remembered that, in young adults, about 50% of the body fat is found subcutaneously; with increasing age, more is deposited internally. Skinfold measurements do not indicate fat distribution. Thus, a similar fatfold reading will represent a greater total body fat content in an older person than a younger one. Tables of typical skinfold results in population groups are available as standards.

Arm muscle circumference can be calculated by subtracting the thickness of the fatfold from a mid-arm circumference measurement. This can indicate muscle development or wasting and can be a useful indicator in clinical situations of change in muscle mass, for example, during illness and rehabilitation.

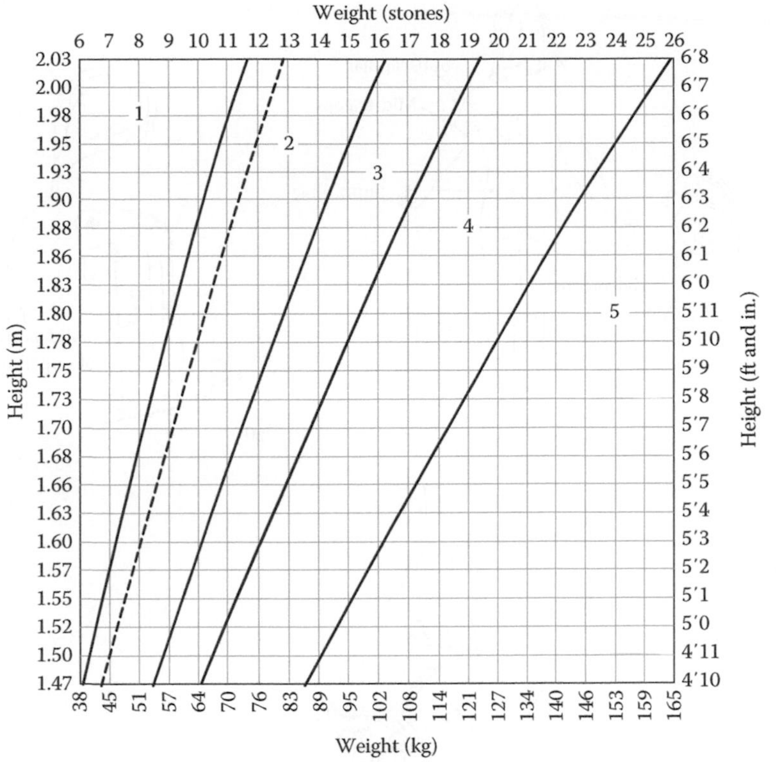

FIGURE 18.3 Weight assessment chart for adults. Take a straight line across the chart from your height and a straight line up from your weight. Make a note of where the two lines meet. This will indicate if you are within the desirable weight for your size. 1, underweight; 2, desirable weight; 3, overweight; 4, fat; 5, obese.

Demispan is a measurement of skeletal size, which can be used as an alternative to height measurement, where it is difficult to obtain an upright posture in a subject. Demispan is the distance between the sternal notch and the roots of the middle and third fingers with the arm stretched out at shoulder height to the side of the body. It is particularly useful in elderly people, in whom height might have been lost due to vertebral collapse. The demispan value can then be used to produce two alternative indices which show good agreement with BMI. These are demiquet, which uses weight/demispan^2 and mindex which is weight/demispan. As an alternative to demi-span, the Lower Leg Length, from knee to ground when sitting can also be used as a reliable proxy for height, to estimate BMI.

Anthropometry

The accuracy of equations using skinfold to predict total body fat was confirmed in a validation study in a separate population, in a study which also found that waist circumference gave an equally good prediction. Waist circumference is also sensitive to differences in fat distribution, for example with age, and much easier and cheaper to use (Lean et al., 1995). Waist circumference measurements (alone) have been shown to correlate well with total body fat ($r = 0.8$ better than BMI), and also to indicate the intra-abdominal fat mass in thinner people.

A non-elasticated tape of adequate length is required for the measurement of waist circumference. The correct position for measuring waist circumference is midway between the uppermost border of the iliac crest and the lower border of the costal margin (rib cage). The measurement

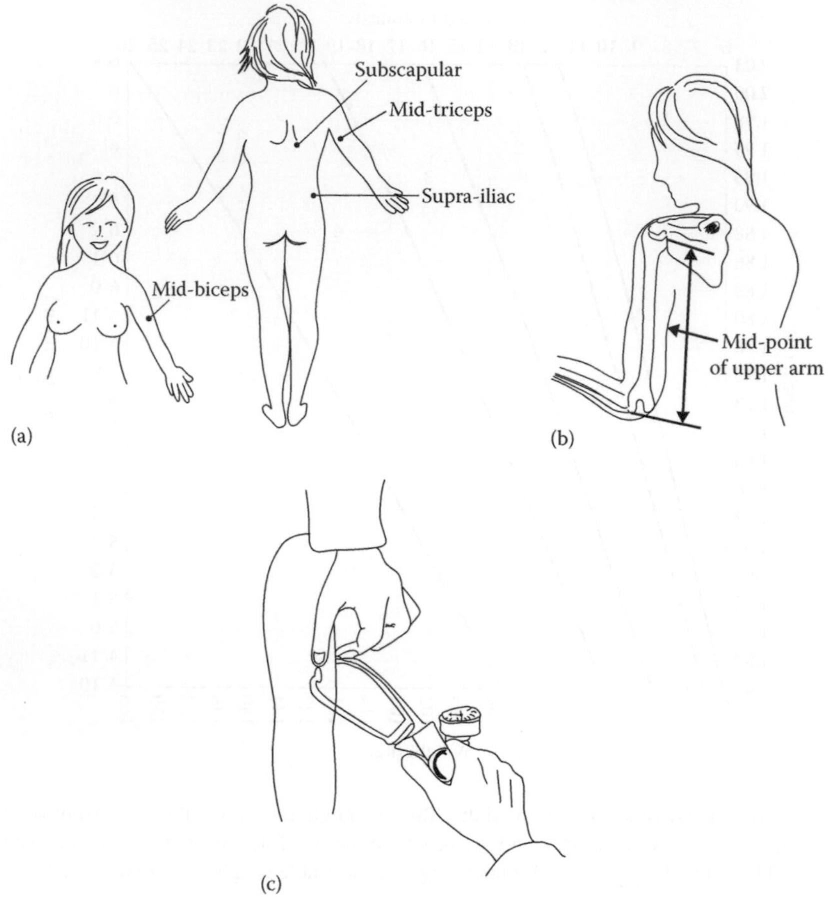

FIGURE 18.4 Measurement of skinfold for assessment of body fat content. (a) The four sites used are subscapular, supra-iliac, mid-biceps and mid-triceps. Measurements from all four sites are added together for use in formulae to obtain fat mass. (b) For mid-triceps measurement, the mid-point of the upper arm is found. (c) The callipers in use. The skinfold is taken lengthways along the arm, grasped firmly between thumb and forefinger, avoiding underlying muscle. The callipers are applied about 1 cm below the operator's fingers and the fold is held throughout the measurement. Three measurements are made and the results averaged.

should be taken when the tape is snug but not squeezing the waist. In practice, it is difficult to accurately palpate those bony landmarks for very overweight patients and therefore to accurately place the tape.

Waist is a useful predictor of multiple health problems (see Table 17.3, previous chapter) and may be used in the future as a quick indicator of risk from overweight. Other ratios, such as waist to height, have also been suggested as useful, as they tend to be 'unisex' and, therefore, a single figure can be used as a cut-off point, but the use of ratios adds complexity. The waist-to-hip ratio performs less well than waist alone.

Recent research has generated and validated new equations based on simple anthropometry (waist, hips, height) with weight, age and sex, to estimate whole body fat mass, and skeletal muscle mass, as measured by MRI. These estimates both have value for identifying different people with health risks from type 2 diabetes and hypertension. Low muscle mass i also relevant to falls and fractures in older people.

Underwater Weighing

This method is based on Archimedes' principle, which states that an object's loss of weight in water is equal to the weight of the volume of water it displaces, because the object in the water is buoyed up by a counterforce, which equals the mass of water it displaces. In applying this to human body composition measurements, the body's volume is determined by the difference between body weight measured in air and measured when completely submerged in water. The density of the body can, therefore, be calculated using the following equation.

$$\text{Density of the body} = \text{Weight in air} - \text{Weight in water}$$

The body weight and density are composed of a mix of fat and fat-free tissue (together with a small correction for gases in the lungs and intestinal tract, which may be added to the calculation). It is assumed that fat has a density of 0.9 g/cm^3 and fat-free tissue a density of 1.1 g/cm^3. Errors may arise from assumptions about bone density and the water content of the body, but these are assumed to be small.

The body density can then be used in the equation derived by Siri, to calculate percentage body fat:

$$\text{Body fat}\,(\%) = \left(\frac{495}{\text{Body density}}\right) - 450$$

A convenient way to make these measurements is to suspend the subject seated on a chair from a spring balance, and to lower it into a pool – for example, a hydrotherapy pool.

Clearly, this technique is not suitable for some people, for example, those with a fear of immersion, the sick and elderly people. Obese subjects, whose overall body density is below 1.0, tend to float; hence, it is necessary to add an equal weight of say 10 kg to keep them submerged.

Other Indirect Methods

A variety of techniques can be used to determine the internal composition of the body from external measurements.

Bioelectrical Impedance

This is based on the flow of electricity through the body, which is conducted by the fat-free tissue and extracellular water because of the electrolyte content. The resistance (or impedance) to the flow of current is related directly to the level of body fat. Attaching electrodes to the hand and foot of a subject and passing a localized electrical signal allows impedance to be measured quickly and painlessly. The results obtained will vary with the level of hydration of the subject and with skin temperature. Details about age, weight and height are entered, and the machine gives a quick read-out of percentage body fat, which generally correlates at least crudely with more robust measures such as underwater weighing, or deuterium dilution. However, it is sometimes unclear whether bio-impedance provides a better estimate of body composition than BMI. Anthropometric estimates of body composition, and even, skinfold or waist circumference may give more reliable results.

Ultrasound

This can be used to measure the thickness of the fat layer at various points of the body, as the ultrasound beam is deflected at each interface between different tissues. A similar method is the use of near-infrared interactance, which records the absorption and reflection of an infrared light beam, and computes fat thickness from the readings obtained.

Other Techniques

Other techniques that require expensive equipment and are not generally available for routine use include computerized tomography, magnetic resonance imaging (MRI) and dual-energy x-ray absorptiometry (DEXA). The DEXA technique has been used most widely in the measurement of bone density, which can help refine the assessment of lean body mass. Some DEXA machines can estimate total, and regional, body fat and the results are very reproducible. They need to be validated against measurements using a robust method such as underwater weighing or deuterium dilation. In research studies, MRI is often used to quantify total and regional fat, and even the fat content of specific organs such as liver or pancreas.

WHAT ARE THE AVERAGE VALUES FOR BODY COMPOSITION?

Various attempts have been made to represent the 'standard body', not necessarily as a goal for individuals to strive for, but to provide a reference for generally healthy body composition, against which variations could be compared. The terms 'reference man' and 'reference woman' describe these hypothetical individuals. There are clear gender differences in body composition with a higher lean body mass in males (and consequently higher body water content) than in females. Females have a greater body fat content. These gender differences become apparent at puberty, when girls gain a greater proportion of fat than lean tissue, whereas boys gain predominantly lean tissue, and may actually lose fat during the teenage years.

Average values are as follows:

	Reference	
	Man	Woman
Weight (kg)	70	60
Lean body mass (kg)	60	48
Body fat (%)	15	25–28

Total body fat exists as essential and storage fat. The essential fat is needed for normal physiological functioning and is believed to represent 3% of total body mass in males, but 10%–12% in females. Highly trained athletes of both genders may have fat levels approaching these minimum values. The gender-specific fat in females is related to the reproductive role and hormone activity. At puberty, the growth spurt generally begins at a body weight of 30 kg. A minimal level of body fat appears to be needed to achieve (13%–17%) for menstruation to begin (perhaps signalled by a rise in leptin secretion from adipose tissue), and a body fat content of up to 22% may be needed to maintain menstrual regularity. If levels fall below these thresholds, menstruation will become erratic or cease.

WHAT WE CAN DO: FUNCTIONAL CAPACITY

Functional capacity can be assessed at every possible level, from molecular activity, through organ functions to whole body activities and capacity to cope with challenges. Functional capacity of groups and populations clearly also depends on the food intakes, and body composition of the individuals, as well as our food security at population and international levels.

If nutritional intake is restricted, then functional capacity will be compromised. If functional capacity is limited, there may be secondary impairment in dietary intake, and/or in the digestion, assimilation and metabolism of nutrients. This will also impact on body composition, and so on.

The starting point for this cycle can be malnutrition, or illness. When nutrient supply drops, the first functional response is conservation, by down-regulating metabolism, or activity, which requires that nutrient. The next stage is adaptation, to optimize overall function in a malnourished state. This commonly involves reducing all activities. In some situations, alternative metabolic functions can be recounted, but at a cost – will reduce efficiency. Examples include adaptation to a low carbohydrate diet, the body switches to fat oxidation, but this cannot provide glycogen for high-energy physical activities, so there tends to be sleepiness and inactivity as a secondary adaptive response. During selenium deficiency, selenium-dependent enzymes will accept sulphur instead, and this allows some function to continue. Zinc-dependent enzymes may be able to use copper as a second-best alternative during dietary deficiency, or if the body loses large amounts of zinc after severe burns. During heart, kidney or liver failure, the body accumulates sodium and/or potassium, sodium/potassium ATP enzymes operate less efficiently – and then is compensatory tiredness and weakness. In this case, it is restricting dietary sodium intake which brings benefit, to maintain a more healthful balance and improve function.

Functional capacity can be assessed biochemically and clinically.

BIOCHEMICAL INDICATORS

Biochemical indicators can include assessment of blood and urine samples for levels of a variety of nutrients and/or their by-products or for levels of nutrient-linked enzyme activities.

Blood (plasma, cells or serum) can provide a great deal of information. Analysis can be used to determine

- Actual levels of a nutrient in relation to expected levels (e.g. vitamin B_{12}, folate, carotenes, vitamin C in white blood cells)
- The activity of a nutrient-dependent enzyme (e.g. transketolase for thiamine)
- The activity of a nutrient-related enzyme (e.g. alkaline phosphatase for vitamin D)
- The rate of a nutrient-dependent reaction (e.g. clotting time for vitamin K)
- The presence of a nutrient carrier or its saturation level (e.g. retinol-binding protein, transferrin [iron])
- Levels of nutrient-related products (e.g. lipoprotein levels reflecting saturated fatty acid intake)

Urine samples may be used to monitor the baseline excretion of a water-soluble nutrient or to follow its excretion after a loading dose. Metabolites of nutrients also appear in the urine and their levels can be monitored. Twenty-four-hour urine collections can be assayed for creatinine to indicate muscle turnover rates or for nitrogen content to check protein intakes.

Analyses of bone include bone marrow biopsies, which will show the blood-forming cells, and radiographic examination, which can detect stages of bone development or rare-faction in ageing.

A large amount of research is currently directed at finding new and sensitive biomarkers for the activity of nutrients in the body. Developments in molecular biology have opened up possibilities of assessments at gene level to provide much more precise indicators of the exact role of the nutrient and the optimum level needed. A major challenge is to translate *in vitro* findings from laboratory studies to meaningful measures of nutritional status in humans.

CLINICAL INDICATORS

Both history (i.e. symptoms) and clinical examination (i.e. signs) can provide clues about nutritional status. Overall malnutrition causes tiredness and depression, coldness, suppressed immune function and amenorrhoea.

Clinical indicators are used to detect changes in the external appearance of the body. A number of nutritional deficiencies may cause functional changes which result in alterations in superficial structures, although many are non-specific. In addition, changes in appearance may also be unrelated to nutritional state. Signs occur most rapidly in those parts of the body where cell turnover is frequent, such as hair, skin and digestive tract (including mouth and tongue). Therefore, a clinical examination may include the hair, face, eyes, mouth, tongue, teeth, gums, glands (such as the thyroid), skin and nails, subcutaneous tissues to detect fat thickness, oedema, and the musculoskeletal system to note bone deformities, muscle wasting. There is very rapid loss of function with muscle wasting. This is often visible, for example in the hands, and in major leg muscle groups, but may be less easy to detect in obese people. 'Sarcopenic obesity' is a particular problem for the elderly. A number of classical nutrient deficiency syndromes affect the neuro system, for example with altered sensation or motor function, and the eyes.

WHAT CAN WE LEARN FROM NUTRITIONAL ASSESSMENT?

The aforementioned techniques can be combined to obtain a more detailed picture of the dietary intake and nutritional status of a population. Food intake at the household level has been monitored in the United Kingdom for over 50 years in the National Food Survey produced by the Ministry of Agriculture, Fisheries and Food (MAFF). However, this does not collect information about health. In the mid-1980s, a new approach was adopted in the United Kingdom, with the introduction of a series of studies organized by the Department of Health and MAFF. The first of these was the Dietary and Nutritional Survey of British Adults (commissioned in 1986–1987, published as Gregory et al., 1990). This collected information about food intake using 7-day records, together with blood and urine analyses, anthropometry and lifestyle features. The Health Survey for England and the Scottish Health Survey were set up in 1991 and 1995, respectively, to monitor trends in the nation's health, using a health and socio-economic questionnaire, physical measurements and blood analysis. These are now running continuously and provide an ongoing picture that includes key nutrition-related health indicators to assess changes towards government targets for health.

The National Diet and Nutrition Survey (NDNS) is a rolling programme of cross-sectional surveys of the food consumption, nutrient intakes and nutritional status of the general population, in age subgroups from 18 month and above, living in private households in the United Kingdom. Surveys have been published on pre-school children, older people over 65 years and the 4–18 age group. Other groups, such as vegetarians, people living on a low income and pregnant women are likely to be studied. Monitoring of people's diet was an essential part of the work of the Food Standards Agency, set up in 2000 in the United Kingdom. This remit is now shared with the Department of Health (DoH) in the UK.

Diet is dynamic and, for this reason, ongoing programmes of study and surveillance are necessary, to monitor both what people are eating and the effects of any dietary changes on the patterns of disease. The NDNS programme provides an example of this, aiming to

- Provide detailed quantitative information about intakes and sources of nutrients, and the nutritional status of the population
- Measure blood and other indices that give evidence of nutritional status, and relate these to dietary, physiological and social data
- Monitor the diet for its nutritional adequacy
- Monitor the extent to which dietary targets are being met

Other countries approach the monitoring of nutrition in similar ways. In the United States, the National Health and Nutritional Examination Survey (NHANES) collects data about food intakes, anthropometric indices, blood pressure and blood levels of minerals and vitamins. Surveillance of the diets of populations occurs in Australia, Canada and several European countries.

Cross-population studies are also performed; the SENECA (Survey in Europe on Nutrition and the Elderly, a Concerted Action) study is one such example.

HOW IS NUTRITIONAL STATUS INFORMATION USED?

The declared purpose of any nutritional surveillance programme is to identify links between diet and disease, and thereby to formulate policy and advice aimed at minimizing the risk of disease, by altering the diet.

Countries have food policies, primarily to promote a profitable food industry, and to some extent relate to the provision of a safe food supply. They incorporate a wide range of measures relating to production, taxation, trade, politics and social and consumer issues. In some cases, food policies may run counter to health policies, for example, by the promotion of fats, dairy produce and meat. These policies may also concentrate on public concern and legislation on pesticide residues, additives or food processing. Incorporating a nutrition policy into a food policy is, however, more problematic as there may be conflicting interests between food producers and the health professionals. Where nutrition is supported at government level, it is necessary for the government to facilitate the nutrition policy by changes to legislation, taxation, food labelling or other measures. Without such changes, a nutrition policy might not be workable. It is, therefore, important that government policy-making is based on solid nutrition surveillance information and that appropriate policy decisions are made.

The UK Food Standards Agency works with the Departments of Health to encourage and facilitate the adoption of a healthy balanced diet, through the Nutrition Strategic Framework to achieve the following objectives:

- Secure a sound evidence base for action to promote a healthy diet.
- Develop appropriate means of informing the general public.
- Identify and address barriers to changing dietary behaviour.
- Evaluate and monitor the effectiveness of the action taken.

In order to achieve these objectives, the FSA and DoH work with many other key players, including the Scientific Advisory Committee on Nutrition (SACN), an independent committee of experts, other government departments including Education, local authorities, the food industry and the scientific community.

See Chapter 19 for more on public health nutrition and food policy, pp. 363–381.

SUMMARY

1. The nutritional status is defined by (1) what we eat (our diet composition), (2) what we are (our body composition) and (3) what we (can) do (our functional capacity).
2. We can perform dietary assessment to obtain information on what people eat. The advantages and disadvantages of each method are important to consider.
3. Several techniques are available to measure body composition, each with advantages and disadvantages. They should be selected according to the purpose of the study, and the resources available.
4. The dietary information collected must be supported by the information about health. Both need continual monitoring, as neither remains static.
5. Information on nutritional status is used in making policy decisions about dietary advice to improve health, and this should be an important driver for food policy.

STUDY QUESTIONS

1. Which methods of obtaining information about food intakes would you use in each of the following examples, and for what reason:
   a. A study to identify groups in a population who have a high, or low, intake of dietary fibre (non-starch polysaccharide; NSP)
   b. An investigation into iron intakes in a group of children who do not eat meat
   c. A comparison of food intakes between two populations who have different disease patterns
   d. A pregnant woman who needs advice about her diet
2. What factors, apart from nutrition, might play a role in the health of a population? How could these be taken into account in results of nutritional assessment?
3. Discuss the different methods of nutritional assessment used in the following scenarios:
   a. Adults versus children
   b. Epidemiological studies, versus healthy individual versus hospitalized patients
4. Describe and evaluate the different approaches to nutritional assessment applicable and relevant to clinical and public health nutrition.
5. Discuss the methods available for measuring body composition in terms of principles, precision, accuracy and practical utility.

ACTIVITY

18.1 1. With a partner, try out a diet history interview on one another.
   a. Go through all of the times in the previous day when your partner might have eaten something, and ask him or her questions about it.
   b. Try to find out how much of everything they ate, how it was prepared, what brand name they had.
   c. Did they eat all of it, or were there any leftovers?

2. Reflect on how easily you managed to complete this activity.
   a. Did you and your partner have a pattern of eating?
   b. How easy was it to assess amounts of food eaten?
   c. Did you have the same ideas about what was a small/medium/large serving of a food?
   d. Could you remember everything you had to eat 2 days ago, 3 days ago, etc.? How far back would your memory of your diet be reliable?

BIBLIOGRAPHY AND FURTHER READING

Ackland, T.R., Lohman, T.G., Sundgot-Borgen, J., Maughan, R.J., Meyer, N.L., Stewart, A.D. and Müller, W., 2012. Current status of body composition assessment in sport. *Sports Medicine*, 42(3), 227.

Al-Gindan, Y.Y., Hankey, C., Govan, L., Gallagher, D., Heymsfield, S.B. and Lean, M.E. 2014. Derivation and validation of simple equations to predict total muscle mass from simple anthropometric and demographic data. *The American Journal of Clinical Nutrition* 100(4), 1041–1051.

Al-Gindan, Y.Y., Hankey, C., Govan, L., Gallagher, D., Heymsfield, S.B. and Lean, M.E. 2015. Derivation and validation of simple anthropometric equations to predict adipose tissue mass and total fat mass with MRI as the reference method. *British Journal of Nutrition* 114, 1852–1867.

Bates, C.J. 1999. Diagnosis and detection of vitamin deficiencies. *British Medical Bulletin* 55(3), 643–657.

Beghin, I., Cap, M. and Dujardin, B. 1988. *A Guide to Nutritional Assessment.* Geneva, Switzerland: WHO.

Black, A. E., & Cole, T. J. (2001). Biased over-or under-reporting is characteristic of individuals whether over time or by different assessment methods. *Journal of the American Dietetic Association*, 101(1), 70–80.

Bingham, S.A., Welch, A.A., McTaggart, A. et al. 2001. Nutritional methods in the European Prospective Investigation of Cancer in Norfolk. *Public Health Nutrition* 4(3), 847–858.

Cade, J., Thompson, R., Burley, V. et al. 2002. Development, validation and utilisation of food-frequency questionnaires – A review. *Public Health Nutrition* 5(4), 567–587.

Colhoun, H. and Prescott-Clarke, P. (eds.). 1996. *Health Survey for England 1994*. London, UK: HMSO.

DoH (UK Department of Health). 1992. *The Health of the Nation. A Strategy for Health in England*. London, UK: HMSO.

Ferro-Luzzi, A., Sette, S., Franklin, M., and James, W. P. 1992. A simplified approach of assessing adult chronic energy deficiency. *European Journal of Clinical Nutrition* 46(3), 173–186.

Food Standards Agency. 2002b. *McCance and Widdowson's the Composition of Foods*, 6th summary edn. Cambridge, UK: The Royal Society of Chemistry.

Frid, H., Adolfsson, E.T., Rosenblad, A. and Nydahl, M. 2013. Agreement between different methods of measuring height in elderly patients. *Journal of Human Nutrition and Dietetics* 26(5), 504–511.

Gavriilidou, N.N., Pihlsgård, M. and Elmståhl, S. 2014. High degree of BMI misclassification of malnutrition among Swedish elderly population: Age-adjusted height estimation using knee height and demispan. *European Journal of Clinical Nutrition* 69(5), 565–571.

Gregory, J., Foster, K., Tyler, H. et al. 1990. *The Dietary and Nutritional Survey of British Adults*. London, UK: HMSO.

Illner, A.K., Freisling, H., Boeing, H., Huybrechts, I., Crispim, S.P. and Slimani, N. 2012. Review and evaluation of innovative technologies for measuring diet in nutritional epidemiology. *International Journal of Epidemiology* 41(4), 1187–1203.

Jackson, M.J. 1999. Diagnosis and detection of deficiencies of micronutrients: Minerals. *British Medical Bulletin* 55(3), 634–642.

Jebb, S.A. and Elia, M. 1993. Techniques for the measurement of body composition. *International Journal of Obesity* 17(11), 611–621.

Kuhnle, G.G. 2012. Nutritional biomarkers for objective dietary assessment. *Journal of the Science of Food and Agriculture* 92(6), 1145–1149.

Lazarte, C.E., Encinas, M.E., Alegre, C. and Granfeldt, Y. 2012. Validation of digital photographs, as a tool in 24-h recall, for the improvement of dietary assessment among rural populations in developing countries. *Nutrition Journal* 11(1), 61.

Lean, M.E.J., Han, T.S., & Morrison, C.E. 1995. Waist circumference as a measure for indicating need for weight management. BMJ 311(6998), 158–161.

Livingstone, M.B.E. and Robson, P.J. 2000. Measurement of dietary intake in children. *Proceedings of the Nutrition Society* 59, 279–293.

Lombard, J.L., Steyn, N.P., Charlkon, K.E. and Senekal, M. 2015. Application and interpretation of multiple statistical tests to evaluate validity of dietary intake assessment methods. *Nutrition Journal*, 14, 40.

Ransley, J.K., Donnelly, J.K., Khara, T.N. et al. 2001. The use of supermarket till receipts to determine the fat and energy intake in a UK population. *Public Health Nutrition* 4(6), 1279–1286.

Stumbo, P.J. 2013. New technology in dietary assessment: A review of digital methods in improving food record accuracy. *Proceedings of the Nutrition Society* 72(1), 70–76.

Tabacchi, G., Amodio, E., Di Pasquale, M., Bianco, A., Jemni, M. and Mammina, C. 2014. Validation and reproducibility of dietary assessment methods in adolescents: A systematic literature review. *Public Health Nutrition* 17(12), 2700–2714.

Trichopoulou, A. and Naska, A. (eds.). 2001. The DAFNE initiative. Assessment of dietary patterns across Europe using household budget survey data. *Public Health Nutrition* 4(5B), 1135–1141.

Welch, A.A., McTaggart, A., Mulligan, A.A. et al. 2001. DINER (Data Into Nutrients for Epidemiological Research) – A new data-entry program for nutritional analysis in the EPIC-Norfolk cohort and the 7-day diary method. *Public Health Nutrition* 4(6), 1253–1265.

Section VI

Applied Nutrition

19 Introduction to Public Health Nutrition and Health Promotion

AIMS

The aims of this chapter are to

- Review and link some of the issues discussed in earlier parts of the book in relation to increasing health through improved nutrition.
- Consider some of the obstacles to improving nutrition that may exist.
- Describe strategies for health promotion and nutrition education that have been developed in recent years.
- Consider future directions.

To develop and implement policies for the prevention of a disease, it is important at the outset to make a realistic assessment of its prevalence and the extent to which it impacts on morbidity and mortality statistics in the population. Further, if these policies are to relate to dietary intake and nutritional goals, it is also important to make an assessment of the role of the diet in the aetiology of these diseases and how much gain can be expected from changes in the diet.

These are areas of controversy, often generating polarized opinions. At one extreme, it is suggested that, because we cannot be certain that diet plays a role in a particular disease, we should do nothing, with the implication that change could do more harm than good. On the other hand, others suggest changes based on very weak evidence, coming from a small database. However, between these extremes, there is a broad consensus on desirable dietary change, based on evidence from a large number of studies. Many of these have been re-evaluated using the technique of 'meta-analysis', which allows a number of studies with similar research criteria to be combined to increase the statistical power of the results.

Since its formation in 1948, the World Health Organization (WHO) has been working to improve the health of all the people of the world. In the last two decades, it has become clear that there have been changes in patterns of morbidity and mortality in many countries. These have arisen from

- Reductions in maternal and infant mortalities
- Better control of infectious diseases through immunization and environmental improvements, although the spread of HIV infection has run counter to this trend
- Increased population life expectancies owing to advances in medical technology and lifestyle changes
- Improvements in diets in some areas

However, in parallel with these, there has been a persistent rise in chronic non-communicable diseases, such as cardiovascular disease, cancers, diabetes, chronic respiratory diseases and osteoporosis. In the Western industrialized countries, these diseases have been well established for over 40 years and, in many of these countries, there have been decreases, especially in coronary heart disease incidence. However, there has been an upward trend in the countries of Eastern Europe and, most notably, in the developing countries.

Many countries whose traditional diet and lifestyle had been associated with a low incidence of non-communicable disease have been experiencing a period of food transition. This is typified by an increased consumption of animal protein and reduction in vegetable protein sources, generally associated with a higher fat intake. In addition, the intake of carbohydrate from starchy staples and minerals and vitamins from vegetables may begin to decrease. This has been noted in Japan, where the prevalence of obesity and coronary heart disease, both previously relatively rare conditions, has begun to increase. Countries such as China and those in South America are also experiencing this trend. In some of the poorer countries in the world, the gradual transition to a more Western diet, accompanied by rapid increasing urbanization and lower levels of physical activity (as well as smoking), is causing a rapid rise in chronic diseases. Because of the greater number of people in these countries than in the developed countries, mortality from chronic diseases has now outstripped on a numerical basis that in the developed world. There is also concern about the spread of overweight and obesity in these countries, and the potential for associated health problems, as has already happened in the industrialized world. These trends have been monitored by the INTERHEALTH programme of WHO, which studies the risk of the major non-communicable diseases in a number of populations around the world, as well as trends in diet and nutrition, and aims to promote and monitor community-based strategies for intervention.

In Europe, the WHO has developed the European Food and Nutrition Action Plan 2015–2020. This is an update to the Action Plan for Food and Nutrition Policy 2007–2012 and establishes a mission to achieve universal access to affordable, balanced, healthy food with equity and gender equality in nutrition for all citizens of the WHO European Region through intersectoral policies in the context of Health 2020. The guiding principles underlying this mission are as follows:

- Reduce inequalities in access to healthy food, as stated in Health 2020.
- Ensure human rights and the right to food.
- Empower people and communities through health-enhancing environments.
- Promote a life-course approach.
- Use evidence-based strategies.

The strategic goal is to avoid premature deaths and significantly reduce the burden of preventable diet-related non-communicable diseases, obesity and all other forms of malnutrition still prevalent in the WHO European Region, which are strongly influenced by social determinants of health and have a profound negative impact on well-being and quality of life. This reinforces the approach inherent in many nutrition policies in that it incorporates concepts of social justice and the importance of fair access to food for all.

The Action Plan stresses the importance of taking integrated, comprehensive action in a range of policy areas through a whole-of-government, health-in-all-policies approach. The key objectives will contribute to improving food system governance and the overall quality of the population's diet and nutritional status and will ultimately promote health and well-being:

- Create healthy food and drink environments.
- Promote the gains of a healthy diet throughout life, especially for the most vulnerable groups.
- Reinforce health systems to promote acceptability of changing to more healthful diets.
- Support surveillance, monitoring, evaluation and research.
- Strengthen governance, alliances and networks to ensure a health-in-all-policies approach.

The European Community has also enshrined human health protection as a part of all its policies. This has led to the formulation of a public health framework, including an action programme, public health policies and legislation. The EURODIET project has been one aspect of this and aims to contribute towards a coordinated European Union (EU) and member-state health promotion programme on nutrition, diet and healthy lifestyles. Progress has been made on European dietary guidelines. Other objectives of this project include the following:

- Translating these into food-based dietary guidelines within member states
- Promoting these to the population
- Identifying and overcoming barriers
- An European Food Safety Authority to oversee the food supply from its production to consumption

Despite some improvements in the incidence of coronary heart disease, it is estimated that, across Europe, the demand for treatment related to chronic diseases will continue to increase, because of the increases in the elderly population. It is, therefore, essential that changes in lifestyle and diet are introduced to reduce the incidence of these diseases, as clearly health services will not be able to cope with such huge increases in demand. There is, therefore, an economic benefit to be gained as well as the social gain for individuals.

Measures to prevent chronic diseases are needed, and these are the goals of many strategies around the world. It is recognized that such strategies must take into account all aspects of the food chain:

- Production policies
- Social policies determining access to the foods
- Education policies to increase awareness
- Dietary guidelines to inform choice

They must, therefore, involve the governments as well as all those concerned with food. Policy-makers also need to examine health impact effectiveness and cost-effectiveness in their decision-making. In addition, there needs to be a commitment to the strategy, which is translated into action. Much has been learned in the last decade about public health approaches that are likely to result in changes in attitudes, behaviour, risk factors, morbidity and mortality. Attention is needed to public health nutrition, which is the promotion of good health through nutrition and physical activity, and the primary prevention of related illness in the population.

The WHO (2010) Tackling Chronic Disease in Europe report (Busse, 2010) reveals that chronic diseases are the leading causes of mortality and morbidity in Europe and it is still increasing.

Currently, there are interventions to work towards tackling chronic disease in Europe. These include

- *Tobacco and alcohol interventions*: For example, pricing policies such as taxes, packaging such as minimum size of packs of cigarettes and consumption such as smoking bans in public places.
- *Sugar interventions*: Several countries have introduced a tax on sugar-sweetened beverages, and there is at least short-term evidence of reduced purchasing. The health benefits would be reduced dental caries, and a possible small reduction in weight gain of children.
- *Obesity interventions*: There are various approaches including public information and disclosure, targeting children and adolescents and taxing unhealthful food, but no country has ever established a sustainable effective intervention.
- *Hypertension interventions*: It is agreed that effective approaches to hypertension should be combined with other strategies aimed at reducing risk factors for ischaemic heart disease. Such programmes in Europe and elsewhere include weight loss, healthy diet, physical activity and moderate alcohol consumption.

WHAT IS THE BASIS OF HEALTH-PROMOTING POLICIES AND WHAT IS PROPOSED?

There exists public concern in Europe about potential hazards associated with recent developments in a complex food chain. This concern focuses on new infections, such as bovine spongiform encephalopathy (BSE), *Escherichia coli* 0157, novel viruses, and perceived environmental hazards from the use of genetically modified plants and food. Yet this concern is out of proportion to the effects on health from these sources, compared to the impact of dietary imbalances, which account for at least 100-fold more premature deaths and considerably more ill health. About one-third of all premature deaths in Europe are diet related and many are preventable. The cost of this burden of ill health is in excess of that caused by tobacco use. Despite this, the budget in most European countries for health promotion is, on average, less than 1% of the total health budget.

DIETARY LINKS

Over 100 expert reports, produced throughout the world over the previous 20 years, have been in broad agreement about both the major chronic diseases threatening health and the dietary changes that are needed to reduce their incidence. The change in disease incidence over the last 40 years has made it increasingly clear that changing environmental factors, including diet, are involved in their aetiology. Although we are now discovering more about the role of genes in the susceptibility to disease, these are rarely the sole factor in its development and, at present, are believed to play a much less important role than other environmental factors, such as activity and diet. It is also unlikely that genetic changes or mutations would have produced such major changes in a relatively short time span. The dietary trends seen around the world point to alterations in the balance of nutrients in the diet, which parallel, in most countries, the changes in disease incidence. Inevitably, there are exceptions that need explanation. In some cases, a satisfactory explanation can be proposed; in others, it awaits further research. Additional dietary concerns are also emerging, as our understanding of disease increases. Table 19.1 shows some of the proposed linkages between chronic disease and dietary factors.

Specific nutritional problems are also important. Anaemia is increasingly recognized as a problem among the female population, affecting adolescent girls in particular. Consumption of foods with low bioavailability of iron contributes to this problem and can result in reduced physical performance and cognitive function. In addition, where it exists in pregnant women, poor iron transfer to the fetus will impact on its early development.

The increasing number of older adults results in a higher prevalence of low vitamin D status. This appears to be associated with low sunshine exposure, even in Southern European countries. Bone pain, difficulty in walking and accelerated bone demineralization may all occur.

In Europe, there is still a problem with iodine deficiency, affecting populations in the central parts of the landmass and in mountainous regions. The use of iodized salt is an important public health measure, but education about its need is required. The consequences for maternal health and, in particular, the normal development of the fetus are profound, if deficiency exists.

LIFESTYLE AND SOCIAL FACTORS

In addition, other aspects of lifestyle are important. There is convincing evidence that physical activity is an essential component of health and interacts with dietary aspects in a number of ways including

- Activity increases energy expenditure and is, therefore, crucial for the maintenance of energy balance and normal weight.
- Activity increases physical fitness and the sense of well-being and may be important in the control of blood pressure, prevention of colon cancer, regulation of blood glucose levels and lowering of blood lipid level.

TABLE 19.1
Summary of Chronic Diseases and Other Health Problems with Possible Dietary Links

Disease	Dietary Excess	Dietary Lack
Heart disease	Saturated fats	Antioxidant nutrients
	Total fats	*n*-3 fatty acids
	Trans fatty acids	Dietary fibre
		Folate
Hypertension	Salt	Calcium
	Total fat	Potassium
	Alcohol	
Diabetes (Type 2)	Energy intake (via obesity)	
Cancers	Total fat/energy	Antioxidant nutrients
	Meat	Fruit and vegetables
	Salt	Dietary fibre
		Dairy products
Gallstones	Energy intake (link via obesity)	Dietary fibre
Osteoporosis	Salt	Calcium
	Animal protein	Vitamin D
		Fruit and vegetables
Dental disease	Sugar	Fluoride
		Dietary fibre
Arthritis	Total energy (linked to obesity)	
Liver cirrhosis	Alcohol	General dietary deficiency
Dementia		Folate
		Vitamin C

- Weight-bearing activity maintains bone health and limits demineralization of bone in later life.
- Activity helps to maintain muscle mass and sense of balance, which is important with increasing age to preserve independence and prevent falls.

The most prevailing social factor that impacts on diet and health is that of poverty. This has increased substantially throughout Europe in the last two decades, as a result of rising unemployment, more insecure and low-paid work and pressures experienced by governments in providing social security. All the evidence shows that the health experience of these groups is worse than in the better-off, with an average of 5 years lower life expectancy. This is attributable to many factors, including dietary choices, lack of physical activity, access to shops and leisure facilities, stressful life experiences and an increased burden of illness. Many dietary goals have now recognized the need to address such social inequalities; for example, the 5 a day programme was introduced to prevent ill health and also to reduce health inequalities.

On the basis of existing evidence, the EURODIET team has put forward population goals for nutrients, some foods and lifestyle features, consistent with the prevention of major public health problems. These are based on a review of the scientific literature and represent the consensus view. These population goals are intended to form the basis for food-based dietary guidelines to be developed, or that have already been developed within individual countries, which reflect the national diet. The population goals for Europe are shown in Table 19.2.

There has been debate about who should be the target population for dietary goals. Those individuals with most risk factors and the most severe risk factors will be in greatest need of intervention. However, they represent only a small proportion of the total population and, therefore, reducing their risk will make little impact on overall population morbidity and mortality. On the other hand, the

TABLE 19.2

Population Goals for Nutrients, Foods and Lifestyle Factors, Consistent with the Prevention of Major Public Health Problems in Europe

Component	Population Goal	Background Information
Physical activity level (PAL)	PAL > 1.75	Maintenance of energy balance and cardiovascular health.
Adult body weight	Body mass index (BMI) 21–22	An optimal individual BMI may be 20, and Asians may be susceptible to weight-related diseases above BMI 23–24.
Dietary fat (% energy)	<30%	The goal is for the prevention of overweight. Higher fat intakes up to 35% may be consumed with high levels of physical activity.
Fatty acids (% energy)		These intakes are recommended in relation to blood lipid levels. Stearic acid has little effect on these. A lower ratio of *n*-6:*n*-3 acids than at present is recommended.
Saturated	<10%	
Trans	<2%	
MUFAs	10%–15%	
n-6 PUFAs	4%–8%	
n-3 PUFAs	2 g linolenic 200 mg very long chain	
Alcohol (where consumed) (g/day)	24–36 (men) 12–24 (women)	The lower values are optimum.
Carbohydrates (% energy)	>55%	Rich in non-starch polysaccharides and of low glycaemic index.
Dietary fibre (g/day)	>25 (or 3 g/MJ)	Based on Southgate method of analysis.
Sugary foods (occasions/day)	<4	To reduce the risk of dental decay; frequency of consumption is a major factor. Important for lifelong oral health.
Fruit and vegetables (g/day)	>400	These have many health-promoting properties, including non-nutritional components.
Folate from food (μg/day)	>400	Bioavailability from food is only 50% of that of folic acid; needed for pregnancy and for normal homocysteine levels.
Sodium (as sodium chloride; g/day)	<6	Population benefits are greater than those obtained if only hypertensive subjects adopt the guideline.
Iodine (μg/day)	150	Essential for normal development.
Exclusive breastfeeding	About 6 months	Promotes immunological responses, lower risk of infection and atopic disease, reduced risk of breast cancer in mother.

Source: Eurodiet Core Report, *Public Health Nutr.*, 4(2A), 265, 2001.
MUFAs, monounsaturated fatty acids; PUFA, polyunsaturated fatty acids.

majority of the population will have moderate levels of risk. Improvement in these risk factors will have less success on an individual basis (because the original risk is less) but, taken for the population as a whole, will amount to a greater reduction in the population's risk of morbidity and mortality.

Hence, many strategies, such as the European goals shown here, are now targeted at the whole population, because this will bring the greatest reduction in risk. It also provides more social support for changes in dietary patterns. This does not, however, exclude an additional policy directed at those most at risk, with more intensive and specific targeting at this group. Of course, before this can happen, the problem of identifying those with greatest risk must be overcome!

Undernutrition, Malnutrition and the Double Burden of Disease in Developing Countries

Public health policy-makers face a particular challenge in developing countries where undernutrition, malnutrition and deficiency diseases remain a serious problem. Serious problems include protein energy malnutrition (PEM), and deficiencies in key micronutrients such as vitamin A, iron and iodine. The WHO estimates that almost 30% of the world's population are suffering from some form of malnutrition. The consequences of malnutrition include death, disability, stunted mental and physical growth, and as a result, retarded national socioeconomic development.

Iodine deficiency is the greatest single preventable cause of brain damage and mental retardation worldwide and is estimated to affect more than 700 million people. Over 2000 million people have iron deficiency anaemia and vitamin A deficiency remains the single greatest preventable cause of childhood blindness and increased risk of premature childhood mortality from infectious diseases. Intrauterine growth retardation, arising from poor maternal nutrition, influences growth and survival of the baby, as well as physical and mental capabilities in childhood. There are also major public health implications arising from the increased risk of developing diet-related chronic diseases later in life.

The double burden of disease refers to the fact that while many developing countries still experience high levels of undernutrition, at the same time, changes to traditional diets and lifestyles, arising from western influences, are resulting in a rise in chronic diseases including obesity, heart disease, hypertension, stroke and type II diabetes. Historically, undernutrition and chronic diseases were seen as separate problems, despite the fact that they coexist. This can lead to the full extent of the public health problem being underestimated, for example, using weight-for-age as the indicator for underweight children can lead to an underestimation of the levels of obesity in a population where there is a high level of stunting. All aspects of nutrition-related problems in a population must be considered as a whole when developing public health strategies and interventions in developing countries.

From Goals to Guidelines

In order to achieve the population goals, practical advice must be developed. It is recognized that across Europe, there are different dietary patterns, so national guidelines must take into account the existing culturally determined diet. Of course, there are many differences between intakes of individuals within any one country and these can provide an opportunity to study which existing dietary pattern comes closer to the desirable goals. In recent years, dietary guidelines have moved from being nutrient based to being food based. In other words, instead of recommending that consumers 'eat more fibre' and 'eat less fat', foods that contain these nutrients are used in the recommendations. Clearly, this is easier for the consumer to understand, as it coincides with how we buy and select our daily food.

Many countries are now publishing food-based guidelines, with the emphasis on foods and the numbers of servings to be eaten; these can also be used to develop advice for populations at higher risk, such as those produced by the American Heart Association in 2000. These recommend the inclusion of fruits and vegetables, whole grains, low-fat dairy products, legumes, fish and low-fat meats. Achieving and maintaining a healthy body weight through physical activity are included as a guideline.

Several stages have been identified in compiling food-based dietary guidelines. These include identification of

- The major food sources of the nutrients recommended (e.g. from tables of food composition)
- The foods contributing substantially to the intake of the population (e.g. from national food surveys)

- Existing food patterns that show differing levels of intake of key nutrients (e.g. from individual dietary intakes studies)
- Key foods that explain the major variation in intakes of specific nutrients in the diets of high and low consumers

With this information, it should be possible to identify the most important foods or eating patterns that could be targeted for change in order to move all dietary intakes towards achievement of a dietary goal. If this can be done for several key nutrients or foods, then many goals can be achieved. Guidelines can be formulated to include choice of products, menu planning, portions and frequencies of eating that have a sound basis within the target population. A further strategy may be to change the supply of food, by modifications to existing products (e.g. lowering the fat content, fortifying with a nutrient) or introducing new products.

Consideration of the population goals suggests some common themes. Reduction of fat intake and attention to the balance of fats with a reduction of saturated fat, and attention to polyunsaturated fats, especially those of the *n*-3 family, addresses a number of health issues. The reduction in energy intake that will ensue may be beneficial for weight loss, but, in many people, it will have to be counterbalanced by an increase in other energy sources. Most appropriate is an increase in complex carbohydrates from cereals, grains, pulses, roots, vegetables and fruits. These will provide not only starch, but also intrinsic sugars, dietary fibre and a wide range of micronutrients. Among these will be folate, the antioxidant nutrients and other non-nutritional factors, such as the phytonutrients, which are considered to be important as protective factors. A shift in the diet to fewer or at least lower-fat animal products may also occur as fat intakes are reduced.

The antioxidant roles of certain vitamins are covered further in Chapter 14, pp. 287–288, in relation to coronary heart disease and in Chapter 15, pp. 303–304, in relation to cancer.

Thus, a series of nutrient goals may be achieved by the same changes in the diet. In theory, this should make the giving of dietary advice more straightforward, as the basis of a 'healthy diet' will apply irrespective of the client's needs. Clearly, there will be differences in emphasis, for example, if weight needs to be lost, or if the appetite is small, as in older sedentary people or in young children.

In Britain, the Nutrition Task Force devised a National Food Guide (the Eatwell Guide), which has been adopted throughout many areas of nutrition education as the basic framework for achieving the nutrient goals.

The role of the Nutrition Task Force cannot, however, be viewed in isolation. It was part of an overall strategy, emanating from the 'Health of the Nation' paper, which has involved many in the move towards actually 'adding years to life' and 'life to years'. Since its publication, public health initiatives related to nutrition have remained on the political agenda. The Department of Health has recognized the importance of nutrition in a series of National Service Framework documents, published since 2000. These indicate the standards of service and care in relation to coronary heart disease, mental health, older people and diabetes, and, in each case, include a role for nutrition. The Food Standards Agency (FSA), created in 2000, became responsible for the public's health and consumer interests in relation to food and now shares this remit with the Department of Health (DoH). One of the key aims is to secure long-term improvements in the health of the population by working to reduce diet-related ill health, within the UK Strategic Framework for Nutrition. The main elements of this are as follows:

- Securing a sound evidence base for action to promote a healthy diet
- Developing appropriate means of informing the general population
- Identifying and addressing barriers to changing dietary behaviour
- Evaluating and monitoring the effectiveness of action taken

This framework is intended to form the basis for developing realistic and effective programmes for the future.

It is possible to illustrate how this might work by considering the Nutrition Strategy developed by the Food Standards Agency Wales. The strategy aims to improve the diet of all the people in Wales, but certain groups have been prioritized, owing to their poor diet and health, and, therefore, have the greatest potential gain from improved nutrition.

The top priority groups were identified as infants, children and young people and socially disadvantaged and vulnerable groups. The second priority groups were women of childbearing age, especially pregnant women, and men, especially middle aged men.

The main recommendations include the following:

- Increase the uptake of a healthy balanced diet to meet recommended levels for nutrients and micronutrients.
- Increase fruit and vegetable intake.
- Develop and manage initiatives to prevent and manage obesity and overweight.
- Ensure that schemes and policies are in place to assist improvement in healthy eating.
- Provide information and training to key players.
- Ensure that the public is well informed about the need for dietary improvement.
- Ensure that local initiatives are in place to tackle the main barriers to improving nutrition.
- Develop and promote initiatives with the food industry to improve healthy eating, especially relating to access to specific foods.
- Evaluate the impact of activities resulting from the strategy.

Key players in delivering the strategy will include policy- and decision-makers, health, nutrition and catering professionals, practitioners and educators at national and local levels, and the food production and the retail industry. Recruiting and training volunteers to become involved with local projects is important. The approach is, therefore, multi-dimensional and flexible, and able to focus on specific targets and develop local initiatives suited to the needs of particular communities. Settings for the interventions can be very diverse. They may include schools, workplaces, health care locations, the commercial sector (e.g. supermarkets), local clubs or day centres or even street markets.

A systematic review of interventions to promote healthy eating in the general population has shown that the most effective appear to the following:

- Adopt an integrated, multidisciplinary comprehensive approach
- Involve a complementary range of actions
- Work at individual, community, environmental and policy levels

Information provided by itself is insufficient to produce change. Thus, any attempt to implement food-based dietary guidelines needs to learn from previous work and adopt the lessons from other interventions. In doing so, the difficult challenge of changing diets to improve health will make progress.

WHAT IS HEALTH PROMOTION?

The aforementioned discussion illustrates some of the principles of health promotion, and these will now be considered in their own right.

The Ottawa Charter for health promotion, developed by the WHO (1986), outlines an approach to health promotion that includes

- Building healthy public policies
- Creating supportive environments
- Developing the personal skills of the public and practitioners
- Re-orienting health services
- Strengthening community action

It, therefore, demonstrates that health promotion involves more than just providing people with knowledge about the functions of the body and ways of preventing illness, and thus helps them to maintain well-being. This part of the process can be better described as health education, or if it is carried out in the nutritional context, then it is nutrition education.

Nutrition education, in turn, has been described as the process that assists the public in applying knowledge from nutrition science, and the relationship between diet and health to their food practices. Having the knowledge, however, is insufficient in itself to effect change. This can be witnessed all around us most vividly in the context of smoking. Almost everyone knows that smoking is injurious to health, yet a substantial proportion of the population continues to smoke. For knowledge to be translated into action, the environment must be supportive of the change and thereby enable it to happen. This includes the political context, the social environment and the individual's personal environment. In addition, the person making the change must have the desire and the belief that this is achievable, by the means available to them.

Thus, health promotion must be seen in a wide context. It includes the following:

- Having in existence the political and community structures that can make health-promoting changes possible
- Providing the information about health-promoting measures to all interested and involved parties
- Developing in the individual the desire to want to change towards a healthier set of practices
- Showing the individual that they have the ability to do this

Briefly, health promotion has been described as 'making healthier choices the easier choices'.

In the context of nutritional improvements, the introduction of nutritional goals is accepted as the responsibility of governments in most countries of the world. This was not always so. The first advice formulated about reducing fat intakes for the prevention of coronary heart disease was developed by the American Heart Association. This government-led approach had been perceived by some as unwarranted interference by the state in food intake, which is a purely personal matter. Nevertheless, without appropriate support from the government in establishing food production policies and legislation, for example, for clear nutritional labelling, the consumer is left without adequate information to make a choice.

Health promotion incorporates a number of related phases:

- Planning
- Intervention
- Evaluation

The public health nutrition cycle is used when considering new interventions for a population. It involves the following seven steps:

1. Identify key nutrition-related problems.
2. Set goals.
3. Define objectives for goal.
4. Create quantitative targets.
5. Develop programme.
6. Implement programme.
7. Evaluate programme.

Planning

This is arguably the most important stage and can determine the success or failure of the programme. Most importantly, the issue that is to be addressed must be identified. In coming to this decision,

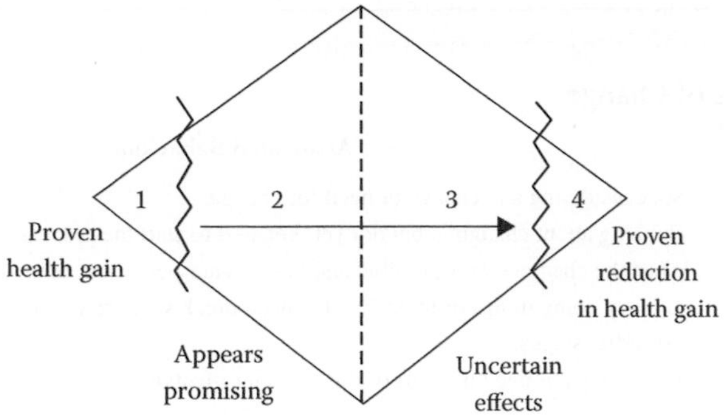

FIGURE 19.1 The health gain rhomboid.

the planners balance the perceived needs with the possible benefits. This may be illustrated in the form of the 'health gain rhomboid' (shown in Figure 19.1). At the two extremes, there are very few interventions that have been assessed and shown definitely to provide health gain, or to diminish it (i.e. at 1 or 4, respectively). Interventions classified as 2 would generally be considered worthwhile, but there may be an equal number at 3 that have not been fully evaluated and whose benefits to health promotion are uncertain. Where decisions have to be taken about the use of a finite amount of resources, most planners will choose interventions in the area 2, rather than 3.

A further element of the planning process is to identify the target group, since particular interventions may be more appropriate and relevant to certain groups. This type of planning and consultation was undertaken in the preparation of the 'Health of the nation' paper. During this period, a very large number of possible goals and targets were discussed, with supporters of each putting forward strong arguments. Eventually, only a small number of goals were identified, although these were chosen, because they were believed to be the most appropriate to achieve the maximum health gain. This has also been described in the case of the Food Standards Agency Wales Nutrition Strategy.

A further aspect of planning includes taking account of the nature of the problem, for example, by collecting data about morbidity and mortality statistics. Perhaps also at this stage, it is important to consider the lifestyle aspects of the target community. When this is being done at national level, the variation among communities within the country makes this more difficult.

Finally, general aims and specific objectives are formulated, taking into account the nature of the existing problem and the potential change expected. This, in turn, depends on existing knowledge, attitudes and behaviours of the target group. A very important consideration is the readiness to change on the part of the target. This has been studied extensively and a model developed that shows change as a process comprising several stages (Table 19.3). It will be necessary to consider what aspects of the programme will facilitate people moving from one stage to the next in the change process.

In the United Kingdom, the information about food intakes is available from Living Costs and Food Survey, published by the Office for National Statistics (ONS) and from National Dietary and Nutrition Survey data.

Intervention

An obvious but important element of this stage of the process is the decision on the methodology to be used. This should take into account information about previous uses of this methodology and their level of success. Constraints that might exist must be taken into account. For example, if the promotional material is presented in a written form, this necessitates that the target group can, and wants to, read. Computer-based images may be more appealing to young

TABLE 19.3
Model for Stages of Change

Stage of Change	Associated Behaviour
Pre-contemplation	Not considering any change or need for change.
Contemplation	Thinking about changing, but not yet prepared to start the process.
Preparation	When the change seems possible and benefits are perceived, ready to change.
Action	Actually doing things differently. May need much support and reassurance; may slip back to earlier stages.
Maintenance	New behaviour becomes part of the healthier lifestyle.

Source: Adapted from Prochaska, J.O. et al., *Am. Psychol.*, 47, 1102, 1992.

people than the written word. Thus, the methodology must be flexible and adaptable to meet the objectives with all of the targets.

The FSA Wales is employing a variety of interventions. Breakfast clubs have been set up in some schools, which can provide a healthy start to the day and encourage children to interact. Nutrition and health education activities in the workplace are increasing awareness of the links between diet and cancer in middle-aged men. Midwives working with vulnerable groups are teaching about meal planning and budgeting to reduce the numbers of low birthweight babies. Local grocers are involved in delivering fruit to schools as part of a school tuck shop scheme. Fitness training in a local club for young people is being linked with some nutrition education as well as smoking, drugs and alcohol education.

Evaluation

The process of health promotion may be seen as cyclic. The evaluation of one programme may generate questions and proposals for an improved programme, which can start with another planning stage. No programme can be brought to a conclusion without evaluating what it has achieved. In the case of health promotion, changes in some of the measures that were used at the planning stages may be indicative of success. These may include morbidity data, measures of quality of life or, in the case of nutrition programmes, changes in patterns of food purchasing. On the other hand, outcomes may be programmes and policies that need to be taken up in subsequent interventions. In its 'Eat well II' report, the Department of Health (1996) published an evaluation of the first 2 years of operation of the Nutrition Task Force initiatives. Follow-on initiatives have since been introduced, so the original outcomes have been superseded by new interventions.

The FSA Wales Nutrition Strategy is aiming for some quantitative outcomes, for example, in terms of knowledge about portions and increased consumption of fruit and vegetables in priority groups, as well as a balance of the diet closer to recommendations by 2010.

The national progress towards a healthier diet in the United Kingdom is more difficult to follow. However, there are indications that intakes of fat are falling, although rates of obesity are increasing. Intake of fruit has increased, although vegetable intakes are static. There is increased knowledge about recommendations to increase fruit and vegetable intake and reduce intakes of fat. Yet, generally food intake patterns remain resistant to change. Many studies demonstrate that people are not making changes for a number of reasons. These include the following:

- Confusion over the message (e.g. what is a portion)
- Perception that the messages are frequently changing and the professionals cannot agree
- Belief that the subject's diet is already healthy, so the messages do not apply to them
- Inadequate/incorrect knowledge about which foods contain particular nutrients

- Concern that healthy food is unappealing
- Perceptions about the cost of healthy food
- Beliefs about the availability of healthy foods, both in local shops and in catering venues
- Lack of interest

For all of these reasons, progress is inevitably slower than nutritionists and other health professionals would like it to be. However, if goals are made specific, measurable, achievable and realistic, then after a set time, some progress is generally found to have occurred. It is important to recognize that such small steps will eventually add up to more substantial change. Trends in the incidence of chronic disease will take longer to become apparent. Evaluation is, therefore, essential to ensure that all changes are recorded and lessons learned from them.

HEALTH-PROMOTION INITIATIVES AND THE INDIVIDUAL

Most individual consumers may know little about national initiatives and are dependent on changes in their own immediate environment to provide them with opportunities to improve their nutrition. This section will consider what difference health-promotion initiatives might make to the individual.

Information and Education

The *Eatwell Guide* in the UK is an example of food-based dietary guidelines and, as such, should be readily understood by consumers. It is used widely by retailers and health professionals and has been adapted for use with groups, such as ethnic minority groups and diabetics.

The Eatwell guide is covered in more detailed in Chapter 2, pp. 24–26.

Past advice had tended to focus on single nutrients. Thus, consumers heard the message that they should 'eat more fibre', for example. They follow this advice by buying wholemeal bread and eating a wholegrain breakfast cereal but continue as before with their previous diet. This may still be high in fat, low in fruit and vegetables, high in salt, or even all of these, but the consumer may believe that he/she is now eating 'a healthy diet'.

This focus on single nutrients has also led to an enormous increase in consumption of supplements, with up to 30% of some groups in the population taking supplements regularly. This again reflects the message about 'antioxidant nutrients', which are being consumed in tablet form rather than by amending the diet. It is possible that it is the chemical substances found alongside these antioxidants that may actually be the biologically important agents.

The Eatwell Guide moves away from this approach and provides a whole diet picture. It can be used in many ways, both as an educational tool in settings ranging from schools to antenatal clinics, a meal-planning guide or even a shopping list; and provides a non-verbal illustration of the balanced diet, which can be very useful in allowing each person to understand the guide in their own way.

Although we are exposed to many messages about nutrition and health throughout the week, some are more likely to persuade us than others. The effectiveness of a message is determined by the wording. Messages need to be the following:

- Reasonable (we should understand the message, and the reason for it)
- Practical (we should find the change possible)
- Compelling (we should want to do it)

We are more likely to be influenced by messages that fit in with existing belief systems, rather than those which seem alien to us. In devising messages, the health promoter must be sure that he or she understands the belief systems of the target group, so the messages will be understood and acted on. A common failing is that health promoters make assumptions about their target group's level of understanding; this can lead to misunderstanding of the message.

Schools

A network of 'School Nutrition Action Groups' has been set up as school-based healthy alliances among schoolchildren, staff and caterers, together with a community dietician. These groups aim to develop a health-promoting environment in the school, establishing, monitoring and evaluating a consistent food policy with health as the main objective, and providing healthy options on the school menu, at lunchtime and for snacks. It allows pupils, caterers and teachers to have involvement and ownership of school meals provision. The existence of good examples of healthy food aims to serve as an educational model. There is now more teaching of food and nutrition in schools, and computer-based packages to facilitate this have been produced by the British Nutrition Foundation. The introduction of new guidelines on school meals in 2008/2009 should help to integrate the educational and food-based messages.

The NHS and Health Professionals

It is recognized that the majority of people will turn to members of the primary health care team if they want specific nutritional advice. However, many studies have indicated that doctors may be uncertain about nutritional advice and, although they appreciate that it is important, often have not included nutrition in a consultation. This may be influenced by a number of factors, including lack of time, inadequate teaching materials, low confidence and patient's non-compliance. The practice nurse in the primary health care setting is more likely to provide nutritional advice and may have more time to do so. The importance of training in nutrition for many groups of health professionals is now widely recognized and included in the curriculum. A recent report by the Royal College of Physicians (2002) confirmed that nutrition of patients was a doctor's responsibility and should be supported by appropriate training in nutrition. A study of nutrition intervention in primary care (Moore and Adamson, 2002) found that there were good levels of nutritional knowledge among members of the primary care team. Diet was discussed with a proportion of patients, although practical aspects of food were not well covered. There is thus evidence of progress in widening the availability of nutritional information to patients. Multi-disciplinary nutrition teams have been established in many hospitals to ensure adequate feeding of at-risk patients in this setting. The WHO (2010) Tackling chronic disease in Europe report has stated that chronic diseases increase the complexity of health problems and the provision of care, requiring changes in professional activities, qualifications and care settings. It further supports that physicians play a key role in guiding patients through the health system, therefore need to be trained to coordinate activities. Some countries, including the United Kingdom, train physicians to play a guiding role and moreover, a new profession of nurse practitioner has been established in the United Kingdom and some other countries. There are also frameworks designed to help support the NHS and health professionals to improve nutritional advice, such as Improving Maternal and Infant Nutrition: A Framework for Action (The Scottish Government, 2011) was recently produced. This can be taken by NHS boards, local authorities and others to improve the nutrition of pregnant women, babies and young children in Scotland.

Media/Advertising

A major source of information for the layperson is the media and advertising. Because the most eye-catching news items are the ones that aim to surprise or shock, it is the sensational aspects of nutrition that tend to reach prominence in the media. An expert opinion, which apparently disagrees with the accepted viewpoint, becomes newsworthy and is published in the press. Where a number of experts have agreed, however, this is often not considered important and so receives no publicity. Thus, the overall impression given is that 'experts' always contradict one another, and there is no point in following any advice, as it is inevitably contradicted within the next few months. Regrettably, this is believed by many and frequently cited as the reason for not following any dietary advice. Information from professionally accredited nutritionists and state-registered dieticians is sound and based on scientific evidence. Unfortunately, a proportion of the information provided by the media is not.

The Food Chain

The food industry is in a very powerful position to determine the nutritional quality of the diet consumed. It is, therefore, essential that health promoters work with the industry. The potential for the development of modified products or new products with a healthier nutritional profile is there, and whether they appear on the supermarket shelves depends on the manufacturers.

In the United Kingdom in recent years, there has been a huge growth in the consumption of ready-made and convenience food products, and, therefore, a great responsibility rests with the food industry with respect to these. The provision of comprehensive nutritional labelling can help the consumer decide whether products are healthy or not. Eating a diet containing many pre-prepared meals makes it difficult to achieve the holistic view of the diet, as many complete dishes span various segments of the Eatwell Guide and make it impossible to gauge exactly how much of each component has been eaten. It is probably easier to achieve the balanced diet using more basic foods than predominantly composite dishes. Unfortunately, many people have little time and/or perhaps ability to do this, and may resort to eating a largely pre-prepared diet. There is evidence that cooking skills are gradually declining in parallel with the more hectic lifestyle and the use of ready meals. This highlights the importance of the food industry in making sure that this type of diet is balanced and healthy. A further challenge for the food industry is to respond to the drive for an increase in fruit and vegetable intake. Traditionally, there has been very little profit margin for the sale of fruit and vegetables, as minimal processing is required. However, if public health is to be improved and the food industry is to be involved, new and more creative ways of promoting plant-based foods will need to be developed.

Catering outlets also have a great responsibility, as over one-third of the meals now consumed in the United Kingdom are eaten away from home. Guidelines on healthy catering practice for hospitals, restaurants, fast-food outlets and in the workplace are available, with awards for good practice. Recommendations for the training of caterers have been drawn up. These initiatives should make it easier for consumers to be able to choose healthy eating in all outside venues, although, in practice, this is not always the case.

Constraints

Change is difficult for most people. Even if the health promotion is well designed and appropriately targeted, there may be some for whom it is not appropriate or for whom it is not possible to change. Some groups that are more difficult to reach by health-promotion programmes are as follows:

- Those on a low income
- The elderly
- People in minority ethnic groups
- Single men
- Children – who need specifically focused programmes

A Targeted Policy

It is useful to consider a more targeted policy as an illustration of how the aforementioned process described can be applied within a more specific health promotion context. The Folic Acid Campaign

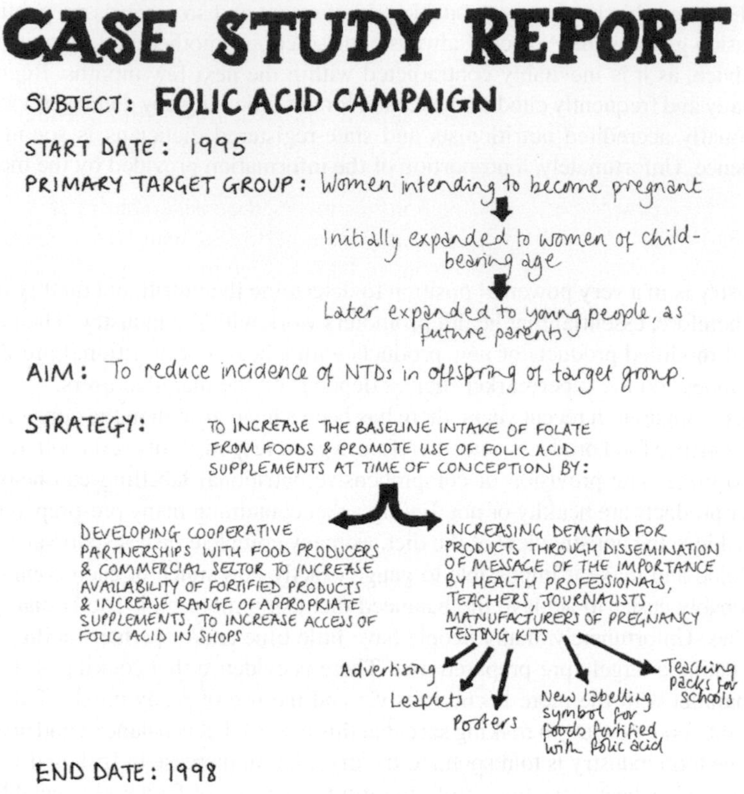

CASE STUDY REPORT
SUBJECT: FOLIC ACID CAMPAIGN
START DATE: 1995
PRIMARY TARGET GROUP: Women intending to become pregnant
Initially expanded to women of child-bearing age
Later expanded to young people, as future parents
AIM: To reduce incidence of NTDs in offspring of target group.
STRATEGY:
TO INCREASE THE BASELINE INTAKE OF FOLATE FROM FOODS & PROMOTE USE OF FOLIC ACID SUPPLEMENTS AT TIME OF CONCEPTION BY:
DEVELOPING COOPERATIVE PARTNERSHIPS WITH FOOD PRODUCERS & COMMERCIAL SECTOR TO INCREASE AVAILABILITY OF FORTIFIED PRODUCTS & INCREASE RANGE OF APPROPRIATE SUPPLEMENTS, TO INCREASE ACCESS OF FOLIC ACID IN SHOPS
INCREASING DEMAND FOR PRODUCTS THROUGH DISSEMINATION OF MESSAGE OF THE IMPORTANCE BY HEALTH PROFESSIONALS, TEACHERS, JOURNALISTS, MANUFACTURERS OF PREGNANCY TESTING KITS
Advertising
Leaflets
Posters
New labelling symbol for foods fortified with folic acid
Teaching packs for schools
END DATE: 1998

FIGURE 19.2 The folic acid campaign. NTDs, neural tube defects. A health economist might wish to compare the costs (C) of a programme to reduce obesity, against the potential saving in the treatment of diabetes (D) associated with obesity. If C is greater than D, then clearly the programme would appear not to be cost-effective as it stands. However, if one also could show that reducing obesity would cause a potential saving in treatment for arthritis and hypertension (A + H), it is now possible that the combined savings (D + A + H) could be greater than the cost C. In this way, a multiple benefit can make the programme cost-effective.

in the United Kingdom, initially commissioned by the Department of Health in 1995, is an example of a policy that was specifically targeted (see Figure 19.2).

The planning stage reviewed the evidence in the literature that the estimated risk of neural tube defects (NTDs) was progressively reduced with an increasing dose of folic acid intake and that supplementation with folic acid would significantly impact on the risk of NTD in the population. A daily dose of 400 µg folic acid was indicated as appropriate to achieve a reduction in NTD incidence of at least 50%. The primary target group for the campaign were women intending to become pregnant, and the aim was to reduce the incidence of NTDs, such as spina bifida, in their offspring. However, since almost half of the conceptions in the United Kingdom are reported to be unplanned, the target audience was initially expanded to all women of childbearing age, and later to young people, as future parents. It was thus intended that, as an outcome, all women would gain an awareness of the importance of folic acid supplementation.

The intervention stage of the campaign was designed to increase the baseline intake of folate from foods, as well as promote the use of folic acid supplements at the appropriate time before conception and during early pregnancy. This entailed developing cooperative partnerships with food producers and the commercial sector to increase the availability of fortified products, as well as an increased range of appropriate supplements in order to increase access to the vitamin in shops. The increased demand was to come as a result of dissemination of the message about the importance of folate, by health professionals, teachers and journalists. Manufacturers of pregnancy testing kits were also involved at this stage. Many diverse strategies were used to disseminate the message about folate. These included leaflets and posters, a new labelling symbol for foods fortified with folic acid, promotion of fortified products by advertising, and development of teaching packs for use in schools.

The campaign finished in 1998, although many elements of the promotion of folic acid remain in place as part of health promotion. Initial evaluation of results indicated an increase in awareness about the issue among women, wider availability of folic acid supplements and fortified products and an increased usage of folic acid supplements. However, women whose pregnancies are unplanned remain at risk as a result of low uptake of folic acid at the critical time around conception. The campaign can thus be viewed as only partly successful and demonstrates that the challenge of achieving change, with a simple supplement and at a highly vulnerable time of life, is enormous. Following 2003 SACN report guidance on salt intake were no more than 6 g/day, Food Standards Agency and the Department of Health took action to work towards the goal of reducing high blood pressure in the population. A Public Awareness Campaign has been running since 2004 to raise awareness of salt as a public health issue and to inform consumers how to lower their salt intakes.

- Phase 1 of this campaign was launched in September 2004: the key aim was to ensure that consumers were aware of why too much salt is bad for their health.
- Phase 2 of this campaign was launched in October 2005: the main focus was on encouraging consumers to check food labels for information on salt content and to raise awareness of the aim to eat no more than 6 g of salt per day.
- Phase 3 of this campaign was launched in March 2007, the main focus was to inform consumers that 75% of the salt we eat is already in everyday foods and to encourage and enable them to choose products with lower salt levels.

All three phases of this campaign focused on women aged between 35 and 65 years in lower social class. The focus was on women as they are the 'gatekeepers' of the house.

A variety of media has been used to deliver messages including TV advertising, posters, articles and news coverage. A salt website and materials such as leaflets were produced in all three phases of the campaign.

Evaluation of this campaign found that the number of consumers cutting down on salt has increased by around one-third, there was a 10-fold increase in the awareness of 6 g a day message and the number of consumers trying to cut down on salt by checking labels has doubled.

Working towards this goal also involved working with the food industry to reduce the levels of salt in foods as around 75% of the salt we eat is already in the everyday foods that we buy. Front-of-pack labelling was also encouraged to provide additional information to consumers on the levels of salt and other nutrients in food. The Food Standards Agency set, in 2009, targets for the year 2012 for salt reduction targets for industries. The challenging targets set across 80 food categories to ensure a commitment to reducing salt levels by food retailers and manufacturers.

ECONOMICS OF HEALTH PROMOTION

It is generally assumed that health promotion is inexpensive and will reduce health care costs. Thus, many see health promotion as a way of saving money. However, although it is possible that money may be saved through health promotion, this cannot be the primary objective. Health promotion involves various cost inputs, most obviously in the form of resources, such as health professionals, their time and materials. There generally needs to be an input in the form of government action whether through legislation or financial 'pump priming'. In addition, better health is also achieved by efforts on the part of individuals, which are more difficult to evaluate economically.

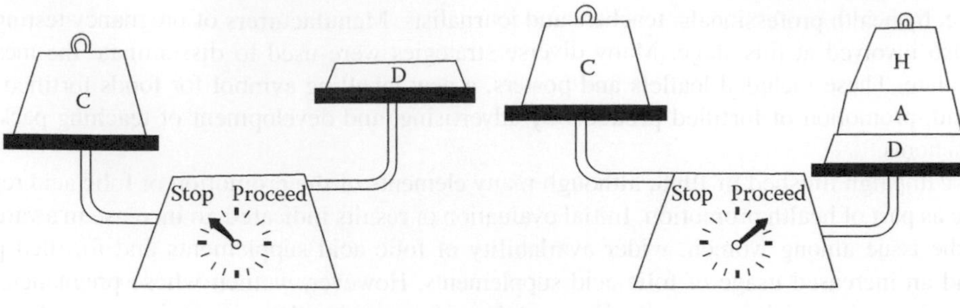

FIGURE 19.3 Economics of health promotion.

To evaluate the cost–benefit of health promotion, it is necessary to identify what is gained as a result of the programme and what has been forgone by diverting these resources from elsewhere (see Figure 19.3).

Because the outcomes of nutritional health promotion are often difficult to measure, decisions of this nature are rarely straightforward. Various measures of health gain may need to be used that show incremental advantages, rather than simply the ultimate goal of reducing chronic disease incidence. Balanced against this are the costs of treating these diseases and the loss of earnings that chronic disease can cause. Each case may need to be evaluated separately and on its merits. However, the more information is provided about nutrition and health and the more that people can be empowered to make their own choices in an informed way, the greater will be the potential benefit for health.

SUMMARY

1. Nutrition plays an important part in the causation of chronic disease. It is, therefore, essential that dietary change be introduced to reverse the high prevalence of some diseases.
2. Guidelines have been established by various national and international bodies that propose change.
3. The consensus on change recommends reductions in fat, and increases in starchy carbohydrates, fruits and vegetables.
4. Health promotion, that involves partnerships between the various players in the food system and the citizen, in a process of education and empowerment, can facilitate change.

STUDY QUESTIONS

1. Improving health involves more than just an awareness of dietary guidelines. What other aspects of life must be considered and changed to make dietary improvements possible?
2. List the major participants in the food chain and indicate how you think each could be involved in promoting healthier eating.
3. Discuss with colleagues:
   a. Where they have obtained information about healthy eating (if at all)?
   b. Have they understood the information?
   c. Have they acted on the information? If not, why?

4. Do you believe that nutrition information available generally to the public is adequate and/or an appropriate way of producing changes in the diet?
5. Survey newspaper articles describing nutritional issues over a period of 3–4 weeks. Try to look at a *popular* newspaper and one which is considered to be of higher 'quality'.
   a. Are issues handled differently and, if so, in what way?
   b. Do you find either of the article types more credible?
   c. As a result of reading the articles are you encouraged to change your diet?
   d. What can you conclude from this investigation?
6. Design a food policy for (1) a small island state with fish but no agriculture and (2) a northern European state with population 7 million.

ACTIVITIES

19.1 What common themes are apparent in Table 19.1 that could form the basis for coordinated dietary advice?
If you were presented with this group of suggested links between diet and disease, what specific dietary changes might you recommend?
Check these with the targets suggested in Table 19.2.

19.2 Applying this in the nutrition context, the nutritionist or dietician wants people to adopt healthier eating practices. Ways must be found to make these 'the easier choices'.
a. Who will need to be involved? Think of all the parties concerned in the food production chain.
b. What does the consumer need to know about the healthier choice?
c. How will the consumer be convinced to try this out?
d. What might the obstacles be and how can they be tackled?
In working through this activity, you should find yourself referring back to the key points made earlier about health promotion.

BIBLIOGRAPHY AND FURTHER READING

Busse, R. Tackling chronic disease in Europe: strategies, interventions and challenges. No. 20. WHO Regional Office Europe, 2010.

DoH (UK Department of Health). 1994. *Eat well!* An action plan from the Nutrition Task Force to achieve the Health of the Nation targets on diet and nutrition. Wetherby, UK: Department of Health.

DoH (Department of Health). 1996. *Eat well II.* A progress report from the Nutrition Task Force on the action plan to achieve the Health of the Nation targets on diet and nutrition. Wetherby, UK: Department of Health.

DoH (Department of Health). 2000. Folic acid and the prevention of disease. Report on Health and Social Subjects 50. London, UK: The Stationery Office.

Eurodiet Core Report. 2001. Nutrition and diet for healthy lifestyles in Europe: Science and policy implications. *Public Health Nutrition* 4(2A), 265–273.

Eurodiet Working Party 2. 2001. A framework for food-based dietary guidelines in the European Union. *Public Health Nutrition* 4(2A), 293–305.

Food and Agriculture Organisation/World Health Organisation (FAO/WHO). 1998. *Preparation and Use of Food-Based Dietary Guidelines.* Geneva, Switzerland: WHO.

Food Standards Agency Wales. 2002. Nutrition strategy for Wales, Consultation document. London, UK: FSA.

Gillespie, A.H. and Shafer, L. 1990. American Dietetic Association position paper on nutrition education for the public. *Journal of the American Dietetic Association* 90, 107–110.

Gregory, J., Foster, K., Tyler, H. and Wiseman, M. 1990. *The Dietary and Nutritional Survey of British Adults.* London, UK: HMSO.

Jackson, A.A. 2001. Human nutrition in medical practice: the training of doctors. *Proceedings of the Nutrition Society* 60(2), 257–263.

James, W.P.T. 1988. Healthy nutrition: Preventing nutrition-related diseases in Europe. WHO Regional Publications, European Series, No. 24. Copenhagen, Denmark: WHO Regional Office for Europe.

Margetts, B.M., Thompson, R.L., Speller, V. et al. 1998. Factors which influence 'healthy' eating patterns: Results from the 1993 HEA health and lifestyle survey in England. *Public Health Nutrition* 1(3), 193–198.

Moore, H. and Adamson, A.J. 2002. Nutrition interventions by primary care staff: A survey of involvement, knowledge and attitude. *Public Health Nutrition* 5(4), 531–536.

Office for National Statistics (ONS). 2014. *Living Costs and Food Survey*. London, UK: Office for National Statistics (ONS). Available at: http://www.ons.gov.uk/ons/rel/family-spending/family-spending/2014-edition/art-chapter-1.html#tab-abstract.

Posner, B.M., Franz, M., Quatromoni, P. and the INTERHEALTH Steering Committee. 1994. Nutrition and the global risk for chronic diseases: The INTERHEALTH Nutrition Initiative. *Nutrition Reviews* 52(6), 201–207.

Prochaska, J.O., DiClemente, C.C. and Norcross, J.C. 1992. In search of how people change. *American Psychologist* 47, 1102–1114.

Roe, L., Hunt, P., Bradshaw, H. et al. 1997. *Health Promotion Interventions to Promote Healthy Eating in the General Population – A Review*. London, UK: Health Education Authority.

Royal College of Physicians. 2002. *Nutrition and Patients: A Doctor's Responsibility*. London, UK: Royal College of Physicians.

Scottish Government. 2011. Improving Maternal and Infant Nutrition: A Framework for Action. Edinburgh: Scottish Government. www.gov.scot/resource/doc/337658/0110855.pdf.

World Health Organization. 1986. *The Ottawa Charter: Principles for Health Promotion*. Copenhagen, Denmark: WHO Regional Office for Europe.

World Health Organization. 1990. Diet nutrition and the prevention of chronic diseases. WHO technical report no. 797. Geneva, Switzerland: WHO.

World Health Organization. 2000. A global agenda for combating malnutrition: Progress report. Geneva, Switzerland: WHO.

World Health Organization. 2014. *European Food and Nutrition Action Plan 2015–2020*. Copenhagen, Denmark: WHO Regional Office for Europe.

20 Introduction to Obesity and Weight Management

AIMS

The aim of this chapter is to

- Provide an overview of the main factors behind the development of obesity and the components of effective weight management.
- Discuss the factors behind different likelihood of obesity developing in people from different backgrounds.
- Outline the components which need to be put in place for a weight management service.

OBESITY: WHAT ARE THE REASONS?

For a deeper understanding of this chapter, refer to the section on energy needs and energy balance in Chapters 16 and 17.

There is an enormous amount of literature on the complexity of the problem of obesity. The terminology used is sometimes tricky, because some words (such as 'energy') have multiple meanings in lay language, as well as precise scientific definitions. Obesity is a disease, with an ICD code like any other disease. It is best not considered as the state of having a particular size or shape, but defined as *a disease process, characterized by excessive body fat accumulation with multiple organ-specific consequences.*

Obesity is one of a relatively small number of diseases which is often on plain view to the public. The sufferer cannot conceal the problem. Moreover, it is also in most societies a value-judgement, a diagnosis which carries major personal stigmata. The word 'obese' is a perfectly ordinary adjective, from the noun 'obesity', whose latin derivation tells a causal story: *ob* – on account of, *esum* – having eaten. Although that remains entirely correct in every case, there are many other factors which give some people greater likelihood of predisposition to weight gain. So the victim-blaming approach to obesity, still evident in the way the disease is viewed and treated in may settings, is very wrong, and alienating if it is detected among healthcare staff. Surveys have shown that members of the general public associate obesity with a wide range of negative concepts, often including laziness, lack of self-control and untrustworthiness. People who are obese know very well that they are, but the lay associations are largely negative and accusatory, so it is a diagnosis they often prefer to ignore or try to blame on some route other than over-eating. In the English language, there are huge numbers of words and euphemisms used to refer to obesity itself, many invoking cynical humour. The term 'obese' is routinely used by professionals, in scientific research and public health statement, with 'overweight' as an intermediate pre-obese stage. However, with individual patients, the less provocative catch-all word 'overweight' is used to include the obese. Oddly, many obese people, and patients themselves, however, are often more comfortable using the simpler lay term 'fat'. To break the ice, it is helpful to ask individuals which term they are most comfortable with.

It is surprisingly difficult to determine at what point or on what criteria an individual is obese, or should be formally diagnosed as overweight or obese. The arbitrary but conventional body mass index (BMI) criteria (normal = 18.5–25, overweight = 25–30, obese ≥ 30 kg/m^2, were developed for epidemiology and adopted by WHO to describe the overall fatness or populations. However, BMI correlates only modestly with body fat content, so these criteria can be very misleading if applied to individuals. For example, athletes such as rugby players with large muscle masses commonly have a BMI above 30, with very little body fat. A slightly better correlate of total body fat is the waist circumference, with cut-offs introduced primarily for health promotion. Waist 'Action level 1' indicates the need for an individual to take note and make diet and lifestyle changes to prevent further increases (80 cm for women and 94 cm for men). 'Action level 2' indicates the point where health risks are high and professional help should be sought, and provided, to produce sustained weight loss (88 cm for women, 102 cm for men) (Table of waist cut-offs). These criteria are aimed at Caucasian people, and the equivalent figures for people of Asian origin are somewhat lower: for the same BMI or waist circumference, an Asian has more body fat, and greater metabolic health risk, than Caucasian. As well as correlating a little better then BMI with total body fat, a high waist circumference reflects metabolic health risks (e.g. for diabetes and heart disease) better than BMI. These waist circumference cut-offs form the key diagnostic criteria for 'metabolic syndrome', as a indicator for weight loss to reduce multiple risks, but still should not be used alone to diagnose obesity in any individual. The diagnosis for an individual should instead be made on the basis of their BMI and/or waist category, together with clinical features. A clinical staging for the diagnosis, similar to the sort of staging used to diagnose cancers, has been proposed by Canadian researchers, and this approach is gaining support internationally (Figure 20.1).

See body composition and waist circumference measurement in Chapter 18, pp. 348–354, and Table 17.3 p. 339.

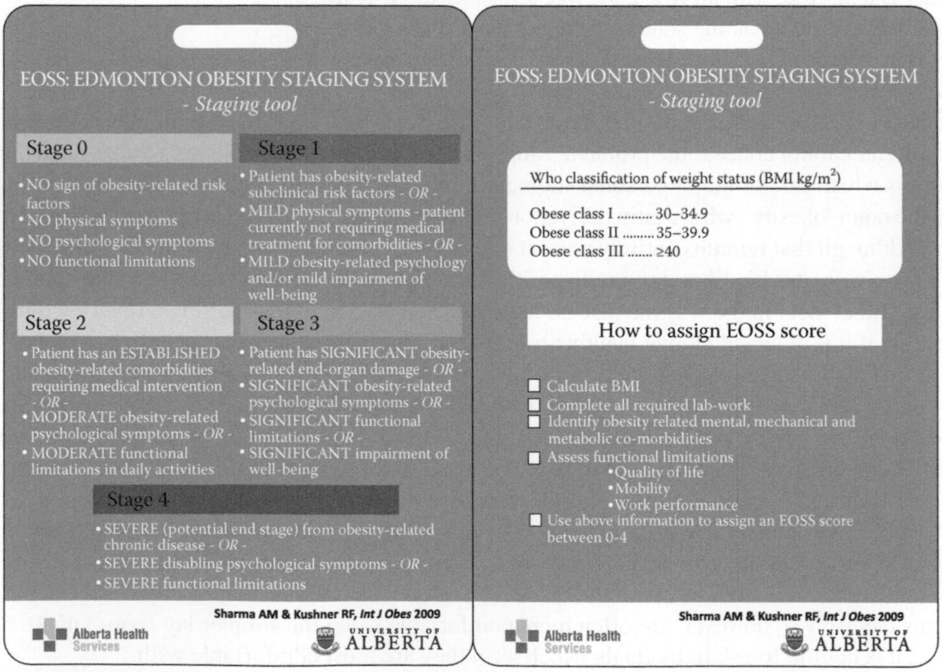

FIGURE 20.1 The Edmonton obesity staging system. (From Edmonton Obesity Staging System Pocket Card, University of Alberta, Edmonton, Alberta, Canada, available at: http://www.drsharma.ca/wp-content/uploads/edmonton-obesity-staging-system-pocket-card.pdf.)

Fundamentally, the problem is that at some stage, each obese individual has been in 'positive energy balance'. Weight gain, or more correctly an increase in body fat, can only occur if there is 'positive energy balance', when the rate of dietary energy intake (measured in calories or Joules) exceeds the rate of energy expenditure in metabolism and physical activity. Once overweight or obese, he or she then has adopted as habitual (or 'normal' to that person), eating habits which provide the extra calories necessary to remain at the higher weight. This chapter considers the reasons for this within an individual, and also why an epidemic of obesity has swept almost the entire world over the last 40 years.

Dietary Intake: Energy Consumption and Obesity

Data collected routinely for health surveys, for example in Britain, show that the average reported energy consumption has fallen steadily over 40–50 years. Over the same period, public interest in personal health, concern about weight gain and 'healthy eating' has resulted in colossal marketing and availability of 'low-calorie' or 'low-fat' products. Yet the weight of the population is increasing. As metabolic rate and energy requirement rises with body weight, a greater average weight of the population means, given that people are not expending more calories in physical activity now than 40 years ago (indeed they expend less), the population must be consuming more energy than previously, in order to avoid losing weight.

Over the years, a number of prominent scientists, encouraged by the food industry, have published influential papers in journals such as the *British Medical Journal*, suggesting that there is some mysterious adaptation in obesity such that people need less and less food as they gain weight, or that the entire obesity epidemic is down to reduced physical activity. However, metabolic research tells us very consistently that metabolic rate, thus energy (calorie) requirement, rises with weight gain. Long-term studies under totally supervised conditions show that obese people cannot survive on the same energy (calorie) intakes as thinner people without losing weight. There is no mystery. The explanation is that when questioned for surveys or in clinical settings, overweight and obese people report and record much lower food consumptions than they really eat. This 'misreporting bias' is seen in all populations across the world. It is an interesting phenomenon, psychologically (many aspects of personal behaviour are misreported – alcohol, smoking, sexual activity, wealth, etc., depending on the perceived reasons for asking the questions), but it means that self-reported food consumption or purchase data cannot be used to indicate actual food intakes. In population surveys, self-reported intakes give results which are the opposite of the truth in relation to body weight or BMI.

If instead of asking people what they eat, observations are made about food sales, they tell the opposite story. Painstaking 'food disappearance' data collection in United States over many years has shown that the population consumption of all food commodities and macronutrient categories has steadily increased and that is over a period when food wastage, at least for higher-calorie items, has generally fallen. Social eating patterns have also changed, to encourage greater energy consumptions. Over the last 30–40 years, starting in United States, there has been a profusion of new food outlets, from petrol stations to sports clubs, which add consumption in between normal meals. It has become normal to eat snacks between meals. Eating meals out of the home has become frequent, notably with aggressive marketing from huge and hugely successful fast-food restaurants. It is difficult, even for thinner people whose food consumption records tend to be more honest, to know exactly what they have eaten from restaurants, but we do know that the catering industry has been quick to absorb the fat skimmed from milk, or trimmed from carcases, and to sell these high-calorie industrial waste-products at a profit. It is also easy for people to forget, in their self-reporting, a cup of coffee which can add 300 kcal if it is a cappuccino or latte. So modern patterns of eating make food consumption surveys more difficult.

One of the main problems with the typical Western diet, in relation to weight gain and obesity, is its high fat content, which is affecting the control of energy balance. Within the fat, Western diets contain high amounts of saturated fatty acids, which promote diabetes and heart disease. It is clear from data on national commodity consumptions, and even from diet records and food purchase data over the last 50 years that the percentage of fat (and saturated fats) in our diet has increased, at the expense of falling carbohydrate content. However, interpretation of the fall in carbohydrate has been complicated by changing proportions of sugars increasing as starchy and complex carbohydrates have fallen.

Over 50 years ago, 53% of dietary energy was derived from carbohydrates and 35% from fats. Thus, for every 1 kJ from carbohydrates, the UK diet provided only 0.6 kJ from fats. By the early 1990s, carbohydrate intakes provided only 44% of energy and 42% came from fats, so that for each 1 kJ from carbohydrates, intakes now provided 0.95 kJ from fat. This represents an increase of 50% in the relative intake of fats. By 2000, the ratio had improved a little to 0.8 kJ of fat for each 1 kJ of carbohydrates. This is the result of a fall in fat intakes. More recent NDNS data show that mean fat intake met the DRVs, with the exception of women and men aged 65 years and over where it was slightly over the DRVs. The extra carbohydrates that are being consumed are frequently more refined than those eaten 50 years ago, with a resulting fall in the non-starch polysaccharide (NSP) and micronutrients which accompany carbohydrate in 'whole' foods that were normally eaten by previous generations. Figure 20.2 shows the results of a large study which suggest that a high fat intake is most likely to result in overweight. The results of four separate meta-analyses, reviewed by Astrup et al. (2000), consistently show that advice directed towards a reduction in dietary fat, rather than directed at reducing total energy intake, causes a reduction of energy intake and weight loss in a dose-dependent manner in overweight patients, with a typical weight loss of 3–4 kg over 6 months.

The metabolic fate of macronutrients is covered in more detail in Chapter 11, pp. 215–233.

Studies on the metabolic fate of dietary macronutrients reveal an oxidative hierarchy, with metabolism extremely well matched to intake in the case of alcohol, proteins and carbohydrates (none of which can be stored to any major degree), but not for fats. Alcohol must be broken down and eliminated quickly from the body because of its toxic nature and absence of storage site. Therefore, it dominates metabolic pathways and suppresses metabolism of other substrates. Most dietary protein is metabolized, after amino groups are removed, in the same way as glucose, and amino acid oxidation matches protein intake effectively. The only carbohydrate storage in the body is as glycogen, in small amounts in muscle as a source of immediate fuel through glycolysis for sudden exertion, and in liver where it serves a vital function, regulated by hormones and autonomic nervous system to maintain blood glucose levels. The brain and nervous system is normally fuelled entirely by glucose. When the direct supply of glucose from dietary carbohydrate falls, it is released from the liver and glucose oxidation is reduced in other tissues, to maintain circulating levels and the obligatory needs of brain and nervous system. Conversely, a high carbohydrate intake will promote its immediate oxidation and its storage as glycogen and will inhibit fat oxidation and promote conversion of excess glucose into fat stores (de novo lipogenesis). The regulation of substrate metabolism, and its matching with appetite and dietary intake is highly complex. Carbohydrate and protein appear to have the greatest influence, inducing satiety and its own oxidation through the release of several satiating hormones, including insulin, noradrenaline and gastric-inhibitory polypeptide, to produce very precise autoregulation of carbohydrate metabolism. This makes it easier for individuals on higher fat (lower carbohydrate) diets to overconsume energy without reaching satiety. After consuming excess fat, subsequent food intake is not reduced, so continued overconsumption can occur, almost without the subject being aware of it. Adjustments made to the macronutrient mixture being used are reflected in changes in the respiratory quotient (RQ), which rises as more carbohydrate is used in metabolism. In addition, a fat-rich diet has a high energy content per gram and consequently is of a small bulk

However, there appears to be little autoregulation of fat metabolism to match intake, and fat consumption has little effect on appetite to generate satiety, probably because the capacity for storage of fat is so large. Thus, an increase in fat intake does not trigger an increase in fat oxidation;

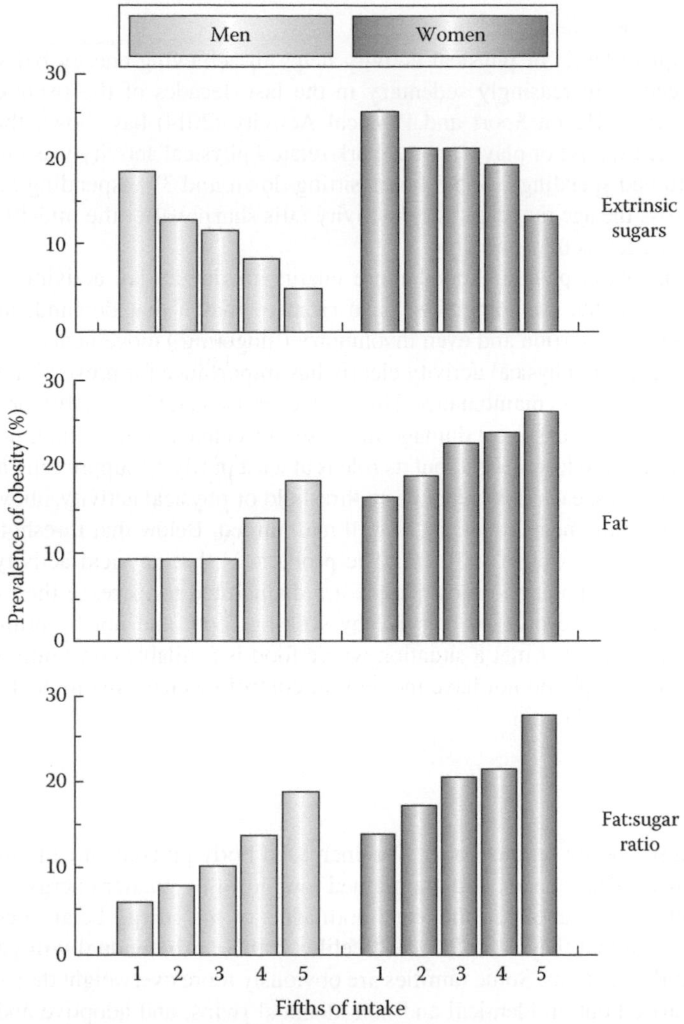

FIGURE 20.2 The relationships between fat and sugar intakes and body weight. (Reprinted by permission from Macmillan Publishers Ltd. *Int. J. Obes.*, Bolton-Smith, C. and Woodward, M., Dietary composition and fat to sugar ratios in relation to obesity, 18, 820–828, copyright 1994.)

instead, any fat that is in excess of immediate needs is stored. Thus, fat metabolism 'fills the gap' between the amount of energy available from the other macronutrients and the total required to meet energy output needs.

This is not a problem if the total intake of energy from the macronutrients equals the total energy expenditure. In this situation, the metabolic mixture reflects the proportions of macronutrients in the diet. Thus, in steady state of energy balance (when body weight and composition is stable), there is not only exact balance between energy intake and expenditure, but balance for all the macronutrients: the oxidations of carbohydrate, fat and protein all must equal their intakes.

When total energy intake is in excess of needs, the excess is stored as fat in preference to the other metabolic products. Dietary fat itself is stored very efficiently, with only 4% of its energy content being wasted in the process. If carbohydrate is stored, the initial conversion into fat wastes, as heat, up to 25% of the total energy, making this a much less energy-efficient process. Hence, in a positive energy balance state, dietary fats are more 'fattening' than carbohydrates or proteins.

Physical Activity

Maintaining adequate levels of physical activity helps in achieving energy balance. Societies in the West have become increasingly sedentary in the last decades of the twentieth century. The Eurobarometer survey 412 on Sport and Physical Activity (2014) has shown that an average of 42% of adults never exercise or play a sport. Work-related physical activity was also low, with 43% the population studied spending 2.5–5.5 hours sitting down and 37% spending 5.5 or more hours sitting down. Across the age range, physical activity falls sharply after the mid-1930s, contributing further to increasing levels of overweight.

Overweight and obese people expend more energy in day-to-day activities, simply through carrying more weight, but their appetites have risen to match that demand, and they become economical in reducing exertion and even involuntary ('fidgeting') movements.

In weight management, physical activity clearly has importance for preventing weight gain, and thus for long-term weight-loss maintenance. However, exercise is seldom useful for achieving weight loss, and can add to musculoskeletal damage in obese individuals. Some young men, in particular, can use physical activity to lose weight, but its role is at least partly by suppressing appetite. It seems that, as in animal studies, each individual has a threshold of physical activity, above which appetite is well matched to requirement, so weight is well maintained. Below that threshold, appetites tend to exceed energy need, so weight will rise. The problem is that physical activity in modern life seldom reaches that threshold, and most people are disinclined to increase their physical activity sufficiently. Humans have evolved to survive by seeking food, and not by minimizing physical activity, and historically never met a situation where food is available constantly without need for physical activity. We simply do not have the natural control mechanisms to deal with the modern environment without weight gain.

Genetic Predisposition

Genes cannot cause obesity on their own. The increased body fat content can only come from an excess of consumed dietary needs and maintained long-term by greater energy consumption than thinner people. However, genes can influence both arms of the energy balance equation, appetite and metabolism, such that they can alter the likelihood that an individual will gain weight under give environmental conditions. Some families are obviously more overweight than others, and much work has been carried out on identical and non-identical twins, and adoptive and natural parents to quantify the hereditary component. It is clear that there is a strong relationship between parents' weights (or BMI or waists) and those of their children, most obvious when their children have gained adulthood. Some of that is inherited genetically, and some through shared and parentally led behaviour patterns. The patterns of fat distribution in individuals also show familial characteristics.

It is clear that obesity is not the result of a simple genetic defect, but is determined by an interplay among factors that include genetic, epigenetic, environmental, nutritional, psychological and social variables. About 200 different genetic variants have been found to be associated with weight gain, or slightly greater BMI, but few if any have significant roles in causing obesity. Although a handful of single-gene defects has been identified as causing severe obesity in a few families, worldwide, ordinary obesities are not caused by conventional genetic factors. Obesity is more likely to be influenced by variations in gene expressions, and animal studies are leading the way to point to epigenetic effects arising from environmental and maternal factors in pregnancy (including overeating) which appear to direct the offspring's metabolism and body weight trajectory.

From the research base, it has been estimated that between 40% and 70% of overweight may be 'heritable'. The contribution of environmental factors may account for a further 30% of the cases of obesity. The importance of the environment has become clearer in recent decades, as prevalence of obesity has increased rapidly, from a constant gene pool in the population. The epidemic of obesity has grown without any change to the genes.

Genetic and epigenetic researches may yet have value at a population/public health level in identifying reversible, or avoidable, factors which modify gene expression and predispose to obesity. However, even subjects with a strong genetic predisposition to put on weight and become obese are able, with education, will power and support, to maintain their weight within a normal range.

Age and Gender

Body fat can only accumulate over time, so it is obvious that overweight and obesity will be more prevalent in older age groups. Patterns of weight gain vary, and at any age, an individual can arrest or reverse weight gain, but in general, an upward drift in weight becomes rather predictable for people whose weights are already above average from early teens onwards. The tracking of obesity, as defined by BMI centiles, is weak in children below the age of 11: the more overweight young children commonly revert to normal weight, and others only reveal their tendency to weight gain later. There is constant debate about the tracking of obesity from childhood into adulthood. Certainly, an overweight child has a greater risk of becoming an overweight adult. However, most overweight adults were not overweight as children, and have experienced positive energy balance in adulthood, as a result of factors operating later in life. When children leave school and enter adult life, the prevalence of BMI>30 is still only 5–6%, but that rises rapidly to reach about 30% by middle life, and now 40% by th age of 65. The most critical time for any intervention to prevent obesity is thus in adolescence and early adulthood.

Across the life course, there are several critical periods for obesity development. These include pregnancy and adolescence when altered hormonal factors may operate to promote fat accumulation, periods of enforced inactivity such as following injury or illness, and other times when social and psychological influences are operating, such as marriage and cohabitation, changes in employment and income.

The period with the most rapid weight gain is in adolescents and early adulthood, with trajectories flattening out in the 7th and 8th decades. In general, women tend to put on weight more rapidly at younger ages, and men catch up a little later. In United Kingdom, obesity is now present in 10% of men and 28% of women aged 20, and ~30%–38% of all adults aged 65. These figures have been rising steadily over recent years, and prevalences of high waist circumference even more rapidly, indicating that older people now have far greater body fat contents, but less muscle. This has worrying implication for health and social care in our aging population.

SOCIO-ECONOMIC STATUS

In Westernized societies, there are greater prevalences of obesity and overweight among communities with more social deprivation and low socio-economic status. In cross-sectional studies, this is seen consistently and markedly for children and for women, but less strongly for men. The more severe categories of obesity, for example BMI > 40 and >50 kg/m^2 show much more marked social gradients. Longitudinal studies also demonstrate a consistent relationship between poorer socio-economic status of origin and adult obesity. This finding awaits full explanation but suggested reasons include: a poorer intrauterine or early life environment, increased likelihood of bottle-feeding rather than breastfeeding and psychological/behavioural factors relating to social norms. These may include poorer self-esteem and attitudes to weight transmitted by obese parents. In addition, variations in environmental factors such as food availability and selection are critically important, with evidence consistently showing that low income creates barriers to obtaining a healthful, weight-maintaining diet. In the past, variations in food types available were considered possible important, but modern food retailing has largely evened out the types of foods supplied to different localities, tending to provide 'obesogenic' profiles of foods to all. There do remain some cheap high-fat foods which seem to be particularly culpable and whose sales are largely restricted to the poorest communities – examples include lard, 'meat-pies' made largely with animal carcase fat imported into United Kingdom as a waste-product from other counties, and the 'mutton flaps' sold to Pacific Islanders in New Zealand. Lifestyles in poorer communities may include low activity levels, where the environment precludes outdoor exercise, and costs prevent the use of leisure centres or gym facilities. Culturally acceptable body size will determine how much an individual may want to change their weight and, therefore, their acceptance of current weight or success in weight loss.

Many of the factors described earlier apply to people from the ethnic minority groups within British society, who in some areas are disproportionately represented among lower income groups. The National Audit Office report (2001) identified women of Black Caribbean and Pakistani origin as groups in whom there is a high rate of obesity. Asian men and women also have a greater prevalence of central adiposity that carries greater health risks at the same BMI or weigh as others.

Psychological Factors

It has been suggested that some individuals overeat and become obese for psychological reasons. Both emotional disturbances and personality disorders have been proposed as a cause of obesity, although in both cases, there is little good scientific evidence to support the theory. Depression and anxiety may occur among some obese individuals, especially those who binge eat. In addition, emotional distress and low self-esteem appear to be higher among the obese. It is difficult to separate cause and effect in these cases, as there can be improvement on weight loss. Stress has been linked to weight gain, both through a consumption of higher fat foods, but also raised levels of cortisol that is involved in regulation of abdominal fat stores. Those subjects who give up smoking are particularly vulnerable to an increase in weight, and the effects may be both psychological and physical in this case. An addiction to carbohydrate has been proposed, with the addict craving carbohydrates (e.g. chocolate) in the way others crave alcohol or drugs. There is little sound scientific evidence to support this.

Overweight may also be the result of abnormal dietary restraint and disordered eating, with characteristics similar to those seen in the psychiatrically defined 'eating disorders', anorexia or bulimia nervosa. These may be associated with poor or distorted body image, and greater sensitivity to external eating cues. In women, an inability or reluctance to achieve the ideal female stereotypical body shape created by society is believed to play a part in the aetiology of these disorders. It is widely believed that the current media preoccupation with idealized, thin and successful women in film, fashion or music industries is driving greater body dissatisfaction among young women in the West. This also impacts on the willingness of some young women in particular to engage in physical activity owing to reluctance to expose their bodies in sports settings. This demonstrates an interaction between social and psychological factors, resulting in poor control of energy balance.

If psychological factors are contributing to energy imbalance, it must be remembered that they are likely to play a major role in any attempts to normalize weight and should, therefore, be addressed in any weight loss programme. These contributory factors are summarized in Figure 20.3.

HEALTH RISKS AND COSTS OF OVERWEIGHT AND OBESITY

Many people still have the impression that being overweight or obese is only an aesthetic issue, linked simply to the appearance of the individual. As such, then, it is considered to be up to the individual to determine if they are content with their appearance. However, this is not the whole picture – overweight and obesity bring with them major health risks that can become life threatening. In population studies, ealth risk increases with BMI in a J-shaped relationship. Below a BMI of 18, there is increased mortality, linked to diseases that may have caused loss of weight, such as cancers and the consequences of smoking. However, as BMI rises above 25 and especially above 30, there is a progressive and accelerating increased risk of mortality. This has been recognized for almost a century when life insurance companies used body weight as a predictor of the 'risk'

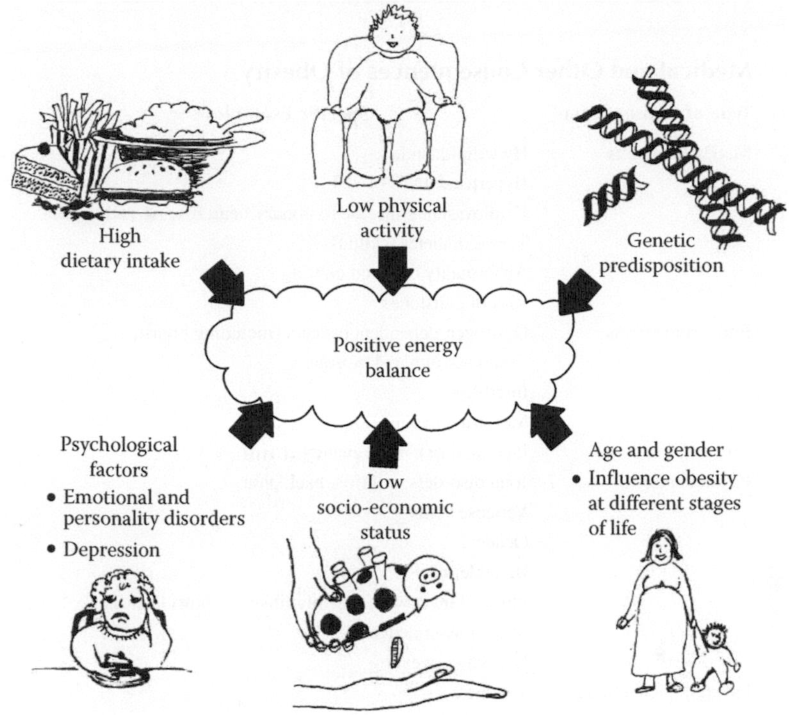

FIGURE 20.3 A summary of factors contributing to positive energy balance.

that a particular client might represent. Obese people die younger, mainly through cancers and cardiovascular disease. They lose on average 4–5 years of healthy life that loss being greater for those who become obese younger.

In addition to a greater risk of death, overweight and obesity carries increased morbidity, often starting at lower levels of BMI than for mortality. The physical and metabolic consequences of obesity increase with its duration, as organs and systems fail to cope with the increased demand put on them. Obesity itself has been classified by the WHO as a disease, but also brings a host of medical consequences. Those that have received particular attention are cardiovascular disease, diabetes and cancers. Cardiovascular disease has received particular attention, as there is striking interaction between obesity and the known risk factors, such as smoking, hypertension and raised blood lipids. In addition, Type 2 diabetes is also a risk factor and is, in turn, strongly associated with obesity. In fact, the risk of Type 2 diabetes is 110–20 times greater in an obese woman and 5–10 times greater in a man than in non-obese individuals. This potentiating effect between risk factors makes it particularly difficult to separate the many aspects of metabolic consequences of obesity. There are, however, also many other effects, some of which are listed in Table 20.1. Many of the consequences listed develop slowly and insidiously and are relatively uncommon in people below the age of 40. However, with the increased prevalence of obesity in younger adults and children, it is likely that the age of first presentation will fall, as it already has in the United States.

The National Audit Office report (2012) attempted to quantify the economic costs of obesity in England. It was estimated that obesity costs £2 billion from the national economy, including at least £0.5 billion in treatment costs to the NHS. Life expectancy is shortened by an average of 9 years; there are 18 million sick days taken each year from work and the overall mortality related to obesity accounts for 6% of all deaths annually. An alternative way to assess the healthcare costs from obesity is to collate all the costs incurred by individuals over a period from the records held

TABLE 20.1
Medical and Other Consequences of Obesity

Type of Consequence	Specific Examples
Metabolic effects	Hyperlipidaemia
	Hypertension
	Cardiovascular disease (coronary heart disease and stroke)
	Type 2 diabetes mellitus
	Abnormality of blood clotting
	Risk of gallstones
Endocrine effects	Oestrogen-dependent cancers (including breast, endometrium and prostate)
	Infertility
	Menstrual dysfunction
	Increased risk in pregnancy
Physical effects	Joint disorders, arthritis, back pain
	Varicose veins
	Oedema
	Breathlessness
	Physical inactivity (possibly linked to bowel cancer)
	Stress incontinence
	Excessive sweating
Psychological effects	Tiredness
	Low self-esteem
	Depression
	Agoraphobia
Social effects	Isolation
	Unemployment
	Family problems/marital stress
	Discrimination
Surgical risk	Poor wound healing
	Chest infections
	Anaesthetic risk
	Venous thrombosis
	Sleep apnoea

Source: Adapted from Lean, M.E.J., *Proc. Nutr. Soc.*, 59, 331, 2000.

by general practitioners. This analysis showed that the costs of both men and women rise steadily with each BMI unit, so the total cost of a person with BMI 40 kg/m^2 is approximately double that at BMI 20 kg/m^2.

TREATMENT OF OBESITY/OVERWEIGHT

Whatever the genetic, social and personal reasons for weight gain, excess weight can be only lost by reverting to a negative energy balance, that is by having energy intake lower than expenditure. And negative energy balance will *always* cause weight loss. Obviously that can be achieved either by cutting down energy intake, or by increasing energy expenditure through physical activity, or both. If the aim is to improve health, maintaining or increasing physical activity is most important, but in practice, few patients are able to achieve and maintain weight loss purely by increasing physical activity.

The big problem in weight management is not losing weight, but maintaining a lower weight, and preventing regain. Most obese people consider their lifelong habitual diets as normal, as do everybody else. Whilst most are able to lose weight, and know how to do that, it is hard for them to adopt eating habits with the lower energy contents (specifically lower fat contents) necessary to maintain a lower weight. Many still assert vigorously their belief that they eat very little, and they may go further to claim that they can live on very low calorie intakes, for example, 1200 kcal/day or even less, without losing weight. That is completely impossible: because metabolic rate is increased, no obese person can avoid weight loss if they consume under about 2000 kcal/day.

Studies performed in carefully controlled metabolic ward environments have shown that even subjects who claim that they cannot lose weight on very small energy intakes when at home will start to lose weight when their food intake is monitored and regulated. Unfortunately, there is a tendency among a large proportion of the population to mislead both themselves and researchers about their food intakes. Overweight and obese subjects are particularly likely to do this, with consistently under-reporting food intakes by around 20% – up to 3.3 MJ (800 cal) per day. This may not be a deliberate intention to deceive; indeed, foods and drinks are forgotten about as they are consumed without thought, or considered 'not to count', but as many as 50% of obese people may provide deliberate under-reporting. Many are prepared to admit this after successful weight loss, but the problem is pervasive and can undermine the therapeutic relationship.

The common objective of weight management is to reduce the amount of energy taken as food and/or to increase the amount of energy expended by the body.

More specifically, and to be acceptable, this should have as clear aims:

- To provide a diet that meets all the nutritional requirements to maintain good health, with the exception of total energy
- To satisfy the individual subjects dietary preferences, religious, financial and lifestyle constraints
- To have a realistic goal for weight loss, within a specific time scale
- To aim for a long-term strategy to maintain the target weight through appropriately chosen diet, behaviour and physical activity

Taking the focus away from weight loss alone as a target, modern guidelines for weight management in health services (e.g. the Scottish NHS guidelines SIGN 115) have established a broader set of health-directed aims:

- Improve health and reduce risk factors irrespective of weight change.
- Prevent further weight gain, and weight regain after loss.
- Optimize weight loss for the maximum number of individuals.

The major factor that will determine success is the motivation of the individual; hence, it is vitally important to assess the expectations as well as the willingness to adopt change. Dietary intervention needs to be accompanied by practical advice on eating patterns, exercise or other physical activity and long-term planning. Weight loss targets can be modest, especially if management is started at an early stage, as quite modest losses (e.g. 5–10 kg) will bring major health benefits. Also, success in a small weight loss can be more satisfying than a failure in a large one. Even maintaining weight stability for a person who is struggling with a weight problem can be seen as a successful outcome.

Energy-Controlled Diets

The energy contents of weight loss diets may be exactly specified or more flexible and can be constructed in many different ways. They generally restrict or exclude the most energy-dense items in the regular diet, that is those which provide the most calories per unit weight or per mouthful (such as spreading fats, cheese, sugar and alcohol.).

The actual energy content to be prescribed for a weight loss regimen depends on the individual, but as a starting point, diets with a modest energy restriction tailored to individual needs, for example, 500–600 kcal below energy requirement, are better accepted and followed than more restricted and fixed diets (e.g. 1000 kcal/day). The energy requirements of individuals can be estimated simply from standard prediction equations, as set out in the 1991 Dietary Reference Value book.

An alternative approach, to achieve much more rapid weight loss if they are followed correctly, is to use 'total diet replacement' (TDR), with commercial diets which are formulated as sachets and shakes to contain all the micronutrients needed for health. These diets are proving acceptable and safe. There is little difference in the weight loss achieved over 8–12 weeks (about 15 kg on average) using a very-low-energy diet (400–800 kcal/day) or better tolerated low-energy TDRs which contains over 800 kcal/day, so the latter are now preferred. They must also contain enough fat to avoid gallstones and enough fibre to avoid constipation.

With any energy-restricted diet, there is need to prepare the patient well for the transition back onto eating 'normal' foods and eating patterns which will maintain the weight loss. If the patient reverts to what they, and their families, have always regarded as normal, their weights will soon climb back. They commonly find it hard and threatening, particularly after a period of 8–12 weeks on a TDR regimen, to start eating food-based meals without introducing the various extras which were previously part of normal life.

Pharmacological Agents

Over the years, a range of anti-obesity drugs have been used, but, largely for political and economic reasons, they have mostly been withdrawn. Some had worrying but very rare side effects. Two types of drugs are currently used.

Orlistat is a pancreatic lipase inhibitor that decreases fat digestion and absorption from foods in the gastrointestinal tract. It reduces fat absorption by about 30%. The drug, therefore, causes steatorrhoea if large amounts of fat are consumed, with undigested fat appearing in the faeces, often as loose and oily stools. To be tolerated without unpleasant symptoms, meals must not contain over about 20 g of fat, as 7–8 g per meal can be passed in the stools without symptoms. The total loss of fat per day is therefore about 21 g, so close to 200 kcal/day. Most subjects do achieve some weight loss with the drug, an average of 4–7 kg, although this may in part be as a result of changes made spontaneously to the diet, to limit some of the unpleasant consequences when fat has been eaten.

The other group of anti-obesity drugs are centrally acting agents that act to promote serotonin and noradrenaline action, or to block their reuptake, and, therefore, promote satiety. Examples such as fenfluramine and dexfenfluramine, and more recently sibutramine, have been withdrawn owing to concerns about their safety, but it is likely that more drugs will be developed in the near future. The new class of glucagon-like peptide-1 (GLP-1) analogues is licensed to manage Type 2 Diabetes, by regulating insulin release, and have few side effects. In slightly larger doses for larger patients, they are also very effective for augmenting and maintaining substantial weight loss of around 8–11 kg. They have recently been licensed in US, Europe and elsewhere for weight control in non-diabetic subjects. A combination product with low doses of naltrexone and buprenorphine is also newly licenced in US, Europe and various other countries. It effectively reduces the drive to eat and leads to increased and sustained weight loss.

It is most important to recognize that no drug can ever generate optimal weight loss without active efforts by the patient, and results are best with the input of trained professionals to support diet and lifestyle modifications. Anti-obesity medications should only be prescribed as adjuncts to these other measures.

In addition to drugs that have been tested through proper scientific procedures, there are a large number of other weight loss agents in the market that claim to be the 'new answer' to weight loss. These have not been properly tested and do not come under the auspices of any legal protection as drugs. Unfortunately, people spend money on these, with little chance of obtaining the promised results. If weight loss does occur, it is likely to be as a result of better attention to diet than to the 'therapy' being taken. In some cases, the treatments may actually be harmful. For all pharmacological treatment, there remains the challenge to re-educate the subject to better eating habits, for long-term maintenance.

Surgical Intervention ('Bariatric Surgery')

Various approaches are used, all of them designed to assist in a weight-loss plan, in conjunction with diet and physical activity, and possibly drugs, rather than as the only means of weight loss. Some surgeons have been guilty in some parts of offering a simple permanent solution to obesity, with apparently little need for patients to do the hard work. The reality is rather different, so good patient selection and preparation for bariatric surgery is now recognized as important. These procedures may attempt to restrict feeding (jaw wiring, gastric banding), mimic satiety (intra-gastric balloon, gastric sleeve resection) or reduce absorption and modify gut hormone secretion (gastric and intestinal bypass operations). All these operations carry immediate risks in obese patients, with operative mortalities of about 0.2%–0.5%, and then a range of post-operative complications. About 20% require repeat surgery or attempts at reversal of the original procedure, and that is even more complicated and costly. Intestinal bypass surgery has now been abandoned because of the frequency of fatal liver failure, and gastric bypass incurs frequent problems with 'dumping syndrome' (dizziness and blackouts through low blood pressure and/or low blood glucose an hour or two after eating), and subsequent nutrient deficiencies caused by dietary limitations and malabsorption in patients whose habitual diets are often bizarre to start with.

In the past, surgeons have attempted to solve obesity by removing fatty tissue, for example, from morbidly obese patients in whom large amounts of fat hang down from the abdomen. The fat reaccumulates rapidly unless there is a substantial and permanent reduction in energy intake and the long-term result is a scarred mess. Liposuction is offered as a part of cosmetic surgery, to draw subcutaneous fat deposits, often from the buttocks or thighs. However, the amount of fat removed this way is minimal and makes little difference to overall body fat content. Again it will reaccumulate with ugly new shapes unless there is a permanent reduction in energy content of the diet.

Psychological and Behavioural Therapy

This may be formal or informal. The use of a psychologist together with a dietitian may help to uncover some of the reasons for the initial eating disorder and perhaps address the causes. However, there is very little evidence to suggest that psychological counselling, either alone or together with trained dietetic input, improves outcomes. A good dietitian will have some input in behavioural change methods during their training and will usually employ elements of techniques such as cognitive behavioural therapy. Much informal behaviour therapy occurs in slimming groups, where peer pressure and encouragement from the group leader may achieve better results than those seen in individual dieters. Motivation is a key aspect of group settings and may help the subject to continue with the process rather than relapsing. A group setting can help some patients by providing the societal support that may be absent in the subject's home environment, and can make them feel more 'normal'. Others are uncomfortable in group settings.

Physical Activity

This is often perceived as a useful method of weight loss. However, the energy deficit that can be achieved by exercise alone does not bring about significant loss of weight, except for some very energetic young men. For example, jogging for 45–60 minutes, three times a week, would use up to 4.2 MJ (1000 kcal) in a week and it would, therefore, take up to 2 months to lose 1 kg of body fat.

This can be contrasted with the possible loss of 1 kg within 1 week by a dietary intake deficit of 6.3 MJ (1500 cal) per day. The usual obstacle is fatigue and pain in joints for obese people who try to increase physical activity significantly.

However, exercise can be beneficial in maintaining long-term energy balance. Endurance muscles, such as those used in walking and gentle jogging, preferentially enhance fat rather than carbohydrate oxidation. This may allow energy balance to be maintained with higher dietary fat intakes. Exercise also tends to promote a dietary preference for higher carbohydrate foods, which are a little less likely to promote body fat accumulation. The net effect of exercise on appetite and food consumption is only to increase appetite (to oppose negative energy balance) at rather high levels of exertion seen among athletes in training. Within the more usual ranges of physical activity in the general population and especially among obese people, physical activity actually reduces appetite and leads to negative energy balance and weight loss. The mechanisms responsible are poorly understood but may include better activation in the brain of the hormone leptin, which reduces appetite. Regular exercise has been shown to increase insulin sensitivity, reduce plasma triglyceride and very-low-density lipoprotein (VLDL) levels, raise high-density lipoprotein (HDL) levels and lower mildly elevated blood pressure in overweight people.

Overall, the effect of exercise on changes in total body weight may be small. However, exercise may make it easier to achieve energy balance and, once weight is lost, it is definitely helpful in the maintenance of the new weight. Importantly there will also be protection of lean tissue during the period of weight loss, if the energy restriction is accompanied by exercise. Endurance muscles (with Type 1 muscle fibres) are specifically increased by regular physical activity. This is the type of muscle that oxidizes fatty acids, a valuable factor for preventing Type 2 diabetes.

Perhaps most importantly, regular physical activity produces feelings of well-being, by a range of neuroendocine mechanisms which may include the release of serotonin and endogenous opiates in the brain. This effect may be particularly beneficial to a subject attempting to lose weight. A restricted food intake may induce feelings of dissatisfaction, possibly even depression for some, which could be counteracted by the stimulation produced by exercise. Physical activity is a powerful but rather neglected antidepressant.

Unsafe Methods of Weight Loss

There are very many dietary regimes that offer rapid weight loss, often linked to the consumption of particular 'wonder remedies'. They may require the dieter to eat more of a particular food (grapefruit is a classic example), or a specific product, which has to be bought from the 'counsellor'. These are unproven, possibly unsafe, and should be avoided. There is no 'magic wand' remedy.

Summary

1. The disease process of obesity, which leads to excessive body fat accumulation and subsequently multiple organ-specific pathologies and symptoms, has complicated causation.
2. Like all diseases there are endogenous and environmental factors, but obesity can only develop through a period of positive energy balance.
3. Conversely, obesity can always be prevented or reversed by interventions which produce a period of negative energy balance (whatever may be the causes in the individual case).
4. Modern weight management follows evidence-based guidelines and recognizes the needs for sustained professional support for individual patients as well as societal and political interventions for primary prevention.

STUDY QUESTIONS

1. Should national public health policy focus more on obesity prevention or treatment?
2. Think about the strategies that could be implemented to prevent childhood obesity. Which approach would you prioritize and why?
3. Can modifications to the food system and the food environment be effective to tackle obesity in Western countries?

ACTIVITY

17.1 You read the following article in your local paper:

Amazing Weight Loss Breakthrough!!

Doctors at the University of Nirvana have made a revolutionary new discovery, which will change the life of literally millions of people. Volunteers in their laboratories have been eating only three different foods a day and have lost an astonishing 30 lbs in a month! The secret of their success is eating just one food at each meal. It doesn't matter what food you eat, but it must never be eaten with anything else. So, if you feel like ice cream for breakfast, chocolate for lunch and a steak for dinner – go ahead, the weight will still fall off and you will emerge a slimmer, fitter person.

Doctors claim that anyone can get the same results, as long as they stick to the diet regime of only one food at each meal. They explain that the body needs other foods to help the digestion process. When we eat only one food at a time, food breakdown stops, and so the calories can't pile on! Results like this have never been obtained before, and it is likely that the whole country will become 'One Food a Meal' crazy. The scientists do offer a word of caution, however. The weight loss is so astonishing that you should not need to stay on the diet for more than 4 weeks at a time. It may be dangerous if you continue on it for longer than this.

- What effect would you expect this article to have if it were published in the national newspapers?
- What alternative explanations for the findings might there be?
- Why might an article like this be nutritionally dangerous?
- Try to find some articles in newspapers or magazines that you feel are misleading and potentially harmful.
- Attempt to identify what it is about the article that concerns you.
- Try to think of an explanation for the way the article has been written.

BIBLIOGRAPHY AND FURTHER READING

Astrup, A., Ryan, L., Grunwald, G. et al. 2000. The role of dietary fat in body fatness: Evidence from a preliminary meta-analysis of ad libitum low-fat dietary intervention studies. *British Journal of Nutrition* 83(Suppl. 1), S25–S32.

Bolton-Smith, C. and Woodward, M. 1994. Dietary composition and fat to sugar ratios in relation to obesity. *International Journal of Obesity* 18, 820–828.

Bouchard, C. and Perusse, L. 1993. Genetics of obesity. *Annual Review of Nutrition* 13, 337–354.

British Nutrition Foundation. 1999. Obesity. The report of the British Nutrition Foundation Task Force. London, UK: Blackwell Science.

Clydesdale, F.M. (ed.). 1995. Nutrition and health aspects of sugars. Proceedings of a workshop. *American Journal of Clinical Nutrition* 62(1S).

Davies, J. 1994. Review of fad diets. *Nutrition and Food Science* 5, 22–24.

DoH (UK Department of Health). 1995. Obesity: Reversing the increasing problem of obesity in England. A report from the Nutrition and Physical Activity Task Forces. Wetherby, UK: Department of Health.

Edmonton Obesity Staging System Pocket Card. Edmonton, Alberta, Canada: University of Alberta. Available at: http://www.drsharma.ca/wp-content/uploads/edmonton-obesity-staging-system-pocket-card.pdf.

European Commision. 2014. Special Eurobarometer 412 – Sport and Physical activity. ec.europa.eu/health/nutrition_physical_activity/docs/ebs_412_en.pdf.

Great Britain National Audit Office. 2001. Tackling obesity in England. House of Commons papers 2000–01 220. London, UK: The Stationnary Office.

Great Britain National Audit Office. 2012. An update on the government's approach to tackling obesity – A report by the Controller and Auditor General. London, UK: The Stationery Office.

Kirk, T.R. 2000. Role of dietary carbohydrate and frequent eating in body weight control. *Proceedings of the Nutrition Society* 59, 349–358.

Lean, M.E.J. 2000. Pathophysiology of obesity. *Proceedings of the Nutrition Society* 59, 331–336.

Lean, M.E.J., Han, T.S. and Morrison, C.E. 1995. Waist circumference as a measure for indicating need for weight management. *British Medical Journal* 311, 158–161.

Lissner, L. and Heitmann, B.L. 1995. Dietary fat and obesity: Evidence from epidemiology. *European Journal of Clinical Nutrition* 49(2), 79–90.

McCombie, L., Lean, M.E. and Tigbe, W.W. 2015. Cost-effectiveness of obesity treatment. *Medicine* 43(2), 104–107.

Moloney, M. 2000. Dietary treatment of obesity. *Proceedings of the Nutrition Society* 59, 601–608.

Moore, M.S. 2000. Interactions between physical activity and diet in the regulation of body weight. *Proceedings of the Nutrition Society* 53, 193–198.

Parsons, T., Power, C., Logan, S. et al. 1999. Childhood predictors of adult obesity: A systematic review. *International Journal of Obesity* 23(Suppl. 8), 1–107.

Prentice, A.M. and Jebb, S.A. 1995. Obesity in Britain: Gluttony or sloth? *British Medical Journal* 311, 437–439.

Scottish Intercollegiate Guidelines Network (SIGN). 1996. *Obesity in Scotland: Integrating Prevention with Weight Measurement*. Edinburgh, UK: Royal College of Physicians.

Sharma, A.M. and Kushner, R.F. 2009. A proposed clinical staging system for obesity. *International Journal of Obesity* 33(3), 289–295.

Singhal, A., Farooqi, I.S., O'Rahilly, S. et al. 2002. Early nutrition and leptin concentration in later life. *American Journal of Clinical Nutrition* 75, 993–999.

Stewart, L. 2015. Childhood obesity. *Medicine* 43(2), 108–111.

Vlassopoulos, A., Combet, E. and Lean, M.E. 2014. Changing distributions of body size and adiposity with age. *International Journal of Obesity* 38(6), 857–864.

World Health Organisation. 1998. *Obesity: Preventing and Managing the Global Epidemic*. Geneva, Switzerland: WHO.

21 Introduction to Clinical Nutrition

AIMS

The aim of this chapter is to

1. Explain what is meant by 'nutritional status' and how it interacts with illnesses.
2. Outline measures which should be taken by all health professionals, with an awareness that an illness can affect nutritional status, and that nutritional status will affect the course of any illness.
3. Provide an overview of optimal nutritional provision during illness, with consideration of the route of administration (oral or artificial, enteral or parenteral) and of diet composition (quantity and quality).
4. Introduce the concepts around intolerance and allergy to foods and nutrients, and how these may compromise health.

Clinical nutrition is the application of nutritional science within a clinical setting. It is therefore relevant for all health professionals involved in the management of patients with, or at risk of, disease.

- Treatment of patients with an existing medical condition that is caused, precipitated or aggravated by nutritional insufficiency. This includes individuals with the classical single-nutrient deficiency diseases, but also those who experience major weight gain or loss, and those with multifactorial diseases such as type 2 diabetes and heart disease
- Treatment of patients with conditions that put them at risk of secondary medical conditions through a nutritional deficit, for example, those with dietary restrictions (either advised and self-imposed), those with metabolic defects of nutrient handling (e.g. inborn errors and liver diseases), those with altered metabolic/nutrient demands (including pregnancy) and those with conditions which result in abnormal nutrient losses, including limited gastric or intestinal function with vomiting and malabsorption syndromes, some kidney diseases and transdermal losses

Clinical nutrition is distinct from dietetics. A dietician is a trained, registered professional with a legally protected title. A state registered dietician (SRD) in United Kingdom (RD in United states) must meet a defined set of statutory criteria, to ensure that their clients/patients receive reliable advice; a bachelor's degree with an accredited nutrition curriculum; satisfactory performance on the registration exam and a supervised internship at an approved health-care facility, foodservice organisation or community agency. A dietician directs the provision of special diets for medical reasons, including the use of nutritional supplements, and advises people how to eat as part of a healthy lifestyle or to achieve a specific health-related goal. Dieticians work in a range of settings from clinical to community, public health policy and food industry. Clinical nutrition, as a specialty, is not defined by statute and includes individuals from a variety of health-care backgrounds who form multidisciplinary teams. It is studied at post graduate level. Dieticians are always involved when there is a need to integrate specific nutritional demands with the overall dietary adequacy of individuals, but clinical nutritionists include a range of trained health professionals: doctors, nurses, pharmacists and indeed registered dieticians. Clinical nutritionists do not simply provide dietary advice to patients. They are involved in determining complex artificial or 'prosthetic' feeding regimens (i.e. intravenous or enteral feeding), and in the detailed metabolic investigations which define specific nutrition support protocols for sick individuals. Clinical nutritionists are involved in research to generate evidence for improved management, including the interactions between diet or nutritional status and other aspects of management – drugs and surgery. Professionals with experience and training in clinical nutrition can be found employed by many sectors, such as the food and pharmaceutical industries, within health improvement and policy departments, and in non-governmental organisations.

Clinical nutrition always needs to consider both the quantity, and the quality, of nutritional provision. Both affect health, and they be compromised together or singly. In practice, malnutrition almost always involves both quantity and quality of the diet. It is traditional to consider quantity, that is, energy (calorie) status first.

NEGATIVE ENERGY BALANCE

Weight loss (not happening as part of a weight management strategy) can only occur when there is negative energy balance – that is, when calorie intake is less than output over a prolonged period. It often entails deficiencies of other specific nutrients as well as energy and can occur for a number of reasons. It is important to consider all when trying to diagnose weight loss, as more than one may coexist:

For a deeper understanding of this chapter, refer to the section on energy needs and energy balance in Chapters 16 and 17.

- Initially deliberate but becoming out of control, in the eating disorder of anorexia nervosa
- In association with an addiction, perhaps to alcohol or drugs, which impair appetite and replace normal food intake
- A consequence of illness, through
  - Loss of appetite, commonly in the context of inflammatory disease (including many cancers)
  - Nausea/loss of appetite from drug treatments
  - Psychological reasons (depression, dementia)
  - Physical obstacles to eating and swallowing
  - Failure to absorb nutrients normally: intestinal malabsorption (without compensatory increase in intake)
  - Losses of nutrients, for example from vomiting, protein-losing enteropathy, renal failure

It is vitally important to base diagnosis and judgements on reliably measured weights, and heights. Many people report weight loss, in themselves or in others, where there is in fact none. Conversely, weight loss is often missed, and an important diagnosis delayed, if weights are not measured and recorded regularly and at every contact with a health professional.

A negative energy balance may be evidenced by a failure to grow rather than by a loss of weight; this may be particularly true during early childhood or adolescent growth spurt, when energy and nutrient needs are high. If these are not satisfied, the growth rate will alter and this can be demonstrated on a growth chart, which will show the deviation from the predicted pattern. This might happen in a young child who becomes ill and consequently has a reduced food intake, or perhaps in an adolescent who is using a great deal of energy in physical activity, for example, training for sport, so that insufficient is left for normal growth.

Change in lean body mass \ Change in fat	Increase	Decrease
Increase	Obesity Overfeeding Pregnancy Puberty (in girls)	Exercise Puberty (in boys) Use of androgens
Decrease	Ageing Bedrest Zero gravity	Underfeeding Anorexia/bulimia nervosa Malnutrition Hibernation

FIGURE 21.1 The relationship between changes in lean body mass and in fat.

Weight Loss Due to Illness

Nutritional assessment and body composition measurement are covered in Chapter 18, pp. 343–358.

During illness, the inflammatory response (mediated by pro-inflammatory cytokines, catecholamines and corticosteroids) tends specifically to cause loss of muscle mass, with rapid weight loss. Muscle contains only about 1000 kcal/kg, compared to 7000 kcal/g in adipose tissue. A week of illness, with an energy deficit of 7000 kcal, could result in loss of 1 kg of adipose tissue, or about 7 kg of muscle. There is usually a mixture, and assessing change requires careful repeated examinations. Generally, changes in lean body mass and fat go in the same direction, both falling during weight loss. However, there is commonly greater loss of lean tissue (muscle) when the weight loss is metabolic, through illness, then when it is simply through dietary restriction. In some cases, changes in lean body mass and fat can oppose one another: for example, in older people, there is often a loss of lean tissue but gain in body fat, with the result that total body weight (and BMI) shows little overall change (Figure 21.1). There is no simple way to measure these changes in body composition in a clinical setting. MRI is the gold-standard method. Proxy methods such as bioelectrical impedance are a poor substitute. It is therefore necessary to incorporate other aspects of nutritional status when assessing patients, importantly including functional capacity.

Correcting Weight Loss

The aim is to increase weight and at the same increases the components of body composition in the correct proportion, not just to increase energy intake if that merely increases body fat. The underlying metabolic state is vitally important. If there is continuing inflammation (with raised CRP, etc.), muscle synthesis is impaired and fat deposition may be abnormal. Providing extra calories by artificial nutrition support can quite quickly lead to fat accumulation in the liver, with damage to liver function and even death. It is therefore most important to correct, or minimizes, the inflammatory process before attempting to refeed. As a general rule, it is safer to underfeed energy slightly, rather than to overfeed, until the underlying illness has resolved.

A second set of problems can develop from nutritional replacement after a period of severe restriction, because certain nutrients are not stored in the body and refeeding, with tissue repair, places very high demands. The key signal of 'refeeding syndrome' is a fall in serum phosphate, and there are commonly falls in serum potassium and magnesium. All of these can potentially be fatal. So it is essential to start refeeding gently, and to monitor their serum concentrations for 2–5 days as refeeding is established. If the serum concentrations dip, they should be replaced intravenously to be certain.

The final essential need during refeeding is to provide adequate vitamin B_1 (thiamin), without which refeeding can cause sudden, potentially permanent, brain damage. The clinical signs of thiamin deficiency, affecting both the nervous and cardiac systems, can develop rapidly, and are often misdiagnosed, with serious consequences. The most feared consequence is Wernicke's encephalopathy, which includes characteristic paralysis of the optic muscles, with nystagmus, plus confusion, loss of balance and staggering. Heart failure develops with enlarged heart on x-ray and abnormal cardiograph. Death can then occur, but all these features resolve rapidly if thiamine is administered intravenously. Serum levels can be measured, but intravenous thiamine should be administered in every case on suspicion, without waiting for results. Thiamin is not stored in the body, so deficiency can develop quite fast, especially amongst alcoholics who avoid cereal foods. Giving excess is safe and can avoid very serious consequences. If deficiency develops more slowly, particularly in alcoholics, Korsakoff's psychosis is the outcome, with permanent loss of the ability to make new memories.

Once underlying disease has been excluded or treated, it may be useful to assess energy expenditure and thereby obtain an indication of energy needs, but estimates based on standard equations are usually adequate, especially as the aim is not to match requirement exactly, until normal appetite takes over. A record of food intake for several days can be kept to establish where specific changes could be made. If poor appetite is a problem, it is important to identify foods that are liked. Other possible courses of action include

- Adding energy supplements to these foods if possible
- Reducing low-energy and low-fat foods in the diet and replacing them with high-energy snacks and meals containing some fat (preferably of vegetable origin)
- Avoiding drinking with meals, as fluids can induce earlier satiety
- Reducing the amount of dietary fibre (or NSP) in the diet, as this has a satiating effect and will reduce total energy intake
- Reducing physical activity (if appropriate) and perhaps including some muscle-building activity, such as work with weights

Starvation and Refeeding

See Chapter 17 for more on the control of energy balance, pp. 331–341.

A healthy human has enough energy stores to survive about 40–50 days of total starvation, provided there is access to water. Death from starvation in famine situations is usually through infection as a result of diminished immunity and defences – commonly pneumonia, but multiple infections contribute. Severe negative energy balance through food deprivation certainly incurs deficiencies of micronutrients, but the effect of insufficient calories dominates the clinical deterioration. The obvious loss of body fat and then muscle mass, gut mucosa and skin atrophy and the immune system shut down, so infections are more likely and less well combated. If infection is avoided, heart function ultimately collapses, with 'pump failure' progressing through oedema and respiratory failure, or ceasing to beat normally and sudden death from arrhythmia. A failure in starvation to maintain normal ion gradients across membranes, with loss of potassium, phosphate and magnesium, is an important cause of death, especially when the weight loss has been rapid, such as through illness. Thus, infections aggravate the functional decline, and hasten death, in many ways.

It is vitally important to recognize the depletion of body potassium, phosphate and magnesium, which occurs when lean tissue (mostly muscle) is lost during illness and starvation, and to replace them. As soon as energy is provided, there is secretion of insulin, which tends to drive potassium, phosphate and magnesium back into the body cells, reducing their blood concentrations which can be life-threatening through sudden cardiac arrest: thus, well-meaning attempts to feed starved individuals rapidly can kill. This is a completely understandable physiological response known as 'refeeding syndrome'. Once electrolyte imbalances, and membrane integrity have been restored, re-feeding of starved people needs to proceed at a rate which they body's damaged metabolic capacity can manage. It is best to work up gradually to a level of modest positive energy balance – perhaps an extra 500 kcal/day above energy expenditure. Above this, there tends to be fat accumulation in the liver, with tissue damage, and even jaundice and severe liver failure. Overfeeding can kill.

When positive energy balance is established by refeeding, extra energy leads to a rapid restoration of some fat storage in adipose tissue. This has obvious survival value – one famine could easily follow the first. However, refeeding alone does little to restore lost muscle mass or its function. Gradually, under the action of anabolic hormones, insulin, growth hormones, IGF-1, testosterones, muscle mass increases again but the critical factor is exercise training, which is difficult after profound underfeeding for both psychological and physical reasons. If weight loss has been the result of an inflammatory process, from a range of diseases, there is often rapid and excessive loss of muscle, and the body's capacity to re-grow muscle is very low if the inflammatory process continues, indicated by raised serum CRP or ESR.

MALNUTRITION SCREENING AND DIAGNOSIS

Chronic malnutrition is poorly recognized and often remains undiagnosed and untreated, both in hospitals, care homes and the wider community, with serious clinical and financial implications. In 2007, it was estimated that the cost of disease-related malnutrition in the United Kingdom was £13 billion (equivalent to 10% of all public spending on health and social care) (Elia et al., 2010). The majority of the estimated 3 million people in the United Kingdom affected by malnutrition are in the community. Those most at risk of malnutrition are the very old and the very young, those who are hospitalized or institutionalized, poor and marginalized populations (for under-nutrition) and affluent populations (for over-nutrition and chronic diseases). It is well understood that malnutrition predisposes people to disease, delays recovery from illness and increases mortality, and is therefore of particular concern in a clinical setting.

In order to treat malnutrition one must first be able to identify and diagnose it. There is no simple method or test. The consequences of malnutrition reflect altered 'nutritional status' and that involved three interacting components: (1) body composition – 'what we are', (2) diet quality and quantity – 'what we eat' and (3) functional capacity – 'what we can do'. It is relatively easy to measure body composition, at least in terms of height and weight. Diet quantity is assessed from weight change. Diet quality can be estimated by a trained dietician, but nearly always depends on memories and impressions of patients or carers. Functional capacity requires a multi-component assessment, but some judgement can be made from clinical observations and some biochemical tests of enzyme activities, etc.

SCREENING TOOLS

The purpose of screening is to identify individuals at high risk, who then need more detailed diagnostic assessment. Most screening tools address four basic questions: current body mass index, recent weight loss, recent food intake and appetite, and disease severity or some other measure for predicting future risk of malnutrition (Barendregt et al., 2008). The use of BMI is easy to criticize, as it is not recommended for categorizing individuals. It is inappropriate for diagnosis, but useful as part of a screening tool. There has been a proliferation of published nutrition screening tools for use with different populations. For example:

- General population: Short nutritional assessment (SNAQ), nutritional risk score (NRS), universal malnutrition screening tool (MUST)
- Geriatrics: Nutrition screening initiative (NST), mini-nutritional assessment (MNA)

In the United Kingdom, the most commonly used tool is the malnutrition universal screening tool (MUST). This has advantage of being valid, reliable and practical (Stratton et al., 2004); it is simple to use and objective in nature. Individuals are scored on the basis of their risk of malnutrition, and there must be an action plan recommendation which is linked to their MUST score.

For a more complete understanding of an individual's nutritional status in a clinical setting, Barendregt recommends an assessment which covers the following:

- *History and examination:* To define all the factors leading to malnutrition and the likely natural history of the patient's condition. Weight loss, appetite, gastro-intestinal symptoms, fever, medical and drug history. A diet history also examines qualitative and quantitative aspects of diet to assess energy, protein and micronutrient intake.
- *Disease status:* This will be revealed not only by history, examination, and bedside measurements such as temperature, pulse rate and blood pressure, but also by laboratory tests of inflammation including full blood count, albumin and C-reactive protein. Additional nutrient losses from wounds, fistulae, etc., should be assessed.
- *Functional assessment:* The mental and physical dysfunction associated with malnutrition may be identified at the bedside. Muscle strength may be assessed qualitatively by the examiner or quantitatively using hand dynamometry, which correlates very well with clinical outcome in surgical patients. The patient should be asked about exercise tolerance and breathing. A validated mental scoring system can be used to assess mood status.
- *Laboratory tests:* as well as quantifying inflammation and disease severity, these are valuable in identifying important changes in minerals, and the levels of vitamins and trace elements where the underlying disease may result in deficiencies.
- *Fluid balance:* This is an intrinsic part of nutritional assessment. Examine for dehydration or oedema. Monitor daily weight to record changes in fluid balance. Keep fluid balance charts and measure creatinine, urea and electrolyte levels in the blood as clinically indicated.

A useful guide for assessing nutritional status is in Table 21.1.

TABLE 21.1

Top 10 Tips for Assessment of Nutritional Status

1. No single measure that captures all aspects of nutritional status.
2. Every patient's nutritional status should be considered with screening as a minimum standard, when admitted to hospital/care-home.

Assessment of dietary intake (what we eat)

3. Consider diet and nutrition during history taking.
4. Consider whether specialist referral is needed.

Assessment of body composition (what we are)

5. Weigh every patient at each new medical contact. Calculate BMI and compare to agreed reference ranges, and review changes since last assessment.
6. Consider the need for more detailed assessment of body composition or of the composition of specific tissues.

Assessment of nutrition-related functional capacity (what we can do)

7. Include assessment of physical activity, and cognitive and social functions in history-taking.
8. Poor nutrition can lead to functional deficit, and illness can compromise nutritional state.

Impact of medical treatments on nutritional status

9. Many medications can influence the nutritional status.

Evidence-based practice

10. Any assessment must include a forward plan to review and optimize nutritional status when appropriate.

Source: Adapted from Royal College of Physicians, Ten top tips for nutritional assessment, available at: https://www.rcplondon.ac.uk/file/1772/download?token=5HJYWGdM, accessed on July 2015.

For paediatric practice, practices vary greatly between the needs in post-industrial and developing countries, with very different healthcare and community services. Malnutrition in all its forms is much more frequent in poorer developing countries, where the drivers sadly include season, drought and war, and large numbers may be affected in the same area simultaneously. In the post-industrial wealthier countries, childhood malnutrition still occurs, usually in isolated cases, where equally sadly the main drivers are psychiatric and substance abuse in parents. In general, four main areas for action must always be considered:

1. Definition and classification of malnutrition, the visible and invisible changes caused by malnutrition as it affects growth and development, and why malnourished children need different care from other children
2. Screening children for risk of malnutrition
3. Diagnosing and managing children with malnutrition, integrating community- and facility-based approaches for long-term support and surveillance, and considering whether common conditions such as gastroenteritis, pneumonia and malaria may have to be treated differently when the child is also malnourished
4. Community-based actions to identify and correct factors which have led to malnutrition, and to identify and assess other family and community members who may be at risk

NUTRITIONAL SUPPORT: ENTERAL AND PARENTERAL FEEDING

Common sense and first principles tell us that all aspects of life, including protection against infection and injury, and recovery and tissue repair after injury or illness, all require the provision of nutrients from outside the body, usually obtained from foods. Evidence from large studies shows that clinical outcomes, including mortality, are improved by optimal nutrition. In many clinical situations, normal food intake is not possible, and in some, the nutritional requirements are altered – usually increased. In other cases, the clinical state places restrictions on the types of foods, or nutrients that can be given. In these situations, there is need for 'nutritional support' in order to optimize outcome. In hospitals, nutritional support is best provided by a multidisciplinary team of trained individuals, with professional skills in dietetics, nursing, medicine, clinical biochemistry and surgery. In the community, it is only dieticians who are trained to assess patients and to define their needs, while doctors and nurses need to be alert in identifying individuals who should be referred to a dietician.

The simplest form of nutritional support involves oral 'sip-feed' dietary supplements, in small cartons. Oral supplements are required by patients who are underweight or experiencing weight loss, and can eat but are unable to eat enough normal foods. A wide range of supplements are available commercially and can be prescribed by doctors. The need is then to provide calories in as concentrated form as is palatable, including some fat in order to avoid biliary stasis and gallstone development, together with all the essential micronutrients necessary to be able to metabolize and use the extra calories. Some commercial supplements simply provide extra calories, usually in the form of sugar: here are few, if any, clinical situations when these supplements are indicated. Sip-feed supplements are expensive and should not be used to replace meals. They are appropriate as supplements between meals, but they are generally less palatable than foods or snacks, and not well accepted in the long term. Efforts to provide palatable, nutritionally appropriate, snacks should always be made before prescribing sip-feed supplements.

Enteral and parenteral feeding are both forms of artificial feeding (or 'prosthetic feeding') used for critically ill patients, particularly for those with pre-existing malnutrition. They must only be used for patients who have some obstacle to using the gastro-intestinal/digestive system, or for those whose oral intake is expected to be inadequate for 7 days or more.

Parenteral nutrition (PN) involves feeding a person intravenously, bypassing the usual process of eating and digestion.

Enteral nutrition (EN) involves administering nutrients via an artificial route into the gastrointestinal tract. EN usually involves gastric introduction either via a naso-gastric tube in the nasal passage or a tube leading directly through the abdominal wall to the stomach, commonly placed while the patient is undergoing gastroscopy, as a percutaneous endoscopic gastrostomy (PEG) as the preferred option for those whose stomach and lower GI tract are working normally. If the stomach is not available, or to try to reduce reverse flow and aspiration, the tube may be placed in the jejunum.

Enteral feeding is not an option for every patient. For many it can be used safely and effectively for prolonged periods; however, it is increasingly being recognized that it often fails to achieve targeted calorie requirements, particularly in critically ill patients where fluid administration needs to be limited. Aspiration pneumonitis is a relatively common and serious complication. It can be minimized by using intermittent feeding, only when the patient is sitting up, but can still occur, potentially fatally. For people who with little or no intestinal capability, for example, post-surgical short-bowel syndrome, or in syndromes where bowel motility has been lost, PN (in extreme cases total parenteral nutrition [TPN]) is necessary. This involves inserting a venous catheter, to provide nutrients directly into a major vein. Many nutrients normally found in foods cannot safely be supplied in this way (especially proteins), so the nutrients for TPN must be in an elemental form: amino acids or very small peptides can be given but not intact proteins. This imposes osmotic limits such that to avoid causing blood clots, they can only be given with rather large amounts of water. Parenteral feeding carries high risks of introducing bacterial infections, because the nutrient mix is ideal for bacteria, and crossing the skin is a potential route for contamination. Thus, parenteral feeding must only be delivered by trained experts under strict sterile conditions. Maintaining parenteral feeding for prolonged periods is possible but very time-consuming and burdensome for both patients and carers.

CLINICAL MICRONUTRIENT DEFICIENCIES

Function of vitamin and minerals, as well as deficiencies are covered in Chapter 12, pp. 235–252.

It is important to distinguish between micronutrient deficiency, which causes classical diseases, and dietary or serum insufficiency – that is, low levels which can be accommodated or compensated for, without specific illness. Diagnosing clinical micronutrient deficiencies requires the integration of clinical/functional data (e.g. night blindness for vitamin A, lipid peroxidation for vitamin E, mean corpuscular volume for iron), dietary data (reported intakes, taking into consideration the risk of under/over-reporting) and biochemical data (e.g. plasma retinol for vitamin A, urinary iodine excretion). Comparison of intake with population thresholds (especially lower reference nutrient intake [LRNI]) is a first indicator of potential deficiencies and may guide subsequent investigations. However, poor absorption or excretion can trigger deficiency in the presence of adequate intake (e.g. vitamin B_{12} deficiency). Infection and stress may also impact on nutritional status. Biochemical analysis relies on collection of biological samples, most often plasma or serum, but also blood cells, urine, or hair. The impact of storage and handling of the stability of the analyte must be considered, and the analytical technique used should be specific, sensitive over the range of interest, robust, with normative data and quality controls available for interpretation and quality assurance.

ADVERSE REACTIONS TO FOOD

Since the earliest times, people have attributed unfamiliar or unexplained illnesses to their foods, usually unusual or short-season foods. There is now massive media and public interest in possible adverse reactions to food, often (mistakenly) referred to as 'food allergy'. The extent of these problems is difficult to ascertain precisely, as levels of self-reporting are invariably greater than can be confirmed by rigorous testing. Most cases of self-diagnosed, or commercially diagnosed, allergy or intolerance are for conditions which come and go, so withdrawing a particular food when a person is experiencing bad symptoms is often followed by a spontaneous improvement – nothing to do with the nutrient or food under scrutiny. Formal testing, with blinded reintroduction of the food, seldom confirms any food-related problem, but disproving an adverse reaction to a food is extremely difficult, especially if the patient believes the reaction is sporadic or variable.

Illnesses attributed to adverse reactions to food may be of three types: there are variations in their classifications within Europe and the United States.

- Food poisoning – resulting from contaminants within the food
- Food aversion – psychological reactions and beliefs, which may not be reproduced on covert introduction of the food
- Food intolerance – reproducible adverse reactions to foods, including true allergies

The first of these occurs as a result of triggers from outside the individual. The remaining two types relate to responses that are initiated within the individual in response to the food eaten and are considered to be less common.

Food Poisoning

This occurs as a result of the consumption of contaminated food or water that results in disease of an infectious or toxic nature. The most frequent causative agents are microorganisms. However, food poisoning may also occur as a result of chemical contamination, or from toxins which are naturally present in the food or acquired within the food. Bacterial food poisoning occurring includes gastroenteritis, with vomiting and diarrhoea, caused by *Campylobacter*, *Salmonella*, *Shigella* and pathogenic varieties of *Escherichia coli*. Some bacteria produce toxins, which cause the symptoms; these include *Staphylococcus aureus*, *Bacillus cereus* and *Clostridium botulinum*. Foods that may be contaminated include eggs, poultry, cold meats, rice, unwashed vegetables and spices. Among the viral causes of food poisoning, the most widespread are highly infectious, small round structured viruses (SRSVs), which may contaminate shellfish, but more probably are introduced into food from infected food handlers. Consumers in semi-closed communities, such as hospitals, hotels and schools, are particularly vulnerable. The timescale of symptoms in relation to exposure may help identify the causal agent: for example staphylococcal toxins commonly cause illness in 2–4 hours, while bacteria such as *Campylobacter* usually take longer to cause symptoms. Most commonly, food poisoning causes rapid vomiting and diarrhoea, although a few of the agents can cause serious damage to the liver, kidneys, nervous system and may even be fatal. The young, sick and elderly are the most vulnerable to serious consequences from bacterial food poisoning.

Contamination of food can occur, for example, from use of dirty water, sewerage overspill, and agricultural chemicals. Some plant foods may contain natural toxins, for example, uncooked red kidney beans or some fungi, or may be contaminated with moulds, for example, aflatoxins, which affect groundnuts (peanuts). Crop contamination with industrial fall-out containing selenium has caused widespread toxicity in the western United States. Some organic pesticides on foods can be toxic, and may accumulate in the body, and in the bodies of animals which become food, particularly the liver. Heavy metals, such as mercury, from industrial pollution are toxic and may also accumulate in animals and in fish.

Food Aversion

Many people may be able to list foods that they avoid, generally because of a sensory preference or dislike. This may be taken to an extreme avoidance of almost all foods in the case of anorexia nervosa. In some cases, an individual believes that the food causes them unpleasant symptoms, perhaps as a result of an experience in the past where the food was temporally associated with sickness or gastro-intestinal upset. In this case, the food is avoided because of an aversion to it and an associated psychological belief that the food is harmful. When tested blind, however, it is generally not possible to reproduce any alleged symptoms, and the conclusion must be drawn that this is a psychosomatic adverse reaction rather than one that has a true physiological basis.

Aversion may also be applied to foods that are believed to affect other aspects of health, for example, tiredness, sleep problems, palpitations, bloatedness and flatulence. The individual excludes particular foods to correct these symptoms, although double-blind testing generally fails to find any scientific basis for this practice. The commonly blamed foods include gluten, milk and citrus fruits (all of which do have the capacity in certain individuals to cause true allergy) depending on culture and the degree of promotion by media personalities and stories. In most of these cases, there is no evidence to support a link between the food and the symptoms. Avoiding foods or food-groups can result in weight loss, with symptoms like fatigue, and in specific micronutrient deficiencies.

Food Intolerance

This is the only group of adverse reactions to food for which reproducible responses can be produced on challenge. Precise figures for prevalence are difficult to obtain because

- Questionnaires are unreliable because of bias from respondents.
- Diagnosis is time-consuming (e.g. use of elimination diets followed by challenge).
- There are no simple reliable tests and these also may not be particularly sensitive.
- There is an almost unlimited number of foodstuffs and additives that can provoke a response.
- Reactions vary between individuals and, especially in children, may change over time.
- Responses may occur immediately or after a considerable period after ingestion; these are poorly understood and difficult to diagnose.

Although many studies have attempted to quantify the extent of food intolerance, a lack of consensus over definitions and methodologies has made it difficult to arrive at reliable data on prevalence. Food intolerance may be subdivided into

- Allergic reactions – immunoglobulin E (IgE)-mediated and non-IgE-mediated
- Pharmacological reactions
- Enzyme reactions

The clinical presentation of food intolerance varies widely, and onset may be immediate or delayed, commonly affecting the following tissues and systems (see Figure 21.2 for a summary). Diagnosis is difficult, and often distorted by manifestations of anxiety (understandable in some cases). The clinical presentation of anxiety as hyperventilation is particularly problematic as its symptoms (perceived difficult breathing, tingling fingers, toes and mouth, light-headedness) can resemble those of food allergy and anaphylactic shock.

- *Gastro-intestinal system*: Symptoms include mouth tingling or swelling, abdominal pain, bloating of the abdomen, vomiting and diarrhoea or constipation. In chronic intolerance, there can be bleeding or loss of plasma protein into the gut lumen, with damage to the gut mucosa.
- *Skin*: Dermatitis, urticaria, angio-oedema and eczema are common consequences.
- *Respiratory system*: Rhinitis, laryngeal oedema and asthma (including wheezing, breathlessness) may occur.
- *Central nervous system*: Symptoms include migraine and possibly some behavioural abnormalities (including hyperactivity and depression), although the evidence for these is controversial.

Food allergy is a form of specific food intolerance that causes reproducible symptoms and includes an abnormal reaction by the immune system. Our diet contains a variety of substances that can stimulate immune responses. They are usually proteins or simple chemicals bound to proteins and are termed

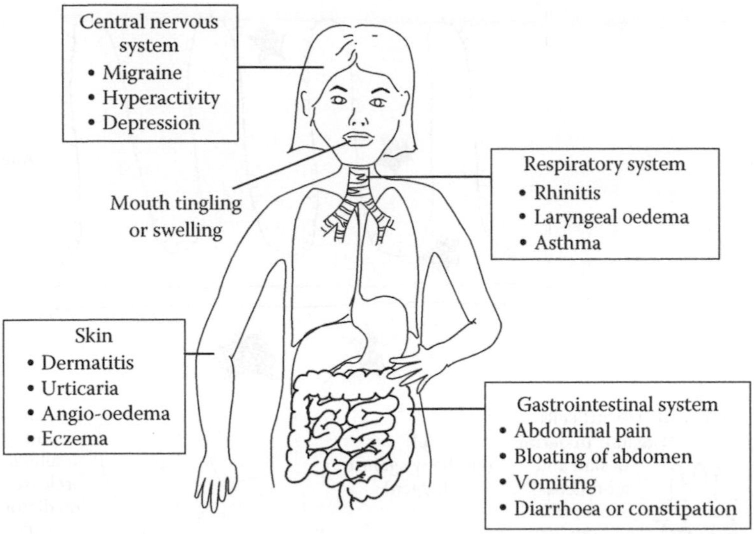

FIGURE 21.2 Symptoms of food intolerance.

allergens. Usually, these allergens are prevented from being absorbed by secretory immunoglobulin A (IgA) lining the gut. However, IgA is absent in the first months of life, so that allergens can be absorbed. Breast milk contains IgA and may offer some protection. Avoidance of contact with potential allergens is important at this age, especially where there is a family history of allergy, although complete protection is unlikely. However, in general, our immune system has evolved responses that allow it to be tolerant to the antigen burden represented by ingested food. This is known as oral tolerance. In some cases, these allergens induce an immune response, usually producing antibodies, which can be detected in the serum, but which are not pathogenic – known as immunological acceptance.

In a minority of individuals, however, this response is abnormal and results in pathological changes when the allergen is ingested, resulting in a food allergy. The immune system responds inappropriately against the allergen to stimulate IgE antibodies sensitized to the particular allergen. These are mainly attached to mast cells and on stimulation cause immediate degranulation of the mast cells and the release of a range of chemical mediators. These include histamine and prostaglandins, which have potent effects. The consequent reaction depends on the size of the dose, the speed of absorption and the distribution of the allergen in the body.

The response to the release of histamine and prostaglandins generally includes some or all of the following:

- Dilation of small blood vessels (redness)
- Increased permeability of blood vessels (swelling/oedema)
- Contraction of smooth muscle in the airways (breathing difficulties) or intestines (causing abdominal pain)
- Stimulation of nerve endings in the skin (itching and pain)

Reactions may be seen in the following:

- The mouth, immediately following ingestion
- The gastro-intestinal tract, when the allergen reaches this area
- One of many other sites, including the skin and respiratory system, including the nose and airways
- Several other sites, causing a widespread and possibly life-threatening reaction (see Figure 21.3)

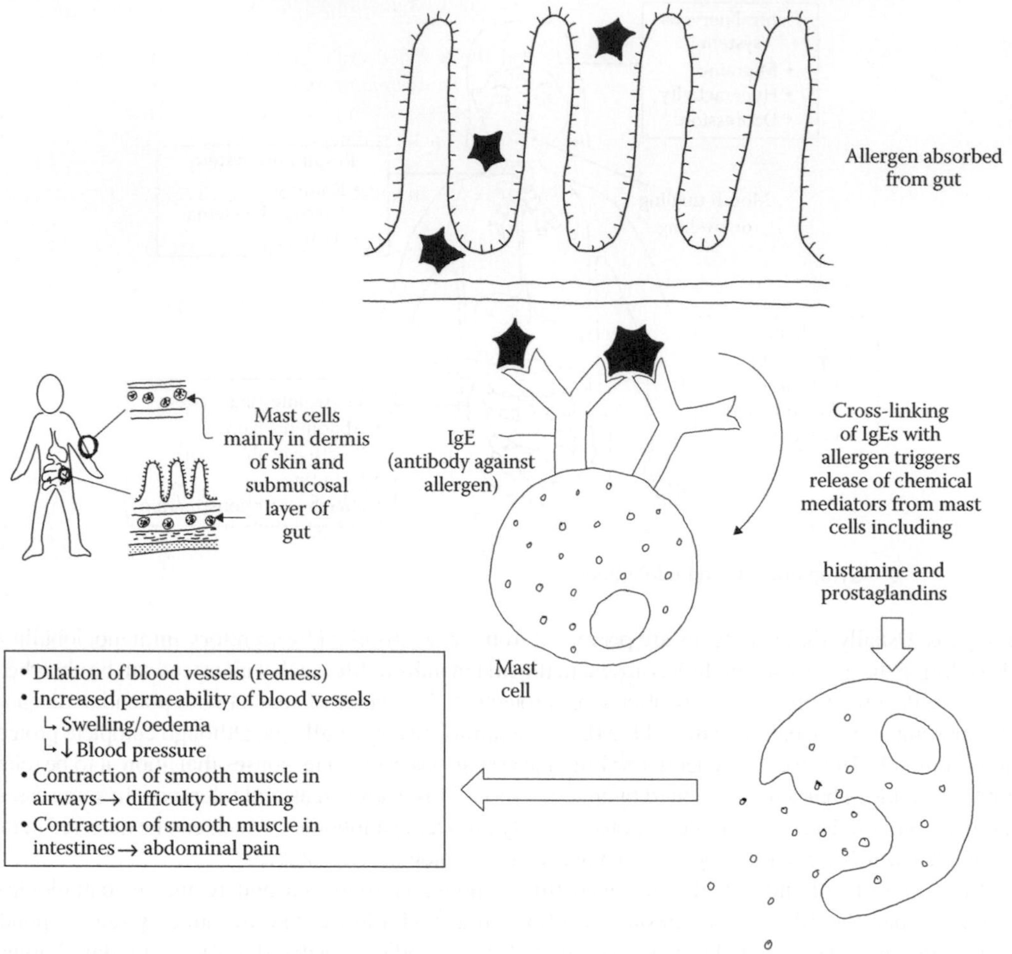

FIGURE 21.3 IgE-mediated food allergy.

The severity of the reaction varies between individuals and may range from mild to life threatening (anaphylactic shock), resulting from a severe fall of blood pressure and possibly difficulties in breathing. Immediate help in the form of an adrenaline injection is required for anyone suffering from such a major allergic reaction. Fortunately, most are not so extreme and recovery follows, resulting from the body's own homeostatic mechanisms, which cause endogenous adrenaline release.

Why Do Some Individuals Develop Food Allergy? Atopy

Genetic predisposition is an important determinant of susceptibility to allergic disease, also called atopy: almost 30% of all people have atopy, and that high proportion suggests that it must have had survival value at some stage of our evolution. The susceptibility is more likely to be inherited from the mother than the father but, with two atopic parents, the likelihood is greatly increased. However, although the susceptibility is inherited, the actual allergens to which a child is sensitive are not necessarily the same as its parents. Babies that are born small for gestational age are more at risk of developing allergies in their first year. This suggests that growth faltering in the womb may play a role in poorer immunocompetence. The skin of people with atopy contains abnormalities of collagen which make it more porous and so allow immune reactions to develop against potentially damaging molecules such as a viral products on the skin (but also against some on-dangerous ones).

Studies have suggested that the risk of atopy in a child can be reduced by avoidance of potential allergens in the mother's diet from very early pregnancy. However, the 'Learning Early About Peanut' (LEAP) study was the first randomized trial to show prevention of peanut allergy in a large cohort of high-risk infants, after early sensitization to the allergen.

In addition, breastfeeding for more than 4 months can reduce the development of atopic disease. Delaying the introduction of solids until after 6 months is also recommended, as well as the use of low allergen foods, such as baby rice, potatoes, fruit and vegetables.

There has been a general increase in the incidence of food and other allergies over the last 30 years. An explanation that is gaining acceptance is that modern children are exposed to fewer infectious diseases and live in a generally clean environment. This does not challenge the immune system, which is less well developed as a result, and reacts inappropriately when presented with harmless antigens, resulting in an allergic reaction.

A further explanation offered for the rising incidence of allergy is the change in balance between *n*-6 and *n*-3 fatty acids in our diets. The *n*-6 fatty acids are more predominant and fewer *n*-3 acids are consumed. The former are associated with more pro-inflammatory eicosanoids, including prostaglandins, which have an important role in allergic responses.

Diagnosis

To obtain a reliable diagnosis, strict criteria must be adhered to. An adverse reaction to a food can only be confirmed if the symptoms disappear when the food is removed from the diet and re-appear when it is re-introduced. Great care must be taken if there is any risk of anaphylaxis, and patients who believe they are at risk may refuse to undergo testing. Because of the risk of a severe reaction on re-introduction, this should be carried out under supervision. A careful history of diet and symptoms needs to be taken to identify possible triggers. The testing procedure should be performed by a double-blind technique, so that neither the clinician nor the subject knows when the suspect food is introduced, within a range of food testing. If several foods are involved and if the reaction is delayed, the procedure may take many weeks to complete. Where there is a suspected allergy, skin prick tests or assay of IgE levels – radioallergosorbent test (RAST) method – may be used as laboratory tests. Even with these, failure to obtain a positive result may not necessarily indicate the absence of hypersensitivity. Intestinal biopsy or intestinal permeability may also be measured in the clinical setting, if this is considered appropriate (see Table 21.2).

A large number of other tests are available directly to the public. Most of these have not been scientifically validated and, therefore, are not considered to be of value in the diagnosis of food allergy. They are potentially dangerous as they are likely to result in misdiagnosis of food allergy and potential harm from restricted diets. Even without testing, individuals may be tempted to use

TABLE 21.2
Diagnosis of Food Intolerance

History of diet and symptoms taken to identify possible triggers
Double-blind food testing
Skin prick-tests or assay of IgE levels (RAST method)
Intestinal biopsy or intestinal permeability measured, if appropriate

self-diagnosis and elimination of foods from the diet. This can readily result in omission of key foods and nutrients, which can produce deficiencies and is particularly hazardous in children. Dietary manipulation should only be undertaken under the supervision of a dietician.

Effect of Infection on Nutritional Status

The presence of infection has a potential impact on nutritional state. This can be as a consequence of

- Loss of appetite and poor dietary intake
- Failure to digest or absorb nutrients, either through loss by vomiting or diarrhoea, or loss of digesting/absorbing ability through lack of enzymes, damage to the mucosa of the gut or intestinal hurry caused by infestation with parasites
- Increased requirements owing to raised metabolic rate consequent on fever, increased utilization of certain nutrients, such as amino acids and antioxidants, or a redistribution of nutrients between different body compartments as part of the immune response

Therefore, nutritional status may decline during an infection and compromise the body's ability to combat it and recover. This is one of the reasons for a higher mortality from infections in poorly nourished individuals, compared to those with better nutritional status. This is summarized in Figure 21.4.

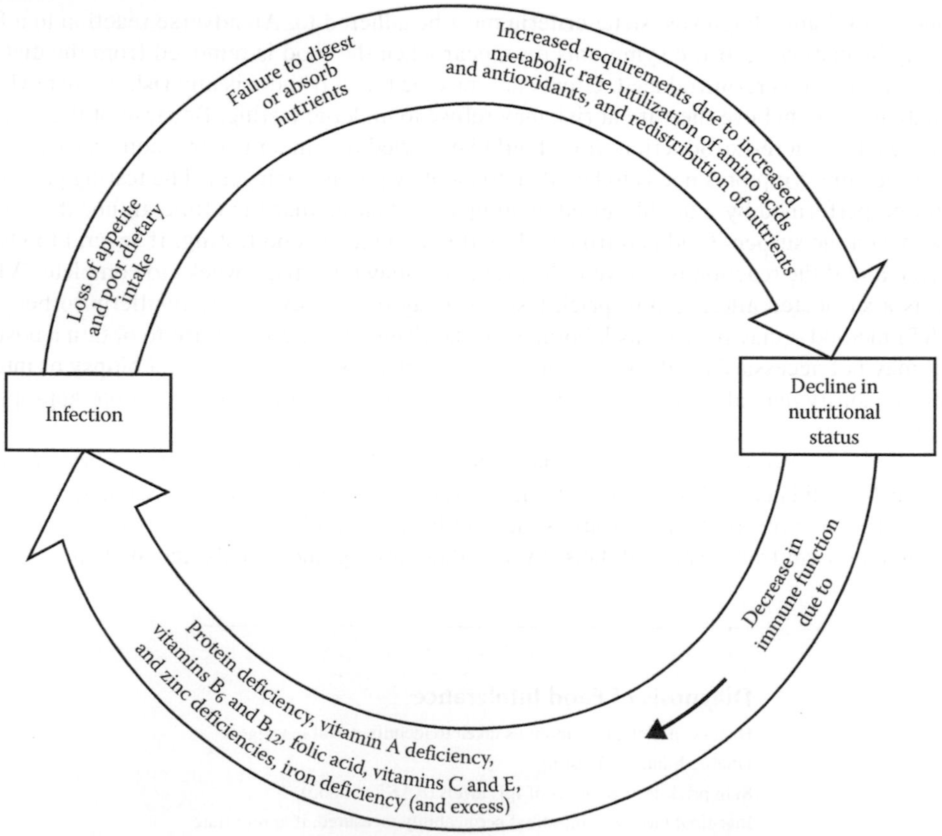

FIGURE 21.4 The relationship between infection and nutrition.

Effect of Nutritional Status on Immunity

The most studied aspect of this relationship is that between 'protein energy malnutrition' and immune function. Almost all aspects of the immune system depend on adequate protein status. This includes the organs of the immune system, such as the thymus, spleen and lymph nodes, which produce phagocytic white blood cells. In addition, the biologically active proteins, such as immunoglobulins, acute-phase proteins and cytokines, are dependent on adequate protein status. Cytokines are a large and diverse group of proteins secreted by cells for the purpose of altering its own function or that of adjacent cells; cytokines may have multiple activities, and include tumour necrosis factor and interleukins. It is, therefore, not surprising that protein deficiency makes the individual vulnerable to almost all infections. Specific amino acids have also been identified as particularly important in sustaining an immune response during acute infections, and following trauma or surgery. These are the sulphur-containing amino acids (methionine and cysteine), arginine and glutamine. Some enteral feeds have been developed, containing these amino acids for use in hospital patients.

The role of dietary fat in immune function has received considerable interest. In experimental studies, a reduction of total dietary fat intake, from 40 to less than 30% of energy, resulted in improved immune activity in a variety of subjects. This has led to the suggestion that high-fat diets may have a suppressing effect on human immune function. Polyunsaturated fatty acids (PUFAs) of the *n*-6 series, when consumed in amounts typical of the Western diet, have no clear effects on immune function. However, *n*-3 PUFAs, such as those found in fish oils and linseed oil, have been reported to have a suppressing effect on immune responses. For this reason, there is interest in their role as potential anti-inflammatory agents for use in conditions where the immune system is responding inappropriately to triggers and causing chronic disease states. These include rheumatoid arthritis, Crohn's disease, ulcerative colitis and psoriasis. Results of trials to date are inconclusive, and further work is still needed.

Among the micronutrients, both vitamins and minerals are important in immune function. Vitamin A deficiency is closely linked with susceptibility to infection, especially of the respiratory system in malnourished children. The role of vitamin A appears to be widespread, in maintaining the integrity of epithelial surfaces as well as in the production and function of both cellular and humoral aspects of the immune system. Other vitamins that have been proposed and studied with regard to an immune function role are vitamins B_6 and B_{12}, folic acid and vitamins C and E.

The most important mineral in relation to immune function is zinc and subjects who are zinc deficient have immune impairment. Supplementation with zinc of malnourished children decreases the risk of diarrhoea and increases the number of T lymphocytes. In infants small for their gestational age, a supplement of zinc (5 mg/day), given for 6 months, increased immune function. However, it should also be noted that excess intakes of zinc (300 mg/day) can also impair immune function.

Iron deficiency has also been associated with impaired immune function. However, excess iron may inhibit immune function, although the mechanisms are unclear. Selenium is concentrated in tissues involved in the immune system, such as lymph nodes, spleen and liver, and various components of the immune system have been shown to be impaired in selenium deficiency. The bactericidal activity of phagocytes is impaired. There have been reports also of benefits of selenium supplementation in HIV-infected subjects.

Overall, it is clear that adequate nutritional status is needed for correct immune function. Supplementation with multi-nutrient mixtures can improve immune function in those individuals whose previous intakes were poor. However, there is little evidence to support enhancement of immune function by the use of supplements in those who are adequately nourished. Indeed, there is a possibility that for some nutrients, an excess intake may result in suppression of immune action. More research is needed in this area.

Nutrition Management and Cancer

Nutritional management in cancer patients is important from a number of perspectives. Most importantly, unless clear advice is offered to all patients, they are likely to be led towards following non-evidence-based dietary practices (often excluding major food groups, which causes weight loss and impairs survival, or to spend money on the so-called complementary medicines, usually expensive dietary supplements which have no effect at all). Eating a nutritionally balanced, healthful, diet may enable the patient to cope with their condition and the treatment more effectively, and there is often a need to promote more energy-dense foods to prevent weight loss. Food safety is also critical as people undergoing chemotherapy often have a compromised immune system and are therefore be more susceptible to infection. Some individuals may need to follow a specialist diet: for example, those with a sore mouth or difficulty in swallowing may need to follow a 'soft' diet, and such a limited diet has the potential to result in a reduced calorie and nutrient intake. People may need nutritional management in dealing with specific symptoms and side effects such as weakness and fatigue, dry or sore mouth, sensory changes, diarrhoea, nausea, constipation, poor appetite and undesirable weight loss (cancer cachexia), bowl problems (such as obstructions). Patients may also need specific advice following cancer surgery such as gastrectomy. McMillan Cancer Support, in the UK provides a range of useful information for healthy eating, preventing weight loss, managing weight gain and keeping active.

Nutrition Management and Metabolic Disorders

The metabolic syndrome is a combination of metabolic disorders, including dyslipidemia, high blood pressure, type II diabetes and the tendency to develop abdominal fat. People with metabolic disorders have a higher risk of developing atherosclerosis and consequently cardiovascular disease. The importance of diet in treating people with metabolic syndrome is supported by evidence from many clinical and epidemiological studies (Pitsavos et al., 2006). The WHO and the National Cholesterol Education Program Adult Treatment Panel suggest that lifestyle changes can reduce the prevalence of the metabolic syndrome. Increasingly scientific studies have focused on the benefits of diets that are rich in fruits, vegetables, legumes and whole grains and which include fish, nuts and low-fat dairy products as well as maintaining a healthy energy balance. It has been suggested that, for people with the syndrome, long-term weight loss can reverse their condition. A recent review of the evidence found that sustained weight loss had positive benefits for those with metabolic syndrome for insulin resistance, hyperglycaemia, lipid and lipoprotein profiles and hypertension (Ferland and Eckel, 2011). Conventional dietary guidance along with advice on physical activity was found to help in reducing the health complications associated with metabolic disorders; however, in the long term, benefits seem to relate to the amount of weight lost. Many different diets can produce clinically significant weight reduction; however, it is the actual methods used to sustain this weight loss that are of particular importance, given the difficulty that many overweight individuals experience in maintaining a calorie controlled regime.

DRUG–NUTRIENT INTERACTIONS

Drugs used in medical treatment may affect nutritional status by influencing food intake or metabolism; similarly, their action and effectiveness may be altered by a person's pre-existing nutritional state. Interactions can occur within the gastro-intestinal tract, in the blood or at the cellular site of action of the drug. The consequence of any interaction will vary with the drug, its formulation, the timing of food intake and the nutritional status and disease state of the individual concerned.

Effects of Diet on Drugs

Most drugs are taken into the body by mouth and, therefore, are processed by the gastro-intestinal tract. Many drugs have to be solubilized by the digestive secretions before they can be absorbed. In a fasting subject, drugs will pass quickly through the stomach, reaching the small intestine within minutes. Drugs taken with food or after meals are likely to be more slowly absorbed than those taken following a period of fasting. The presence of food and fluid also facilitates the solubility of solid drugs. The increased flow of blood in the splanchnic circulation associated with eating may enhance the bioavailability of some drugs, for example, some of the beta-blockers.

Nevertheless, there are some drugs that are better absorbed in the fasting state, such as penicillin and tetracycline. In particular, tetracycline is less well absorbed when taken with foods containing calcium, magnesium, iron or zinc, and should, therefore, not be taken within 2 hours of food containing dairy products or protein.

Dietary Factors Affecting Drug Metabolism

Adequate protein intake is required for normal drug metabolism, and a low protein status may be linked with prolonged drug action. Fat-free diets may also reduce the activity of drug-metabolizing enzymes. Vitamin C is required for hepatic cytochrome P450, a key component of the microsomal oxidizing system, which metabolizes drugs. Many of the other enzymes involved in the phase I (oxidation, hydroxylation, reduction or hydrolysis) reactions, which alter the functional groups on the drug molecules, require vitamins, especially the B complex, and minerals to act as cofactors. Dietary factors are also needed to supply the groups needed to conjugate drugs in phase II reactions. These include glucuronate, glutathione, acetate and sulphate, all of which facilitate the solubilization and excretion of drugs.

This presents a potential problem for individuals with a chronic disease. If the disease affects their food intake, yet is treated by drugs, the effectiveness of the drugs and their potential side effects may be significantly influenced by the nutritional status. In other words, those who require the drug therapy may well be in the most nutritionally vulnerable state and might not be able to metabolize the drugs.

Dietary Factors Affecting Drug Excretion

A low-protein diet may alter urinary pH, decrease renal blood flow and reduce the excretion of certain drugs. Some drugs are preferentially excreted in acidic conditions and reabsorbed when the pH of the urine becomes more alkaline. Lower clearance via the kidney may increase levels in the blood, resulting in side effects. This has been reported in patients with gout, who are taking allopurinol and a low-protein diet. When several drugs are taken, there may be competition between drugs for renal excretion, with higher levels remaining in the blood.

Drug Effects on Food Intake

One of the most important influences of many drugs is their effect on appetite. In some cases, this may be the main aim of using the drug, when weight loss is required. However, other drugs may induce nausea or cause oral ulceration, which makes food intake unpleasant, notably those used in cancer chemotherapy. Effects further along the gastro-intestinal tract, such as abdominal pain, bloating or diarrhoea, may also reduce the desire to eat.

Some drugs can increase appetite as an unwanted side effect.

Gastro-Intestinal Function

Drugs may affect absorption from the digestive tract. Examples of such effects include

- An alteration in pH (by antacids) and thus a change in the solubility of minerals for absorption
- Inhibition of folate deconjugating enzymes by sulphasalazine, which is used in inflammatory bowel disease, thus preventing liberation of folate from foods or competition with carrier molecules for folate transport

- Induction of catabolism of 25-OH vitamin D by anticonvulsants, reducing circulating levels and interfering with calcium absorption
- Binding of fat-soluble vitamins to mineral oil laxatives
- Destruction by long-acting antibiotics, such as neomycin, of gut flora that synthesize some vitamins
- Reduced vitamin B_{12} absorption owing to interaction with peptic ulcer drugs (H_2 antagonists)
- Damage to mucosal surfaces of the gut and small intestinal enzymes by excessive intakes of alcohol

Metabolic Effects of Drugs on Nutrients

Some drugs may be specific antagonists of the metabolic role of vitamins and may result in alterations in mineral status by specific effects on excretion. Specific vitamin antagonists include those that are intended to inhibit the vitamin or those that affect the vitamin as a side effect. The most important of the specific antagonists are those for folic acid, which are used in cancer chemotherapy, against *Pneumocystis carnii* infection in AIDS, and as antimalarial and anti-inflammatory agents. Coumarin derivatives, used as anticlotting agents, are vitamin K antagonists.

Nitrous oxide, used as an anaesthetic, and the antituberculosis drug isoniazid, however, have unwanted side effects, interfering with B_{12} and B_6, respectively.

Drugs may also lead to excessively high levels of sodium, potassium, calcium and magnesium by interfering with normal regulatory mechanisms. This may be a particular problem with drugs used in cardiac patients receiving diuretic therapies or when several drugs are used together. Diuretics can also result in mineral depletion. In both these cases, the mineral intake of the diet may need to be monitored.

The group in the population most at risk from these many interactions are the elderly. It has been reported that nursing home residents consume on average eight different medications per day. This may also be seen in elderly people living elsewhere, who may take a range of both prescribed and non-prescribed drugs. Interactions between the pharmacological effects of these substances are inevitable. If, at the same time, the physiological processes to cope with the metabolism of the drugs are beginning to be less efficient and maybe the nutritional intake is not as good as it could be, there is potential for undesirable side effects. These may take the form of excessively large or inadequate therapeutic effects, both of which have medical implications.

INFLUENCE OF DISABILITY ON NUTRITION

People who suffer chronic disability, especially those severe enough to require residential care, are at particular risk of nutritional problems. The term 'disability' is used to cover a very wide range of physical or mental conditions that may influence the ability of an individual to function in an otherwise healthy world. The disability may be present from birth, or may have affected the person as a result of an accident or disease (such as Parkinson's disease, multiple sclerosis or stroke). The degree of disability will be reflected in the extent to which these functions are compromised. The disability may be progressive and deteriorating, or there may be a gradual improvement. The perception of change may influence the person's willingness to look after themselves, and take an interest in their health and possible rehabilitation.

Some disabilities will have very little impact on nutrition; others may have profound effects. Those having the greatest effects will be those that affect food intake, digestion and absorption and metabolic needs.

Food intake may be influenced by

- Factors affecting appetite
- Factors affecting the ability to obtain and prepare the food
- Factors affecting the ability to ingest, chew and swallow the food

Appetite

Appetite will be influenced by mental state and thus can be affected by anxiety or depression. Physiological factors will also have an influence; for example, dulled sensation of taste, nausea, constipation or pain after eating will reduce appetite. A common side effect of drug therapy is a dry mouth, which makes food ingestion difficult and unpleasant, and depresses the appetite for eating. Physical factors, such as lack of exercise and immobility, may also mean that the individual does not feel hungry.

Environmental factors, including monotonous menu presentation, especially if the diet has to be soft or purèed, and unpleasant surroundings may be off-putting. Eating snacks or sweets between meals may also be a major factor contributing to a lack of appetite at mealtimes.

In a non-verbal individual affected by any of these factors, their unwillingness to eat and the carer's desire to provide food for eating may result in conflict and frustration.

Ability to Obtain and Prepare Food

In the situation where the individual is responsible for his/her own food supply, both the mental and physical capabilities are important. Understanding what to buy to produce a meal is essential. The process of going out and buying the food may be compromised in many ways, including mobility, ability to communicate, to see/hear and to carry the food. All of these will determine the range of foods that are actually available to eat. Cooking skills and capabilities are also important.

Where a carer is responsible for all of these functions, the autonomy of the individual must be taken into account. The question of whether the food that is being prepared is actually what is desired needs to be addressed. Food is a very personal issue and another person's choice may not be our own.

Ability to Ingest, Chew and Swallow Food

Ingestion, biting, chewing and swallowing of food may be difficult in some disabilities. There may be tongue thrusting, spitting out, choking and dribbling. These may be linked, for example, to a lack of coordination, involuntary movements, lack of lip closure or cleft lip and palate. Careful techniques are required to provide useful nutrition. Appropriate modification of texture may be needed, with the use of thickeners to improve the appearance of meals and make them easier to eat. If the individual is responsible for his/her own feeding, hand to mouth coordination is needed.

Appropriate positioning is essential to facilitate swallowing and prevent regurgitation. Special feeding utensils are available to help the process; occupational therapists can help to develop skills required for feeding and advise on modified equipment. Becoming an independent feeder can lead to marked improvements in nutritional status.

Impact on Digestion and Absorption

Some individuals with disabilities may tend to regurgitate food. Food that has been swallowed may later be brought back into the mouth and spat out. If this is continuous and severe, nutritional status will be threatened.

Drugs used to manage an underlying condition, such as tranquillizers, anticonvulsants, antibiotics, analgesics and antihypertensive drugs, may all affect the digestion and absorption of food from the gut. It is important that potential drug–nutrient interactions are anticipated and avoided by suitable timing of drugs and meals, wherever possible.

Laxatives may be used to treat constipation. A form of laxative that has no impact on nutrient absorption should be chosen and, if possible, dietary fibre and fluid intakes should be increased.

Impact on Metabolism

Nutritional needs may be altered by increased or reduced energy expenditure, drug-induced alterations in metabolism and specific nutritional requirements related to the underlying condition. It is, therefore, important to monitor the nutrient needs of each individual. In children, growth should be monitored regularly, including height and weight; in adults, weight is a useful indicator of adequate energy intake. However, other assessments of nutritional status may be required, particularly micronutrient status.

Nutritional Consequences

If total food intake is small, there is a risk of malnutrition, resulting in poor physical and mental well-being, increased risk of infection and, in children, delayed growth. More often, however, sufficient food is eaten, but it may be low in nutrient density, perhaps because of the foods chosen or if it is diluted during purée production. Attention should also be paid to nutrient retention during preparation. Foods that are kept hot for periods of time lose vitamin content, and modification of texture may result in significant losses of water-soluble vitamins. If specific groups of food are omitted entirely, the individual may be left vulnerable to deficiencies; for example, if few fruit and vegetables are included, they may lack trace elements and folate. Constipation may be a problem if non-starch polysaccharide (NSP) intake is low. Laxative use, on the other hand, may deplete the body of fat-soluble vitamins.

Infection and the associated physiological stress will increase nutritional needs, especially for vitamins B and C, zinc and protein.

Involuntary muscle spasms or tremors (e.g. with Parkinson's disease) may increase energy expenditure and result in weight loss. This is particularly common in children with athetoid cerebral palsy and autism, and with oral motor defects.

Specific drug–nutrient interactions should be anticipated by adjusting food intake. If appetite is very poor, a nutritional supplement may be needed to improve well-being to a point where adequate nutrition can be obtained through the diet.

In summary, there are many threats to the nutritional status of a person experiencing some disability. If these can be identified and anticipated, they should not result in nutritional deficiency. However, the most important criterion is to judge each case in the context of the specific circumstances.

EATING DISORDERS

The eating disorders anorexia and bulimia nervosa are defined as psychiatric illnesses. Despite considerable research on both of these disorders, no effective way of preventing them has been discovered. Both conditions are much more prevalent among females (90%–95%) than males. Patients are commonly of higher than average intelligence and may have particular conflicts with their mother. The key elements of both disorders are a distorted body image, which perceives the body weight to be greater than it is in reality, and a horror of food and its caloric content.

Anorexic patients try to eat very little, with foods chosen carefully to include only those with very low energy content. In addition, the sufferer may exercise frequently and compulsively. There may be mood swings and a denial of the problem, with baggy clothing being worn to disguise thinness. In girls, a diagnostic sign is amenorrhoea and fine 'lanugo' hair may grow on the face and body. People with bulimia nervosa tend to be older and may have a body weight in the normal or overweight range, and some are obese. The pattern of eating involves binges, during which abnormally large amounts of food are consumed. These are then almost immediately followed by deliberately induced vomiting. In both cases, laxatives and diuretics may be used in an attempt to reduce weight.

With prolonged weight loss, and abnormal nutrient intake, plus nutrient losses associated with purging and/or self-induced vomiting, anorexic patients may die – mainly the result of electrolyte disturbances (including refeeding syndrome) and cardiac arrhythmias. If weight loss is not quite so drastic, other changes will still be present, which include loss of muscle and bone mass which reflect negative energy balance, and other features which may relate to micronutrient deficiencies: anaemias, dry and itchy skin, hair loss, digestive tract irregularities (including constipation or diarrhoea), loss of tooth enamel due to vomiting, fainting and cardiac arrhythmias. Treatment requires both clinical and psychiatric intervention, but often takes a long time and may not be entirely successful. There has to be a wish on the part of the sufferer to get better; this is sometimes easier to achieve in the case of bulimic patients than in those with anorexia.

SUMMARY

1. Clinical nutrition involves understanding what determines 'nutritional status' and how it interacts with illnesses.
2. All health professionals need to be aware that an illness can affect nutritional status, and that altered nutritional status affects functional capacity and health.
3. Monitoring of health and weight is vital, at every clinical contact.
4. Screening for malnutrition should be routine in all new medical contacts, and for older and institutionalized people.
5. Optimal nutritional provision during illness needs consideration of the route of administration (oral or artificial, enteral or parenteral) and of the composition of diet (quantity and quality).
6. Overfeeding is liable to cause more clinical problems than underfeeding.

STUDY QUESTIONS

1. What is meant by 'nutritional status'? How can it be assessed in a clinical setting?
2. Is a food allergy diagnosis straightforward? How can it affect health?
3. When should artificial nutrition support be considered? What determines the methods used?
4. In what clinical situations is there a need for emergency nutritional intervention?

BIBLIOGRAPHY AND FURTHER READING

Barendregt, K., Soeters, P.B., Allison, S.P. and Kondrup, J. 2008. Basic concepts in nutrition: Diagnosis of malnutrition – Screening and assessment. *European e-Journal of Clinical Nutrition and Metabolism* 3, e121–e125.

British Dietetic Association. 2014. *Dietician, Nutritionist, Nutritional Therapist or Diet Expert? A Comprehensive Guide to Roles and Functions*. Available at: https://www.bda.uk.com/publications/dietician_nutritionist.

Buttriss, J. (ed.). 2002. *Adverse Reactions to Food. The Report of a British Nutrition Foundation Task Force*. Oxford, UK: Blackwell Science.

Calder, P.C. 2013. Omega-3 polyunsaturated fatty acids and inflammatory processes: Nutrition or pharmacology? *British Journal of Clinical Pharmacology* 75(3), 645–662.

Chafen, J.J.S., Newberry, S.J., Riedl, M.A. et al. 2010. Diagnosing and managing common food allergies: A systematic review. *JAMA* 303(18), 1848–1856.

DoH (UK Department of Health). 1995. Sensible drinking. The report of an interdepartmental working group. Wetherby, UK: Department of Health.

Du Toit, G., Roberts, G., Sayre, P.H. et al. 2015. Randomized trial of peanut consumption in infants at risk for peanut allergy. *New England Journal of Medicine* 372(9), 803–813.

Elia, M., Russell, C.A. and Stratton, R.J. 2010. Conference on 'Malnutrition matters'. Symposium 2: The skeleton in the closet: Malnutrition in the community. Malnutrition in the UK: Policies to address the problem. *Proceedings of the Nutrition Society* 69, 470–476.

Ferland, A. and Eckel, R.H. 2011. Does sustained weight loss reverse the metabolic syndrome? *Current Hypertension Reports* 13(6), 456–464.

Gowland, M.H. 2002. Food allergen avoidance: Risk assessment for life. *Proceedings of the Nutrition Society* 61, 39–43.

Grimble, R.F. 2001. Nutritional modulation of immune function. *Proceedings of the Nutrition Society* 60, 389–397.

Gruchalla, R.S. and Sampson, H.A. 2015. Preventing peanut allergy through early consumption – Ready for prime time? *New England Journal of Medicine* 372(9), 875–877.

Ho, M.H.K., Wong, W.H.S. and Chang, C. 2014. Clinical spectrum of food allergies: A comprehensive review. *Clinical Reviews in Allergy and Immunology* 46(3), 225–240.

Hughes, D.A. 2000. Dietary antioxidants and human immune function. *British Nutrition Foundation Nutrition Bulletin* 25, 35–41.

Leslie, W.S., Hankey, C.R. and Lean, M.E.J. 2007. Weight gain as an adverse effect of some commonly prescribed drugs: A systematic review. *QJM* 100(7), 395–404.

MacFie, J. and McNaught, C. 2015. The ethics of artificial nutrition. *Medicine* 43(2), 124–126.

Mara, J., Gentles, E., Alfheeaid, H.A. et al. 2014. An evaluation of enteral nutrition practices and nutritional provision in children during the entire length of stay in critical care. *BMC Pediatrics* 14(1), 186.

McKee, R.F. 2015. Artificial nutrition and nutritional support and refeeding syndrome. *Medicine* 43(2), 119–123.

McKenna, L.A., Drummond, R.S., Drummond, S., Talwar, D. and Lean, M.E. 2013. Seeing double: The low carb diet. *BMJ* 346, f2563.

Pitsavos, C., Panagiotakos, D., Weinem, M. and Stefanadis, C. 2006. Diet, exercise and the metabolic syndrome. *Review of Diabetic Studies* 3(3), 118–126.

Royal College of Physicians. Ten top tips for nutritional assessment. Available at: https://www.rcplondon.ac.uk/file/1772/download?token=5HJYWGdM (accessed on July 2015).

Salomon, J., De Truchis, P. and Melchior, J.-C. 2001. Nutrition and HIV infection. *British Journal of Nutrition* 87(Suppl. 1), S111–S119.

Saunders, J., Smith, T. and Stroud, M. 2015. Malnutrition and undernutrition. *Medicine* 43(2), 112–118.

Schneider Chafen, J.J., Newberry, S., Riedl, M. et al. 2010. Prevalence, natural history, diagnosis, and treatment of food allergy. A systematic review of the literature. Available at: http://www.rand.org/pubs/workingpapers/2010/RAND_WR757-1.pdf (accessed on 19 December 2014).

Stratton, R.J., Hackston, A., Longmore, D., Dixon, R., Price, S., Stroud, M., King, C. and Elia, M. 2004. Malnutrition in hospital outpatients and inpatients: Prevalence, concurrent validity and ease of use of the 'malnutrition universal screening tool' ('MUST') for adults. *British Journal of Nutrition* 92(5), 799–808.

Thomas, J.A. 1995. Drug–nutrient interactions. *Nutrition Reviews* 53(10), 271–282.

Tsiountsioura, M., Wong, J.E., Upton, J. et al. 2014. Detailed assessment of nutritional status and eating patterns in children with gastrointestinal diseases attending an outpatients clinic and contemporary healthy controls. *European Journal of Clinical Nutrition* 68(6), 700–706.

University of Southampton. Malnutrition online course. Nutrition portal. Available at: https://www.som.soton.ac.uk/learn/test/nutrition/.

Ware, L.J., Wootton, S.A., Morlese, J.M. et al. 2002. The paradox of improved antiretroviral therapy in HIV: Potential for nutritional modulation? *Proceedings of the Nutrition Society* 61, 131–136.

World Gastroenterology Organisation (WGO); The WGO Foundation (WGO-F). 2014. *WGO Handbook on Gut Microbes. World Digestive Health Day WDHD*. Milwaukee, WI: World Gastroenterology Organisation (WGO).

22 Introduction to Sport Nutrition

AIMS

The aim of this chapter is to

- Outline the energy needs in sport, before, during and after exercise.
- Consider the requirements for protein and vitamins in the context of exercise and fatigue.
- Review the importance of hydration in the context of sport and exercise.

The goals of diet for an athlete, or any individual who practices a sport, are simple and mirror recommendations for the general population:

- Follow the healthy eating principles which apply to all adults (caution must be exercised for the child athlete, who is still growing).
- Maintain energy balance while securing the adequate range of micronutrient.
- Maintain hydration levels at all time.
- Identify potential risk of nutrient deficiencies and correct them as applicable.

The child athlete is discussed in Chapter 7, p. 148.

The diet will, in particular, be tailored not only to enhance performance, but also limit fatigue, and potential injuries. When nutrition has such a potential role in influencing the well-being of athletes as well as those engaging in recreational sport activities, it is not surprising that a large market has developed, focusing on nutrition supplements, targeted at strength and endurance enhancement. Various dietary strategies are also advocated, and a sound understanding of nutrition principles is required in order to decipher the evidence-based information from the unsubstantiated commercial solutions. Perhaps not surprisingly, studies have found that athletes have a nutrition knowledge on par with non-athletes, if sometime slightly better, but not to the level of nutrition students.

NUTRITION AND THE ATHLETE

High levels of energy expenditure impose unusual physiological demands on the body. There is an increased need for energy and associated nutrients for increased metabolism as well as adequate fluids to maintain body temperature in the face of large amounts of heat production in exercising muscles. Exercise generates large amounts of free radicals because of the increase in oxidative processes. Thus, there is an increased need for antioxidant factors in the body. First and foremost, the endogenous antioxidant defence systems (with its large array of enzymes including catalase, superoxide dismutase, glutathione peroxidise) are very important, supported by dietary components with antioxidant capacity (including vitamins, minerals as co-factors and possibly some phytochemicals). These should be secured principally from a nutritionally balanced diet, rather than multi-vitamin supplements.

See Chapter 22 for an introduction to sport nutrition, pp. 421–430.

To enable the body to make the most of its nutrient supplies, regular training facilitates the development of a more profuse blood supply in the muscle and shifts metabolism to more energy-sparing pathways. In addition, physical activity confers a number of health advantages. A large follow-up study of 1800 British male civil servants showed that those who took vigorous exercise in their leisure time had less than a quarter of the fatal heart attacks seen in the inactive group. That study design cannot offer proof, but is an encouraging association.

In addition, exercise promotes a sense of well-being, believed to be related to altered levels of neurotransmitters in the brain. There is generally less body fat and more lean body mass than in comparable non-exercisers and a healthier blood lipid profile, with higher levels of high-density lipoproteins (HDLs). Those who exercise can consume more fat in their diet without increasing their adipose tissue levels. People who exercise regularly may also adopt other aspects of a healthier lifestyle, particularly not smoking.

The dietary needs of the athlete are, in essence, very similar to those of the average individual. Differences may arise, however, because of increased energy needs, the timing of meals to ensure an adequate intake around a busy schedule and the importance of maintaining a high intake of carbohydrate during training and after competition. Fluid balance is also crucial.

Athletes can be very vulnerable to suggestions about their diet and may follow a succession of dietary fads and ideas, often spending a huge amount of money on pills and potions. When dietary advice is proposed, they may be reluctant to change what they believe to be a 'winning' diet, even if this is not nutritionally sound. If an athlete can be persuaded to adopt a sound healthy diet, it could remove a whole area of worry from the training programme and allow the focus to be concentrated on the physical training regime. In addition, careful attention to nutrition can make the difference between winning and coming second. It is the responsibility of the nutritionist to work with the athlete, to identify specific nutritional goals that are achievable and to provide strategies that match individual circumstances.

Energy Needs in Sport

The key consideration in any sports performance is the need for energy that is additional to that required for maintaining normal metabolism and everyday physical activity. Not all individuals undertaking sport have high energy requirements: in some sports, energy expenditure may be little more than is found in a moderately active person. Total amount of energy used is also dependent on body size, so a lightweight athlete will use less energy than one with a large body size. Exercising intensively on an energy-restricted diet can cause increased protein breakdown and may cause physiological stress. This, in turn, can result in a suppression of immune function. It is also very important to remember at this point that energy needed for growth must also be met. In teenage athletes, high levels of activity and inadequate intakes will compromise growth. Thus, adequate levels of energy must be provided (Figure 22.1).

Energy as Adenosine Triphosphate (ATP)

At the cellular level, the muscles use adenosine triphosphate (ATP) in their contraction. A constant supply of this must, therefore, be maintained. In the first moments of exercise, the body will use its store of ATP, contained in the muscles, but after 3 seconds, this has been exhausted. The next source is generation of ATP from creatine phosphate, also stored in the muscle, which can provide about 15 seconds' worth of ATP. This may be enough for a short burst of activity, such as a single jump, throw or lift. After this, ATP must come from other metabolic substrates, namely, carbohydrates, proteins and fats. All of these can be transported to the muscle cell and broken down for energy; however, they are not used in equal amounts. Proteins do not usually contribute much to total energy expenditure in exercise except in very prolonged, endurance events or in very intense exercise, when they may supply about 10% of the total energy. The major supply comes from fats and carbohydrates. The choice of fuel is made on the basis of several aspects of the exercise, of which the most important is the intensity.

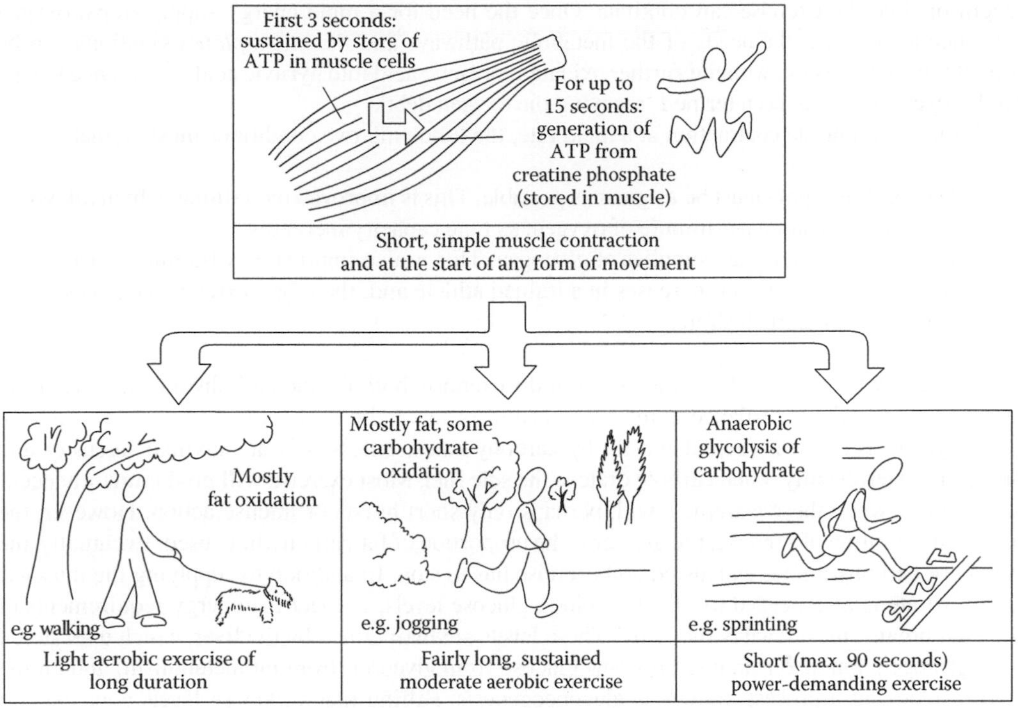

FIGURE 22.1 The provision of energy in sport.

Energy from Fat and Carbohydrates

> The storage and mobilisation of carbohydrates and fats is covered further in Chapter 11, pp. 215–233.

Energy from the diet is stored as glycogen (in the liver and muscles) or adipose tissue. At rest, almost all the body's energy is supplied from fat oxidation (many mistakenly think carbohydrate is the principal source of energy at rest, when in fact, the primary fuel would be alcohol, then fat, then carbohydrate). This is the most efficient source of energy, providing 80–200 units of ATP per molecule. Its main drawback, however, is that it is a slow producer of energy and uses more oxygen than carbohydrate metabolism. Energy obtained from fat is similar to a steam engine – it can use up fuel for long periods of time and maintain a steady pace. Even at low rates of exercise, the body has to use a small amount of carbohydrate to complete the oxidation of fats. Thus, stores of carbohydrate in the form of glycogen are important.

As exercise intensity increases, ATP must be produced more quickly to maintain energy supplies. This can be achieved by using increasingly more carbohydrate, which can produce 38 units of ATP per molecule of glucose as long as the oxygen supply is adequate, that is under aerobic conditions. If the intensity of exercise becomes so great that the production of energy outstrips the supply of oxygen, glucose can still be broken down, albeit very inefficiently (no other substrate can be broken down in this way), but will only produce two units of ATP per molecule of glucose, by anaerobic metabolism. Such a burst of energy can be harnessed for a short and intense exercise, such as a 100 m race or a power lift. However, it is an incomplete metabolic process and lactic acid is produced. This has several consequences, particularly in the production of fatigue. A build-up of lactic acid reduces the pH in the muscle to the point where contraction can no longer occur. This terminates the exercise, so anaerobic exercise of short duration is necessary (a maximum of about 90 seconds). The body's tolerance to lactic acid also increases with training, increasing the length of time the exercise can continue. Once the need for a rapid energy supply stops, oxygen can once again meet the needs of the metabolic pathways and the *incomplete* oxidations can be brought to a conclusion, with the further oxidation of lactic acid into pyruvic acid, and thence via the Kreb's cycle. This has been termed 'repaying the oxygen debt'.

To maintain muscle contraction at a rapid rate, the following two conditions must be met:

1. The oxygen supply must be as great as possible. This is improved by training, which allows a greater utilization per minute of oxygen, as lung capacity increases.
2. There must be adequate supplies of glycogen. This is also improved by training, since the ability to use fat as fuel increases in a trained athlete and, therefore, extends the period of availability of carbohydrate.

In summary, whatever may be the intensity of the exercise, both fat and carbohydrate are generally used. At low levels, the balance is mostly in favour of fats, with little carbohydrate used. At high intensity, the exercise is fuelled mostly by carbohydrates, unless it is at maximal intensity and proceeds anaerobically, when carbohydrate is the sole fuel. Most exercise will predominantly occur at a level between these extremes, with perhaps only short bursts of intense action. However, the longer the duration of exercise, the greater is the proportion of fat:carbohydrate used. Eventually, the supply of carbohydrate is exhausted and exercise has to stop. In addition to supplying the muscles, carbohydrate is also needed to maintain blood glucose levels, to meet the energy requirements of the vital organs, most notably the brain. These levels are maintained by the liver, which uses stored liver glycogen, but also manufactures new glucose from glycerol (from fat metabolism) and amino acid residues, in a process known as gluconeogenesis. Falling blood glucose levels contribute to fatigue. Low blood glucose levels also cause physiological stress, which results in the release of hormones, such as cortisol, which in turn have a negative effect on immunity.

From the aforementioned texts, it can be seen that maintaining a high level of stored glycogen in the muscle is important to extend duration of exercise. Many studies on exercising subjects, first carried out

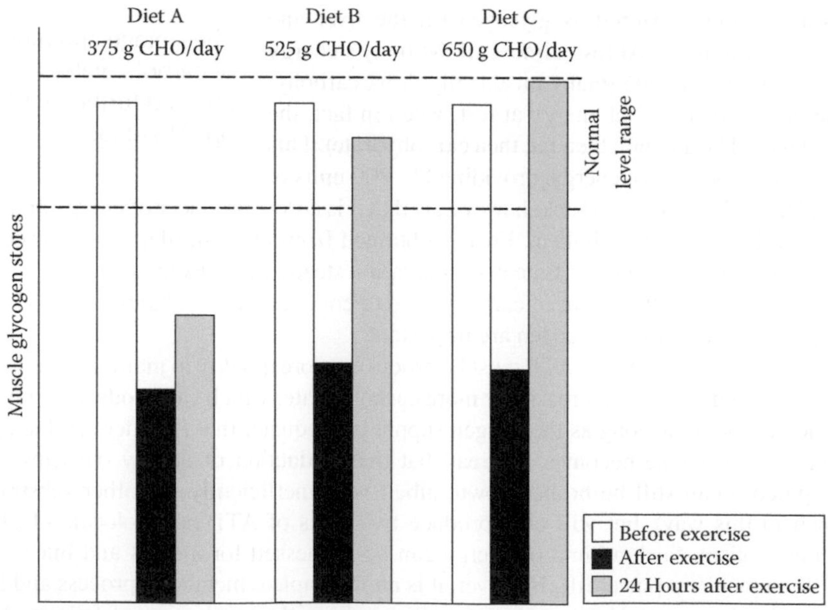

FIGURE 22.2 Effects of different amounts of carbohydrate in the diet on the refuelling of muscle by glycogen reaccumulation in the 24–48 hours after exercise. (Reproduced from Wootton, Simon & Schuster, London, UK, 1988. With permission.)

in the 1930s, have shown that exercise time to exhaustion can be lengthened in subjects consuming a diet containing a high proportion of carbohydrate. This increases exercise times compared with times achieved by subjects on normal diets, which in turn are greater than those in subjects fed a high fat/protein diet with low levels of carbohydrate. It has subsequently been shown that exercised muscle is capable of taking up carbohydrate in increased amounts in the first 1–2 hours after activity, which helps to replenish stores and permits exercise to be repeated on the following day (Figure 22.2). This increased capacity to store carbohydrate is believed to be at least partly the result of increased blood flow to muscles in the post-exercise period. Cell volume, influenced by osmotic changes, is also a determinant of carbohydrate synthesis after exercise. These two findings highlight the importance of carbohydrate in the diet of the athlete.

During Training

In practical terms, the diet during training should be based on carbohydrates, ideally supplying 55%–60% of the energy. This means that, if levels of protein are 10%–15% of energy, the amount of fat is 25%–35%. This is clearly very close to the general healthy eating guidelines. The carbohydrate should be a mixture of both simple and complex sources. In reality, an athlete who has very high energy needs would find it very difficult to consume the volume of complex carbohydrate this would represent. This would be exacerbated by the usual lack of time for eating, which is common among amateur athletes. Nevertheless, adequate intake of carbohydrate is essential if daily exercise is taken (Figure 22.3). A daily requirement of 8–10 g carbohydrate/kg body weight is recommended during periods of hard training. For training sessions that last for more than 60 minutes, it is also important to take carbohydrate at intervals starting after the first 30 minutes. This helps to maintain circulating blood glucose levels and prevents depletion of liver glycogen stores. Once these have been depleted, they cannot be replaced until exercise has stopped.

After Exercise

When exercise stops, the muscles need to be refilled as quickly as possible with glycogen, to be ready for the next bout. The first priority after exercise is thus to consume some carbohydrate-containing food, which will be readily absorbed and deliver its glucose content to the muscles. The food chosen should have a high glycaemic index, which will cause a quick rise in blood sugar. During this time, it is recommended that at least 50–100 g carbohydrate is consumed (1–2 g/kg) within the first hour (foods grouped according to glycaemic index are given in Table 22.1).

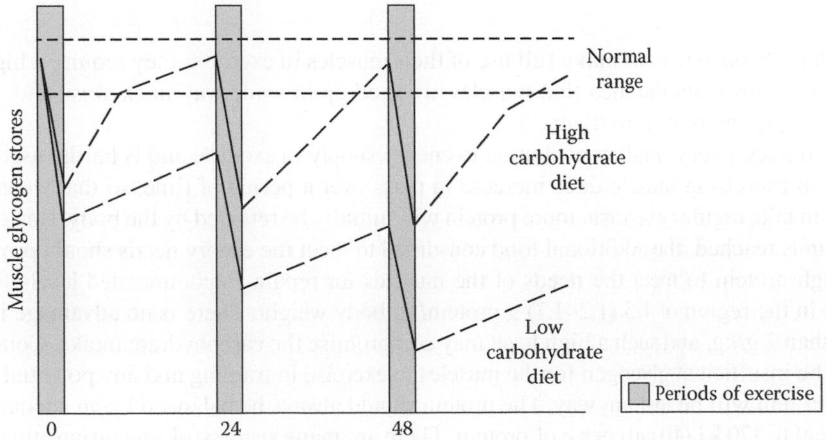

FIGURE 22.3 Effects of different amounts of carbohydrate in the diet on muscle glycogen levels during three consecutive periods of exercise over 72 hours. (Reproduced from Wootton, Simon & Schuster, London, UK, 1988. With permission.)

TABLE 22.1

Grouping of Some Commonly Eaten Foods According to Glycaemic Index

Foods with High Glycaemic Index (above 85)	Foods with Moderate Glycaemic Index (less than 60)	Foods with Low Glycaemic Index (60–85)
Bread (white or wholemeal)	Pasta and noodles	Apples, grapefruit, peaches, plums
Rice	Porridge	Beans
Breakfast cereals (e.g. cornflakes, muesli, Weetabix)	Grapes, oranges	Milk, yogurt and ice cream
Raisins, bananas	Crisps	Fructose
Potato, sweetcorn	Biscuits	Tomato soup
Glucose, sucrose, honey		
Soft drinks		
Maltodextrin drink (20%)		

Source: Adapted from Williams, C. and Devlin, J.T., eds., *Foods, Nutrition and Sports Performance*, E & F Spon, London, UK, 1992. With permission.

Many athletes find that they do not want to eat immediately after exercise; in this case, a carbohydrate-containing drink is useful. This helps to achieve the goal of replenishment of carbohydrate stores, as well as providing some rehydration. Small carbohydrate-containing snacks eaten at frequent intervals are also helpful. It should be remembered, however, that too many high-sugar foods may pose problems for dental hygiene and appropriate advice should also be given on this. Where possible, a meal or large snack high in carbohydrate should be consumed within 2 hours.

Later on, foods with a lower glycaemic index are acceptable, as they cause a slower but more sustained increase in blood glucose levels, which can enter the muscles over a longer period of time to maintain the refuelling process. Protein supply is also important at this time to ensure sufficient levels of amino acids in the circulation for tissue repair and protein synthesis. This does not need to come from special protein supplements but can readily be supplied from normal foods, such as a sandwich with cheese, lean meat or fish, a baked potato with beans, or a pasta dish with a meat- or cheese-based sauce. All of these provide a combination of protein and carbohydrate.

Protein Needs

Many athletes believe that, to make full use of their muscles in exercise, they require a high protein intake. This stems from the idea that muscles are used up in some way in exercise and, therefore, require extra protein to restore them.

Protein makes a very small contribution to energy supply in exercise and is hardly used up at all. However, an exercising muscle does increase in mass over a period of time, so that when a person first starts to take regular exercise, more protein will initially be retained by the body. However, when equilibrium is reached, the additional food consumed to meet the energy needs should provide more than enough protein to meet the needs of the muscles for repair. Recommended levels for protein intake are in the region of 1.5 (1.2–1.7) g protein/kg body weight. There is no advantage in exceeding more than 2 g/kg, and such a high level may compromise the carbohydrate intake. Consequently, there will be insufficient glycogen for the muscles to exercise in training and any potential benefit of the extra protein will be lost anyway. The protein should always be balanced by an adequate energy intake, equal to 170 kJ (40 cal) per g of protein. There are many successful vegetarian athletes whose protein intakes are derived only from plant foods, and also athletes whose protein intakes do not exceed 10% of the energy intake. It is the training that increases muscle size, strength and exercise capacity, and not the increased protein intake. Many athletes from developing countries do not have access to such high levels of protein, yet compete effectively on the world stage.

Dietary Supplements

Athletes use a wide range of supplements, and surveys from various countries indicate that over 90% of casual athletes studied are currently using, or have used dietary supplements in the past. Usage varies with the particular sport, level of competition and gender of the athlete, and on the extent of local marketing which often depends on providing incentives by marketing companies to sports clubs, supermarkets etc to stock and sell their products.

Very few of the supplements used by athletes have been scientifically evaluated for efficacy to enhance performance, although, if the diet is inadequate, there may be a valid case for using the supplement. Professional athletes in general do not use special supplements, because they do not actually work. The enormous current market for protein supplements, and others, is an indication of the ignorance and gullibility of consumers.

Vitamin and Mineral Supplements

There is little evidence that vitamin supplements are of any benefit in an adequately nourished athlete. Studies that have claimed to show an improvement often give no indication of the initial nutritional status of the athlete and, therefore, their findings prove little.

> The metabolism and function of vitamins and minerals is covered in detail in Chapters 4 and 5.

The following two points are, however, important:

- Athletes who consume very little food in an attempt to maintain a low body weight appropriate to their particular sport may not meet their nutritional requirements for all micronutrients. A supplement may be indicated in this case.
- Intense physical activity produces free radicals, which may represent a health risk to the individual, if insufficient levels of antioxidant nutrients are present. Attention should be paid particularly to vitamin E and C intakes to ensure adequate status. There is some evidence that immune status is poorer in athletes who undertake heavy training. This may be linked to low levels of certain micronutrients needed for the components of the immune response, although stress responses may also be an important factor.

Mineral status is of concern in terms of calcium and iron, especially in female athletes, who may consume diets deficient in both of these nutrients. Low calcium status in young women, together with a low body weight, which results in amenorrhoea (loss of menstrual periods), may compromise bone density and lead to fractures and early osteoporosis. This condition has been described as 'fit but fragile'. The drive to maintain a low body weight may be so intense that a type of anorexic behaviour is seen, with obsessive avoidance of food that might cause weight gain, compulsive exercise and amenorrhoea with resulting low bone density that may lead to frequent fractures. This is sometimes described as 'the female athlete triad'. When competitive sport participation stops, normal menstrual activity is likely to return, but it is possible that bone density does not recover to that expected for age. Most at risk are young females in whom high levels of exercise delay menarche and disrupt the phase of most rapid bone mass accretion.

Iron needs are higher in women because of menstrual losses; low-weight female athletes may cease to menstruate and thereby conserve some iron. However, evidence exists of a higher turnover of iron in athletes, possibly owing to increased destruction of red blood cells. This may result in increased needs and, if these are not met, then stores will decline and anaemia can develop, which will affect performance.

Creatine

Creatine phosphate is an important energy source for muscles during intense exercise. However, the content in muscle is limited. Creatine is obtained from the diet, predominantly in meat and animal products, but is also synthesized in the body from amino acid precursors, such as glycine and arginine. Vegetarian athletes have to rely on endogenous synthesis, which can provide enough creatine. However, since the early 1990s, creatine supplements have been available, which have been shown to enhance the content in muscle by up to 50%. The scientific evidence supports a positive effect of creatine supplementation in repeated short bursts of intense activity. It does not enhance duration of prolonged effort. Creatine supplementation can result in an initial gain in muscle bulk of 1–2 kg after a loading dose (4 × 5 g doses daily) for 4–5 days. This is probably due to swelling of cells, which may be accompanied by increased protein synthesis. A maintenance dose of 1–2 g daily is recommended. Subjectively, heaviness of muscles may be a reported side effect. No clinically significant negative effects have been reported to date. There are many other dietary supplements which are used by athletes.

Fluid

Fluid is also an important consideration for athletes. Sweating is essential to lose heat and maintain body temperature during prolonged exertion, and hyperventilation entails extra fluid loss by evaporation in expired breath. Extra fluid is therefore always required, even in cool conditions without heavy sweating. For most activities, that extra fluid is provided from the liver, because glycogen is stored with 4 g of water for each 1g of glycogen. Water is thus released as glycogen is used up. Depending on degree of training, extra drinking water is needed after about 1 hour of sustained exertion. Sweat contains electrolytes, most notably sodium, potassium and chloride ions, derived from the plasma. However, the concentration of electrolytes in the sweat is different from that in the plasma, with the result that the remaining plasma may actually have higher concentrations of some electrolytes at the end of the exercise. Consequently, the top priority for replacement after exercise is water, to restore normal concentrations in plasma. Dehydration and sodium losses are key contributors to fatigue – however, thirst alone is not a sufficient indicator to prevent dehydration.

The issue is complicated by the observation that the best way to increase water absorption from the gut is to include some electrolytes in solution. This enhances water uptake and speeds rehydration. Many rehydrating solutions are available; most of them contain electrolytes (at less than 2.6 g/dL), together with varying amounts of carbohydrate. The carbohydrate is present in amounts that may be

- Lower than concentrations in body fluids (hypotonic solutions)
- The same as body fluids (isotonic solutions)
- Greater than body fluids (hypertonic solutions)

Absorption of these is most rapid from the hypotonic solution and slowest from the hypertonic solution. Drinking a hypertonic solution will not provide rapid rehydration and may actually aggravate matters, as fluid from the body is drawn into the digestive tract. However, hypotonic and isotonic solutions are useful in providing quick rehydration. The added benefit of the carbohydrate content when taken at the end of exercise is its contribution to refuelling the glucose stores. These solutions are also useful during prolonged exercise, when they help to maintain blood glucose levels and prevent dehydration, thus enabling performance to continue at an optimal level. Solutions that contain glucose polymers are now available; this enables more glucose to be contained in the drink without compromising the tonicity and, therefore, provide more potential energy in the drink.

Over-consumption of fluid is not advisable, however. Those who consume large volume of fluids may suffer from bloating and pains, and performance is impaired. A serious consequence of over-drinking is exercise-associated hyponatremia (low sodium levels in the blood). This condition is serious, as it creates an osmotic imbalance. While it manifests itself with headache and nausea, it can quickly progress to cardiac arrest and death if the sodium stores are not rapidly replenished.

TABLE 22.2
Functional Foods in Sports Nutrition

Dietary Constituent	Suggested Role	Strength of Evidence
Amino acids		
Arginine, lysine, ornithine	Promote growth hormone secretion and aid muscle development	Weak
Glutamine	Prevents immunodepression, reduces infections	Some experimental evidence
Caffeine	Promotes fatty acid release, sparing glycogen stores	Can be beneficial, in extreme performance
Carnitine	Central role in energy production, could enhance aerobic performance	Weak
Coenzyme Q_{10}	Needed for generation of ATP	Weak
Creatine	Increases capacity for repeated bouts of high-intensity exercise	Good
Ginseng	Increases mental energy and stamina	Weak
Sodium bicarbonate	Increased alkaline reserve to buffer lactic acid produced in anaerobic exercise	May be effective in specific circumstances. Gastrointestinal effects unpleasant

Sports Products

The sports nutrition market contains a wide range of functional foods for athletes that are promoted as supplying specific benefits over and above basic nutrition.

The development of sports drinks containing glucose polymers allowed more carbohydrate to be consumed, without undesirable effects in terms of sweetness and palatability as well as excessive osmotic effects. Products, such as high-energy bars, also provide a large amount of energy in a very small volume of food, allowing energy needs to be met. Glycerol is now included in some sports drinks as research has suggested that this can promote hyperhydration, although the evidence is equivocal.

A huge range of products that have potential use as ergogenic aids are marketed and can be considered as functional foods. Some of these are summarized in Table 22.2.

Although there is a theoretical potential for a metabolic effect for some of the functional products available for athletes, the actual ability of the substances to reach the target site and be incorporated into the cellular or subcellular metabolic machinery is usually not proven. Much more research is needed to examine possible beneficial effects of putative ergogenic agents, as well as their safety.

SUMMARY

1. While athletes need to follow the healthy eating recommendations for the general population, their specific nutritional requirements need to be considered, and their diet adapted in order to meet the increased needs.
2. Low nutritional knowledge can put athletes in a vulnerable position, considering the large commercial set-up promoting diet aids and supplements.
3. During exercise, muscle need energy to contract, in the form of ATP.
4. While (stored) fat is the primary source of energy at rest, reliance on carbohydrates as a source of energy increases with exercise intensity, leading to depletion of muscle glycogen.

5. In the later stage of exercise, there is a shift towards fatty acids as a source of energy.
6. After exercise, glycogen stores need to be replaced (2 hours after exercise is adequate, since it coincides with increased glycogen synthase activity and insulin sensitivity).
7. While exercise leads to increase free radical production, there is little evidence supporting the use of vitamin supplement, since endogenous antioxidant system is usually up-regulated in athletes.
8. Maintaining fluid balance is essential for performance, since dehydration and sodium loss are the principal factors contributing to fatigue.

STUDY QUESTIONS

1. a. What do you consider to be the main difficulties encountered by an athlete that might prevent the consumption of an adequate diet?
   b. How can some of these difficulties be tackled and overcome?
2. What is the influence of body composition on energy needs?
3. What are the main sources of energy stored in the body, and how are they mobilized?
4. Is there any value in adding carbohydrate and electrolytes to drinks consumed during exercise?

ACTIVITIES

22.1 An athlete requires a daily intake of approximately 21 MJ (5000 cal). Calculate the amount of carbohydrate this would represent according to the aforementioned guidelines.
Devise a day's menu to supply this amount of carbohydrate:
- using predominantly sources of complex carbohydrate;
- including some simple carbohydrate.

Repeat the calculation using a target energy intake of 10.5 MJ (2500 cal).
Compare the practicalities of consuming the two diets.

22.2 List the key nutritional considerations that need to be taken into account for a child endurance athlete.
- What diet plan would you devise?
- Are there challenges associated with the implementation of this diet?

BIBLIOGRAPHY AND FURTHER READING

British Nutrition Foundation. 2001. Nutrition and sport. Briefing paper. London, UK: British Nutrition Foundation.

Close, G.L. and Jackson, M.J. 2014. Antioxidants and exercise: A tale of the complexities of relating signalling processes to physiological function? *The Journal of Physiology* 592(8), 1721–1722.

Coombes, J.S. and Hamilton, K.L. 2000. The effectiveness of commercially available sports drinks. *Sports Medicine* 29(3), 181–209.

Heaney, S., O'Connor, H., Michael, S., Gifford, J. and Naughton, G. 2011. Nutrition knowledge in athletes: A systematic review. *International Journal of Sport Nutrition and Exercise Metabolism* 21(3), 248–261.

Jeukendrup, A. 2014. A step towards personalized sports nutrition: Carbohydrate intake during exercise. *Sports Medicine* 44(1), 25–33.

Johnson, N.A., Stannard, S.R. and Thompson, M.W. 2004. Muscle triglyceride and glycogen in endurance exercise. *Sports Medicine* 34(3), 151–164.

Laursen, P.B. and Rhodes, E.C. 2001. Factors affecting performance in an ultraendurance triathlon. *Sports Medicine* 31(3), 195–209.

Maughan, R. 2002. The athlete's diet: Nutritional goals and dietary strategies. *Proceedings of the Nutrition Society* 61, 87–96.

Williams, C. and Devlin, J.T. (eds.) 1992. *Foods, Nutrition and Sports Performance*. London, UK: E & F Spon.

Wootton, S. 1988. Nutrition in Sport. London: Simon & Shulster.

23 Improving Foods for Better Nutrition

AIMS

The aims of this chapter are to

- Discuss the concept of nutrition improvement to foods for consumers health.
- Describe some of the 'smart foods' that are available to the consumer designed to optimize health.
- Describe the evidence to support the use of these foods.
- Explain the concepts of food reformulation and nutrient profiling.

In the last few decades, there has been a shift in perception of the possible roles of food and nutrition. The fundamental role of food is to supply the basic nutrients required for the maintenance of physiological function and growth, while also satisfying sensory needs. Such basic requirements give rise to the dietary reference values used for population recommendations. However, as the science of human nutrition has grown, our knowledge of the role of nutrients in the body has developed and increased our understanding on how the intake of specific nutrients may impact on health and the prevention and development of disease states. Thus, there has been a shift from discussing 'adequate' nutrition to considering 'optimal' nutrition. This presents a challenge to nutritional scientists to decide, where relevant,

- how much is enough (to minimize deficiency)?
- how much is best (to meet biochemical, physiological and other functions for normal health)?
- how much can provide other benefits in non-nutritional ways?
- how much is too much and may cause harmful effects?

The dietary reference values are covered in Chapter 2, pp. 18–20.

Suitable indices are required in order to be able to define these limits, and this brings considerable methodological, practical and ethical challenges. Traditional approaches have included balance studies, tissue saturation studies, measurement of body stores and functional studies. However, many of these methods are used to determine minimal rather than optimal requirements for nutrients.

The function of a nutrient within a specific target tissue or pathway can be used to determine its level of activity, and to explore the effects of changes in intake or circulating levels of the nutrient. It would be expected that increases in intake, or circulating levels up to a certain point, would cause a dose–response change in activity of the measured function. At the point where activity ceases to increase, it can be assumed that maximal physiological (or optimal) function has been achieved. However, with the current state of knowledge, the role of a nutrient is likely to be assessed in a more general way: for example, in terms of its effect on antioxidant status, muscle strength or blood clotting. This is because, in most cases, the precise biochemical point at which deficiency of a particular nutrient becomes limiting may not be known. With developments in molecular biology, it may be possible, in the future, to explore the effects of nutrients on gene expression and determine their role precisely. A general function is also likely to be used to assess possible health benefits of a nutrient, perhaps in amounts greater than those needed to meet functional needs.

Even if it were possible to precisely determine optimal levels of nutrients for particularly physiological processes, it is difficult to translate such results obtained in the laboratory into guidelines or targets for dietary intakes of a particular nutrient. These include

- Interactions between nutrients and other chemical components in food
- Uncertainties about the bioavailability of nutrients at the gut level
- Efficiency of transport to the target site
- Inter-individual variation
- Potential interaction between nutrients at different stages in the life cycle

Research on optimal levels for the majority of nutrients is at an early stage. The Food Standards Agency in the United Kingdom has an Optimal Nutritional Status research programme (renamed the Nutritional Status and Function Research Programme in 2004), designed to understand the links between optimal nutrition status and the maintenance of good health, including the potential interactions between micronutrients at different life stages in the reduction of specific diseases. A secondary objective is to develop accurate measures of bioavailability of nutrients from foods; the processing of nutrients at the gut level and their transport to cellular sites.

FOODS, FOOD COMPONENTS AND HEALTH CLAIMS

The growth of interest in the use of food to promote a state of health and well-being, and reduce the risk of disease, has led to the rapid development of an industry that produces foods that claim to possess these characteristics. A health claim describes a positive relationship between a food substance in the diet and a disease or other health-related condition. This may include a lessening of the condition or a reduction in the risk of that condition.

Early research on these foods started in Japan in the 1980s, with the purpose of developing foods for specific health use (FOSHU). These were defined as 'processed foods containing ingredients that aid specific bodily functions in addition to nutrition'. Legislation allowed claims to be made about specific health effects of foods in certain categories. In the United States, the Nutrition Labelling and Education Act, enforced in 1994, allowed health claims to be made for ingredients for which there was recognized evidence of a correlation between intake and cure or prevention of certain diseases, although this does not necessarily mean that the evidence can be applied to the food itself.

The promotion of foods with health claims is much more restricted in the United Kingdom, where the law separates foods and medicines so that foods cannot be described as providing a medical health benefit. Therefore, foods cannot be labelled as 'preventing' or 'curing' a specific disease. As a result of growing concern about the unregulated market in the United Kingdom, the Food Advisory Committee produced a set of guidelines. These have been developed into a Code of Practice by the Joint Health Claims Initiative (JHCI), a panel of representatives from consumer, food industry and enforcement groups. This aims to help the food industry to make health claims that are within current legislative constraints. An expert committee is to review all claims to ensure that they are supported by scientific evidence, with the aim of producing a list of approved generic health claims for use by food manufacturers whose products meet the criteria. New submissions for products will also be considered. It is anticipated that this will allow consumers to receive information about health benefits without infringing current UK legislation.

There is a relatively high degree of public suspicion of processed foods in the United Kingdom, due to a number of food-related health scares in recent years. A meeting with consumers by the Foresight Task Force, set up by the Government in the United Kingdom in 2001, indicated that there is cynicism among consumers about the need for new products developed by the food industry. Clear consumer communication on the value of products designed to optimize nutrition is essential in promoting their use. This puts the onus on the food industry to follow the principles of scientific research and on regulatory authorities to ensure that systems are in place to protect the consumer. There is a clearly defined process that must be followed by food companies in the development of such products or food components:

- Fundamental research techniques should be used to identify possible interactions between a food component and a function relevant to health, thus generating hypotheses for study. Appropriate markers of this function need to be developed for the assessment. This is problematic, as few such markers exist.
- The hypothetical effect needs to be tested in appropriate models, including human studies, and safety assessments carried out. Trials should be carried out in a manner similar to drug testing, with the potential to demonstrate a dose–response relationship, and any potential risk be evaluated. The cost–benefit analysis of the use of the food component should be made.
- The food component being studied should be able to be included in a variety of normal diets, in amounts sufficient to produce the desired effects, that is, they should remain 'foods'.
- Possible adverse effects of an excess intake of the component must also be examined (e.g. if the same component is included in a number of products, will this still be safe?).
- The differential effects of the component in people of different ages and states of health should be considered.
- The evidence relating to the product must be evaluated by an independent authority, which is empowered to approve the use of the product, and which can determine the nature and content of the health claim being made. This is a fundamental part of any food safety and labelling regulations that exist in a country.
- The information to the consumer about the product must be both clear and informative. It should include information about the target group or condition (if this is specific), the benefit claimed and the amount to be consumed.

Terminology

There is a confusing range of terms given to foods that have been specifically developed by the food industry to meet the demand for healthier foods.

SMART FOODS

Smart foods is the term being used in schools in the United Kingdom as part of the design and technology curriculum. The food industry uses the term 'modern' or 'novel' food materials. These are foods that have been developed through new or improved processes, generally by human intervention and, therefore, not through naturally occurring changes. This classification includes

- Foods with novel molecular structures, including fat substitutes and sweeteners
- Meat analogues, including novel proteins
- Foods produced by biotechnology
- Functional foods (also known as pharmafoods or nutraceuticals)

Foods with Novel Molecular Structures

In relation to healthy eating initiatives, the most important components in this group are fat replacers and sweeteners. Both are useful in reducing the energy content of the diet. Fat replacers can be derived from carbohydrate or protein, or be lipid based. In the case of carbohydrate- or protein-derived products, these can be used to substitute fat in the production of low-fat meals, and additionally act as stabilizers to prevent separation of ingredients. Lipid-based fat replacers are fatty acid esters with sugars, which are not absorbed from the digestive tract. These have the advantage of being stable at high temperatures and can, therefore, be used in fried or baked products, such as crisps and biscuits. An example of this group is Olestra, licensed for use in the United States.

Sweeteners are a well-established item in the diet of people wishing to reduce their energy intake. The main products used in the United Kingdom are saccharin, aspartame, acesulfame and cyclamate. All the intense sweeteners provide the sensation of sweetness in very small amounts because of their molecular structure and can, therefore, mimic the effect of sucrose, without supplying the associated energy. Aspartame is composed of phenylalanine and aspartic acid and, therefore, yields these amino acids when digested. However, the quantity consumed produces a negligible amount of energy. Because it contains phenylalanine, aspartame should not be used by people with phenylketonuria (PKU) who cannot metabolize it. Over 2000 products available in Europe contain aspartame.

This group of smart foods also contains modified starches, which are used in many food products that need to be stabilized or thickened, and has extended the range of 'instant' and 'ready to eat' products on the market.

Meat Analogues

This group of smart foods includes products made from soya protein (textured vegetable protein, tofu) or fungal proteins (Quorn) that have been extruded, spun, coagulated and moulded into products that resemble meat in texture. Flavours and additional nutrients may be added as part of the processing. These products are included in the diet of people who prefer not to eat meat, but may also be considered by some to be a healthier alternative to meat. This may not necessarily be the case, as levels of fat may be comparable to those in similar meat dishes and micronutrient levels may be lower.

Foods Produced by Biotechnology

Plant and animal breeders have for centuries tried to breed in the best characteristics of the species, and breed out the least advantageous ones. Biotechnology is the use of biological processes to make useful products. The use of yeast to make bread and beer, and microorganisms to make yogurt and vinegar are all traditional examples. In recent years, developments in molecular biology and genetics have made it possible to manipulate the genes of plants and animals to an extent that specific characteristics have been transferable. This has made it possible to produce new varieties of certain plants having desirable characteristics. Disease resistance can be enhanced by genetic modification so that insect- or virus-borne diseases no longer destroy the crop. This has been achieved for a substantial proportion of maize grown in the United States. Work is under way to increase disease resistance in the sweet potato, which could enhance yields three fold.

One of the most successful 'genetically modified' (GM) plants has been the soya bean, which carries resistance to particular herbicides, thus allowing more effective treatment of the cultivated land with less herbicide and hence more efficient crop growth and less environmental damage. Varieties of maize and rice have also been developed, which have advantages in terms of nutrient composition or yield over the more traditional varieties. For example, the protein and vitamin A content of rice has been enhanced to improve dietary balance. It is anticipated that, in the future, more beneficial amino-acid profiles or higher meat yields can be engineered into animals. Higher levels of antioxidants are being bred into tomatoes. The removal of potential allergens from foods, such as wheat, is another area of research, which would help individuals who are unable to consume gluten. Similarly, research on allergens in peanuts may yield a non-allergenic product. Slower ripening allows crops to be preserved better with fewer losses.

There is concern that introducing alien genes into plants may have adverse consequences for the humans who consume these, and a considerable amount of resistance to the introduction of foods containing GM components. Careful testing for safety and long-term trials are necessary to ensure that these products are safe. Clear labelling of products that contain GM ingredients is also called for by consumers, and European legislation has been reviewed in the light of concerns and will be monitored in the future.

Functional Foods

This is the largest category of smart foods and also the most diverse. The world market for functional foods and drinks is expected to reach $130 billion by 2015. Market growth is fuelled by product innovation and increasingly health-conscious consumers with higher disposable incomes. A functional food is defined as one having health-promoting benefits, and/or disease-preventing properties over and above the usual nutritional value. This definition can cause difficulties in that some common foods could be considered to be covered by this definition. For example, many vegetables provide non-nutritive phytochemicals, which are believed to have health-promoting benefits but do not contribute to the accepted nutritional value of the vegetable. It has been suggested that functional foods might be better viewed as a concept that can help to optimize nutrition rather than a means to categorize them.

Nevertheless, it is useful to consider the different types of products that could come into this group.

- Foods containing added (1) or reduced levels of nutrients – these can be nutrients that may or may not normally be found in the food.
- Foods containing phytochemicals, that is, components with no known nutritional role that are promoted as such in the diet, or have added levels of some phytochemicals.
- Foods containing added components that do not occur generally in the typical diet, with the specific aim of producing a functional effect.
- Foods containing bacteria that are used to promote gastrointestinal tract function.

The following sections will consider examples of foods/food components in each of these categories and some of the evidence for their use as functional foods.

Fortified Foods

This group includes foods that have been fortified with macronutrients or micronutrients. On a global basis, food fortification is an important strategy for combating specific nutrient deficiency that may be prevalent in a community. Notable examples of this include fortification of salt with iodine and the addition of iron to breakfast cereals. In such national schemes, it is important to choose both an appropriate food for fortification, which represents a regular item in the diet, as well as the best form of the mineral or vitamin to maintain the stability of the food product, and maximize bioavailability of the nutrient.

There is no widespread single nutrient deficiency in the United Kingdom, yet there are a great number of fortified foods available aimed at promoting health rather than preventing deficiency. These include white bread and flour, which are required legally to have thiamin, iron and calcium added to restore the content to that found in wholemeal flour. This was introduced to protect the health of the population following World War II, but has been maintained ever since, although the nutritional need for this is arguable. In the United States, folate is added to flour; but this is not the case in the United Kingdom, following a decision taken by the Food Standards Agency in 2002, after a wide-ranging consultation. Margarine is required by law to be fortified with vitamins A and D, to provide levels of these vitamins that are comparable to those in butter. Many of the other spreading fats are also fortified with these vitamins. Breakfast cereals are voluntarily fortified with a wide range of nutrients; however, this is not a legal requirement. The range of nutrients added, and the level of fortification, varies between products and from time to time in the same product.

Infant milks and foods contain various added nutrients to enhance their nutritional value. There are guidelines on the levels of nutrients that should be provided in foods for infants. Other products that are fortified include instant mashed potato, bedtime drinks, yogurts, soft drinks, condensed milk and dried milk powder. The range of fortified foods available is not consistent, and it is therefore important to read the nutritional labels on products. Most of the examples mentioned contain added nutrients that would be found in a more *natural* form of the food. However, there are now exceptions to this, with nutrients being added that would not be found associated with the product, for example, the addition of calcium to orange juice. Currently, it is difficult to add some nutrients to foods because of the technological difficulties of dispersal, taint and stability of the products. However, micro-encapsulation of nutrients may expand this field further in the future. One group of nutrients being considered in this context is the *n*-3 fatty acids, which could be added to some foods in the future in this way. Similarly, calcium can be added to soya milk in an encapsulated form that avoids precipitation of the soya protein.

Reduced Content of Nutrients

This group contains foods mostly for the weight-reduction market, with a wide range of products that are 'low calorie' and, therefore, to be used 'as part of a calorie-controlled diet'. These include individual products, such as drinks, biscuits, yogurts and whole meals, available as 'ready meals' that have been 'calorie counted'. A further range of foods are 'low-fat' products, which represent a separate area of the market. These are not necessarily lower in energy content than a corresponding regular product, as they may contain other energy-containing constituents within the formulation, but do meet regulations of having lower percentage fat than the regular product.

Specific alterations to other constituents may include reduced sugar or salt content. A number of specific dietary products are marketed to meet the demand for foods that are free from a specific component, such as gluten-free products for people with coeliac disease. Other examples may include products that are free from lactose, sucrose, milk or egg.

Foods Containing Phytochemicals

Digestion and absorption of phytochemicals is covered in Chapter 10, p. 212.

In general, the phytochemicals are produced by the plant as a defence against predators, and are bitter, acrid or astringent in an attempt to make the plant unpalatable or toxic. As a result, humans too may find these substances unpleasant, and this may be a strong disincentive to consume foods that could be good for our health but may not agree with our palate. A challenge to the food industry, both in the past and future, has been to breed varieties of plants in which the bitter taste is reduced, while at the same time attempting to ensure that the beneficial effects of the phytochemicals are preserved or enhanced by selective breeding. Extracting the active agent and adding it to other products is a possible developmental step. This has already happened with the use of isoflavones from soya in some types of bread.

The interest in phytochemicals stems from the strong link between diets rich in plant foods and lower rates of cancer and coronary heart disease. The diversity of these compounds creates an enormous task to study the roles of individual phytochemicals in disease prevention or risk reduction and, at present, the evidence often relates to groups of related compounds. Several different mechanisms of action have been identified, usually by *in vitro* study.

Foods with Added Components

Designing foods with a specific health purpose may involve adding an ingredient that is not usually present in foods, or present in only small amounts in the food.

Phytosterols are compounds that are structurally similar to cholesterol and are currently being used in a range of products as cholesterol-lowering agents. Phytosterols are thought to have been present in the diet of our ancestors in much greater amounts than occurs currently. Intakes of naturally occurring plant sterols are higher in vegetarians than in omnivores. The plant sterols currently used are extracted from soya bean oil or pine tree oil and are esterified to increase solubility. The most common are sitosterol, campesterol and stigmasterol. Products may contain plant sterol (unsaturated) or plant stanol (saturated) esters, and evidence shows that both have a similar capacity to lower circulating total and LDL cholesterol levels. The phytosterols reduce the absorption of cholesterol from the small intestine by forming insoluble particles with cholesterol, and by competing with cholesterol for bile that would facilitate absorption. Thus, a greater proportion of dietary cholesterol is excreted, although some of the phytosterol is absorbed. Absorption is estimated as no more than 5% of the phytosterol. The liver does compensate for reduced cholesterol absorption by increasing synthesis of endogenous cholesterol, but the net effect is a reduction of total cholesterol in the body.

These effects are achieved with relatively small doses of the phytosterols. As little as 1 g/day may have an effective lipid-lowering effect, although a dose of 1.6 g/day of plant sterol is recommended. There appears to be a plateau effect with no further reduction of cholesterol seen at intakes above 3 g/day. The average reduction in cholesterol levels is in the region of 5%–8% from spread alone and, when combined with other lipid-lowering measures in the diet, or drug treatments, levels of cholesterol may be reduced by 10%–15%. The dispersal of the phytosterol within the food product appears to be the key determinant of its effectiveness.

There has been some concern expressed about the potential for reduced absorption of fat-soluble vitamins, as a consequence of phytosterol ingestion. Lower plasma levels of vitamin E and carotenoids have been reported, but these effects are considered to be marginal.

Although developed as an aid to the management of blood lipids levels in cardiovascular disease reduction, new evidence suggests that the plant sterols may also have a role in inhibition of tumour growth.

Plant sterols and stanols are currently marketed as a range of spreads, dairy goods, such as yogurt and cream cheese, and salad dressing.

Omega-Enriched Eggs

A range of eggs are on sale in the United Kingdom from chickens that have been fed on a vegetarian seed-rich diet containing *n*-3 fatty acids. This results in eggs enriched with these fatty acids. This illustrates how manipulation of the nutritional content of a product can be achieved. The eggs form a small part of the total egg sales in the United Kingdom, but can provide up to 70% of the currently recommended level of *n*-3 fatty acids in one egg.

Clinical Usage

In clinical nutrition, feeds are being produced to contain 'functional' components for which there is believed to be an additional need in particular circumstances. Glutamine is an important fuel source for rapidly dividing cells: for example, those lining the gastrointestinal tract and blood cells. Severely ill patients may be at risk of receiving insufficient glutamine to meet their increased demands. Supplemental glutamine may improve gut mucosal and immune functions, and reduce episodes of clinical sepsis. Trials have shown reduced mortality, lower infection rates and shorter hospital stay.

Arginine is also a conditionally essential amino acid in states of trauma and sepsis, and arginine-containing formulas may reduce complications in surgical patients.

Foods Containing Bacteria

The contribution to human health of bacteria resident in the gut is increasingly recognized. More than 500 different bacterial species inhabit the human gut, amounting to about 1 kg in weight.

Some of these are considered to be beneficial and health promoting, some benign and some harmful or pathogenic. The balance of these bacteria is important and a predominance of one group over another can alter the risk or progression of disease, and the health and function of the colon. Longevity had been noticed among groups of the world population who consumed fermented dairy products that were believed to reduce levels of toxin-producing bacteria, thus suggesting that the dietary intake may have an influence on the health of the bowel and the organism.

Far from being a passive excretory route, the bowel is now understood to be a metabolically active organ that provides a protective barrier for the host through effects on the immune system. The protection exists at various levels, in terms of physical exclusion of the antigen, elimination of antigens that have penetrated the mucosa and finally control of any antigen-specific immune reactions. In order to be able to perform these functions, the gut depends on both appropriate nutrients as well as a beneficial microbial balance.

In addition, metabolism in the bowel may provide between 7% and 10% of the daily energy supply through the fermentation of carbohydrates and proteins (to a lesser extent). Some 60–80 g of the food ingested each day reaches the colon; the microbiota degrade this by fermentation to lactic acid and short-chain fatty acids, as well as carbon dioxide, hydrogen, methane, phenolic compounds, amines and ammonia (see Figure 23.1).

In the past, there was a frequent challenge to the gastrointestinal tract by microorganisms present in the environment and in food, and this primed the immune system to function normally. Our increasingly clean and processed environment, with foods containing artificial sweeteners, preservatives and even antibiotic residues, reduces the microbial challenge and results in an underperformance of the immune system. Modern lifestyle, with poor eating habits, stress and use of antibiotics, can all contribute to alterations in the microflora. It is believed that this may be one of the mechanisms whereby there has been an increase in chronic inflammatory diseases, including eczema, asthma, allergies, Crohn's disease, inflammatory bowel disease and ulcerative colitis.

The gut of the newborn infant is sterile but becomes colonized soon after birth. The method of feeding determines the bacterial flora, with lactobacilli, coliform bacteria and bifidobacteria prevailing in the breastfed infant. Formula feeding induces a wider microflora, which additionally includes *Bacteroides*, *Clostridia* and *Streptococci*. After weaning, the microflora becomes similar to that of the adult, with a predominance of anaerobic bacteria, which die in the presence of oxygen. Among these, the *Bifidobacteria* and *Lactobacilli* are considered to be beneficial to health, and some, such as certain *Eubacterium* spp., are benign but suppress the growth of harmful bacteria. Examples of the latter include proteolytic *Bacteroides* spp., many *Clostridium* spp. and pathogenic species of Enterobacteriaceae. Many other microorganisms are present in the bowel, some of which have not yet been characterized, and there is more research required.

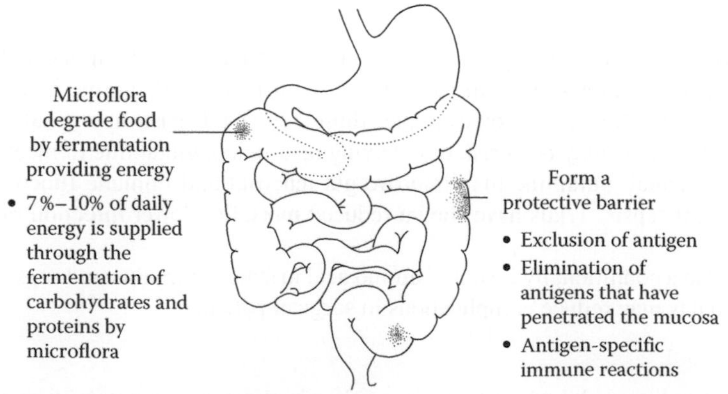

Microflora degrade food by fermentation providing energy
• 7%–10% of daily energy is supplied through the fermentation of carbohydrates and proteins by microflora
Form a protective barrier
• Exclusion of antigen
• Elimination of antigens that have penetrated the mucosa
• Antigen-specific immune reactions

FIGURE 23.1 How microflora are used in the bowel?

Probiotics have been developed, therefore, as an aid to restore the immune function of the gut and to reduce the incidence or symptoms of associated clinical conditions. Thus, probiotics can be described as products that contain live micro-organisms in fermented foods, which could promote good health by establishing an improved balance in intestinal microflora. The main organisms currently used are various species of *Lactobacilli* and *Bifidobacteria*, together with a non-pathogenic yeast, *Saccharomyces boulardii*.

The impact of carbohydrate fermentation on gut health is covered in more detail in Chapter 11, p. 231.

A probiotic product must fulfil several criteria including safety, ease and reproducibility of production, and stability during storage. Furthermore, the organisms should be able to survive in the digestive tract and colonize the bowel in adequate amounts to be able to provide benefit to the host. Although there is evidence from *in vitro* and animal experiments of beneficial effects of probiotics, clinical studies in humans are still at a relatively early stage. Most evidence exists for the reduction of diarrhoea and prevention of gastroenteritis, especially in infants and young children. In adults, antibiotic-induced and hospital-acquired diarrhoea has been shown to be better controlled with the use of probiotics as part of the treatment. Probiotics containing *Lactobacilli* have also been used successfully in cases of lactose malabsorption. A study in older adults showed an improvement in several aspects of cellular immunity after 3 weeks of probiotic use, especially in those with low immune status at baseline. Some evidence of an immune system–stabilizing effect has also been found in inflammatory bowel conditions and atopic eczema. There is still a lack of good evidence, however, that probiotics can prevent cancer, reduce plasma cholesterol levels or reduce levels of *Helicobacter pylori* infection in the stomach. Major advances in studying the mechanisms of action of probiotics, and gut structure and function *in vivo* are needed to further clarify the potential benefits and better target specific organisms for particular health needs.

Microorganisms require a substrate on which to grow and multiply. If this is not provided in the diet, the microflora can be compromised. This is the basis of the use of prebiotics, which are non-digestible food components that reach the colon where they can selectively stimulate the growth of beneficial microorganisms. In many ways, this definition is similar to that for components of dietary fibre, although these do not support the growth of one type of microorganism alone. Candidates for prebiotics are the oligosaccharides containing fructose (fructans). A naturally occurring example of this group is inulin, although other fructans are found in wheat, onions, bananas and chicory. Oligosaccharides containing xylose, galactose and mixtures of these sugars have also been studied. The most promising results have been obtained with fructo-oligosaccharides (FOS), which were shown to stimulate growth of *Bifidobacteria* in the colon and change the balance of microflora. Lactulose (containing galactose and fructose) has also been used in a number of clinical trials and found to promote growth of *Lactobacilli*. Prebiotics may be useful in the management of constipation, owing to the osmotic effect associated with increased bacterial fermentation. Increased acidity in the bowel has been suggested to be beneficial in the absorption of a number of minerals, most notably calcium.

As with all of the other functional foods, however, more randomized controlled trials are needed to confirm this effect and any associated health benefits.

Prebiotics are found in a range of foods in Europe, including dairy products, infant formula and bakery products.

FOOD REFORMULATION

Reformulation for health benefit, also known as health-by-stealth, is the deliberate manipulation of the composition of food products in order to give them a healthier nutrient profile. Opportunities to improve the nutritional content of food exist throughout the food chain, from the farm to the manufacturer to the retailer to our homes. Governments and those with a public health responsibility recognize this as a key strategy with the potential to improve health at a population level. In 2003, a joint WHO/FAO Expert Consultation provided population goals for nutrients consistent with the prevention of major public health problems in Europe. These goals included a reduction of total dietary fat, in particular of saturated fat, a reduction in trans fatty acids, an increase in polyunsaturated fatty acids, a reduction in sugar consumption and a reduction in salt intake. Reformulation of commonly eaten foods was thought to be one of the key options to achieve these goals (World Health Organisation, 2004). Recent attempts to evaluate the effectiveness of policy interventions to promote healthy eating suggest that reformulation may be more effective than general public health education; however, there is still a lack of studies examining their effects on healthy eating and the prevention of chronic noncommunicable diseases in the long term.

Reformulation with the intention of providing a healthier nutrient profile can mean limiting nutrients associated with negative health effects or maintaining nutrients associated with a positive health effect, for example

- Reducing energy density (kJ/g food)
- Reducing the amount of fat, saturates, sugar or salt
- Changing the fat or carbohydrate profile, e.g. by choice of oil/fat, changing the diet of ruminants, use of structured lipids and blending of oils
- Removal of trans fatty acids
- Improving the nutrient profile through choice of ingredient
- Replacement of nutrients normally removed during processing (e.g. bran and germ removed when flour is milled)

Food reformulation is distinct from functional foods (addition of 'positive' nutrients and ingredients in substantial quantities with purported health-promoting effects); food enrichment (addition of nutrients to foods in accordance with a standard of identity as defined by food regulations); food supplementation (addition of nutrients that are normally not present in the food or only in minimal quantities); and food fortification (addition of nutrients and the carrier food chosen have met certain criteria, so that the fortified product will become a good source of the nutrient for a targeted population). Reformulation can be applied to a range of foods, including those considered as 'junk food' such as pizzas; however, acceptability and palatability needs to be assessed.

In the United Kingdom, an initiative from the Department of Health, The Public Health Responsibility Deal, focusses on working in partnership with the food industry to improve the healthfulness of food products (DoH, 2011) and there has been some success arising from this initiative. For example in 2012/13:

- *Tesco*: Reduced the number of calories sold in its own brand soft drinks by over 1 billion in 2012.
- *Sainsbury's*: Reduced the sugar content of its own brand high juice squashes by between 4% and 10%, removing over 600 million cal from customers' baskets per year; as well as removing 23 tonnes of saturated fat from the pastry in its biggest selling mince pies.
- *Coca-Cola*: Sprite now contains 30% fewer calories.
- *JD Wetherspoon*: Reduced the calories in 12 dishes.
- *Nestlé*: Over half (54%) of Nestlé confectionery now contain less than 110 cal per serving.
- *Mars*: On way to reducing the calories in all its chocolate products to no more than 250 cal per portion (by end 2013); with further reductions in some leading products, including Twix (from 284 to 248 cal). Has also launched the Maltesers Teasers chocolate bar (186 cal per bar).
- *Burton's Biscuits*: Changes to the ingredients across all its brands will result in an estimated national reduction of 700,000 kcal/day for its customer in 2013.

- *Subway*: In 2012, Subway spent around 65% of its promotional budget on healthier eating, and launched a new range of low fat flatbreads.
- *Morrisons*: Launched a new healthier range, NuMe, which includes lower calorie options on an extended range of products.

However, the food industry continues to face significant challenges in implementing food reformulation. The emphasis remains almost exclusively on nutrients that are in excess in the diet and is therefore on weight control rather than providing a healthy balance of nutrients. Additionally, the choice of which products to buy and consume and in what quantities remains firmly in the hands of the consumer and is therefore subject to their acceptance of the concept of reformulated foods and perceptions of taste and acceptability.

Most commercial reformulation is aimed at making health claims, and it tends to focus on just a few prominent nutrients in foods. An alternative approach is to address the meal, as the smallest unit of human nutrition, and to reformulate entire meals so that they meet all nutritional guidelines. That has been done with the EatBalanced pizzas (Combet et al, 2014), in collaboration with an innovative start-up company (EatBalanced Ltd.). A traditional pizza recipe was adjusted in order to provide 27 essential nutrients in the required amounts, without compromising appearance or taste, and without significantly greater production costs. The pizzas are now being provided for some 30,000 schoolchildren in their school lunches.

NUTRIENT PROFILING

Nutrient profiling of foods is defined as the science of characterizing foods based on their nutrient composition. Measures of nutrient density, once used exclusively to assess total diets, are being adapted for use with individual foods. In the United Kingdom, a nutrient profiling tool was developed which allows individual foods and drinks to be assessed against specific scientific nutrition criteria, designed to assess combinations of macronutrients, vitamins and minerals (FSA, 2012). The tool, originally used to provide Ofcom with a tool to enable the regulation of marketing and advertising to children, is fast becoming the basis for regulating health claims for food. Similar models have also been developed in the United States, France and the Netherlands (Drewnowski and Fulgoni, 2008). The UK model is slightly simpler than others as it considers the overall fruit, vegetable and nut content of the food rather than considering specific selected micronutrients.

The UK NP model is a simple scoring system where points are allocated on the basis of the nutritional content of 100 g of the food or drink. 'A' points are awarded for the levels of energy, saturated fat, sugars and sodium and 'C' points for levels of fruit, vegetables, nuts, fibre ad protein. The overall score is then calculated by subtracting 'C' points from 'A' points.

Total 'A' points = (energy) + (saturated fat) + (sugars) + (sodium)

Total 'C' points = (fruit, veg and nut content) + (fibre [either NSP or AOACI]) + (protein)

The calculation of the overall score then depends on the detailed mix of points scored, that is

Food Scores:	Overall Score Calculation:
<11 'A' points	OS = (total 'A' points) – (total 'C' points)
≥11 'A' points and ≥5 points for fruit, veg and nuts	OS = (total 'A' points) – (total 'C' points)
≥11 'A' points and <5 points for fruit, veg and nuts	OS = (total 'A' points) – (fibre points + fruit, veg and nuts points) i.e.: not allowed to score 'C' points for protein

A food is classified as 'less healthy' where it scores 4 points or more and a drink is classified as less healthy where it scores 1 point or more. This apparently simple scoring system is somewhat complicated when applying it to processed foods and substantial effort has gone into defining and providing guidance on quantifying the fruit, vegetable and nut content of such foods.

Nutrient profiling may have multiple applications. Although not designed for use by consumers, assigning foods into categories based on their nutrient composition would permit consumers to identify and select nutrient-dense foods, while permitting some flexibility where discretionary calories are concerned, thus significantly simplifying nutritional labelling of foods. Nutrient profiling may also have implications for policy makers in the design of nutritional labelling, dealing with food health claims and the regulation of marketing and advertising.

ORGANIC FOOD

The concept of organic food is in many ways the opposite end of the spectrum from the functional foods discussed earlier. Organic foods represent more traditional food production methods, without the use of man-made chemical agents to potentiate the yield or reduce pest damage. Organic farming systems rely on traditional concepts of crop rotation, the use of animal and plant manures and biological methods of pest control. The market in organic foods has increased rapidly in the last 20 years, as consumers have become concerned about the perceived safety of mass or intensively produced foods. Such concerns include the presence of pesticide, growth promoter and antibiotic residues. In addition, there may be concerns about the presence of known (such as bovine spongiform encephalopathy [BSE]), or unknown disease-causing factors in the foods.

Although the primary concern may be one of food safety, organic food is also perceived as having superior sensory attributes and being 'healthier'. This is taken to mean that food produced organically has a higher nutrient content. Williams (2002), in reviewing the evidence on nutritional quality of organic food, notes that there is no evidence in the scientific literature to support these claims. There are methodological shortcomings in most of the publications that report on nutritional quality of organic versus conventionally produced foods. Many cover a long time period, during which there have been many changes in the production methods. Comparisons of effects of feeding experiments in animals produce inconsistent and conflicting results. No studies of effects on human health have been performed. Some data show that conventionally produced vegetables, especially green leafy vegetables, may have a lower vitamin C content. This is associated with a higher water content, producing a dilution effect. Conventionally grown plants grow more quickly and are harvested sooner than those grown organically, resulting in a higher water content. Nitrate levels were also higher in the conventionally grown leafy vegetables, probably associated with fertilizer use. There is no evidence of a negative impact on health from these differences. An area of potential interest that has not been studied is the level of various phytochemicals contained in plants. These are produced by plants as a protection against adverse conditions or to combat attack by potentially damaging pests or diseases. It is possible that levels may be higher in organically grown products that are less protected by sprays. However, there has been no study of this area.

It should also be remembered that organic food may carry a higher level of microbial contamination, through the application of manure or the unchecked growth of fungi or bacterial contaminants.

Much of the organic food available for sale in the United Kingdom is imported. This has possible implications for its freshness and associated nutritional content. It is also more expensive than conventional produce. As a result, a substantial proportion of the population is unable to afford organic foods. If they choose to buy organic produce, this may be at the expense of other items in the diet that could have contributed more to a healthy balance. Where money is not an issue, individuals can buy organic produce without fear of compromising the balance of the rest of their diet.

In summary, it is more important to concentrate on consuming a diet in line with healthy eating guidelines, as there is much more good scientific evidence to support this than to worry about any risk to health of conventionally produced foods that might be avoided by eating 'organically'. At present, there is insufficient evidence to support any benefit to health of 'organic' food, and more research is needed to clarify these issues.

CONCLUSIONS

Advances in knowledge about molecular biology and the characterization of the human genome will make it possible at some point in the future to study genetic polymorphisms that are associated with particular diseases. It is likely that these will also characterize individual responses to particular dietary components. We will also have a clearer view of the molecular mechanisms of nutrient action. An understanding of how genetic polymorphisms affect nutrient metabolism may make it possible to design specific dietary regimes to tackle nutritional problems, or disease risk. It is likely to become the responsibility of the food industry to develop products that help to fulfil these goals.

Although progress in recent years has been rapid, the preceding sections have indicated how little is known in some cases about mechanisms at cellular and tissue levels. This is hindered by a lack of biomarkers and specific tools for identification of processes, for example, within the gut mucosa. Properly controlled large-scale clinical trials need to be performed to evaluate the potential benefits of products, and caution needs to be exercised when claims are made that have not been properly evaluated and cause confusion among consumers. Safety aspects must also be addressed, if new products are developed. A focus on reformulating popular meals, to satisfy nutritional needs and guidelines for health, along the lines of the EatBalanced pizzas, probably offers the best prospect.

In the mean time, consuming a balanced diet following healthy-eating guidelines is our best guarantee of optimizing nutrition from food. This, after all, is what has sustained the human race over thousands of years, and should not be forgotten in the rush for new designer foods that offer promises of better health and disease reduction.

SUMMARY

1. Optimal nutrition is a concept that encompasses positive benefits of food in the promotion of health.
2. Foods with altered nutritional contents have been produced to address some issues of 'healthy eating'.
3. Some of the more researched food components have been introduced into foods to produce potentially health-promoting products.
4. There are many other components of food that have no known nutritional role but may modify the risk of disease.
5. The use of bacteria to promote gut health is a novel approach to optimizing nutritional state.

STUDY QUESTIONS

1. Debate with a partner what are the arguments for and against more development of smart foods. You could consider
   a. Are they useful for all people?
   b. Should they be targeted at specific groups? – if so, give examples?
   c. Which foods should be promoted and which allowed to disappear?
   d. Are there other smart foods that you think might be useful?

2. You could imagine that you are an expert committee and have to decide on permission for the development of some new products. What would you need to know?
3. Survey a number of people in your community to discover how many buy organic foods.
   a. Which foods are commonly bought, and what are the perceived benefits of choosing these?
   b. What foods are they replacing in the diet, and does this lead to better or poorer balance of healthy items?
4. Discuss with a colleague the benefits and disadvantages of adding specific nutrients to manufactured foods. Do you think this practice would help or hinder the work of a nutritionist?

ACTIVITIES

23.1 1. Look in the supermarket for examples of 'instant' and 'ready to eat' products. Identify which of these contain modified starch that is acting as a stabilizer or thickening agent.

2. Prepare a number of drinks (e.g. cups of tea) with different sweetening agents – try to use examples of each chemical type, as well as sugar. Test these on several volunteers to study any perceived differences in taste and sweetness detected.

23.2 1. Look at some of the foods mentioned in this section in a grocery store or supermarket. For each of the foods:
   a. Note the added nutrients, how much is added and how this relates to the reference nutrient intake (RNI).
   b. What fraction of the RNI does the food provide?
   c. How much of the food would need to be eaten each day to meet the RNI – is this realistic and feasible?
   d. Is there any indication on the label of the target consumer group for the product?

2. Try to find some examples of foods with added nutrients that would not normally be found in the food (as in the case of orange juice mentioned earlier). Why do you think these foods have been chosen for fortification with these particular nutrients?
3. List the advantages and disadvantages of fortifying foods with nutrients. If possible, think about the different situation in industrialized and developing countries. Discuss your findings with other members of your group.

BIBLIOGRAPHY AND FURTHER READING

Buttriss, J. and Hughes, J. 2000. A review of the MAFF optimal nutrition programme: Aims and objectives. *British Nutrition Foundation Nutrition Bulletin* 25, 79–80.

Buttriss, J.L. 2013. Food reformulation: The challenges to the food industry. *Proceedings of the Nutrition Society* 72, 61–69.

Capacci, S., Mazzocchi, M., Shankar, B. et al. 2012. Policies to promote healthy eating in Europe: A structured review of policies and their effectiveness. *Nutrition Reviews* 70, 188–200.

Cassidy, A. and Faughnan, M. 2000. Phyto-oestrogens through the life cycle. *Proceedings of the Nutrition Society* 59, 489–496.

Combet, E., Jarlot, A., Aidoo, K.E. and Lean, M.E.J. 2014. Development of a nutritionally balanced pizza as a functional meal designed to meet published dietary guidelines. *Public Health Nutrition* 17(11), 2577–2586.

Department of Health (DoH). 2011. Public health responsibility deal. Available at: https://responsibilitydeal.dh.gov.uk/wp-content/uploads/2012/03/The-Public-Health-Responsibility-Deal-March-20111.pdf (accessed on 16 October 2014).

Drewnowski, A. and Fulgoni, V. 3rd. 2008. Nutrient profiling of foods: Creating a nutrient-rich food index. *Nutrition Reviews* 66, 23–39.

Food Standards Agency (FSA). 2012. Guide to using the nutrient profiling model. Available at: http://www.food.gov.uk/northern-ireland/nutritionni/niyoungpeople/nutlab/nutprofmod (accessed on 16 October 2014).

Johnson, I.T. 2001. New food components and gastrointestinal health. *Proceedings of the Nutrition Society* 60, 481–488.

Kolida, S., Tuohy, K. and Gibson, G.R. 2000. The human gut flora in nutrition and approaches for its dietary modification. *British Nutrition Foundation Nutrition Bulletin* 25, 219–222.

Marteau, P. and Boutron-Ruault, M.C. 2002. Nutritional advantages of probiotics and prebiotics. *British Journal of Nutrition* 87(Suppl. 2), S153–S157.

McConnon, A., Cade, J. and Pearman, A. 2002. Stakeholder interactions and the development of functional foods. *Public Health Nutrition* 5(3), 469–477.

Omenn, G.S., Goodman, G.E., Thornquist, M.D. et al. 1996. Effects of a combination of beta carotene and vitamin A on lung cancer and cardiovascular disease. *New England Journal of Medicine* 334, 1150–1155.

Plump, J.A., Rhodes, M.J.C., Lampi, A.M. et al. 2011. Phytosterols in plant foods: Exploring contents, data distribution and aggregated values using an online bioactives database. *Journal of Food Composition and Analysis* 24, 1024–1031.

Rowland, I.R. 2002. Genetically modified foods, science, consumers and the media. *Proceedings of the Nutrition Society* 61, 25–29.

Scarborough, P. and Rayner, M. 2014. When nutrient profiling can (and cannot) be useful. *Public Health Nutrition* 17(12), 2637–2640.

Schrooyen, P.M.M., van der Meer, R. and De Kruif, C.G. 2001. Microencapsulation: Its application in nutrition. *Proceedings of the Nutrition Society* 60, 475–479.

van Raaij, J., Hendriksen M. and Verhagen, H. 2009. Potential for improvement of population diet through reformulation of commonly eaten foods. *Public Health Nutrition* 12, 325–330.

Various authors. 1999. Symposium on optimal nutrition. *Proceedings of the Nutrition Society* 58, 395–512.

Williams, C.M. 2002. Nutritional quality of organic food: Shades of grey or shades of green? *Proceedings of the Nutrition Society* 61, 19–24.

World Health Organisation (WHO). 2004. Global strategy on diet, physical activity and health. Available at: http://www.who.int/dietphysicalactivity/strategy/eb11344/strategy_english_web.pdf (accessed on 16 October 2014).

Index

E

Printed and bound by CPI Group (UK) Ltd, Croydon, CR0 4YY
23/10/2024
01777682-0009